Essential Revision Notes for MRCP Second Edition

edited by

Philip A Kalra MA MB BChir FRCP MD
Consultant Nephrologist and Honorary Lecturer Hope Hospital, Salford Royal Hospitals Trust and The University of Manchester

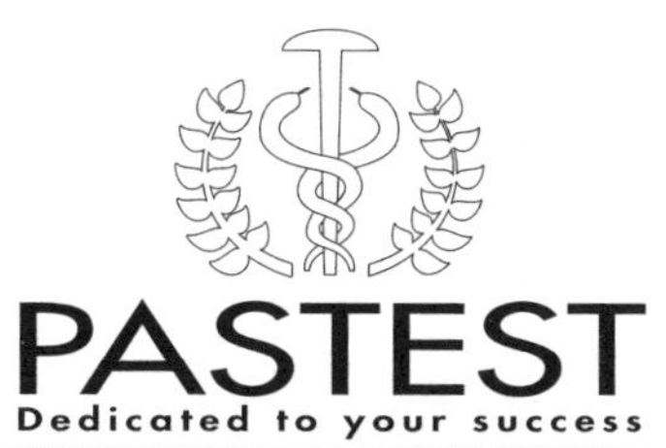

Egerton Court
Parkgate Estate
Knutsford
Cheshire WA16 8DX
Telephone: 01565 755226

First published 1999
Reprinted 1999
Revised edition 2002
Reprinted 2003
Second edition 2004
Reprinted 2007

ISBN: 1 904627 15 3

A catalogue record for this book is available from the British Library.

Original design and typesetting by Editext, Derbyshire (01457 857622).
Second edition prepared by Saxon Graphics Ltd, Derby
Printed and bound by MPG Books Ltd, Bodmin, Cornwall

Contents

Contributors to Second Edition

Professor Philip Baker BMed Sci BM BS DMR FRCOG
Maternity and Fetal Research Director, St Mary's Hospital, Whitworth Park, Manchester *Maternal Medicine*

Louise Byrd MRCOG
Specialist Registrar in Obstetrics and Gynaecology, North West Region *Maternal Medicine*

Colin M Dayan MA MBBS FRCP PhD
Consultant Senior Lecturer in Medicine, Head of Clinical Research, URCN, Henry Wellcome Laboratories for Integrative Neuroscience and Endocrinology, University of Bristol *Endocrinology*

Ben Goorney MBChB FRCP
Consultant Genito-Urinary Physician, Department of Genito-Urinary Medicine, Hope Hospital, Salford *Genito-urinary Medicine and AIDS*

Philip A Kalra MA MB BChir FRCP MD
Consultant Nephrologist, Department of Renal Medicine, Hope Hospital, Salford *Nephrology*

Louise Kenny MBChB Hons, PhD, MRCOG
Clinical Lecturer in Maternal and Fetal Health, Tommy's The Baby Charity funded Maternal and Fetal Health Research Centre, St Mary's Hospital, Manchester *Maternal Medicine*

Mike McMahon BSc MBChB FRCP
Consultant Physician and Rheumatologist, Department of Rheumatology, Dumfries and Galloway Royal Infirmary, Dumfries *Immunology & Rheumatology*

Donal J O'Donoghue BSc MBChB FRCP
Consultant Renal Physician, Department of Renal Medicine, Hope Hospital, Salford *Metabolic Diseases*

John Paisey BM MRCP
Specialist Registrar, Cardiology, Wessex Region *Cardiology*

Keith Patterson FRCP FRCPath
Consultant Haematologist, Department of Haematology, University College London Hospitals, London *Haematology*

Geraint Rees BA BMBCh MRCP PhD
Wellcome Senior Clinical Fellow, Institute of Cognitive Neuroscience, University College London *Neurology*

Helen Robertshaw BSc(Hons) MBBS MRCP
Specialist Registrar in Dermatology, Southampton University Hospitals Trust, Southampton *Dermatology*

Andrew Robinson MA BM BcH FRCP PhD
Consultant Gastroenterologist, Honorary Clinical Lecturer, Hope Hospital, Salford *Gastroenterology*

Elizabeth Sampson MBChB MRCPsych MD
Lecturer in Old Age Psychiatry, Royal Free and University College Medical School, University College London *Psychiatry*

Katherine Smyth MBChB MRCP FRCOpth
Consultant Ophthalmologist, Royal Bolton Hosptial, Bolton *Ophthalmology*

Kevin Talbot MBBS MRCP DPhil
MRC-GlaxoSmithKline Clinical Scientist Fellow/Honary Consultant Neurologist, University of Oxford *Molecular Medicine*

Angie Wade MSc PhD CStat ILTM
Senior Lecturer in Medical Statistics, Institute of Child Health and Great Ormond Street Hospital, London *Statistics*

Deborah A Wales MBChB MRCP FRCA
Consultant Respiratory Physician, Nevill Hall Hospital, Brecon Road, Abergavenny, Monmouthshire *Respiratory Medicine*

Stephen Waring MRCP(UK)
Consultant Physician in Acute Medicine and Toxicology, The Royal Infirmary of Edinburgh *Clinical Pharmacology*

Gary Whitlock BHB MBChB MPH(Hons) PhDFAFPHM
Clinical Research Fellow, Clinical Trial Service Unit, University of Oxford *Epidemiology*

Louise C Wilson BSc MBChB MRCP
Consultant in Clinical Genetics, Clinical and Molecular Genetics Unit, Institute of Child Health, London *Genetics*

Contributors to Revised Edition

Simon Allard BSc MBBS MD FRCP
Consultant Physician and Rheumatologist, Department of Rheumatology, West Middlesex University Hospital, Isleworth, Middlesex *Rheumatology*

Ameet Bakhai MBBS MRCP
Senior Research Fellow and Specialist Registrar in Cardiology, Clinical Trials and Evaluation Unit, Royal Brompton Hospital, London, Imperial College Divison of Medicine, London *Cardiology*

Christopher Bench MBBS MRCPsych
Senior Lecturer, Division of Neuroscience and Psychological Medicine, Imperial College School of Medicine, London *Psychiatry*

Mark Caulfield MBBS MD FRCP
Professor of Clinical Pharmacology, Department of Clinical Pharmacology, William Harvey Research Institute, Bart's and the London, London *Clinical Pharmacology*

Colin M Dayan MA MBBS FRCP PhD
Consultant Senior Lecturer in Medicine, University Division of Medicine, Bristol Royal Infirmary, Bristol *Endocrinology and Diabetes*

Ben Goorney MBChB FRCP
Consultant Genito-Urinary Physician, Department of Genito-Urinary Medicine, Hope Hospital, Salford *Genito-urinary Medicine and AIDS*

Girish Gupta MBChB MRCP
Consultant Dermatologist, Department of Dermatology, Monklands Hospital, Lanarkshire *Dermatology*

Philip A Kalra MA MB BChir FRCP MD
Consultant Nephrologist, Department of Renal Medicine, Hope Hospital, Salford *Nephrology*

Jennifer MacDowall MBChB MRCP (UK)
Specialist Registrar in Gastroenterology, Department of Gastroenterology, Blackburn Royal Infirmary, Blackburn *Gastroenterology*

Mike McMahon BSc MBChB FRCP
Consultant Physician and Rheumatologist, Department of Rheumatology, Dumfries and Galloway Royal Infirmary, Dumfries *Immunology & Rheumatology*

Donal J O'Donoghue BSc MBChB FRCP
Consultant Renal Physician, Department of Renal Medicine, Hope Hospital, Salford *Metabolic Diseases*

Keith Patterson FRCP FRCPath
Consultant Haematologist, Department of Haematology, University College London Hospitals, London *Haematology*

Geraint Rees BA BMBCh MRCP (UK)
Lecturer, Institute of Neurology, University College London *Neurology*

Jon L Shaffer MBBS FRCP
Consultant Physician/Gastroenterologist, Department of Gastroenterology, Hope Hospital, Salford *Gastroenterology*

Katherine Smyth MBChB MRCP FRCOpth
Consultant Ophthalmologist, Royal Bolton Hospital, Bolton *Ophthalmology*

Kevin Talbot BSc MBBS MRCP DPhil
MRC-GlaxoSmithKline Clinical Scientist Fellow/Honary Consultant Neurologist, University Department of Clinical Neurology, Radcliffe Infirmary, Oxford *Molecular Medicine*

Angie Wade BSc MSc PhD CStat
Senior Lecturer in Medical Statistics, Department of Epidemiology and Public Health, Institute of Child Health, London *Statistics*

Deborah A Wales MBChB MRCP FRCA
Consultant Respiratory Physician, Royal Lancaster Infirmary, Lancaster *Respiratory Medicine*

William R C Weir FRCP FRCP (Edin)
Consultant Physician, Department of Infectious and Tropical Diseases, Coppett's Wood Hospital, London *Infectious Diseases*

Louise C Wilson BSc MBChB MRCP
Consultant in Clinical Genetics, Clinical and Molecular Genetics Unit, Institute of Child Health, London *Genetics*

Preface to the Second Edition

Although there have been major changes in the style of the MRCP examination in recent years the fundamental need of the practising physician, namely a core knowledge across all of the sub-specialties of medicine, remains the same. However, as a result of the rapid pace of advances in medicine it is now increasingly difficult to keep abreast. Hence, the aim of the *Essential Revision Notes for MRCP* is to fill the void between the large, detailed comprehensive textbook and those smaller texts which concentrate specifically on how to pass the examinations.

In this 2nd edition we have maintained the successful style of the 1st edition with emphasis upon concise text, bullet points and tables, hopefully making the book easy to read and more useful for facilitating revision. Every chapter has been thoroughly revised and updated, and there are two new chapters, *Epidemiology and Maternal Medicine*, covering topics which are of considerable importance to the general physician. Although *Essential Revision Notes* is primarily aimed at candidates studying for the MRCP, the book will also be of value to final year medical students and to help update the knowledge of all grades of practising physician.

As with all projects of this size, deadlines have been tight, and I would like to thank all of the chapter authors/contributors for their expedient efforts which have ensured that this new edition has been completed on time. Cathy Dickens again deserves special mention for co-ordinating the book production process at Pastest.

Philip A Kalra

Acknowledgement

We are most grateful to Dr M Chaponda (SpR Pharmacology/Infectious Diseases) for his help in updating Chapter 11 Infectious Diseases and Tropical Medicine

Preface to the Revised Edition

Although it is only three years since the publication of *Essential Revision Notes for MRCP* we felt that there was now a need for a revised edition. The practice of medicine is changing all the time, and never more so than in the current era of rapidly advancing science and evidence-based medicine. Several chapters have been expanded to include necessary new material (e.g. the HIV section of Chapter 7, *Genito-urinary Medicine and AIDS*; polycythaemia, Hodgkin's lymphoma and myeloma in Chapter 8, *Haematology*; multiple sclerosis in Chapter 14, *Neurology*) and all chapters have been updated in line with current practice and latest developments. The PasTest team has worked hard in order to complete this revised edition in time for the New Year, and I would especially like to praise Cathy Dickens, with thanks also to Sue Harrison.

Philip A Kalra

Acknowledgements

We are most grateful to Dr FJ Vilar for his help in updating Chapter 7, *Genito-urinary Medicine and AIDS*, and to Dr Paul Kalra and Dr Stephen Dye for similar help with Chapter 2, *Cardiology*, and Chapter 16, *Psychiatry*, respectively.

Chapter 1 Cardiology

CONTENTS

Cardiology

1. CARDIAC INVESTIGATIONS

1.1 Common aspects of the ECG

Both the axis and sizes of QRS vectors give important information. Axes are defined:

- –30° to +90°: normal
- –30° to –90°: left axis
- +90° to +180°: right axis
- –90° to –180°: indeterminate.

The causes of common abnormalities are given below.

Causes of common abnormalities in ECG

- **Causes of left axis deviation**
  Left bundle branch block (LBBB)
  Left anterior hemi block (LAHB)
  Left ventricular hypertrophy (LVH)
  Primum atrial septal defect (ASD)
  Cardiomyopathies
  Tricuspid atresia

- **Causes of right axis deviation**
  Infancy
  Right bundle branch block (RBBB)
  Right ventricular hypertrophy
  (eg lung disease, pulmonary embolism, large secundum ASD, severe pulmonary stenosis, Fallot's)

- **Low voltage ECG**
  Pulmonary emphysema
  Pericardial effusion
  Myxoedema
  Severe obesity
  Incorrect calibration
  Cardiomyopathies
  Global ischaemia
  Amyloid

- **Abnormalities of ECGs in athletes**
  Sinus arrhythmia
  Sinus bradycardia
  1° heart block
  Wenckebach phenomenon
  Junctional rhythm

Clinical diagnoses which may be made from the ECG of an asymptomatic patient

- Atrial fibrillation
- Complete heart block
- Hypertrophic cardiomyopathy (HCM)
- Atrial septal defects (with RBBB)
- Long QT syndromes
- Wolff–Parkinson–White syndrome (delta waves).

Short PR interval

This is rarely less than 0.12 s; the most common causes are those of pre-excitation involving accessory pathways or of tracts bypassing the slow region of the AV node; other causes do exist.

- **Pre-excitation**
  Wolff–Parkinson–White (WPW) syndrome
  Lown–Ganong–Levine syndrome (short PR syndrome)

- **Other**
  Ventricular extrasystole falling after P wave
  AV junctional rhythm (but P wave will usually be negative)
  Low atrial rhythm
  Coronary sinus escape rhythm

Causes of tall R waves in V1

It is easy to spot tall R waves in V1. This lead largely faces the posterior wall of the left ventricle (LV) and the mass of the right ventricle. As the overall vector is predominantly towards the bulkier LV in normal situations, the QRS is usually negative in V1. This balance is reversed in the following situations:

- right ventricular hypertrophy
- RBBB
- posterior infarction
- dextrocardia
- Wolff–Parkinson–White (WPW) **type A** (ventricular conduction starts via a left posterior accessory pathway, ie towards V1)
- hypertrophic cardiomyopathy (septal mass greater than posterior wall).

Bundle branch block and ST segment abnormalities

Complete bundle branch block is a failure or delay of impulse conduction to one ventricle from the AV node, requiring conduction via the other bundle, and the transmission within the ventricular myocardium; this results in abnormal prolongation of QRS duration (≥ 120 ms) and abnormalities of the normally iso-electric ST segment.

- **Causes of left bundle branch block (LBBB)**
  Ischaemic heart disease (recent or old myocardial infarction (MI))
  Left ventricular hypertrophy (LVH)
  Aortic valve disease
  Cardiomyopathy
  Myocarditis
  Post-valve replacement
  Right ventricular pacemaker

- **Causes of right bundle branch block (RBBB)**
  Normal in young
  Right ventricular strain (eg pulmonary embolus)
  Atrial septal defect
  Ischaemic heart disease
  Myocarditis
  Idiopathic

- **Causes of ST elevation**
  Early repolarisation
  Acute MI
  Pericarditis (saddle-shaped)
  Ventricular aneurysm
  Coronary artery spasm
  During angioplasty

- **Other ST-T wave changes (not elevation)**
  Ischaemia
  Digoxin therapy
  Hypertrophy
  Post-tachycardia
  Hyperventilation
  Oesophageal irritation
  Cardiac contusion
  Mitral valve prolapse
  Acute cerebral event (eg subarachnoid haemorrhage)
  Electrolyte abnormalities

Q waves may be permanent (reflecting myocardial necrosis) or transient (suggesting failure of myocardial function, but not necrosis).

- **Pathological Q waves**
  Transmural infarction
  LBBB
  Wolff–Parkinson–White syndrome
  Hypertrophic cardiomyopathy
  Idiopathic cardiomyopathy
  Amyloid heart disease
  Sarcoidosis
  Neoplastic infiltration
  Progressive muscular dystrophy
  Friedreich's ataxia
  Myocarditis (may resolve)
  Dextrocardia
- **Transient Q waves**
  Coronary spasm
  Hypoxia
  Hyperkalaemia
  Cardiac contusion
  Hypothermia

Potassium and ECG changes

There is a reasonable correlation between plasma potassium and ECG changes.

- **Hyperkalaemia**
  Tall T waves
  Prolonged PR interval
  Flattened/absent P waves
- **Very severe hyperkalaemia**
  Wide QRS
  Sine wave pattern
  Ventricular tachycardia/ventricular fibrillation/asystole
- **Hypokalaemia**
  Flat T waves, occasionally inverted
  Prolonged PR interval
  ST depression
  Tall U waves

ECG changes following coronary artery bypass surgery

- Osborne u waves (hypothermia)
- Saddle-shaped ST elevation (pericarditis)
- PR segment depression (pericarditis)
- Low voltage ECG in chest leads (pericardial effusion)
- Changing electrical alternans (alternating ECG axis–cardiac tamponade)
- $S_1Q_3T_3$ (pulmonary embolus)
- Atrial fibrillation
- Q waves
- ST segment and T wave changes.

Electrocardiographic techniques for prolonged monitoring

- **Holter monitoring**: the ECG is monitored in one or more leads for 24–72 h. The patient is encouraged to keep a diary in order to correlate symptoms with ECG changes.
- **External recorders**: the patient keeps a monitor with them for a period of days or weeks. At the onset of symptoms the monitor is placed to the chest and this records the ECG.
- **Wearable loop recorders**: the patient wears a monitor for several days or weeks. The device records the ECG constantly on a self-erasing loop. At the time of symptoms, the patient activates the recorder and a trace spanning some several seconds before a period of symptoms to several minutes afterwards is stored.
- **Implantable loop recorders**: a loop recorder is subcutaneously implanted in the pre-pectoral region. The recorder is activated by the patient or according to pre-programmed parameters. Again the ECG data from several seconds before symptoms to several minutes after are stored; data are uploaded by telemetry. The battery life of the implantable loop recorder is approximately 18 months.

1.2 Echocardiography

Diagnostic uses of echocardiography

Conventional echocardiography is used in the diagnosis of:

- pericardial effusion and tamponade
- valvular disease (including large vegetations)
- hypertrophic cardiomyopathy, dilated cardiomyopathy, LV mass and function
- cardiac tumours and intracardiac thrombus
- congenital heart disease (eg patent ductus arteriosus (PDA); coarctation of the aorta).

Stress echo is used in the diagnosis of infarction and ischaemia.
Contrast echo is used in the diagnosis of atrial septal defects/ventricular septal defects.

Classical M-mode patterns

With M-mode echocardiography, the normal pattern of movement of the mitral cusps creates an M-shaped box pattern during diastole (when the leaflets are open) and a slit line when the cusps close in systole (see figure overleaf). Particular M-mode patterns are associated with certain cardiac conditions:

- **Aortic regurgitation**: fluttering of the anterior mitral leaflet is seen.
- **Hypertrophic cardiomyopathy**: systolic anterior motion of the mitral valve leaflets (SAM) and asymmetrical septal hypertrophy (ASH) (see figure overleaf).
- **Mitral valve prolapse**: one or both leaflets prolapse during systole.
- **Mitral stenosis**: the opening profile of the cusps is flat and multiple echoes are seen when there is calcification of the cusps.

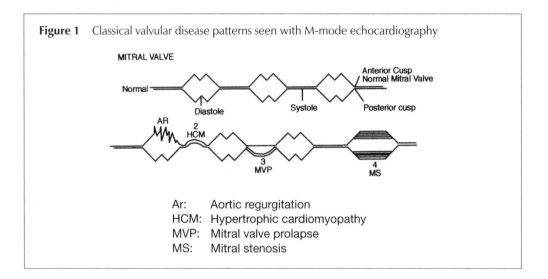

Figure 1 Classical valvular disease patterns seen with M-mode echocardiography

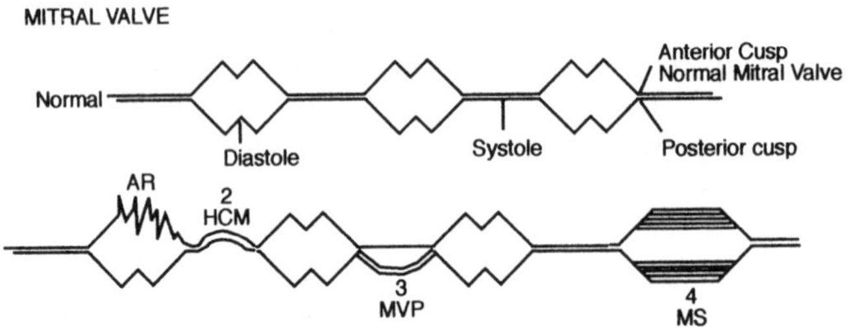

Ar: Aortic regurgitation
HCM: Hypertrophic cardiomyopathy
MVP: Mitral valve prolapse
MS: Mitral stenosis

Potential uses of transoesophageal echocardiography

Transoesophageal echo (TOE) provides much clearer pictures, particularly of posterior structures, and is therefore useful in the following:

- diagnosis of aortic dissection
- suspected atrial thrombus
- assessment of vegetations or abscesses in endocarditis
- prosthetic valve dysfunction or leakage
- intra-operative assessment of left ventricular function
- technically sub-optimal transthoracic echocardiogram.

1.3 Nuclear cardiology: myocardial perfusion imaging (MPI)

Perfusion tracers such as thallium or technetium can be used to gauge myocardial blood flow, both at rest and during stress that is induced by drugs or exercise. Tracer uptake is detected using tomograms and displayed in a colour scale in standard views.

Lack of uptake may be:

- **Physiological**: due to lung or breast tissue absorption.
- **Pathological**: reflecting ischaemia, infarction or other conditions in which perfusion abnormalities also occur (eg HCM or amyloidosis).

MPI may be used to:

- detect infarction
- investigate atypical chest pains
- assess ventricular function

- determine prognosis and detect myocardium that may be re-awakened from hibernation with an improved blood supply (eg after coronary bypass grafting).

1.4 Cardiac catheterisation and complications

Complications are uncommon (approximately 5%, including minor complications); these include contrast allergy, local haemorrhage from puncture sites with subsequent occurrence of thrombosis, false aneurysm or AV malformation. Vasovagal reactions are common. Other complications are:

- Coronary dissection (particularly the right coronary artery (RCA) in women) and aortic dissection or ventricular perforation.
- Air or atheroma embolism: in either the coronary or other arterial circulations with consequent ischaemia or strokes.
- Ventricular dysrhythmias: may even cause death in the setting of left main stem disease.
- Mistaken cannulation and contrast injection into the conus branch of the RCA will cause ventricular fibrillation.
- Overall mortality rates are quoted at <1/1000 cases.

Aortography in cardiac diagnoses

The following conditions can be identified with an aortogram:

- aortic regurgitation
- coarctation of the aorta
- aortic dissection
- patent ductus arteriosus
- aberrant subclavian arteries
- aortic root abscess
- coronary artery anomalies
- paraprosthetic aortic regurgitation
- identification of bypass grafts
- aortic root dilatation (eg Marfan's syndrome).

1.5 Exercise stress testing

This is used in the investigation of coronary artery disease, exertionally induced arrhythmias, and in the assessment of cardiac workload and sinus node function. Exercise tests also give diagnostic and prognostic information post-infarction, and generate patient confidence in rehabilitation after MI.

The main contraindications to exercise testing include those conditions where fatal ischaemia or arrhythmias may be provoked, or those patients in whom cardiac function may be severely and acutely impaired by exertion. These include the following:

- Severe aortic stenosis or HCM with marked outflow obstruction
- Acute myocarditis or pericarditis
- Pyrexial or 'flu'-like illness
- Severe left main stem disease
- Untreated congestive cardiac failure
- Unstable angina
- Dissecting aneurysm
- Adults with complete heart block
- Untreated severe hypertension

Indicators of a positive exercise test result

The presence of each factor is additive in the overall positive prediction of coronary artery disease.

- Development of anginal symptoms
- A fall in BP of >15 mmHg or failure to increase BP with exercise
- Arrhythmia development (particularly ventricular)
- Poor workload capacity (may indicate poor left ventricular function)
- Failure to achieve target heart rate (allowing for beta-blockers)
- >1 mm down-sloping or planar ST segment depression, 80 ms after the J point
- ST segment elevation
- Failure to achieve 9 min of the Bruce protocol due to any of the points listed

Exercise tests have **low specificity** in the following situations (often as a result of resting ST segment abnormalities):

- Ischaemia in young women with atypical chest pains
- Atrial fibrillation
- LBBB
- Wolff–Parkinson–White syndrome
- Left ventricular hypertrophy
- Digoxin or beta-blocker therapy
- Anaemia
- Hyperventilation
- Biochemical abnormalities such as hypokalaemia

1.6 24-hour ambulatory blood pressure monitoring

The limited availability and relative expense of ambulatory blood pressure monitoring prevents its use in all hypertensive patients. Specific areas of usefulness are in the following situations:

- Assessing for 'white coat' hypertension
- Borderline hypertensive cases that may not need treatment
- Evaluation of hypotensive symptoms
- Identifying episodic hypertension (eg in phaeochromocytoma)
- Assessing drug compliance and effects (particularly in resistant cases)
- Nocturnal blood pressure dipper status (non-dippers are at higher risk)

2. JVP, ARTERIAL PULSE AND HEART SOUNDS

2.1 Jugular venous pulse (JVP)

This reflects the right atrial pressure (normal to 3 cm above the clavicle with the subject at 45°). This should fall with inspiration, which increases venous return by a suction effect of the lungs, and with expansion of the pulmonary beds. However, if the neck veins are distended by inspiration this implies that the right heart chambers cannot increase in size due to restriction by fluid or pericardium: **Kussmaul's Sign**. Non-pulsatile JVP elevation occurs with SVC obstruction.

Normal waves in the JVP	
a wave:	Due to atrial contraction – active push up superior vena cava (SVC) and into right ventricle (may cause an audible S4)
c wave:	An invisible flicker in the x descent due to closure of the tricuspid valve, before the start of ventricular systole
x descent:	Downward movement of the heart causes atrial stretch and drop in pressure
v wave:	Due to passive filling of blood into the atrium against a closed tricuspid valve
y descent:	Opening of tricuspid valve with passive movement of blood from the right atrium to the right ventricle (causing an S3 when audible)
Pathological waves in the JVP	
a waves:	Lost in atrial fibrillation, giant in tricuspid stenosis or in pulmonary hypertension with sinus rhythm (atrial septal defect will exaggerate the natural a and v waves in sinus rhythm)
Giant V(S) waves:	Merging of the a and v into a large wave (with a rapid y descent) as pressure continues to increase due to ventricular systole in patients with tricuspid regurgitation

Steep x descents: Occur in states where there is atrial filling only due to ventricular systole and downward movement of the base of the heart, ie compressed atrial states with tamponade or constrictive pericarditis

Rapid y descent: Occurs in states where high flow occurs with tricuspid valve opening (eg tricuspid regurgitation (high atrial load) or constrictive pericarditis) – vacuum effect. A slow y descent indicates tricuspid stenosis

Cannon a waves: Atrial contractions against a closed tricuspid valve due to a nodal rhythm, a ventricular tachycardia, ventricular-paced rhythm (regular), complete heart block or ventricular extrasystoles (irregular). They occur regularly but not consistently in type 1 second degree heart block

2.2 Arterial pulse associations

- **Collapsing**: aortic regurgitation, arterio-venous fistula, patent ductus arteriosus or other large extra-cardiac shunt.
- **Slow rising**: aortic stenosis (delayed percussion wave).
- **Bisferiens**: a double shudder due to mixed aortic valve disease with significant regurgitation (tidal wave second impulse).
- **Jerky**: hypertrophic obstructive cardiomyopathy.
- **Alternans**: severe left ventricular failure.
- **Paradoxical (pulsus paradoxus)**: an excessive reduction in the pulse with inspiration (drop in systolic BP >10 mmHg) occurs with left ventricular compression, tamponade, constrictive pericarditis or severe asthma as venous return is compromised.

Causes of an absent radial pulse

- Dissection of aorta with subclavian involvement
- Iatrogenic: post-catheterisation
- Peripheral arterial embolus
- Takayasu's arteritis
- Trauma

2.3 Cardiac apex

An absent apical impulse

The apex may be impalpable in the following situations:

- obesity/emphysema
- right pneumonectomy with displacement
- pericardial effusion or constriction
- dextrocardia (palpable on right side of chest).

Apex associations

Palpation of the apex beat (reflecting counterclockwise ventricular movement striking the chest wall during isovolumic contractions) can detect the following pathological states:

- **Heaving**: left ventricular hypertrophy (and all its causes), sometimes associated with palpable fourth heart sound.
- **Thrusting/hyperdynamic**: high left ventricular volume (eg in mitral regurgitation, aortic regurgitation (AR), PDA, VSD).
- **Tapping**: palpable first heart sound in mitral stenosis.
- **Displaced and diffuse/dyskinetic**: left ventricular impairment and dilatation (eg dilated cardiomyopathy, myocardial infarction).
- **Double impulse**: with dyskinesia is due to left ventricular aneurysm; without dyskinesia in HCM.
- **Pericardial knock**: constrictive pericarditis.
- **Parasternal heave**: due to right ventricular hypertrophy (eg ASD, pulmonary hypertension, chronic obstructive pulmonary disease, pulmonary stenosis).
- **Palpable third heart sound**: due to heart failure and severe mitral regurgitation.

2.4 Heart sounds

Abnormalities of first heart sound (S1): closure of mitral and tricuspid valves

Loud	Soft	Split	Variable
Mobile mitral stenosis	Immobile mitral stenosis	RBBB	Atrial fibrillation
Hyperdynamic states	Hypodynamic states	LBBB	Complete heart block
Tachycardic states	Mitral regurgitation	VT	
Left to right shunts	Poor ventricular function	Inspiration	
Short PR interval	Long PR interval	Ebstein anomaly	

Continues …

Abnormalities of second heart sound (S2): closure of aortic then pulmonary valves (<0.05 s apart)

Intensity	Splitting	
Loud:	***Fixed:***	***Single S2:***
Systemic hypertension (loud A2)	ASD	Severe PS/AS
Pulmonary hypertension (loud P_2)		Hypertension
Tachycardic states	***Widely split:***	Large VSD
ASD (loud P_2)	RBBB	Fallot's tetralogy
	Pulmonary stenosis	Eisenmenger syndrome
Soft or absent:	Deep inspiration	Pulmonary atresia
Severe aortic stenosis	Mitral regurgitation	Elderly
		Reversed split S2:
		LBBB
		Right ventricular pacing
		PDA
		Aortic stenosis

Third heart sound (S3)

Due to the passive filling of the ventricles on opening of the AV valves, audible in normal children and young adults. Pathological in cases of rapid left ventricular filling (eg mitral regurgitation, VSD, congestive cardiac failure (CCF) and constrictive pericarditis).

Fourth heart sound (S4)

Due to the atrial contraction that fills a stiff left ventricle, such as in left ventricular hypertrophy, amyloid, HCM and left ventricular ischaemia. It is absent in atrial fibrillation.

Causes of valvular clicks

- **Aortic ejection**: aortic stenosis, bicuspid aortic valve
- **Pulmonary ejection**: pulmonary stenosis
- **Mid-systolic**: mitral valve prolapse.

Opening snap (OS)

In mitral stenosis an opening snap may be present and occurs after S2 in early diastole. The closer it is to S2 the greater the severity of mitral stenosis. It is absent when the mitral cusps become immobile, due to calcification, as in very severe mitral stenosis.

3. VALVULAR DISEASE AND ENDOCARDITIS

3.1 Murmurs

Benign flow murmurs: are soft, short systolic murmurs heard along the left sternal edge to the pulmonary area, without any other cardiac auscultatory, ECG or chest X-ray abnormalities. Thirty per cent of children may give an innocent flow murmur.

Cervical venous hum: continuous when upright and is reduced by lying; occurs with a hyperdynamic circulation or with jugular vein compression.

Large A-V fistula of the arm: may cause a harsh flow murmur across the upper mediastinum.

Effect of posture on murmurs: standing significantly increases the murmurs of mitral valve prolapse and HCM only. Squatting and passive leg raising increases cardiac afterload and therefore decreases the murmur of HCM and mitral valve prolapse, whilst increasing most other murmurs such as ventral septal defect, aortic, mitral and pulmonary regurgitation, and aortic stenosis.

Effect of respiration on murmurs: inspiration accentuates right-sided murmurs by increasing venous return, whereas held expiration accentuates left-sided murmurs. The strain phase of a valsalva manoeuvre reduces venous return, stroke volume and arterial pressure, decreasing all valvular murmurs but increasing the murmur of HCM and mitral valve prolapse.

Classification of particular murmurs

- **Mid/late systolic murmur**
  Innocent murmur
  Aortic stenosis or sclerosis
  Coarctation of the aorta
  Pulmonary stenosis
  HCM
  Papillary muscle dysfunction
  Atrial septal defect (due to high pulmonary flow)
  Mitral valve prolapse
  High AV flow states (ASD, VSD, PDA, anaemia, mitral regurgitation, tricuspid regurgitation)
  Atrial tumours (particularly if causing AV flow disturbance)

- **Mid-diastolic murmurs**
  Mitral stenosis or 'Austin Flint' due to aortic regurgitant jet
  Carey Coombs (rheumatic fever)

- **Continuous murmurs**
  PDA
  Ruptured sinus of valsalva aneurysm
  ASD
  Large AV fistula
  Anomalous left coronary artery
  Intercostal AV fistula
  ASD with mitral stenosis
  Bronchial collaterals

3.2 Mitral stenosis

Two-thirds of patients presenting with this are women. The most common cause remains chronic rheumatic heart disease; rarer causes include congenital disease, carcinoid, systemic lupus erythematosus (SLE) and mucopolysaccharidoses (glycoprotein deposits on cusps). Stenosis may occur at the cusp, commisure or chordal level.

- Anticoagulation for atrial fibrillation protects from 17× increased risk of thromboembolism.

Mitral balloon valvuloplasty

Valvuloplasty using an Inoue balloon requires either a trans-septal or a retrograde approach and is used only in suitable cases where echo shows:

- the mitral leaflet tips and valvular chordae are not heavily thickened, distorted or calcified
- the mitral cusps are mobile at the base
- there is minimal or no mitral regurgitation
- no left atrial thrombus is seen on TOE.

Features of severe mitral stenosis

- **Symptoms**
  Dyspnoea with minimal activity
  Haemoptysis
  Dysphagia (due to LA enlargement)
  Palpitations due to atrial fibrillation
- **Chest X-ray**
  Left atrial or right ventricular enlargement
  Splaying of subcarinal angle (>90°)
  Pulmonary congestion or hypertension
  Pulmonary haemosiderosis
- **Echo**
  Doming of leaflets
  Heavily calcified cusps
  Direct orifice area <1.0 cm^2
- **Signs**
  Low pulse pressure
  Soft first heart sound
  Long diastolic murmur and apical thrill (rare)
  Very early opening snap, ie closer to S2 (lost if valves immobile)
  Right ventricular heave or loud P2
  Pulmonary regurgitation (Graham-Steell murmur)
  Tricuspid regurgitation
- **Cardiac catheterisation**
  Pulmonary capillary wedge (PCW) end diastole: left ventricular end-diastolic pressure (LVEDP) gradient >15 mmHg
  Left atrium (LA) pressures >25 mmHg
  Elevated right ventricular and pulmonary artery pressures
  High pulmonary vascular resistance
  Cardiac output <2.5 l min^{-1} m^{-2} with exercise

3.3 Mitral regurgitation

The full structure of the mitral valve includes the annulus, cusps, chordae and papillary musculature, and abnormalities of any of these may cause regurgitation. The presence of symptoms, and increasing left ventricular dilatation are indicators for surgery in the chronic setting. Operative mortalities are 2–7% for valvular replacements in patients with NYHA grade 2–3 symptoms. Valve repair (when possible) has better long-term results in terms of both mortality and morbidity and is most commonly performed for patients with mitral valve leaflet prolapse.

When left ventricular impairment leads to annular dilatation, mitral regurgitation may be functional and this is commonly encountered. The main causes of mitral regurgitation are:

- Chronic rheumatic disease
- Disorders of collagen such as Marfan's syndrome
- Ischaemic (eg papillary muscle dysfunction)
- Mitral valve prolapse (floppy mitral valve)
- Endocarditis
- Connective tissue diseases
- Associated with an atrial septal defect or with HCM
- Annular dilatation (functional regurgitation)

Indicators of the severity of mitral regurgitation

- Small volume pulse
- Left ventricular enlargement due to overload
- Presence of S3
- Mid-diastolic flow murmur
- Precordial thrill, signs of pulmonary hypertension or congestion (cardiac failure).

Signs of predominant mitral regurgitation in mixed mitral valve disease

- Soft S1; S3 present
- Displaced and hyperdynamic apex (left ventricular enlargement)
- ECG showing left ventricular hypertrophy and left axis deviation.

Mitral valve prolapse (MVP)

This condition occurs in 5% of the population and is commonly overdiagnosed (depending on the echocardiography criteria applied). The patients are usually females and may present with chest pains, palpitations or fatigue. Squatting increases the click and standing increases the murmur, but the condition may be diagnosed in the absence of the murmur by echo. Often there is myxomatous degeneration and redundant valve tissue due to deposition of acid mucopolysaccharide material. Antibiotic prophylaxis before dental or surgical interventions should be recommended for those with a murmur. Several conditions are associated with MVP, and patients with the condition are prone to certain sequelae.

Sequelae of mitral valve prolapse:

- embolic phenomena
- rupture of mitral valve chordae
- dysrhythmias with QT prolongation
- sudden death
- cardiac neurosis.

Conditions associated with mitral valve prolapse

- Coronary artery disease
- Cardiomyopathy – dilated cardiomyopathy (DCM)/HCM
- PDA
- Pseudoxanthoma elasticum
- Myocarditis
- Muscular dystrophy
- Polycystic kidney disease
- Secundum ASD
- WPW syndrome
- Marfan's syndrome
- Osteogenesis imperfecta
- SLE; polyarteritis nodosa
- Left atrial myxoma

3.4 Aortic regurgitation

Patients with severe chronic aortic regurgitation (AR) have the largest end-diastolic volumes of those with any forms of heart disease and also have a greater number of non-cardiac signs. AR may occur acutely (as in dissection or endocarditis) or chronically when the left ventricle has time to accommodate.

Causes of aortic regurgitation

- **Valve inflammation**
  Chronic rheumatic
  Infective endocarditis
  Rheumatoid arthritis; SLE
  Hurler's syndrome
- **Aortitis**
  Syphilis
  Ankylosing spondylitis
  Reiter's syndrome
  Psoriatic arthropathy
- **Aortic dissection/trauma**

Eponymous signs associated with AR

- Quincke's sign – nail bed fluctuation of capillary flow
- Corrigan's pulse – (waterhammer); collapsing radial pulse
- Corrigan's sign – visible carotid pulsation
- De Musset's sign – head nodding with each systole
- Duroziez's sign – audible femoral bruits with diastolic flow (indicating moderate severity)
- Traube's sign – 'pistol shots' (systolic auscultatory finding of the femoral arteries)

Continues ...

... Continued

Causes of aortic regurgitation

- **Hypertension**
- **Bicuspid aortic valve**
- **Ruptured sinus of valsalva aneurysm**
- **VSD with prolapse of (R) coronary cusp**
- **Disorders of collagen**
  Marfan's syndrome (aortic aneurysm)
  Hurler's syndrome
  Pseudoxanthoma elasticum

Eponymous signs associated with AR

- Austin Flint murmur – functional mitral diastolic flow murmur
- Argyll–Robertson pupils – aetiological connection with syphilitic aortitis
- Müller's sign – pulsation of the uvula

Indications for surgery

Acute severe AR will not be tolerated for long by a normal ventricle and therefore requires prompt surgery, except in the case of infection where delay for antibiotic therapy is preferable (if haemodynamic stability allows). At 10 years, 50% of patients with moderate chronic AR are alive, but once symptoms occur deterioration is rapid.

Features of AR indicative of the need for surgery

- **Symptoms of dyspnoea/left ventricular failure (LVF)**
  Reducing exercise tolerance
- **Rupture of sinus of valsalva aneurysm**
- **Infective endocarditis not responsive to medical treatment**
- **Enlarging aortic root diameter in Marfan's syndrome with AR**
- **Enlarging heart**
  End systolic diameter >55 mm at echo
  Pulse pressure >100 mmHg
  Diastolic pressure <40 mmHg
  Lengthening diastolic murmur
  ECG: lateral lead T wave inversion

3.5 Aortic stenosis (AS)

Patients often present with the classic triad of symptoms: angina, dyspnoea and syncope. Echo and cardiac catheterisation gradients of >60 mmHg are considered severe and are associated with a valve area <0.5 cm^2. The gradient may be reduced in the presence of deteriorating left ventricular function or mitral stenosis, or significant aortic regurgitation.

- **Causes of AS**: may be congenital bicuspid valve (usually male children, who present in sixth decade), degenerative calcification (common in the elderly) and post-rheumatic disease.
- **Subvalvular**: causes of aortic gradients include HCM and subaortic membranous stenosis, while **supravalvular** stenosis is due to aortic coarctation, or William's syndrome (with elfin facies, mental retardation, hypercalcaemia).
- **Sudden death**: may occur in AS or in subvalvular stenosis due to ventricular tachycardia. The vulnerability to ventricular tachycardia is due to LVH.
- **Complete heart block**: may be due to calcification involving the upper ventricular septal tissue housing the conducting tissue. This may also occur post-operatively (after valve replacement) due to trauma.
- **Calcified emboli**: may arise in severe calcific AS.
- All symptomatic patients should be considered for surgery: operative mortality for AS is predominantly related to the absence (2–8%) or presence (10–25%) of left ventricular failure.

Indicators of severe AS

- Symptoms of syncope or LV failure
- Signs of left ventricular failure
- Soft single S2 or paradoxically split A2
- Presence of precordial thrill
- S4
- Slow rising pulse with narrow pulse pressure
- Late peaking of long murmur
- Valve area <0.5 cm^2 on echocardiography

3.6 Tricuspid regurgitation (TR)

Aetiologies for severe TR include the following:

- Functional, due to right ventricular dilatation.
- Infection, due to intravenous drug abuse.
- Carcinoid (nodular hepatomegaly and telangiectasia).
- Post-rheumatic.
- Ebstein's anomaly: tricuspid valve dysplasia with a more apical position to the valve. Patients have cyanosis and there is an association with pulmonary atresia or ASD and, less commonly, congenitally corrected transposition.

3.7 Prosthetic valves

Valve prostheses may be metal or tissue (bioprosthetic). Mechanical valves are more durable but tissue valves do not require full lifelong anticoagulation. All prostheses must be covered with antibiotic therapy for dental and surgical procedures; they have a residual transvalvular gradient across them.

Mechanical valves

- **Starr–Edwards**: ball and cage – ejection systolic murmur (ESM) in aortic area and an opening sound in mitral position are normal
- **Bjork–Shiley**: single tilt disc – audible clicks without stethoscope
- **St Judes/Carbomedics**: double tilt discs with clicks.

Tissue valves

- **Carpentier–Edwards**: porcine three-cusp valve – 3 months' anticoagulation needed until tissue endothelialisation. No need for long-term anticoagulation if patient is in sinus rhythm
- **Homografts**: usually cadaveric and, again, need no long-term anticoagulation.

Infection of prosthetic valves

- Mortality is still as high as 60% depending on the organism
- Within 6 months of implantation, it is usually due to colonisation by *Staphylococcus epidermidis*
- Septal abscesses may cause PR interval lengthening
- Valvular sounds may be muffled by vegetations; new murmurs may occur
- Mild haemolysis may occur, and is detected by the presence of urobilinogen in the urine
- Dehiscence is an ominous feature requiring urgent intervention.

Anticoagulation in pregnancy

Warfarin may cause fetal haemorrhage and has a teratogenicity risk of 5–30%. This risk is dose-dependent and abnormalities include chondrodysplasia, mental impairment, optic atrophy and nasal hypoplasia. The risk of spontaneous abortion may be increased. At 36 weeks it is advised to switch to intravenous heparin for delivery. Breast-feeding is not a problem with warfarin. In all cases, consideration of the health of the mother should be paramount.

3.8 Infective endocarditis

Groups affected by endocarditis	% of all cases of endocarditis
Chronic rheumatic disease	30
No previous valve disease	40
Intravenous drug abuse	10
Congenital defects	10
Prosthetic	10

- *Streptococcus viridans* (α haemolytic group) are still the most common organisms, occurring in 50% of cases.
- Marantic (metastatic-related) and SLE-related (Libman–Sacks) endocarditis are causes of non-infective endocarditis.

See also Section 3.7 on 'Prosthetic valves'.

Signs of infective endocarditis

As well as cardiac murmurs detected at auscultation, there are several other characteristic features of infective endocarditis:

- **systemic signs of fever and arthropathy**
- **hands and feet**: splinter haemorrhages, Osler nodes (painful), Janeway lesions (painless) and clubbing (late); needle track signs may occur in arm or groin
- **retinopathy**: Roth spots
- **hepatosplenomegaly**
- **signs of arterial embolisation** (eg stroke or digital ischaemia).

- **Poor prognostic factors in endocarditis**
  Prosthetic valve
  Staphylococcus aureus infection
  Culture-negative endocarditis
  Depletion of complement levels

- **Indications for surgery**
  Cardiac failure or haemodynamic compromise
  Extensive valve incompetence
  Large vegetations
  Septic emboli
  Septal abscess
  Fungal infection
  Antibiotic-resistant endocarditis
  Failure to respond to medical therapy

Antibiotic prophylaxis

This is indicated in the following:

Higher risk

- Prosthetic heart valves
- Previous infective endocarditis
- Cyanotic congenital heart disease
- PDA
- VSD
- AR/AS
- Mitral regurgitation (MR)
- Mitral stenosis (MS) and MR
- Coarctation

Intermediate risk

- Mitral valve prolapse with regurgitation
- Pure MS
- Tricuspid and pulmonary valve disease
- Asymmetrical septal hypertrophy
- Bicuspid aortic valve

- Antibiotic prophylaxis is indicated for all dental (including scaling of teeth), surgical, obstetric and gynaecological procedures, rigid bronchoscopy, urethral catheterisation (if urinary infection present) and vaginal delivery (if complicated by infection).
- Prophylaxis is not generally recommended for cardiac catheterisation or for upper GI endoscopy.
- Prophylaxis is not required for patients with isolated secundum ASD or mitral valve prolapse without regurgitation/murmur.

4. CONGENITAL HEART DISEASE

Causes of congenital acyanotic heart disease*

- **With shunts**
  Aortic coarctation (with VSD or PDA)
  VSD
  ASD
  PDA
  Partial anomalous venous drainage (with ASD)
- **Without shunts**
  Congenital aortic stenosis
  Aortic coarctation

Causes of cyanotic heart disease

- **With shunts**
  Fallot's tetralogy (VSD)
  Severe Ebstein's anomaly (ASD)
  Complete transposition of great vessels (ASD VSD/PDA)
- **Without shunts**
  Tricuspid atresia
  Severe pulmonary stenosis
  Pulmonary atresia
  Hypoplastic left heart

*Associated shunts

4.1 Atrial septal defect (ASD)

Atrial septal defects (ASDs) are the most common congenital defects found in adulthood. Rarely, they may present as stroke in young people, due to paradoxical embolus that originated in the venous system and reached the cerebral circulation via right to left shunting. Fixed splitting of the second heart sound is the hallmark of an uncorrected ASD. There may be a left parasternal heave and a pulmonary ejection systolic murmur due to increased blood flow. There are three main sub-types:

- **Secundum (70%)**: central fossa ovalis defects often associated with mitral valve prolapse (10–20% of cases). ECG shows incomplete or complete RBBB with *right* axis deviation. Note that the **patent foramen ovale** (slit-like deficiency in the fossa ovalis) occurs in 25% of the population, but this does not allow equalisation of atrial pressures, unlike ASD.
- **Primum (15%)**: sited above the atrio-ventricular valves, often associated with varying degrees of mitral and tricuspid regurgitation and occasionally a VSD, and thus usually picked up earlier in childhood. ECG shows RBBB, left axis deviation, 1° heart block. Associated with Down's, Klinefelter's and Noonan's syndromes.
- **Sinus venosus (15%)**: defect in the upper septum, often associated with anomalous pulmonary venous drainage directly into the right atrium.

Operative closure is recommended with pulmonary to systolic flow ratios above 1.5:1. Closure of secundum defects may be performed via cardiac catheterisation.

Holt–Oram syndrome: (triphalangeal thumb with ASD) is a rare syndrome (autosomal dominant with incomplete penetration). It is associated with absence (or reduction anomalies) of the upper arm.

Lutembacher's syndrome: a rare combination of an ASD with mitral stenosis (the latter is probably rheumatic in origin).

Investigations for ASDs

Right atrial and right ventricular dilatation may be seen on any imaging technique as may pulmonary artery conus enlargement. Other characteristic features are:

- **Chest X-ray**: pulmonary plethora.
- **Echo**: paradoxical septal motion, septal defect and right to left flow of contrast during venous injection with valsalva manoeuvre.
- **Catheterisation**: pulmonary hypertension: raised right ventricular pressures and step up in oxygen saturation between various parts of the right circulation (eg SVC to high right atrium (RA)).

4.2 Ventricular septal defect (VSD)

Ventricular septal defects (VSD) are the most common isolated congenital defect (2/1000 births; around 30% of all congenital defects); spontaneous closure occurs in 30–50% of cases (usually muscular or membranous types).

- Irreversible pulmonary changes may occur from 1 year of age, with vascular hypertrophy and pulmonary arteriolar thrombosis, leading to Eisenmenger's syndrome.
- Parasternal thrill and pansystolic murmur are present. The murmur may be ejection systolic in very small or very large defects. With large defects the aortic component of the second sound is obscured, or even a single/palpable S2 is heard; a mitral diastolic murmur may occur. The apex beat is typically hyperdynamic.

There is a high risk of subacute endocarditis (SBE) with defects of any size and thus antibiotic prophylaxis is necessary.

Once Eisenmenger's complex develops, the thrill and left sternal edge (LSE) murmur abate and signs are of pulmonary hypertension ± regurgitation and right ventricular failure. Surgery should occur earlier to avoid this situation.

- **Other cardiac associations of VSD**
  PDA (10%)
  Aortic regurgitation (5%)
  Pulmonary stenosis
  ASD
  Fallot's tetralogy
  Coarctation of aorta
- **Types of VSD**
  Muscular
  Membranous
  Atrio-ventricular defect
  Infundibular
  Into right atrium (Gerbode defect)

4.3 Patent ductus arteriosus (PDA)

Patent ductus arteriosus (PDA) is common in premature babies, particularly female infants born at high altitude; also if maternal rubella occurs in the first trimester. The connection occurs between the pulmonary trunk and the descending aorta, usually just distal to the origin of the left subclavian artery. PDA often occurs with other abnormalities.

Key features of PDA

- A characteristic left subclavicular thrill
- Enlarged left heart and apical heave
- Continuous 'machinery' murmur
- Wide pulse pressure and bounding pulse

Signs of pulmonary hypertension and Eisenmenger's syndrome develop in about 5% of cases. Indomethacin closes the duct in about 90% of babies while intravenous prostaglandin E_1 may reverse the natural closure (useful when PDA is associated with coarctation, hypoplastic left heart syndrome and in complete transposition of the great vessels, as it will help to maintain flow between the systemic and pulmonary circulations). The PDA may also be closed thoracoscopically or percutaneously by use of a 'clam shell' or other device.

4.4 Coarctation of the aorta

Coarctation may present in infancy with heart failure, or in adulthood (third decade) with hypertension, exertional breathlessness or leg weakness. This 'shelf-like' obstruction of the aortic arch, usually distal to the left subclavian artery, is 2–5 times more common in males and is responsible for about 7% of congenital heart defects.

Treatment is by surgical resection, preferably with end-to-end aortic anastomosis, or by balloon angioplasty for recurrence after surgery (which occurs in 5–10% of cases). Complications may occur despite resection/repair and these include hypertension, heart failure, berry aneurysm rupture, premature coronary artery disease and aortic dissection (in the third or fourth decade of life).

Associations of coarctation

- **Cardiac**
  Bicuspid aortic valve (and thus AS ± AR) in 10–20%
  PDA
  VSD
  Mitral valve disease

- **Non-cardiac**
  Berry aneurysms (Circle of Willis)
  Turner's syndrome
  Renal abnormalities

- **Signs of coarctation**
  Hypertension
  Radio-femoral delay of arterial pulse
  Absent femoral pulses
  Mid-systolic or continuous murmur (infraclavicular)
  Subscapular bruits
  Rib notching on chest X-ray
  Post-stenotic aortic dilatation on chest X-ray

4.5 Eisenmenger's syndrome

Reversal of left to right shunt, due to massive irreversible pulmonary hypertension (usually due to congenital cardiovascular malformations), leads to Eisenmenger's syndrome. Signs of development include:

- decrease of original pansystolic (left to right) murmur
- decreasing intensity of tricuspid/pulmonary flow murmurs
- single S2 with louder intensity, palpable P2; right ventricular heave

- appearance of Graham–Steell murmur due to pulmonary regurgitation
- 'V' waves due to tricuspid regurgitation (TR) (which may be audible)
- clubbing and central cyanosis.

Eisenmenger's syndrome

- **Causes**
  VSD (termed Eisenmenger's complex)
  ASD
  PDA
- **Complications of Eisenmenger's syndrome**
  Right ventricular failure
  Massive haemoptysis
  Cerebral embolism/abscess
  Infective endocarditis (rare)

4.6 Tetralogy of Fallot

The most common cause of cyanotic congenital heart disease (10%) usually presenting after age 6 months (as the condition may worsen after birth).

Key features

- Pulmonary stenosis (causes the systolic murmur)
- Right ventricular hypertrophy
- VSD
- Overriding of aorta
- Right-sided aortic knuckle (25%)

Clinical features	Possible complications of Fallot's tetralogy
Cyanotic attacks (pulmonary infundibular spasm)	Endocarditis
Clubbing	Polycythaemia
Parasternal heave	Coagulopathy
Systolic thrill	Paradoxical embolism
Palpable A2	Cerebral abscess
Soft ESM (inversely related to pulmonary gradient)	Ventricular arrhythmias
Single S2 (inaudible pulmonary closure)	
ECG features of right ventricular hypertrophy	

- Cyanotic attacks worsen with catecholamines, hypoxia and acidosis. The murmur lessens or disappears as the right ventricular outflow gradient increases.
- Squatting reduces the right to left shunt by increasing systemic vascular resistance; it also reduces venous return of acidotic blood from lower extremities, and hence reduces infundibular spasm.
- The presence of a systolic thrill and an intense pulmonary murmur differentiates the condition from Eisenmenger's syndrome.
- A Blalock shunt operation results in weaker pulses in the arm from which the subclavian artery is diverted to the pulmonary artery.

5. ARRHYTHMIAS AND PACING

Atrial fibrillation remains the most common cardiac arrhythmia, with incidence increasing with age (Framingham data indicate a prevalence of 76/1000 males and 63/1000 females aged 85–94 years).

Use of the term 'supraventricular tachycardia' (SVT) is best avoided as it is imprecise, particularly as radiofrequency ablation is changing the face of treatment in this condition. Ventricular tachycardia and fibrillation are life-threatening conditions, but implantable defibrillators and catheter or surgical ablation are now additional treatments to conventional pharmacological therapy.

5.1 Complete heart block (CHB)

Untreated acquired CHB is associated with mortality that may exceed 50% at 1 year, particularly in patients aged over 80 years and in those with non-rheumatic structural heart disease.

- CHB is the most common reason for permanent pacing.
- It occurs mostly with right coronary artery occlusion, when related to an infarction, as the AV nodal branch is usually one of the distal branches of the right coronary artery.
- CHB rarely (3–7% of patients) requires permanent pacing when it occurs after acute infarction.
- In patients with an anterior infarct CHB is a poor prognostic feature, indicating extensive ischaemia.
- Congenital cases may be related to connective tissue diseases; however, in patients having normal exercise capacities, recent studies show that prognosis is not as benign as was previously thought and pacing is therefore recommended.

5.2 Re-entrant tachycardias

There are two major groups of re-entrant tachycardias:

- **AV nodal re-entry tachycardia (AVNRT)**: this is often referred to as SVT, and involves a re-entry circuit in or around the AV node.
- **AV re-entry tachycardia (AVRT)**: this involves an abnormal connection between the atria and ventricles some distance from the AV node (eg Wolff–Parkinson–White syndrome).

Wolff–Parkinson–White (WPW) syndrome

Occurring in 0.15% of healthy individuals, WPW is associated with an accessory pathway that connects the atrium and ventricle; this mediates the tachycardia by enabling retrograde conduction from ventricle to atrium. More seriously, the accessory pathway may predispose to unopposed conduction of AF from atria to ventricles as a result of anterograde conduction through the pathway. This may lead on to ventricular fibrillation.

- Characteristically produces a delta wave on the ECG due to early pathway-mediated ventricular activation (NB Lown–Ganong–Levine syndrome: accessory pathway without a delta wave) and thus has a short PR interval. The delta wave is lost with tachycardia if conduction via the pathway is retrograde (ventricle to atrium).
- Usually presents in adolescents with a narrow complex tachycardia (AV re-entry tachycardia) with the P wave occurring visibly and shortly after the QRS, rather than buried in the QRS as in AV nodal re-entry tachycardias (where the atria and ventricles depolarise simultaneously). In 90% of cases there is retrograde conduction via an accessory pathway – hence narrow tachycardia.
- Vagal manoeuvres may help, as may beta-blockers, flecainide and amiodarone.
- Digoxin and IV verapamil may accelerate conduction down the accessory pathway by blocking the AV node and **therefore should be avoided**.
- Radiofrequency ablation is the treatment of choice; it incurs a <1% risk of CHB.

Associations with WPW include: Ebstein's anomaly (may have multiple pathways), HCM, mitral valve prolapse, thyrotoxicosis, more common in men.

5.3 Atrial arrhythmias

Atrial flutter

The atrial rate is usually between 250 and 350 beats/min and is often seen with a ventricular response of 150 (2:1 block) beats/min. The block may vary between a 1:1 ratio to 1:4 or even 1:5. Isolated atrial flutter (without atrial fibrillation) is uncommon and has a lower association with thromboembolism; however, at the present time anticoagulation is often recommended with prolonged flutter.

- The ventricular response may be slowed by increasing the vagal block of the AV node (eg carotid sinus massage) or by adenosine which 'uncovers' the flutter waves on ECG.
- This is the most likely arrhythmia to respond to DC cardioversion with low energies (eg 25 volts).
- Amiodarone and sotalol may chemically cardiovert, slow the ventricular response or act as prophylactic agents.
- Radiofrequency ablation is curative in up to 90% of cases.

Atrial fibrillation (AF)

This arrhythmia is due to multiple wavelet propagation in different directions. The source of the arrhythmia may be myocardial tissue in the openings of the four pulmonary veins which enter into the posterior aspect of the left atrium, and this is particularly the case in younger patients with paroxysmal atrial fibrillation. AF may be paroxysmal, persistent (but 'cardiovertable') or permanent, and in all three states is a risk factor for strokes. Treatment is aimed at ventricular rate control, cardioversion, recurrence prevention and anticoagulation. Atrial defibrillators are now available.

Associations with atrial fibrillation

- IHD
- Mitral valve disease
- Hypertension
- Thyroid disease
- Acute alcohol excess/chronic alcoholic cardiomyopathy
- Caffeine excess
- Dilated left atrium (>4.5 cm)
- WPW
- Pericarditis
- Pulmonary embolus
- Atrial myxomas
- Left ventricular hypertrophy
- ASD
- Post-coronary artery bypass graft (CABG)
- Pneumonia
- Bronchial malignancy

The overall risk of systemic emboli is 5–7% annually (higher with rheumatic valve disease); this falls to 1.6% with anticoagulation. **Trans-oesophageal echocardiography** may exclude atrial appendage thrombus but cannot predict development of a thrombus in the early stages post-cardioversion; anticoagulation is therefore always recommended for prolonged atrial fibrillation.

- **Risk factors for stroke with non-valvular AF**
  Previous history of CVA or TIA (risk ↑ ×22.5)
  Diabetes (×1.7)
  Hypertension (×1.6)
  Left ventricular impairment
  Left atrial enlargement

- **Risk factors for recurrence of AF after cardioversion**
  Long duration (>1–3 years)
  Rheumatic mitral valve disease
  Left atrium size >5.5 cm
  Older age (>75 years)
  Left ventricular impairment

5.4 Ventricular arrhythmias and long QT syndromes

Ventricular tachycardia (monomorphic)

Ventricular tachycardia (VT) has a poor prognosis when left ventricular function is impaired. After the exclusion of reversible causes such patients may need implantable defibrillators and anti-arrhythmic therapy.

- Ventricular rate is usually 120–200 beats/min.
- Patients should be DC cardioverted when there is haemodynamic compromise; overdrive (or underdrive) pacing may also terminate VT.
- Amiodarone, sotalol, flecainide and lignocaine may be therapeutic adjuncts or prophylactic agents; magnesium may also be useful.

Associations of ventricular tachycardia

- Myocardial ischaemia
- Hypokalaemia or severe hyperkalaemia
- Long QT syndrome (see overleaf)
- Digoxin toxicity (VT may arise from either ventricle, especially with associated hypokalaemia)
- Cardiomyopathies
- Congenital abnormalities of the right ventricular outflow tract (VT with LBBB and right axis deviation pattern)

Features favouring ventricular tachycardia (VT) in broad complex tachycardia

It is often difficult to distinguish VT from SVT with aberration (disordered ventricular propagation of a supraventricular impulse); VT remains the most common cause of a broad complex tachycardia, especially with a previous history of myocardial infarction (MI). The following ECG observations favour VT:

- capture beats: intermittent SA node complexes transmitted to ventricle
- fusion beats: combination QRS from SA node and VT focus meeting and fusing (causes cannon waves)
- right bundle branch block (RBBB) with left axis deviation (LAD)
- very wide QRS >140 ms
- altered QRS compared to sinus rhythm
- V leads concordance with all QRS vectors, positive or negative
- dissociated P waves: marching through the VT
- history of ischaemic heart disease: very good predictor
- variable S1
- HR <170 beats/min with no effect of carotid sinus massage.

Ventricular tachycardia (polymorphic) - torsades des pointes

Anti-arrhythmic agents (particularly class III) may predispose to torsades as the arrhythmia is often initiated during bradycardia. The VT is polymorphic (QRS complexes of different amplitudes twist around the isoelectric line), with QT prolongation when patient is in sinus rhythm.

- Intravenous magnesium and K^+ channel openers may control the arrhythmia, whereas isoprenaline and temporary pacing may prevent bradycardia and hence the predisposition to VT.
- May be due to QT prolongation of any cause (see later).

Long QT syndromes (including Romano Ward; Jervell–Lange–Neilsen)

Abnormally prolonged QT intervals may be familial or acquired, and are associated with syncope and sudden death, due to ventricular tachycardia (especially torsades des pointes). Mortality in the untreated symptomatic patient with congenital abnormality is high but some patients may reach the age of 50–60 years despite repeated attacks. Causes and associations are shown below.

Causes and associations of prolonged QT intervals

- **Familial**
  Jervell–Lange–Neilsen syndrome
  Romano Ward syndrome
- **Ischaemic heart disease**
- **Metabolic**
  Hypocalcaemia
  Hypothyroidism
  Hypothermia
  Hypokalaemia
- **Rheumatic carditis**
- **Mitral valve prolapse**
- **Drugs**
  Quinidine
  Erythromycin
  Amiodarone
  Tricyclic antidepressants
  Phenothiazines
  Probucol
  Non-sedating antihistamines
  (eg terfenadine)

- The corrected QT is >540 ms (normal = 380–460 ms).
- Ninety per cent are familial, with chromosome 11 defect (Romano Ward is autosomal dominant inheritance, Jervell–Lange–Neilsen is autosomal recessive and associated with congenital deafness).
- Arrhythmias may be reduced by a combination of beta-blockers and pacing.

Cardiac causes of electro-mechanical dissociation (EMD)

When faced with a cardiac arrest situation it is important to appreciate the list of causes of electro-mechanical dissociation (EMD):

- hypoxia
- hypovolaemia
- hypokalaemia/hyperkalaemia
- hypothermia
- tension pneumothorax
- tamponade
- toxic/therapeutic disturbance
- thromboembolic/mechanical obstruction.

5.5 Pacing and ablation procedures

Temporary pacing

The ECG will show LBBB morphology (unless there is septal perforation when it is RBBB). Pacing may be ventricular (right ventricle apex) or atrio-ventricular (atrial appendage and right ventricle apex) for optimised cardiac output.

Complications include:

- Crossing the tricuspid valve during insertion causes ventricular ectopics, as does irritating the outflow tract.
- Atrial or right ventricular perforation and pericardial effusion.
- **Pneumothorax**: internal jugular route is preferable to subclavian as it minimises this risk and also allows control after inadvertent arterial punctures.

Permanent pacing

More complex permanent pacing systems include rate-responsive models which use piezocrystal movement sensors or physiological triggers (respiratory rate or QT interval) to increase heart rates. Although more expensive they avoid causing pacemaker syndrome and they act more physiologically for optimal left ventricular function.

- **Indications for temporary pacing**
  Asystole
  Haemodynamically compromised bradycardia
  Prophylaxis of myocardial infarction complicated by second-degree or complete heart block
  Prior to high-risk cardiac interventions or pacemaker replacement
  Prevention of some tachyarrhythmias (eg torsades)
  Overdrive termination of various arrhythmias (eg atrial flutter, VT)

Continues ...

... Continued

- **Indications for permanent pacing**
  Chronic atrio-ventricular block
  Sick sinus syndrome with symptoms (including chronotropic incompetence – the inability to appropriately increase the heart rate with activity)
  Chronotropic incompetence
  Post-AV nodal ablation for arrhythmias
  Neurocardiogenic syncope
  Hypertrophic cardiomyopathy
  Dilated cardiomyopathy (may pace more than two chambers)
  Long QT syndrome
  Prevention of atrial fibrillation
  Post-cardiac transplantation

Pacing in heart failure

There are several synonymous terms for pacing in patients with cardiac failure. These include cardiac resynchronisation therapy, biventricular pacing or multisite pacing. The indications for pacing in heart failure are all of the following:

- NYHA III-IV heart failure.
- QRS duration >130 ms.
- Left ventricular ejection fraction <35% with dilated ventricle and patient on optimal medical therapy (diuretics, angiotensin converting enzyme (ACE) inhibitors and beta-blockers).

The atria and right ventricle are paced in the usual fashion and in addition to this a pacing electrode is placed in a tributary of the coronary sinus on the lateral aspect of the left ventricle. The two ventricles are paced simultaneously or near simultaneously with a short atrio-ventricular delay. The aim is to optimise AV delay and reduce inter- and intraventricular asynchrony. This therapy is known to improve exercise capacity, quality of life and to reduce hospital admissions.

Implantable cardioverter defibrillators (ICD)

ICD are devices that are able to detect life-threatening tachyarrhythmias and to terminate them by overdrive pacing or a counter shock. They are implanted in a similar manner to permanent pacemakers. Current evidence supports their use in both secondary prevention of cardiac arrest and also as targeted primary prevention (eg individuals with left ventricular impairment and those with familial syndromes such as arrhythmogenic right ventricular dysplasia, Brugada syndrome, long QT variants).

Radio frequency ablation

Radio frequency ablation is heat-mediated (65 °C) protein membrane disruption causing cell lysis without the risk of coagulum forming on the electrode tip. Using cardiac catheterisation (with electrodes in right- or left-sided chambers) it interrupts electrical pathways in cardiac structures. Excellent results are obtained with accessory pathways, His–Purkinje system or for AV nodal ablation. It is technically more difficult in atrial flutter (where a line of block across the atrium is required) and in VT (ventricular myocardium is much thicker than atrial). Ablation for atrial fibrillation is a rapidly developing technique. This involves isolating the pulmonary veins by ablation therapy, and it currently has a modest success rate of around a 60% cure. Complete heart block and pericardial effusions are rare complications of radio frequency ablation.

6. ISCHAEMIC HEART DISEASE

Cardiovascular disease remains the largest cause of death in the UK, accounting for almost 250, 000 deaths (77, 000 from myocardial infarction) in 1994 (compared to 140, 000 deaths from malignant disease). Ischaemic heart disease may present with an acute ischaemic event, heart failure or with arrhythmia.

Risk factors for coronary artery disease (CAD)

- **Primary**
  Hypercholesterolaemia (LDL)
  Hypertension
  Smoking
- **Unclear**
  Low fibre intake
  Hard water
  High plasma fibrinogen levels
  Raised Lp (a) levels
  Raised Factor VII levels
- **Protective factors**
  Exercise
  Moderate amounts of alcohol
  Low cholesterol diet
  Increased HDL:LDL
- **Secondary**
  Reduced HDL cholesterol
  Obesity
  Insulin-dependent diabetes mellitus (IDDM)
  Non-insulin-dependent diabetes (NIDDM)
  Family history of CAD
  Physical inactivity
  Stress and personality type
  Gout and hyperuricaemia
  Race (Asians)
  Low weight at 1 year of age
  Male sex
  Chronic renal failure
  Increasing age
  Low social class
  Increased homocystine levels and homocystinuria

Smoking and its relationship to cardiovascular disease

Smokers have an increased incidence of the following cardiovascular complications:

- Coronary artery disease
- Malignant hypertension
- Ischaemic stroke
- Morbidity from peripheral vascular disease
- Sudden death
- Subarachnoid haemorrhage
- Mortality due to aortic aneurysm
- Thromboembolism in patients taking oral contraceptives

Both active and passive smoking increase the risk of coronary atherosclerosis by a number of mechanisms. These include:

- increased platelet adhesion/aggregation and whole blood viscosity
- increased heart rate; increased catecholamine sensitivity/release
- increased carboxyhaemoglobin level and, as a result, increased haematocrit
- decreased HDL cholesterol and vascular compliance
- decreased threshold for ventricular fibrillation.

6.1 Angina

Other than the usual forms of stable and unstable angina, those worthy of specific mention include:

- **Decubitus**: usually on lying down – due to an increase in LVEDP or associated with dreaming, cold sheets, or coronary spasm during REM sleep.
- **Variant (Prinzmetal)**: unpredictable, at rest, with transient ST elevation on ECG. Due to coronary spasm, with or without underlying arteriosclerotic lesions.
- **Syndrome X**: this refers to a heterogeneous group of patients who have ST segment depression on exercise test, but angiographically normal coronary arteries. The patients may have very small vessel disease and/or abnormal ventricular function. It is commonly described in middle-aged females and oestrogen deficiency has been suggested to be an aetiological factor.
- **Vincent angina**: nothing to do with cardiology; infection of pharyngeal and tonsillar space!

Causes of non-anginal chest pains

- **Pericardial pain**
- **Aortic dissection**
- **Mediastinitis**
  Associated with trauma, pneumothorax or diving
- **Pleural**
  Usually with breathlessness in pleurisy, pneumonia, pneumothorax or a large peripheral pulmonary embolus
- **Musculoskeletal**
- **Gastrointestinal**
  Including oesophageal, gastric, gallbladder, pancreatic
- **Hyperventilation/anxiety**
  Reproduction of sharp infra-mammary pains on forced hyperventilation is a reliable test
- **Mitral valve prolapse**
  May be spontaneous, sharp, superficial, short-lived pain

Symptomatic assessment of angina

The Canadian cardiovascular assessment of chest pain is useful for grading the severity of angina:

- **grade I**: angina only on strenuous or prolonged exertion
- **grade II**: angina climbing two flights of stairs
- **grade III**: angina walking one block on the level (indication for intervention)
- **grade IV**: angina at rest (indication for urgent intervention).

6.2 Myocardial infarction

Myocardial infarction (MI) occurs with an annual incidence of 5/1000 in the UK. The mortality associated with MI remains high, with a 40% out-of-hospital and a 20% in-hospital mortality rate, and an overall mortality of 27% at 28 days post-MI.

Diagnosis of MI

Acute, evolving or recent MI

Either one of the following criteria satisfies the diagnosis for an acute, evolving or recent MI.

- Typical rise and gradual fall (troponin) or more rapid rise and fall (CK-MB) of biochemical markers of myocardial necrosis with at least one of the following:
  ischemic symptoms
  development of pathologic Q waves on the ECG
  ECG changes indicative of ischemia (ST segment elevation or depression) coronary artery intervention (eg coronary angioplasty).

- Pathologic finding of an acute MI (eg at post-mortem).

Established MI

Any one of the following criteria satisfies the diagnosis of an established MI:

- Development of new pathologic Q waves on serial ECGs. The patient may or may not remember previous symptoms. Biochemical markers of myocardial necrosis may have normalised, depending on the length of time that has passed since the infarct developed.
- Pathologic finding of a healed or healing MI.

Distinction between STEMI (ST segment Elevation MI) and NSTEMI

An acute MI should be classified as **STEMI** when there is :

- ST segment elevation (≥2 mm in two or more chest leads, or ≥1 mm in two or more limb leads)
- a chronic MI with Q wave formation
- pathological or imaging evidence of a full thickness scar.

Other MI that do not meet these criteria should be classified as **NSTEMI**.

Cardiac enzymes

A number of markers of cardiac damage are now available. The following table is a guide to the timing of the initial rise, peak and return to normality.

Marker	Initial rise	Peak	Return to normal	Notes
Creatine phosphokinase*	4–8 h	18 h	2–3 days	CPK-MB is main cardiac isoenzyme
Myoglobin	1–4 h	6–7 h	24 h	Low specificity from skeletal muscle damage
Troponin**	3–12 h	24 h	3–10 days	Troponins I and T are the most sensitive and specific markers of myocardial damage available
Lactate dehydrogenase (LDH)	10 h	24–48 h	14 days	Cardiac muscle mainly contains LDH

* Creatine phosphokinase has three isoenzymes of which the CPK-MB isoenzyme is most cardiac-specific, although numerous other organs possess the enzyme in small quantities. A CPK-MB of >2.5% of the total CPK has been suggested as very specific for MI in the context of chest pain. This is inaccurate in situations of significant acute or chronic skeletal injury where CPK levels will be high.

** Troponins are reliably positive from 12 hours after onset of ischaemia, a level greater than the 99th centile for the assay is regarded as positive. Assays may be read only, semi quantitative or quantitative and local laboratory guidelines for interpretation should be adhered to. False positives occur in renal impairment and uncontrolled diabetes mellitus. Myocardial necrosis and hence positive troponins also occur in pulmonary embolus, myocarditis and extreme brady or tachycardia.

Troponin I and T

- There is increased interest in the use of troponin assays (I and T) in the diagnostic and prognostic assessment of patients presenting with acute coronary syndromes (STEMI or NSTEMI and unstable angina).
- Troponin I and T are subunits of the complex that is involved in the regulation of the calcium-mediated contractile process of cardiac muscle.
- Troponin T may take up to 10–14 days to return to normal values after myocardial ischaemia.
- False-positive troponin elevations occur in renal impairment (see later) and in uncontrolled diabetes.

	Stable angina	Unstable angina	NSTEMI	STEMI
ECG changes	None, ST depression	None, ST depression	ST depression, T wave inversion	ST elevation, BBB
Troponin	Normal	Normal or elevated*	Elevated	Elevated
CK	Normal	Normal	Elevated	Elevated
Echo	No new RWMA	No new RWMA	Possible RWMA	Usually RWMA

BBB = bundle branch block; NSTEMI = (non) ST segment elevation MI; RWMA = regional wall motion abnormality; STEMI = ST segment elevation MI.
*Some (including ESC) categorise all troponin-elevated episodes as MI.

Troponin assays in patients with renal failure

The troponin level may be elevated simply because a patient has renal failure. In patients with renal failure who present with chest pain it is helpful to assess the troponin level at baseline as well as at 12 hours after the onset of symptoms, and sometimes at later time points. In these circumstances only a rising troponin level would be suggestive of ischaemic myocardial damage.

- **Posterior infarction** (a tall R wave in V1 with ST depression in leads V1–V3): no clear benefit of thrombolysis has been shown as few patients have been enrolled into major trials, especially as ECG interpretation is often difficult when the presentation is not with inferior infarct. However, the general consensus would still be to give thrombolysis. Sixty per cent are due to right coronary artery disease.
- **NSTEMI (sub-endocardial) infarctions**: have not been shown to benefit from thrombolysis. They have a low in-patient but high (65%) one-year mortality (compared to 34% for STEMI infarcts) and they should be investigated early and aggressively.
- Temporary pacing is indicated in anterior MI complicated by CHB. This presentation is associated with high mortality due to the extensive myocardial damage. The decision as to whether to temporarily pace a patient with inferior infarction and CHB is primarily dictated by the patient's haemodynamic status. Atropine and isoprenaline can also be tried. Narrow complex escape rhythms are more stable. A 2-week post-MI period is appropriate to allow the return of sinus rhythm before considering permanent pacing.

- The right coronary artery (RCA) is the dominant vessel (over left circumflex) in 85% of patients. As this gives off branches to SA and AV nodes, heart block and a larger infarct might be observed if a dominant RCA is occluded.

Although **warfarin** provides no general benefit, it may reduce the overall CVA rate (1.5–3.6%) in those patients with mural left ventricular thrombus on echo after a large anterior MI, and is thus recommended for up to 6 months after the infarction.

Complications of MI

Since the advent of thrombolysis, complication rates have been reduced (eg halved for pericarditis, conduction defects, ventricular thrombus, fever, Dressler's syndrome). All complications may be seen with any type of infarction, but the following are the most common associations.

- **Anterior infarctions**
  Late VT/VF
  Left ventricular aneurysm
  Left ventricular thrombus and systemic embolism (usually 1–3 weeks post-MI)
  CHB (rare)
  Ischaemic mitral regurgitation
  Congestive cardiac failure
  Cardiac rupture – usually at days 4–10 with EMD
  VSD with septal rupture
  Pericarditis and pericardial effusion (**Dressler's** syndrome with high ESR, fever, anaemia, pleural effusions and anti-cardiac muscle antibodies is seen occasionally)

- **Inferior infarctions**
  Higher re-infarction rate
  Inferior aneurysm – with mitral regurgitation (rare)
  Pulmonary embolism (rare)
  CHB and other degrees of heart block
  Papillary muscle dysfunction and mitral regurgitation
  Right ventricular infarcts need high filling pressures (particularly if posterior extension)

Post-MI rehabilitation

After myocardial infarction, a patient should take 2 months off work and 1 month's abstinence from sexual intercourse and driving (see following text). Cardiac rehabilitation is particularly important for patient confidence. Depression occurs in 30% of patients.

Fitness to drive

The DVLA provides extensive guidelines for coronary disease and interventions, but the essential points are:

- Ordinary drivers do not need to inform the DVLA of cardiac events unless a continuing disability results. Driving should be avoided for 1 month after MI, coronary artery bypass grafting (CABG), unstable angina, and for 1 week after percutaneous coronary angioplasty (PTCA) or pacemaker insertion.

- Vocational drivers (HGV, etc) must inform the DVLA. They should not recommence driving until 3 months post-MI or CABG, and they must be symptom free and able to complete the first three stages of a Bruce protocol safely (off treatment for 24 hours), without symptoms, signs or ECG changes.
- Implantation of cardiac defibrillators usually results in loss of licence, although this may be reconsidered if the patient remains shock free for at least 6 months.

6.3 Thrombolysis

Thrombolysis is beneficial up to 6 hours after pain onset but may be given for up to 12 hours in the context of continuing pain or deteriorating condition. Recanalisation after thrombolysis occurs in 70% (15% without) of patients and results in a higher, earlier CPK rise (but a lower total CPK release). Reperfusion arrhythmias are common within the first 2 hours after thrombolysis. Theoretically (but generally impractical at this stage) primary angioplasty is better than thrombolysis for acute MI if performed within the first few hours.

Tissue plasminogen activator (TPA) and similar recombinant agents are five to seven times more expensive than streptokinase (SK) and should be used only in patients to whom SK has previously been administered, those with proven streptococcal throat infections, or in hypotensive patients. The absolute added mortality benefit for large anterior MI in younger patients presenting within 4 hours is only 1% above SK.

Contraindications to thrombolysis

Although there are numerous relative contraindications where the risk/benefit considerations are individual to the patient (eg a large anterior infarct in a patient where access to primary percutaneous coronary angioplasty is unavailable), there are several absolute contraindications to thrombolysis.

Contraindications to thrombolysis

- **Absolute**
  Active internal bleeding or uncontrollable external bleeding
  Suspected aortic dissection
  Recent head trauma (<2 weeks)
  Intracranial neoplasms
  History of proven haemorrhagic stroke or cerebral infarction <2 months earlier
  Uncontrolled blood pressure (>200/120 mmHg)
  Pregnancy
- **Relative**
  Traumatic prolonged cardiopulmonary resuscitation
  Bleeding disorders
  Recent surgery
  Probable intracardiac thrombus (eg AF with mitral stenosis)
  Active diabetic haemorrhagic retinopathy
  Anticoagulation or INR >1.8

Groups particularly benefiting from thrombolysis (determined by the GUSTO, ISIS 2 and ISIS 3 trials) include:

- large anterior infarction
- pronounced ST elevation
- elderly (>75 years)
- poor left ventricular function or LBBB, or systolic BP <100 mmHg
- early administration: within 1 hour of pain onset.

Summary of clinical trials in patients with acute MI†

Agents used for acute MI	Mortality in treated group (%)	Mortality in control subjects (%)	Number treated to save 1 life	Trials involved
Aspirin	9.4 (at 5 weeks)	11.8	42	ISIS 2
Thrombolytics	10.7* (at 21 days)	13.0*	43*	GISSI 1*, ISIS 2, TIMI II, GUSTO
Beta-blockers	3.9 (at 7 days)	4.6	143	ISIS 1
ACE inhibitors	35.2* (after 39-month mean follow-up)	39.7*	22*	SAVE, SOLVD*, AIRE
Lipid-lowering therapy (patients with average cholesterol)	10.2 (after 5 years)	13.2	33	CARE (note endpoints included second non-fatal MI and cardiac deaths)
Heparin with aspirin and any form of thrombolysis	8.6	9.1	200	Meta-analysis of 68, 000 patients
Magnesium: contradictory data but no mortality reduction				LIMIT 1, 2, ISIS 4
Nitrates: no clear benefit				ISIS 4, GISSI 3
Warfarin: no proven benefit above aspirin after thrombolysis				

† See also Appendix 2: 'Summary of important large trials in cardiovascular disease'.
* Data from that particular trial.

6.4 Coronary artery interventional procedures

After **percutaneous coronary angioplasty** (PTCA) the recurrence or re-stenosis rate is 30% within 3 months (without stent insertion) and 40–60% for total occlusions that are successfully dilated. Lesions particularly amenable to PTCA include those that are discrete, proximal, non-calcified, unoccluded, which are away from side-branches and which occur in patients with a short history of angina. While there is an acute occlusion rate of the order of 2.5–3% with angioplasty, many of these can be managed successfully with intra-coronary stenting, such that the need for emergency CABG has fallen to around 1%.

Elective **stenting** is used increasingly (around 70% of all angioplasties) and this appears to have reduced the re-stenosis rates. It is of particular benefit in diabetic patients, during angioplasty of saphenous vein grafts, and for chronic total occlusions. Other important considerations in coronary intervention are:

- Vessels <2.5 mm in diameter have sub-optimal results after stenting whilst vessels >4.5 mm in diameter rarely require it if the flow is good.
- **Ticlopidine**, used for a month, was previously given in addition to aspirin to reduce the rates of acute occlusion and in-stent re-stenosis. However, the combination of choice has now changed to **clopidogrel** and aspirin. Clopidogrel has advantages over ticlopidine, including a much lower incidence of severe neutropenia (*see* Chapter 2, Clinical Pharmacology, Toxicology and Poisoning).
- Elective balloon pump insertion may be useful in particularly high-risk patients.
- In patients with three-vessel disease, PCTA and CABG are comparable in price, but the former requires more repeat procedures.
- **Glycoprotein IIb/IIIa receptor blockers** (inhibit platelet aggregation) are used increasingly in both higher risk angioplasties/stents (eg diabetics, saphenous vein grafts, and in patients undergoing intervention for acute coronary syndromes), and also in the medical management of patients with NSTEMI or unstable angina.
- **Drug eluting stents**: a major complication of bare metal stents is in-stent re-stenosis. The coating of stents with immunosuppressant agents (eg sirolimus) almost abolishes this problem.

Coronary artery bypass grafting (CABG)

Coronary artery bypass grafting (CABG) has clear benefits in specific groups of patients with chronic coronary artery disease (when compared to medical therapy alone). Analysis has previously been limited because randomised trials included small numbers and were performed several decades ago; patients studied were usually males aged <65 years. The population now receiving CABG has changed, but so has medical therapy.

- Prognostic benefits are shown for symptomatic, significant left main stem disease (Veteran's Study), symptomatic proximal three-vessel disease and in two-vessel disease which includes proximal left anterior descending (LAD) artery (CASS data).
- Patients with moderately impaired left ventricular function have greater benefit, but those with poor left ventricular function have greater operative mortality. Overall mortality is <2%, rising to between 5% and 10% for a second procedure. Eighty per cent of patients gain symptom relief.
- Peri-operative graft occlusion is around 10% for vein grafts, which otherwise last 8–10 years. Arterial grafts (internal mammary, gastro-epiploic) have a higher patency rate but long-term data are awaited.
- A 'Dressler-like' syndrome may occur up to 6 months post-surgery.
- Minimally invasive CABG involves the redirection of internal mammary arteries to coronary vessels without the need for cardiac bypass and full stenotomy incisions. Recovery times following this procedure are extremely short.

7. OTHER MYOCARDIAL DISEASES

7.1 Cardiac failure

Cardiac failure can be defined as the pumping action of the heart being insufficient to meet the circulatory demands of the body (in the absence of mechanical obstructions). A broad echocardiographic definition is of an ejection fraction (EF) <40% (as in the SAVE trial, which enrolled patients for ACE inhibitors post-MI). Overall 5-year survival is 65% with EF <40%, compared to 95% in those with EF >50%. The most common cause of cardiac failure in the Western world is ischaemic heart disease.

The ejection fraction is, however, only a guide and is dependent on other pre-load and after-load factors.

- **Pre-load**: will affect left ventricular end-diastolic pressure.
- **After-load**: will affect left ventricular systolic wall tension.

Other echocardiographic features of LV dysfunction include reduced fractional shortening, LV enlargement and paradoxical septal motion.

The New York Heart Association (NYHA) classification is a helpful indication of severity:

NYHA class	Symptoms	One-year mortality (%)
I	Asymptomatic with ordinary activity	5–10
II	Slight limitation of physical activities	15
III	Marked limitation of physical activities	30
IV	Dyspnoeic symptoms at rest	50–60

7.2 Hypertrophic cardiomyopathy (HCM)

Characteristic features of HCM

- Jerky pulse with large tidal wave as outflow obstruction is overcome
- Large 'a' waves in JVP
- Double apical impulse (palpable atrial systole, S4, in sinus rhythm)
- LSE systolic thrill (turbulence) with harsh ESM radiating to axilla
- Often accompanied by mitral regurgitation
- Often paradoxical splitting of second heart sound
- The ejection systolic murmur increases with valsalva manoeuvre and decreases with squatting.

Important points to remember

- Associations with Friedreich's ataxia, WPW, phaeochromocytoma, familial lentiginosis.
- ESM *increases* with: glyceryl trinitrate (GTN), digoxin and standing, due to volume reduction in diastole; ESM *decreases* with: squatting, beta-blockers, valsalva release, handgrip.

- Avoid digoxin (if in sinus rhythm), nitrates, atropine, inotropes, diuretics (unless in left ventricular failure (LVF)).
- Cardiac catheterisation abnormalities include a 'banana' or 'spade-shaped' left ventricular cavity in systole, mitral regurgitation and 'sword fish' narrowing of the left anterior descending artery.
- Autosomal dominant in half the patients, associated with chromosomes 1, 11, 14 or 15. May also result from a gene mutation which leads to myocardial disarray and varying expression of hypertrophy. Prevalence <0.2% of the general population. Life expectancy is variable with symptoms and investigations determining risk of sudden death.
- **Sudden death** may be due to catecholamine-driven extreme outflow obstruction, ventricular fibrillation related to accessory pathway – transmitted AF, or massive MI. Sudden death may occur without hypertrophy. Annual mortality of 2.5% in adults and 6% in children.
- Poor prognostic features include young age of diagnosis, family history of sudden death and syncopal symptoms, but there is no correlation with the left ventricular outflow tract gradient.
- Pregnancy is possible, but haemorrhage, prolonged vaginal delivery effort and epidural analgesia are best avoided; antibiotic prophylaxis and counselling are advised.
- Therapeutic options include beta-blockers, calcium antagonists, amiodarone, dual chamber pacing, internal defibrillators, surgical myomectomy or therapeutic septal infarction.

Echocardiographic features of HCM (none are diagnostic)

- Asymmetrical septal hypertrophy: septum >30% thicker than left ventricular posterior wall
- Left ventricular outflow tract gradient ± turbulence
- Premature closure of aortic cusps
- Almost complete obliteration of left ventricular cavity
- Systolic anterior motion of anterior mitral valve cusp probably due to venturi effect (see on M mode)
- Tip thickening of anterior mitral cusp where it strikes the septum
- Hypertrophy which may only be apical

7.3 Dilated cardiomyopathy (DCM)

Dilated cardiomyopathy (DCM) is a syndrome of global ventricular dysfunction and dilatation, usually with macroscopically normal coronary arteries (if causes of ischaemic cardiomyopathy are excluded). Aetiology is often undetermined and the condition is more common in males and Afro-Caribbeans. There is often LBBB or poor R wave progression on ECG and anticoagulation may be warranted as the incidence of AF and ventricular thrombus is high.

Causes of DCM

- Alcohol
- Undiagnosed hypertension
- Autoimmune disease
- Nutritional deficiency (eg thiamine and selenium)
- Muscular dystrophies
- Viral infections (eg Coxsackie and HIV)
- Peripartum
- Drugs (eg doxorubicin)
- Infiltration (eg haemochromatosis, sarcoidosis)
- Tachycardia-mediated cardiomyopathy (uncontrolled fast heart rates, eg atrial fibrillation)

7.4 Restrictive cardiomyopathy

This produces identical symptoms to constrictive pericarditis (see Section 8.1) but surgery is of little use in restrictive cardiomyopathy. The ventricles are excessively rigid and impede diastolic filling. AF may supervene and stagnation of blood leads to thrombus formation.

- **Myocardial causes**
  Idiopathic
  Scleroderma
  Amyloid (see below)
  Sarcoid
  Haemochromatosis
  Glycogen storage disorders
  Gaucher's disease
- **Endomyocardial causes**
  Endomyocardial fibrosis
  Hypereosinophilic syndromes (including Löffler's)
  Carcinoid
  Malignancy or radiotherapy
  Toxin-related

Cardiac amyloidosis

Cardiac amyloidosis behaves like restrictive cardiomyopathy but it may also be accompanied by pericardial thickening (due to nodular deposition), pericardial effusion and, rarely, tamponade. It is important to avoid digoxin in amyloid cardiac disease because of the risk of heart block and asystole.

7.5 Myocarditis

Myocarditis may be due to many different aetiological factors (eg viral, bacterial, fungal, protozoal, autoimmune, allergic and drugs). It may be difficult to differentiate it from DCM, but the following features may help:

- usually young patient
- acute history
- prodrome of fever, arthralgia, respiratory tract infection, myalgia
- neutrophilia
- slight cardiomegaly on chest X-ray
- episodes of VT, transient AV block and ST/T wave changes
- elevated viral titres
- cardiac enzymes raised (with normal coronary arteries).

Rheumatic fever

This follows a group A streptococcal infection; pancarditis usually occurs and valvular defects are long-term sequelae. The cardiac histological marker is the Aschoff nodule. Patients are treated with penicillin and salicylates or steroids.

Criteria for diagnosis include the need for evidence of preceding α-haemolytic streptococcal infection (raised ASOT, positive throat swab or history of scarlet fever), together with two major (or one major and two minor) Duckett–Jones criteria (see below).

Rheumatic fever (Duckett–Jones diagnostic criteria)

Major criteria	**Minor criteria**
Carditis	Fever
Polyarthritis	Arthralgia
Chorea	Previous rheumatic heart disease
Erythema marginatum	High ESR and CRP
Subcutaneous nodules	Prolonged PR interval on ECG

7.6 Cardiac tumours

Myxomas are the most common cardiac tumours, comprising 50% of most pathological series.

Atrial myxomas

- **Autopsy incidence** of <0.3%; more common in females (2:1) and in the left atrium (75% of myxomas); usually benign and occasionally familial.
- **Signs**: fever and weight loss occur in 25%, and this may be due to release of interleukin-6 (IL-6). There may be transient mitral stenosis, early diastolic 'plop', clubbing, Raynaud's phenomenon (rare), pulmonary hypertension. Usually the rhythm is sinus. Atrial myxomas may present with the classical triad of systemic embolism, intra-cardiac obstruction and systemic symptoms.
- **Investigations**: WCC high, platelets low, haemolytic anaemia or polycythaemia, raised immunoglobulins, raised ESR in 60% (thought to be due to secretion of IL-6).

- Avoid left ventricular catheterisation; use transoesophageal echo (TOE) to diagnose. They occur most commonly on the inter-atrial septum.
- Atrial myxomas grow rapidly with a risk of embolisation and sudden death. Therefore, they should be resected surgically without delay.

Other primary cardiac tumours

These include papillomas, fibromas, lipomas, angiosarcomas, rhabdomyosarcomas and mesotheliomas, which are all rare lesions.

7.7 Alcohol and the heart

Acute alcoholic intoxication is the most common cause of paroxysmal atrial fibrillation amongst younger individuals. Chronic excessive intake over 10 years is responsible for a third of the cases of dilated cardiomyopathy (DCM) in Western populations; alcohol is also aetiologically related to hypertension, CVA, arrhythmias and sudden death. Atrial fibrillation may be the first presenting feature (usually between the ages of 30 and 35 years).

Pathological mechanisms

- Direct myocardial toxic effect of alcohol and its metabolites
- Toxic effect of additives (eg cobalt)
- Secondary effect of associated nutritional deficiencies (eg thiamine)
- Effect of hypertension

Treatment includes nutritional correction and – most importantly – complete abstinence from alcohol, without which 50% will die within 5 years. Abstinence may lead to a marked recovery of resting cardiac function.

Beneficial mechanisms of modest amounts of alcohol

- Favourable effects on lipids (50% of this benefit is due to raised HDL levels)
- Anti-thrombotic effects (perhaps by raising natural levels of tissue plasminogen activator (t-PA))
- Anti-platelet effects (changes in prostacyclin:thromboxane ratios)
- Increase in insulin sensitivity
- Antioxidant effects of red wine (flavonoids and polyphenols)

7.8 Cardiac transplantation

With over 2500 heart-only transplants being performed in the USA each year, most often for intractable coronary disease and cardiomyopathy (44%), survival rates have been estimated at

80% at 1 year, 75% at 3 years and 40–50% at 10 years. Myocarditis is yet another indication; transplantation during the acute phase does not worsen prognosis, but myocarditis may recur in the donor heart.

The major complications encountered after transplantation include accelerated coronary atheroma, lymphoma, skin cancer (and other tumours) and chronic renal failure (CRF) (due to ciclosporin A toxicity).

8. PERICARDIAL DISEASE

8.1 Constrictive pericarditis

Rare in clinical practice, it presents in a similar way to restrictive cardiomyopathy, ie with signs of right-sided heart failure (cachexia, hepatomegaly, raised JVP, ascites and oedema) due to restriction of diastolic filling of both ventricles. It is treated by pericardial resection.

Other specific features include:

- A diastolic pericardial knock occurs after the third heart sound, at the time of the y descent of the JVP and this reflects the sudden reduction of ventricular filling – 'the ventricle slaps against the rigid pericardium'.
- Soft heart sounds and impalpable apex beat.
- Severe pulsus paradoxus rarely occurs and indicates the presence of a co-existent tense effusion.
- Thickened, bright pericardium on echocardiography.

Causes of constrictive pericarditis

- Tuberculosis (usually post-pericardial effusion)
- Mediastinal radiotherapy
- Pericardial malignancy
- Drugs (eg hydralazine, associated with a lupus-like syndrome)
- Post-viral (especially haemorrhagic) or bacterial pericarditis
- Following severe uraemic pericarditis
- Trauma/post-cardiac surgery
- Connective tissue disease
- Recurrent pericarditis

Signs common to constrictive pericarditis and restrictive cardiomyopathy

- Raised JVP with prominent x + y descents
- Atrial fibrillation
- Non-pulsatile hepatomegaly
- Normal systolic function

Some key features distinguish constrictive pericarditis from restrictive cardiomyopathy:

- Absence of LVH in constrictive pericarditis.
- Absent calcification on chest X-ray, prominent apical impulse and conduction abnormalities on ECG, which are features of restrictive cardiomyopathy.

However, a combination of investigations, including cardiac CT, MRI and cardiac biopsy, may be necessary to differentiate between the two conditions.

8.2 Pericardial effusion

A slowly developing effusion of 2 litres can be accommodated by pericardial stretching and without raising the intrapericardial pressure. The classical symptoms of chest discomfort, dysphagia, hoarseness or dyspnoea (due to compression) may be absent. A large effusion can lead to muffled heart sounds, loss of apical impulse, occasional pericardial rub, small ECG complexes and eventually electro-mechanical dissociation.

Other key features are:

- **pulsus alternans**: variable left ventricular output and right ventricular filling
- **pulsus paradoxus**: exaggerated inspiratory fall in systolic BP (mechanism described in Section 2.2)
- **electrical alternans on ECG**: 'swinging QRS axis'
- **globular cardiac enlargement on chest X-ray.**

Causes of pericardial effusion

- All causes as listed for constrictive pericarditis
- Aortic dissection
- Iatrogenic due to pacing or cardiac catheterisation
- Ischaemic heart disease with ventricular rupture
- Anticoagulation associated with acute pericarditis

8.3 Cardiac tamponade

In contrast, if a small amount of intrapericardial fluid (eg <200 ml) accumulates rapidly, it can significantly limit ventricular filling, reduce cardiac output and elevate intracardiac pressures (particularly right-sided initially). Thus the 'y' descent due to right ventricular filling with tricuspid valve opening is lost as right ventricular pressures are high, and the 'x' descent of right atrium filling due to right ventricular contraction is prominent. The right atrium collapses in diastole as a result of impaired filling and high intrapericardial pressures. In early diastole even the right ventricle may collapse.

Occasionally the stretched pericardium may compress the lingular lobe of the left lung, causing bronchial breathing at the left base (Ewart's sign). The QRS axis of the ECG may also be altered (electrical alternans).

Common signs of cardiac tamponade

- Elevated jugular venous pressure
- Kussmaul's sign
- Tachypnoea
- Systolic hypotension
- Pulsus paradoxus
- Tachycardia
- Diminished heart sounds
- Impalpable apex beat

Treatment is by urgent drainage – usually under echocardiographic control. Surgical 'pericardial' windows may be necessary for chronic (eg malignant) effusions.

9. DISORDERS OF MAJOR VESSELS

9.1 Pulmonary hypertension

It is important to determine whether pulmonary hypertension is secondary to an underlying condition as this may be treatable. The most common cause of secondary pulmonary hypertension is chronic obstructive pulmonary disease (COPD).

Causes of pulmonary hypertension

- **Primary pulmonary hypertension**

- **Secondary causes**
  Mitral valve disease
  DCM/IHD
  Chronic parenchymal lung disease (eg COPD)
  Chronic pulmonary thromboembolism
  Left to right shunt (eg ASD, VSD)
  Chronic hypoxia (high altitude, polio, myasthenia)
  HCM
  Cor triatrium
  Constrictive pericarditis and restrictive cardiomyopathy
  Left atrial myxoma

Primary pulmonary hypertension (PPH)

Primary pulmonary hypertension is a rare disease with an incidence of 2 per million per year; it is a disease of children and young adults, with a ratio of females:males of 2:1. PPH constitutes less than 1% of all cases of pulmonary hypertension and is characterised by a mean pulmonary artery pressure of >25 mmHg at rest, in the absence of another demonstrable cause. One in ten cases is familial. PPH is associated with connective tissue disease, vasculitis, HIV infection and also the use of appetite suppressants (eg fenfluramine). The pulmonary arteries become dilated and abnormally thickened; there is dilatation of the proximal pulmonary vessels with thick-walled, obstructed 'pruned' peripheral vessels. As a consequence of the high pulmonary pressure the right ventricle undergoes marked hypertrophy.

Three types of PPH are recognised:

- primary plexogenic pulmonary arteriopathy
- thrombotic pulmonary arteriopathy
- pulmonary veno-occlusive arteriopathy.

Patients present with gradually worsening exertional dyspnoea and, in the later stages, angina of effort and syncope occur. Fatigue is common and haemoptysis may occur.

- Signs include: cyanosis, right ventricular heave, loud P_2, tricuspid regurgitation, peripheral oedema and ascites.
- Untreated, the median survival is approximately 3 years.

Treatment of primary pulmonary hypertension

- Advise avoidance of strenuous exercise and recommend contraception, as pregnancy is harmful.
- Anticoagulation to avoid thrombus formation in situ in the pulmonary arteries and also pulmonary embolism.
- Prostacyclin (PGI_2), a potent pulmonary and systemic vasodilator, is used, particularly to bridge patients to transplantation. The drug has an extremely short half-life and has to be given by continuous intravenous infusion, usually through a tunnelled central venous catheter. It is also very expensive.
- Calcium channel antagonists have been used to lower pulmonary (and systemic) pressure.
- Diuretics are helpful in the management of right heart failure.
- Continuous ambulatory inhaled nitric oxide is being developed, and this would provide good pulmonary vasodilatation, but without systemic effect.

The chief therapeutic option is transplantation, as other treatments are of limited benefit, or are difficult to administer.

Summary of available treatments for pulmonary hypertension

- **General**
  Address secondary causes where possible
  Digoxin even in patients with sinus rhythm
  Diuretics for symptoms
  Ambulatory supplemental oxygen for some
  Anticoagulation

- **Vasodilator therapy (only helps some subjects)**
  PGI_2 or PGE (chronic infusion)
  Adenosine infusions or boluses
  Nitric oxide inhalation, nitrates (chronic infusion)
  Calcium channel blockers

- **Surgical options (in selected cases)**
  Heart-lung or single/double lung transplant
  Atrial septostomy (only if no resting hypoxia)

9.2 Venous thrombosis and pulmonary embolism (PE)

The true incidence of pulmonary embolism (PE) is unknown but PE probably accounts for 1% of all admissions. Predisposing factors are discussed in Chapter 9, Haematology.

One or more predisposing risk factors are found in 80–90% of cases. The oral contraceptive increases the risk of deep vein thrombosis (DVT)/PE two to four times. However, thrombo-embolism is rare in women taking oestrogens without other risk factors.

Clinical features

Nearly all patients have one or more of the following symptoms: dyspnoea, tachypnoea or pleuritic chest pain. With a large pulmonary embolus patients may present with collapse. Hypoxaemia may be present with moderate or large pulmonary emboli.

Investigations

- **Chest X-ray**
  May be normal; pleural-based, wedge-shaped defects described classically are rare and areas of oligaemia may be difficult to detect

- **D-dimer**
  Will be raised in PE but the test is non-specific

- **Helical CT scanning**
  Will demonstrate pulmonary emboli in the large pulmonary arteries but may not show small peripheral emboli

- **ECG**
  May show sinus tachycardia and, in massive PE, features of acute right heart strain; non-specific S-T segment and T-wave changes occur

- **Arterial blood gases**
  Shows a low or normal pCO_2 and may show a degree of hypoxaemia

- **Ventilation/perfusion (V/Q) scanning**
  Shows one or more areas of ventilation/perfusion mismatching

- **Pulmonary angiography**
  Remains the 'gold standard', but this is under-used

In each case a clinical assessment of the probability of PE should be made. As demonstrated in the PIOPED study:

- Cases of high clinical probability combined with a high probability V/Q scan are virtually diagnostic of PE.
- Similarly, cases of low clinical suspicion combined with low probability or normal V/Q scans make the diagnosis of PE very unlikely.
- All other combinations of clinical probability and V/Q scan result should be investigated further.
- Patients who present with collapse need urgent echocardiography, helical CT scan or pulmonary angiogram to demonstrate pulmonary embolus.

Management

In all cases of moderate or high clinical probability of PE, anticoagulation with heparin should be started immediately after baseline coagulation studies have been taken. If unfractionated heparin is used, an initial loading dose of 5000–10, 000 units should be given intravenously followed by a continuous infusion of 1300 IU/hour (adjusted according to the results of the activated partial thromboplastin time (APTT) which should be 1.5–2.5 times the control). Low molecular weight heparin, given as a once-daily subcutaneous injection, has recently been licensed for the treatment of PE; no monitoring is required. Patients should be treated with heparin for at least 5 days; during that time warfarin is introduced and the heparin is discontinued once the INR is two to three times the control.

- Warfarin is continued for 3–6 months in most cases; for PE occurring post-operatively, 6 weeks' anticoagulation is adequate. In recurrent PE, anticoagulation should be for longer periods (eg 1 year) and consideration should be given to life-long treatment.
- In cases of collapse due to massive PE, thrombolysis with streptokinase or recombinant t-PA given by peripheral vein should be considered. This should be avoided when the embolic material is an infected vegetation (eg iv drug abusers).
- Occasionally, pulmonary embolectomy is used for those with massive PE where thrombolysis is unsuccessful or contraindicated.
- Inferior vena caval filters should be considered in patients where anticoagulation is contraindicated or in those who continue to embolise despite anticoagulation.

9.3 Systemic hypertension

A UK population survey in 1994 showed that 19.5% of a sample adult population would be classified as having hypertension using criteria of systolic blood pressure (SBP) >160 mmHg or diastolic blood pressure (DBP) >95 mmHg and/or receiving treatment for hypertension. Guidelines for treatment continually adapt to new clinical evidence, but the British Hypertension Society (BHS) would recommend the following:

- All adults should have their blood pressure measured every 5 years until the age of 80 years.
- Patients who have high normal blood pressure (SBP 135–139 mmHg or DBP 85–89 mmHg) should be monitored annually.
- Non-pharmacological measures (lifestyle) should be initiated in all hypertensive patients and those with borderline blood pressures. These measures include cessation of smoking; appropriate dieting for obesity; reduced cholesterol intake and improvement in exercise.
- Treatment is also indicated for all patients with sustained SBP >160 mmHg and/or DBP >100 mmHg.
- Treatment is also indicated for patients with sustained SBP >140–159 mmHg and/or DBP 90–99 mmHg if there is evidence of target organ damage, established cardiovascular disease, diabetes or if the patient would have an estimated 10-year coronary heart disease risk >15%.

Recommended targets for blood pressure control

Blood pressure treatment targets have changed with evidence from recent large trials. Current recommendations are:

- patients without diabetes mellitus <140/85 mmHg
- patients with diabetes mellitus <140/80 mmHg
- diabetic nephropathy <125/75 mmHg
- chronic renal disease with persistent proteinuria (>1 g/24 hours) <125/75 mmHg.

Stepped antihypertensive therapy is probably outmoded as 50% of patients will be uncontrolled by monotherapy, and therapeutic gains with two- to three-agent low-dose therapy far outweigh the incidence of side-effects. The important recent trials which have underpinned the above treatment rationale are summarised next.

MRFIT (Multiple Risk Factor Intervention Trial)

This involved 350, 000 men, aged 35–75 years, who had no previous history of cardiovascular disease. Follow-up was long (11.6 years) and the outcomes of patients with different baseline blood pressure was noted. When compared with a blood pressure of 120/80 mmHg, all strata of blood pressure above this were associated with an increased risk of cardiovascular death.

HOT (Hypertension Optimal Treatment, 1998) Study

This involved approximately 19, 000 patients, aged 50–80 years, who had diastolic hypertension. They were randomised to receive treatment to achieve one of three diastolic blood pressure targets (<90, <85 or <80 mmHg). The lowest cardiovascular event incidence was seen at a mean DBP of 82 mmHg. In the diabetic patients within the study, cardiovascular events were 51% less in patients randomised to the <80 mmHg compared to the <90 mmHg DBP group.

UK PDS 38 (1998)

This included 1148 hypertensive type 2 diabetic patients who were randomised to receive treatment so as to achieve either tight or sub-optimal blood pressure control. At the end of the 8-year follow-up period, the mean blood pressures achieved in each group were 144/82 mmHg versus 154/87 mmHg. A significant reduction in macro-vascular and micro-vascular complications, as well as mortality, was noted in the patients with better-controlled blood pressure.

SysEur Trial (2000)

This investigated the effects of treatment of sustained **systolic** blood pressure upon outcomes. Active treatment was shown to significantly reduce cardiovascular and cerebral vascular events.

Other considerations in hypertension management

- Investigation of **phaeochromocytomas**: recommend three 24-hour urinary vanillic VMAs on a vanilla-free diet (and off all drugs). Urinary metadrenalines may also be measured.
- Hypertension **increases the risk** (Framingham data) of: stroke (×7); cardiac failure (×4); coronary artery disease (×3); peripheral vascular disease (×2).
- Potassium salt should be substituted for sodium salt where possible.
- **Drugs to avoid in pregnancy**: diuretics, ACE inhibitors, angiotensin II receptor blockers. **Drugs with well-identified risks preferred in pregnancy**: beta-blockers (especially labetalol), methyldopa and hydralazine.
- Young Black men have a poor response to ACE inhibitors, thiazides and beta-blockers as they are salt conservers by background, and so are resistant to renin manipulation and are particularly likely to develop the side-effect of impotence.

9.4 Aortic dissection

Two-thirds of tears occur in the ascending aorta with about one-fifth occurring in the descending aorta. Mortality is highest in the first few hours if the dissection is untreated. The differential diagnosis for ascending dissection includes MI if the vulnerable right coronary ostium is involved (giving rise to an inferior infarct pattern). This is particularly important when considering thrombolysis; aortic regurgitation provides supportive evidence of the diagnosis.

Associations with aortic dissection

- Systemic hypertension (present in 80%)
- Marfan's syndrome
- Cystic medial degeneration (rare in the absence of Marfan's syndrome)
- Noonan's, Turner's syndromes
- Trauma
- Aortic coarctation
- Congenital bicuspid aortic valve (present in 10–15% and dissection is therefore associated with aortic stenosis)
- Giant cell arteritis
- Pregnancy (particularly in patients with Marfan's syndrome)
- Cocaine abuse

Involvement of ascending aorta may cause

- Aortic regurgitation
- Inferior myocardial infarction
- Pericardial effusion (including cardiac tamponade)
- Carotid dissection
- Absent or decreased subclavian pulse

Medical therapy to be considered for

- Old, stable dissections (>2 weeks)
- Uncomplicated dissection of descending aorta
- Isolated arch dissections

Investigations for aortic dissection

- TOE, aortic MRI or contrast-enhanced spiral CT scans all have a high diagnostic sensitivity, but CT rarely identifies the site of tear or the presence of aortic regurgitation or coronary involvement.
- MRI is of the highest quality but is contraindicated in patients with pacemakers, certain vascular clips and metal valve prostheses.
- TOE is probably the most widely used investigation as it is available in the acute situation and has high sensitivity and specificity.
- Aortography is no longer the gold standard and coronary angiography is applicable only when deciding on the need for concomitant CABG.

APPENDIX I

Normal cardiac physiological values

ECG

- PR interval 0.12–0.20 s
- QRS duration >0.10 s
- QTc (males) 380 ms, (females) 420 ms
- QRS axis –30° to + 90°.

Indices of cardiac function

- Cardiac index = Cardiac output/body surface area (BSA) = 2.5–4.0 $l \cdot min^{-1} \cdot m^{-2}$
- Stroke volume index = stroke volume/BSA = 40–70 $ml \cdot m^{-2}$
- Systemic vascular resistance (SVR) = $\frac{80 \times (Ao - RA)}{(\text{Cardiac output})}$ = 770–1500 $dyn \cdot s \cdot cm^{-5}$, where Ao is the mean aortic pressure and RA is the mean right atrial pressure
- Ejection fraction = proportion of blood ejected from left ventricle = 50–70%.

Cardiac catheterisation pressures (mmHg)		Criteria for significant oxygen saturation set up	
Mean right atrial	0–8	SVC/IVC to RA	>7% (eg ASD)
Right ventricular systolic	15–30	RA to RV	>5% (eg VSD)
End diastolic	0–8	RV to PA	>5% (eg PDA)
		Any level:	
Pulmonary artery systolic	15–30	SVC to PA	>7%
End diastolic	3–12	Usual saturations (SaO_2)	
Mean	9–16	Venous	65–75%
Pulmonary artery wedge		Arterial	96–98%
a	3–15		
v	3–12		
Left atrial mean	1–10		
Left ventricular systolic	100–140		
End diastolic	3–12		
Aortic systolic	100–140		
End diastolic	60–90		
Mean	70–105		

APPENDIX II

Summary of important large trials in cardiovascular disease

Table 1 Acute myocardial infarction (AMI)

Acronym	Agent	*N*	Result	Reference
		Thombolytics (streptokinase (SK) and tissue plasminogin activator (t-PA))		
ISIS 2 *International Study of Infarct Survival*	SK and aspirin, either alone or in combination vs placebo	17,187	5-week CV mortality reduced (aspirin 23%, SK 25%, both agents 42%)	*Lancet* 1988; **ii**: 349–60
ISIS 3	SK vs t-PA vs APSAC (anisoylated plasminogen streptokinase activator complex) ± heparin	41,299	No difference in 35-day mortality between the three thrombolysis regimes. Haemorrhagic strokes were higher in the t-PA arm. No additional benefit of heparin	*Lancet* 1992; **339**: 753–70
GUSTO 1 *Global Utilisation of Streptokinase and t-PA for Occluded Coronary Arteries Trial 1*	SK vs t-PA heparin	41,021	No difference between agents except in certain subgroups (eg small benefit of t-PA and iv heparin over SK, but haemorrhagic stroke risk increased in the former arm)	*New Engl J Med* 1993; **329**: 673–82
GISSI 1 *Gruppo Italiano per lo Studio della*	SK vs placebo	11,521	Mortality benefit from SK	*Lancet* 1986; **i**: 397–401
GISSI 2	SK vs TPA	12,490	No difference between agents, no benefit of heparin	*Lancet* 1990; **336:** 65–71
		Beta-blockers		
ISIS 1	Atenolol (iv for 1 day and then oral for 7 days) vs placebo	16,027	15% decrease in 7-day mortality with atenolol. (Most benefit on days 0–2; probably due to reduced cardiac rupture or cardiac arrest.) Trial in the pre-thrombolysis era	*Lancet* 1986; **ii**: 57–66
BHAT *Beta-blocker Heart Attack Trial*	Propranolol vs placebo	3837	Mortality reduction with propranolol	*J Am Med Assoc* 1982; **247**: 1707–14

CAPRICORN *Carvedilol Post-infarct Control in left ventricular dysfunction*	Carvedilol vs placebo	1964	Mortality reduction with carvedilol	*Lancet* 2001; **357**: 1385–90
		ACE inhibitors		
AIRE *Acute Infarction Ramipril Efficacy study*	Post-infarction patients with early clinical or radiological evidence of heart failure received ramipril or placebo (excluded patients with severe or resistant heart failure)	2006	15 months mortality reduced 27% with ramipril (and 31% at 5 years)	*Lancet* 1993; **342**: 821–8
SAVE *Survival And Ventricular Enlargement Study*	Captopril vs placebo	2231	Captopril given to patients with post-MI ejection fraction <40% (vs placebo) had a 19% mortality reduction in 3- to 5-year follow-up period with fewer re-infarctions and re-admissions for heart failure	*N Engl J Med* 1992; **327**: 669–77
GISSI 3	Lisinopril nitrates vs placebo	18, 895	Mortality reduction with lisinopril; nitrates neutral effect	*Lancet* 1994; **343**: 1115–22
TRACE *Trandolapril Cardiac Evaluation*	Trandolapril vs placebo	6676	Mortality reduction with trandolapril	*N Engl J Med* 1995; **333**: 1670–6
CONSENSUS II *Co-operative North Scandinavian Enalapril Survival Study*	Enalapril vs placebo	6090	No improvement in mortality with enalapril (query due to hypotension causing coronary perfusion compromise)	*N Engl J Med* 1987; **316**: 1429–35

Table 2 Heart failure

Acronym	Agent (inclusion criteria)	*N*	Result	Reference
			Beta-blockers	
MERIT-HF *Metoprolol Randomised Intervention Trial in Heart Failure*	Metoprolol vs placebo (NYHA II-IV on ACEI)	3991	Mortality (7.2% vs 11.0% per patient year) hospitalisation and symptom reduction in metoprolol group	*Lancet* 1999; **353**: 2001–7
CIBIS II *Cardiac Insufficiency Bisoprolol Study 11*	Bisoprolol vs placebo (NYHA III-IV)	2647	All-cause mortality significantly lower in the bisoprolol group compared to placebo (11.8% vs 17.3%)	*Lancet* 1999; **353**: 9–13
COPERNICUS *Carvedilol Prospective Randomised Cumulative Survival Trial*	Carvedilol vs placebo (NYHA III-IV)	2289	Mortality, hospitalisation and symptom reduction in carvedilol group	*N Engl J Med* 2001; **344**: 1659–67
			ACE inhibitors	
SOLVD *Studies of Left Ventricular Dysfunction*	Enalapril vs placebo (LVEF <35%)	2569	Mortality and hospitalisation reduction in enalapril group	*N Engl J Med* 1991; **325**: 293–302
ATLAS *Assessment of Treatment with Lisinopril and Survival*	Lisinopril vs placebo (NYHA II-IV)	3164	A dose-dependent reduction in combined mortality and hospitalisation in the lisinopril group	*Circulation* 1999; **100**: 2312–18
CONSENSUS *Co-operative North Scandinavian Enalapril Survival Study*	Addition of enalapril to conventional therapy (NYHA V)	253	Significant benefit in enalapril group, mortality reduction of 40% at 6 months and 31% at 1 year (due to improvement in left ventricular function). Study terminated early	

Devices (Implantable Cardioverter Defibrillators (ICD) and Cardiac Resynchronisation Therapy (CRT))				
MUSTIC *Multisite pacing in intraventricular conduction delay*	Crossover study with CRT (NYHA III-IV, QRS>150 ms)	67	Reduction in heart failure symptoms and hospitalisation in the active pacing mode	*N Engl J Med* 2001; **344**: 873–80
MIRACLE *Multicenter InSync Randomised Clinical Evaluation*	CRT vs placebo (NYHA II-IV, QRS >130 ms)	266	Reduction in combined endpoint of mortality and hospitalisation in the active pacing group	*N Engl J Med* 2002; **346**: 1845–53
MADIT II *Multicenter Automated Defibrillator Implantation Trial*	ICD vs placebo (IHD; LVEF <30%)	1232	Reduction in all-cause mortality in the defibrillator group	*N Engl J Med* 2002; **346**: 877–83
COMPANION *Comparison of Medical Therapy, Pacing and Defibrillation*	CRT vs CRT/ICD vs placebo (LVEF< 30%; QRS>120 ms)	1600	Reduction in all-cause mortality in the combined CRT/ICD group. Morbidity benefit in the CRT group	*N Engl J Med* 2004; **350**: 2140–50
Other agents in heart failure				
RALES *Randomised Aldactone Evaluation Study*	Spironolactone vs placebo (NYHA III-IV on ACEI)	1663	Mortality, hospitalisation and symptom reduction in spironolactone group	*N Engl J Med* 1999; **341**: 709–17
DIG *Digitalis Investigation Group Trial*	Digoxin vs placebo (NYHA II-IV)	6800	Reduced hospitalisations in the digoxin group	*N Engl J Med* 1997; **336**: 525–33

Table 3 Lipid-lowering therapy trials and trials of arrhythmia treatment

Acronym	Agent (inclusion criteria)	*N*	Result	Reference
		Lipid-lowering therapies		
4S *Scandinavian Simvastatin Study*	Simvastatin vs placebo (patients with angina or post-MI with cholesterol 5.5–8.0 mmol/l)	4444	33% reduction of mortality and cardiovascular events at 5 years in simvastatin group, for a mean cholesterol reduction of 25%	*Lancet* 1994; **344**: 1383–9
WOSCOPS *The West of Scotland Coronary Prevention Study* (LDL >252 mg/dl)	Pravastatin vs placebo (men aged 45–65 years with no overt coronary disease and cholesterol >4 mmol/l)	6595	All-cause mortality is reduced by 22% in the simvastatin arm for a 20% total cholesterol reduction. This was a primary prevention study	*N Engl J Med* 1995; **333:** 1301–7
HPS *Heart Protection Study*	Simvastatin vs placebo (cholesterol >3.4 mmol/l and any one of MI, DM, arterial disease or hypertension)	20, 536	Mortality benefit in simvastatin arm	*Lancet* 2002; **360**: 7–22
		Arrhythmias		
CAST *Cardiac Arrhythmia Suppression Trial*	Any one of the following: flecainide/encainide/ moracizine vs placebo (ventricular ectopics post-MI)	1727	Antiarrhythmic use increased mortality	*N Eng J Med* 1989; **321**: 406–12
AVID *Antiarrhythmics vs Implantable Defibrillators*	ICD vs amiodarone (post-cardiac arrest)	1016	ICD reduced mortality	*N Engl J Med* 1997; **337**: 1576–83
SWORD *Survival With Oral d-sotalol*	Sotalol vs placebo (patients with IHD and NYHA II-IV)	3121	Sotalol increased mortality	*Lancet* 1996; **348**: 7–12

AFFIRM *Atrial Fibrillation Follow-up Investigation of Rhythm Management*	Rate control vs rhythm control (patients with AF and high stroke risk)	4060	Mortality and morbidity increased in the rhythm control arm	*N Engl J Med* 1992; **347 (23)**: 1825–33

Chapter 2
Clinical Pharmacology, Toxicology and Poisoning

CONTENTS

5. **Poisoning**

Clinical Pharmacology, Toxicology and Poisoning

1. DRUG METABOLISM AND INTERACTIONS

1.1 Genetic polymorphisms of drug metabolism

Genetic determination of enzyme activity may alter the susceptibility of an individual to adverse drug reactions. For example, the slow acetylator phenotype is possessed by 50% of UK citizens and may be associated with specific adverse effects due to higher drug concentrations:

- drug-induced lupus
- isoniazid-induced peripheral neuropathy.

Drug-induced lupus is associated with slow acetylation and possession of HLA DR4. Unlike autoimmune SLE, male and female incidence are equal. Laboratory findings include antibodies to histones and single-stranded DNA. Clinical features include:

- arthralgia
- butterfly rash
- pleurisy.

Renal involvement (except with hydralazine) or neuropsychiatric manifestations are unusual.

Drugs causing a lupus erythematosus-like syndrome

- Beta-blockers
- Chlorpromazine
- Clonidine
- Flecainide
- Haloperidol
- Hydralazine
- Isoniazid
- Lithium
- Methyldopa
- Penicillin
- Phenytoin
- Procainamide
- Sulfasalazine
- Sulphonamides
- Tetracyclines

Poor metabolisers of particular drugs

- **Debrisoquine**: 6% of the UK population are poor metabolisers of debrisoquine; these patients have reduced activity of another liver enzyme which potentiates the effects of metipranolol and nortriptyline.
- **s-Mephenytoin**: 3–5% of the UK population are poor metabolisers of this anti-epileptic agent.

The metabolism of proton pump inhibitors (eg omeprazole) may be impaired in these patients, leading to excess adverse effects, such as diarrhoea.

Rapid acetylators

Rapid acetylators may be more prone to adverse effects due to the actions of excess drug metabolite. This is seen with isoniazid-induced hepatitis.

1.2 Liver enzyme induction

Many drugs are capable of inducing liver enzyme systems. Increased hepatic enzyme activity can result in more rapid metabolism of other drugs, thereby decreasing their effectiveness. Induction of microsomal enzymes of the cytochrome P450 system occurs over days because it requires transcription and translation of the genetic code to produce more enzyme. This may lead to treatment failure with the following agents:

- hydrocortisone
- oral contraceptive pill
- phenytoin
- warfarin.

The drugs that cause this effect can be remembered by the mnemonic **PC BRAS**:

(**P**henytoin, **C**arbamazepine, **B**arbiturates, **R**ifampicin, **A**lcohol (chronic excess), **S**ulphonylureas)

1.3 Liver enzyme inhibition

A number of drugs are capable of inhibiting hepatic enzyme systems, which can occur immediately. Enzyme inhibition can reduce the rate of metabolism of other drugs, thereby increasing plasma concentrations and increasing the risks of adverse effects. Hepatic enzyme inhibition can potentiate the effects of:

- carbamazepine
- ciclosporin
- phenytoin
- theophyllines
- warfarin.

Drugs that are liver enzyme inhibitors may be recalled by the mnemonic **AODEVICES**:

(**A**llopurinol, **O**meprazole, **D**isulfiram, **E**rythromycin, **V**alproate, **I**soniazid, **C**imetidine (and ciprofloxacin), acute **E**thanol intoxication, **S**ulphonamides)

1.4 Failure of the combined oral contraceptive pill

Any condition that leads to impaired absorption of the components of the contraceptive pill (eg traveller's diarrhoea) may result in its failure as a contraceptive agent. In addition:

- The oestrogenic component of the oral contraceptive may be metabolised more rapidly in the presence of liver enzyme inducers (see previous page), leading to pill failure, but enzyme inhibitors have no clinically significant effect.
- Pill failure may also result from concomitant antibiotic usage. For example, ampicillin, amoxicillin and tetracyclines may damage gut flora that deconjugate bile salts thereby interrupting enterohepatic cycling of the oestrogenic component.

2. PRESCRIBING IN PARTICULAR CLINICAL STATES

2.1 Drugs and breast-feeding

Infants under one month of age are at greatest risk from drugs excreted in breast milk because they have immature metabolism and excretion. Drugs that are definitely excreted in breast milk and are contraindicated during breast-feeding include:

- **amiodarone**: thyroid anomalies
- **cytotoxics and chloramphenicol**: blood dyscrasia.

Other drugs that should not be taken by breast-feeding mothers are:

- **gold**: haematological reactions and renal impairment
- **indometacin**: has been reported to cause seizures
- **iodides**: thyroid disturbance
- **lithium**: involuntary movements
- **oestrogens**: feminisation of male infants.

2.2 Pregnancy and drug therapies

During the first 16 weeks of pregnancy, drugs may exert teratogenic effects on the fetus leading to malformations. Particular associations are:

- **lithium**: cardiac abnormalities
- **phenytoin**: facial fusion abnormalities such as cleft lip and palate
- **sodium valproate** and **retinoids**: neural tube defects
- **warfarin**: abnormalities of long bones and cartilage.

Later in pregnancy some drugs may cross the placenta and harm the fetus:

- **carbimazole**: neonatal goitre (which may even be large enough to obstruct labour)
- **gentamicin**: VIIIth nerve deafness in the newborn.

2.3 Prescribing in liver disease and liver failure

Depressed central nervous system function can result from the accumulation of either high concentrations of drugs normally cleared by the liver, or toxic substances as a result of impaired hepatic metabolism. Patients with liver impairment are more sensitive to the sedative effects of a number of drugs, and the latter may induce hepatic encephalopathy. Opioids in particular may cause coma due to altered brain sensitivity. Similarly, benzodiazepines may accumulate and depress the central nervous system. Thiazides and loop diuretics may cause hypokalaemia, thereby provoking encephalopathy. Other important aspects of drug metabolism in liver disease are listed below:

- Drugs excreted via the bile, such as rifampicin, may accumulate in patients with obstructive jaundice.
- Hypoalbuminaemia, resulting from cirrhosis, may reduce available binding sites for protein-bound drugs (eg phenytoin) to very low levels.
- Reduced clotting factor synthesis means an increased risk of bleeding for patients taking warfarin.
- Patients with advanced liver disease retain salt and water due to secondary hyperaldosteronism; the resulting ascites and oedema can be worsened by non-steroidal anti-inflammatory drugs and steroids.

2.4 Prescribing in renal failure

Consideration of drug metabolism is important in patients with renal failure, as nephrotoxic agents may exacerbate renal damage (especially in patients with acute renal failure), and other drugs, especially those that are water soluble and therefore eliminated largely by the kidneys, may accumulate in patients with a low glomerular filtration rate (GFR), leading to toxic effects.

Drugs that accumulate and cause toxicity in patients with severe renal failure (GFR <10 ml/min) include:

- **digoxin**: cardiac arrhythmias, heart block
- **erythromycin**: encephalopathy
- **lithium**: cardiac arrhythmias and seizures
- **penicillins** and **cephalosporins** (high dose): lead to encephalopathy.

Nephrotoxic drugs may lead to an acute deterioration of renal function in patients with chronic renal failure, and they can severely exacerbate renal damage in acute renal dysfunction. If treatment is considered essential (eg gentamicin or parenteral vancomycin for staphylococcal infections) then levels should be carefully monitored, otherwise such agents should be avoided in these patient groups. Examples of nephrotoxic drugs include:

- aminoglycosides
- amphotericin
- non-steroidal anti-inflammatory drugs.

Other drugs may have more specific nephrotoxic effects, such as gold-induced proteinuria or nephrotic syndrome, which is usually due to membranous glomerulonephritis. (*See also* Chapter 15, Nephrology.)

3. INDIVIDUAL DRUGS AND THOSE USED IN SPECIFIC CLINICAL CONDITIONS

3.1 Cardiology

Abciximab (Reopro)

This chimeric monoclonal antibody irreversibly binds GpIIb/IIIa glycoprotein receptors in platelets, preventing the final common pathway of platelet activation and aggregation. It has a potent long-term anti-platelet effect after intravenous bolus/infusion. Licensed now for high-risk angioplasty (EPIC trial), it prevents acute thrombosis and chronic re-stenosis within coronary arteries and has recently been shown to be beneficial for unstable angina (EPILOG-Stent trial). Risks of thrombocytopenic haemorrhage are low and reversed by platelet administration. Abciximab should be used only once in a particular patient.

Adenosine

Adenosine is a purine nucleoside with a half-life of 8–10 seconds. It acts via specific adenosine receptors, activating K^+ channels, in sinoatrial and atrioventricular nodes to cause sinus node arrest, so terminating supraventricular tachycardia (SVT). Its chief therapeutic use is to distinguish between SVT and ventricular tachycardia. The action of adenosine may be inhibited by aminophylline and potentiated by dipyridamole, which interferes with its metabolism.

Side-effects of adenosine

- Anxiety
- Bronchospasm (avoid in asthmatic patients)
- Chest tightening
- Facial flushing

Amiodarone

Amiodarone has anti-arrhythmic action which spans all categories of the Vaughan–Williams classification. Its main action is to prolong the refractory period, and thus the QT interval, on the ECG. Amiodarone may be used to control supraventricular and ventricular arrhythmias. It may prolong the lifespan of patients with recurrent VT or hypertrophic cardiomyopathy.

- It is iodine-containing and has a very long half-life (26–127 days).
- Protein binding can displace digoxin or warfarin, so increasing their actions.
- Given intravenously, the anti-arrhythmic action occurs within a few hours; given orally this may take 1–3 weeks.
- Amiodarone is the least negatively inotropic anti-arrhythmic with the exception of digoxin.
- Hyperthyroidism may result from enhanced peripheral de-iodination of thyroxine to T_3.

Hypothyroidism arises from increased production of reverse T_3 in the liver.

Side-effects of amiodarone

- arrhythmias (torsades)
- ataxia
- alveolitis
- hepatitis
- hyperthyroidism
- hypothyroidism
- metallic taste
- peripheral neuropathy
- photosensitivity
- pulmonary fibrosis
- reversible corneal microdeposits
- slate grey discoloration of skin.

Angiotensin converting enzyme (ACE) inhibitors

ACE inhibitors reduce mortality in all grades of heart failure and may reduce death after myocardial infarction, probably by reducing deleterious remodelling. They are contraindicated in bilateral renal artery stenosis and should be used with caution in severe renal impairment.

- Dry cough may accompany their use; this may be due to persistence of bradykinin and is more common in women, who have more sensitive cough reflexes.
- Hypersensitivity to ACE inhibitors is manifest as angio-neurotic oedema.
- Potassium may rise during therapy due to inhibition of aldosterone production by ACE inhibitors.

Angiotensin receptor blockers

Angiotensin II receptor (type AT1) antagonists do not inhibit bradykinin breakdown (unlike ACE inhibitors) and so do not provoke cough. They provide more specific AT1 receptor antagonism at tissue level, and are indicated for treatment of hypertension and cardiac failure as an alternative to ACE inhibitor therapy. They may precipitate acute renal failure in patients with reduced renal blood flow (eg bilateral renal artery stenosis, severe cardiac failure, hypovolaemia) in an identical manner to that seen with ACE inhibitors.

Digoxin

Digoxin increases block at the atrioventricular node and so is used to slow ventricular rate in atrial fibrillation and flutter. It has a limited role as a positive inotrope but it may be an effective treatment in patients with co-existent heart failure and atrial fibrillation.

- Eighty-five per cent of a digoxin dose is eliminated unchanged in the urine; it can therefore accumulate in renal impairment.
- The steroid-like structure of digoxin has occasionally caused gynaecomastia in chronic use.
- Digoxin has a narrow therapeutic window, above which toxic effects are often seen.

Digoxin toxicity

Any arrhythmia may occur with digoxin toxicity; the most common is heart block but even atrial fibrillation has been observed. Pulsus bigeminus is indicative of a ventricular ectopic coupled to a normal QRS complex on the ECG and this may herald digoxin toxicity.

- However, note that 'reversed tick' ST segment depression is commonly seen in the inferior and lateral leads on the ECG, and represents a sign of **digoxin therapy** and not specifically toxicity. First-degree heart block is also seen in patients with sinus rhythm who take digoxin.
- Electrolyte imbalances which may predispose to digoxin toxicity include hypokalaemia, hypomagnesaemia and hypercalcaemia.
- Amiodarone may displace digoxin from tissue-binding sites leading to toxicity, whereas quinidine/quinine and calcium antagonists may interfere with tubular clearance of digoxin leading to accumulation and risk of toxic effects.

Toxic effects of digoxin

- Anorexia
- Arrhythmias (eg atrial fibrillation, heart block)
- Diarrhoea
- Nausea/vomiting
- Yellow vision (xanthopsia)

Flecainide

A class 1c agent used for treatment of ventricular arrhythmias, pre-excitation syndromes and for chemical cardioversion of acute atrial arrhythmias. The CAST trial suggested that flecainide is pro-arrhythmic post myocardial infarction; it should be avoided in left ventricular impairment. Its half-life is about 16 hours; other main side-effects are vertigo and visual disturbance.

HMG CoA reductase inhibitors

Statins inhibit the rate-limiting enzyme in cholesterol synthesis (HMG CoA reductase), which is normally predominantly active during sleep (due to fasting and increased hepatic blood flow). They also cause up-regulation of low-density lipoprotein (LDL) receptors thereby reducing LDL by 30% and increasing the clearance of cholesterol, and increasing high-density lipoprotein

(HDL). Most statins have minimal effects on triglycerides. However, although atorvastatin may reduce triglycerides, mortality data are still awaited.

- Statins reduce mortality after myocardial infarction in men who have high cholesterol ('4 S' study).
- They have recently been shown to be effective in reducing primary mortality from ischaemic heart disease (WOSCOP trial).
- Statins rarely cause rhabdomyolysis (frequency 1/100, 000), but this is more likely in patients with renal impairment or when given with a fibrate; drug-induced hepatitis may also occur.
- The joint British recommendations on prevention of coronary heart disease recommend a target total serum cholesterol of <5.0 mmol/l and LDL cholesterol of <3.0 mmol/l.

Nicorandil

A K^+ channel opener that induces arterial vasodilatation, it also possesses a nitrate component that promotes venous relaxation. Used as an anti-anginal agent. Side-effects are transient headache, flushing and dizziness. In large doses it may cause hypotension with a reflex tachycardia.

Thiazide diuretics

Thiazides are capable of lowering blood pressure. The exact mechanism is unclear, but it seems to be independent of the modest diuretic effect provided by these agents. Maximum blood pressure reduction is achieved using low doses (eg bendroflumethiazide 2.5 mg daily). They are associated with a number of dose-dependent metabolic effects:

- Hyponatraemia, hypokalaemia and hypomagnesaemia; a hypochloraemic alkalosis may result.
- Raised plasma urate may occur due to reduction of tubular clearance of urate; rarely, gout may be precipitated.
- Diabetic glycaemic control may worsen on thiazides due to impaired insulin release; tissue-based insulin resistance and cholesterol may rise, at least temporarily.
- Thiazide diuretics may also cause postural hypotension, photosensitivity and impotence (mechanism unclear).

Rare dose-independent side-effects of thiazide diuretics

- Agranulocytosis
- Pancreatitis
- Thrombocytopenia

Ticlopidine

This is a novel anti-platelet agent, which probably acts via GpIIb/IIIa glycoprotein. Its uses include secondary stroke prevention, treatment of unstable angina and post-coronary stent insertion. It is at least as effective as aspirin. Severe (but reversible) neutropenia occurs in 1% of users and diarrhoea in 20%. Intrahepatic cholestasis and marrow aplasia have also been reported.

Clopidogrel

Like ticlopidine, clopidogrel inhibits ADP-mediated platelet aggregation. It is also used to prevent ischaemic heart disease and stroke. Evidence from the CAPRIE trial suggests that it is at least as effective an alternative as aspirin. It may also cause neutropenia, but less frequently so than ticlopidine.

3.2 Endocrinology

Carbimazole

Carbimazole acts by inhibiting a peroxidase which catalyses all phases of thyroid hormone production from the amino acid tyrosine. It takes at least 6 weeks to reduce blood levels of thyroid hormones. Therefore, somatic symptoms of hyperthyroidism, such as tachycardia and anxiety, are best suppressed by beta-blockers (eg propranolol).

- Agranulocytosis may occur within the first 16 weeks of therapy and in the event of a sore throat patients should be advised to seek medical help.
- The drug crosses the placenta; however, if it is given in low dose in pregnancy, fetal hypothyroidism may be prevented.

Hormone replacement therapy

On average, over a third of a woman's life is in the post-menopausal phase, yet only 12% receive hormone replacement therapy (HRT); 60–75% of menopausal women will experience vasomotor symptoms and these will be reduced by HRT.

- Without HRT, women aged 70 years have a 50% reduction in bone mass and one in two will have an osteoporosis-related fracture.
- HRT therefore leads to a 50% reduction in fractures and may reduce ischaemic heart disease by 20% and stroke by 15%; this may be at the expense of an increased risk of breast cancer.
- *See also* Chapter 4, Endocrinology, Section 3.5.

Nateglinide and repaglinide

These agents have a short duration of action and may be used to stimulate insulin release in patients with type 2 diabetes prior to meals. They may also be given alongside metformin. Side-effects include gastrointestinal upset and hypersensitivity reactions.

Acarbose

Acarbose inhibits intestinal alpha-glucosidase and thereby delays absorption of starch and sucrose. It reduces post-prandial hyperglycaemia in type 1 diabetes and is used as an adjunct to metformin or sulphonylurea therapy in type 2 diabetes. Excess flatus is a common adverse effect.

Thiazolidinediones (pioglitazone and rosiglitazone)

Thiazolidinediones reduce peripheral insulin resistance and are used in combination with metformin (or sulphonylureas) to treat patients in whom combined therapy with the latter two agents is inadequate or not tolerated. Thiazolidinediones may delay the requirement for insulin. Hepatic impairment is a recognised adverse effect, and hence regular monitoring of liver biochemistry is required.

3.3 Gastroenterology

Mesalazine and olsalazine

Mesalazine and olsalazine differ from sulfasalazine in being purely 5-amino salicylic acid (5-ASA) molecules which are split for local action in the colon. They suppress local inflammation in ulcerative colitis.

- They have some systemic side-effects including nausea, abdominal pain, headache and sometimes worsening of colitis.
- Rare side-effects of mesalazine and olsalazine include reversible pancreatitis, blood dyscrasias and interstitial nephritis (with mesalazine).

Sulfasalazine

Sulfasalazine consists of a sulphonamide molecule plus 5-ASA. It is used in the treatment of ulcerative colitis, and also as a disease-modifying anti-rheumatic in rheumatoid arthritis. The sulphonamide moiety frequently leads to gastrointestinal upset. Other key features are as follows:

- Oligospermia, leading to male infertility, may occur but this is usually reversible on stopping sulfasalazine.
- Patients may note orange discoloration of body fluids.
- Slow acetylators may experience more toxicity with sulfasalazine due to exposure to higher levels of the sulphonamide constituent.
- Rare side-effects of sulfasalazine include Stevens–Johnson syndrome, blood dyscrasias (especially agranulocytosis and aplasia) and nephrotic syndrome.

3.4 Neurology

Treatment of Parkinson's disease

Enhanced dopaminergic transmission is central to the medical management of Parkinson's disease:

- **Selegiline** is a type B monoamine oxidase inhibitor (MAO-B); inhibition of monoamine oxidase potentiates dopamine and reduces end-dose akinesia. It was thought that selegiline might also retard progression of Parkinson's disease by preserving dopaminergic neurones. This is now known to be untrue.
- **Amantadine** potentiates dopamine by preventing its re-uptake into pre-synaptic terminals.
- **Levodopa** (L-dopa) is absorbed in the proximal small bowel by active transport, but the presence of amino acids (and thus meals) may reduce absorption. It is a pro-drug which must be converted to dopamine within the nigro-striatal pathway. The drug is largely metabolised by catechol-o-methyl transferase. After 8 years of therapy with L-dopa, 50% of patients will have choreo-athetoid dyskinesia and end-dose akinesia. By this time many patients will have deteriorated to pre-treatment levels of disability due to progression of Parkinson's disease.
- **Dopamine receptor agonists** include apomorphine, bromocriptine, cabergoline, lisuride, pergolide, pramipexole and ropinirole. These agents cause less dyskinesia than L-dopa but they are associated with more neuropsychiatric adverse effects. Certain of these agents have been associated with pulmonary and retroperitoneal fibrosis (bromocriptine, cabergoline, lisuride, pergolide). **Apomorphine** is a powerful dopamine agonist which needs to be given by parenteral administration under specialist supervision. It is highly emetogenic and domperidone must therefore be given 2 days prior to the commencement of therapy.

Side-effects of L-dopa

- Cardiac arrhythmias
- Involuntary movements (dyskinesia) occur commonly
- Nausea and vomiting
- Postural hypotension
- Psychosis (depression or mania)
- Somnolescence (including sudden onset)

Orlistat

This agent inhibits the action of pancreatic lipase and may be indicated in obesity where the body mass index is >30 kg/m^2 and where the individual has been able to lose 2.5 kg in weight over a four-week period. It causes liquid, oily stools and may reduce the absorption of fat-soluble vitamins.

Treatment of epilepsy

Recent developments in the therapeutics of epilepsy have concentrated on agents which interact with neurotransmitters.

- **Glutamic acid** is an excitatory central nervous system neurotransmitter; lamotrigine inhibits it, so suppressing seizures. The side-effects of lamotrigine include mood changes, maculopapular rashes, influenza-like symptoms and Stevens–Johnson syndrome.
- **Gamma-aminobutyric acid** (GABA) is an inhibitory central nervous system neurotransmitter. Gabapentin and vigabatrin potentiate GABA and thus may be used to treat seizures.
- **Vigabatrin** is used for refractory epilepsy, potentiating GABA by irreversible inhibition of GABA transaminase. Side-effects of vigabatrin include mood disturbance and psychosis in 5%. Severe visual field defects may occur from one month to several years after initiation of therapy; regular visual field assessment is advised.
- **Diazepam** also terminates seizures by indirectly interacting with GABA transmission. It stimulates the benzodiazepine receptor in the brain which in turn enhances the affinity of the neighbouring GABA receptor for its neurotransmitter.
- **Carbamazepine** is a derivative of the tricyclic antidepressants and is useful for epilepsy and also neural pain (eg trigeminal or post-herpetic neuralgia). Patients commonly experience headaches and diplopia on starting carbamazepine and 5–15% of patients can develop a generalised morbilliform rash.
- **Sodium valproate** is used in absence attacks and temporal lobe epilepsy. It inhibits liver enzymes and may potentiate other anti-epileptics such as phenytoin. It may cause alopecia, with curly regrowth after stopping the drug.

Adverse effects of valproate

- Alopecia
- Amenorrhoea
- Ataxia
- Gynaecomastia
- Hepatitis (sometimes fatal)
- Liver enzyme inhibition
- Thrombocytopenia
- Weight gain

5-HT agonists (sumatriptan and rizatriptan)

5-HT agonists are used during the acute phase of migraine. They are effective only if taken early in the attack, and oral and sublingual preparations are available. They maintain vasoconstriction and prevent headache associated with the vasodilator phase of migraine. They must not be given in hemiplegic migraine, or within 24 hours of ergotamine, as intense vasospasm may lead to permanent neurological damage. Sumatriptan may lead to permanent neurological damage. It may also cause angina due to coronary vasospasm.

Side-effects of sumatriptan

- Chest pain
- Drowsiness
- Fatigue
- Flushing
- Vasospasm

3.5 Psychiatry

Chlorpromazine

Chlorpromazine blocks many different receptors; for example, it acts as a dopamine blocker, an alpha blocker, anti-cholinergic and anti-histamine. Due to prolongation of the QT interval on the ECG, ventricular tachycardia may result (particularly when used in high dose).

Adverse effects of chlorpromazine

- Agranulocytosis
- Contact dermatitis and purple pigmentation of the skin
- Dystonias (including oculogyric crisis)
- Neuroleptic malignant syndrome
- Photosensitivity
- Tardive dyskinesia (chronic use)
- Ventricular tachycardia (prolonged QT)

Lithium

Lithium carbonate is used for prophylaxis in bipolar affective disorder, for treatment of acute mania/hypomania and to augment antidepressants in recurrent or resistant depression. It is also used to treat aggressive behaviour in patients with learning disabilities. It has a narrow therapeutic range (0.6–1.2 mmol/l). Toxic effects occur at levels >2.0 mmol/l.

- **Toxicity** is more likely in renal impairment or when there are imbalances of electrolytes; it may also arise when lithium excretion is impaired by thiazide and loop diuretics, ACE inhibitors and non-steroidal anti-inflammatory drugs.
- Lithium may cause **histological changes** in the kidney and it has been recommended that long-term treatment is reviewed every 2–3 years.
- **Polyuria** arises due to nephrogenic diabetes insipidus; lithium prevents anti-diuretic hormone (ADH) from interacting with the collecting duct receptor, so leading to water loss. There is a compensatory increase in ADH release.

Toxic and side-effects of lithium	Side-effects of lithium*
• **(At 1–2 mmol/l)** Anorexia and vomiting Ataxia and dysarthria Blurred vision Coarse tremor Diarrhoea Drowsiness Muscle weakness	• **Common** Fine tremor (in about 15% of patients) Leukocytosis Loose motions Nausea Oedema Polydipsia Polyuria Weight gain
• **(Severe toxicity >2 mmol/l)** Circulatory failure Coma Convulsions Death Hyper-reflexia Oliguria Toxic psychoses	• **Rare** Goitre Hypothyroidism Interstitial nephritis Worsening of psoriasis and acne

*May arise despite therapeutic range dosing

- Antacids, theophylline and acetazolamide lead to decreased plasma lithium carbonate.
- CNS toxicity has been described with selective serotonin re-uptake inhibitors (SSRIs), carbamazepine and phenytoin, methyldopa, antipsychotics (especially haloperidol), calcium channel blockers and sumatriptan.

3.6 Rheumatology

Penicillamine

Penicillamine is used as a disease-modifying agent in rheumatoid arthritis and also to chelate cysteine in cystinuria and copper in Wilson's disease, respectively. In the first 6 weeks of therapy reversible loss of taste may occur. This may resolve without stopping the drug.

- After 4–18 months of therapy, proteinuria due to membranous glomerulonephritis may ensue.
- Thrombocytopenia and neutropenia may result from penicillamine therapy; patients should be warned to seek medical advice if a sore throat or ready bruising develop.
- Myasthenia, drug-induced lupus and Stevens–Johnson syndrome have also been reported.

Treatment of gout

Allopurinol inhibits xanthine oxidase, the enzyme which converts purines into uric acid, and so prevents gout. However, commencement of therapy will occasionally provoke an acute attack of gout. Established gouty tophi may regress with chronic use of allopurinol.

- Azathioprine, a pro-drug, is converted to 6-mercaptopurine in the body and may accumulate causing bone marrow toxicity in patients receiving allopurinol.
- The renal clearance of cyclophosphamide may also be impeded in patients receiving allopurinol and this again leads to marrow toxicity.

Colchicine inhibits macrophage migration into a gouty joint but its use is limited by the frequent occurrence of diarrhoea. It has therefore been said that with colchicine 'you run before you can walk'!

Urate oxidase enzymatically degrades urate to allantoin. Intravenous administration causes a significant reduction in serum urate concentrations (by up to 95%) and is used to prevent renal impairment in tumour lysis syndrome.

3.7 Miscellaneous

A detailed description of the mechanism of action, important pharmacokinetics and characteristic or serious side-effects of commonly used antibacterial, antiviral and antihelminthic agents is provided in Chapter 11, Infectious Diseases.

Ciprofloxacin

This 4-quinolone inhibits DNA bacterial gyrase, an enzyme which prevents supercoiling of bacterial DNA; it has activity against both Gram-positive and Gram-negative organisms. It is a liver enzyme inhibitor and particularly potentiates theophylline. Ciprofloxacin is not recommended for children under 12 years of age (except in cystic fibrosis) because of the potential for bony anomalies (which have been shown in pre-pubertal animal models).

Side-effects of ciprofloxacin

- Anaphylaxis
- Arthralgia
- Diarrhoea
- Impaired motor function
- Photosensitivity
- Sedation (which may affect driving)
- Seizures

- The **seizures** occur because ciprofloxacin can compete with the inhibitory neurotransmitter, GABA, within the brain.

Ciclosporin A

Ciclosporin A is used to reduce transplant rejection and it has significantly improved graft survival. It causes dose-dependent nephrotoxicity and has a narrow therapeutic range. The risk of toxicity is therefore assessed by therapeutic drug monitoring. (*See also* Chapter 15, Nephrology.)

Gum hyperplasia is common; it is increased in individuals with poor oral hygiene, and also those concomitantly taking dihydropyridine calcium-channel blockers. As with most immunosuppressives, there is an increased risk of skin and lymphoproliferative malignancy with long-term therapy.

Adverse effects of ciclosporin A

- Burning hands and feet (especially during 1st week of therapy)
- Fluid retention
- Gum hyperplasia
- Hyperkalaemia
- Hypertension
- Hypertrichosis
- Liver dysfunction
- Nephrotoxicity
- Oligodystrophy

Cytotoxics

The majority of cytotoxic agents have the potential to cause marrow suppression.

Specific side-effects of cytotoxic agents

- **Bleomycin**
  Causes dose-dependent lung fibrosis; it is one of the least myelotoxic chemotherapeutic agents
- **Cisplatin**
  May cause ototoxicity, nephrotoxicity (interstitial nephritis), hypomagnesaemia and peripheral neuropathy
- **Doxorubicin**
  May cause skin irritation and cardiomyopathy
- **Methotrexate**
  May cause severe mucositis and myelosuppression, which is prevented by the use of folinic acid rescue. During chronic administration pneumonitis and liver fibrosis may occur
- **Vincristine and vinblastine**
  Cause a reversible peripheral neuropathy

Leukotriene antagonists

Agents such as montelukast block the effects of leukotriene in the airways. They are used as add-on therapy in mild to moderate asthma. They should not be used to attempt to relieve acute asthma. Churg–Strauss-like eosinophilic vasculitis and peripheral neuropathy have been reported with these agents.

Retinoids

Oral retinoids are indicated for treatment of severe psoriasis and acne that is resistant to other therapies. They are teratogenic, leading to neural tube defects. Like other vitamin A derivatives they may cause benign intracranial hypertension. Dryness of mucous membranes leading to intolerance of contact lenses has been noted during treatment with retinoids.

High-dose retinoids can rarely cause diffuse interstitial skeletal hyperostosis.

Adverse effects of retinoids

- Alopecia
- Benign intracranial hypertension
- Dry mucous membranes
- Hepatitis
- Hypertriglyceridaemia
- Mood changes
- Photosensitivity
- Reduced night vision
- Skeletal abnormalities (with high doses)
- Teratogenicity
- Thrombocytopenia

4. SPECIFIC ADVERSE EFFECTS

4.1 Secondary amenorrhoea due to drugs

Dopamine inhibits prolactin release and so dopamine-blocking drugs, such as chlorpromazine and cimetidine (but not ranitidine), may provoke hyperprolactinaemia and hence amenorrhoea. Sodium valproate may also cause amenorrhoea.

4.2 Bronchospasm

Bronchospasm may be induced by **aspirin** and **non-steroidal anti-inflammatory drugs**, particularly in patients with late-onset asthma. Sensitivity to these agents is thought to relate to pharmacological effects on prostaglandin metabolism; the effect is not immunological, and thus it is termed 'pseudoallergic'.

- **Adenosine** should be avoided in asthma, as it may cause bronchoconstriction via stimulation of adenosine receptors found in bronchial smooth muscle.
- Even **cardioselective beta-blockers**, such as atenolol, may provoke bronchospasm.
- **Sodium chromoglycate** is a mast cell stabiliser; it is an inhaled, preventative agent in asthma. However, bronchospasm has occasionally been reported, because chromoglycate is administered as a dry powder.
- *N*-Acetyl cysteine may cause bronchospasm and anaphylaxis when given as an antidote to paracetamol overdose.

4.3 Dyskinesia and dystonia

Both dopamine agonists and antagonists can lead to movement disorders.

- Drugs with **dopamine-like effects** that are used to treat Parkinson's disease may cause dyskinesia (L-dopa, bromocriptine, lysuride and pergolide).
- **Dopamine-blocking agents** such as phenothiazines (chlorpromazine) or butyrophenones (haloperidol) may also cause dyskinesias. This is a recognised complication of treatment with dopamine antagonists such as domperidone. It is less common with metoclopramide due to poorer uptake of this agent across the blood–brain barrier.
- Fluoxetine and paroxetine, **serotonin re-uptake inhibitors** used in the treatment of depression, have both been associated with dystonias.

4.4 Gynaecomastia

Gynaecomastia can complicate treatment with drugs that are oestrogen-like in action or anti-androgens.

Oestrogen-like action

- Digoxin
- Spironolactone
- Stilboestrol

Anti-androgen action

- Cimetidine
- Cyproterone acetate
- Luteinising hormone releasing hormone (LHRH) analogues (eg goserelin)

4.5 Hypothyroidism

Impaired thyroid hormone production may result from:

- amiodarone
- carbimazole
- lithium
- propylthiouracil
- radio-iodine.

4.6 Drug-induced liver disease

Drug-induced liver disease may represent either dose-dependent or dose-independent effects.

- Dose-dependent liver disease includes paracetamol poisoning, fatty change due to tetracyclines and alcoholic hepatitis.

- Dose-independent liver disease usually involves either **hepatitis** or **cholestasis**; it generally has an allergic basis and may on occasion be associated with liver failure.

Drug-induced hepatitis occurs with

- Amiodarone
- HMG CoA reductase inhibitors
- Isoniazid metabolite
- Methyldopa
- Paracetamol
- Phenytoin
- Pyrazinamide
- Valproate

Causes of drug-induced cholestasis

- Carbamazepine
- Chlorpromazine
- Co-amoxiclav (combination of amoxicillin and clavulanic acid)
- Erythromycin
- Sulphonylureas

- Liver tumours may be associated with use of androgens and oestrogens (which can also cause Budd–Chiari malformations); liver fibrosis may accompany methotrexate treatment.

4.7 Drugs provoking myasthenia

- **Aminoglycosides**, certain **beta-blockers** (propranolol, oxprenolol), **phenytoin**, **lignocaine**, **quinidine** and **procainamide** may all impair acetylcholine release, leading to worsening or unmasking of myasthenia.
- **Penicillamine** may cause formation of antibodies against the acetylcholine receptor, and a syndrome indistinguishable from myasthenia results. This resolves in two-thirds of cases after penicillamine withdrawal.
- **Lithium** may also cause myasthenia-like weakness by impairing synaptic transmission.

4.8 Photosensitivity

Drugs causing photosensitivity

- Amiodarone
- Ciprofloxacin
- Griseofulvin
- Loop and thiazide diuretics
- Oral contraceptives
- Piroxicam
- Psoralens
- Retinoids
- Sulphonylureas
- Tetracyclines

4.9 Drug-induced vasculitis

Drug-induced vasculitis can affect the skin or internal organs.

Drugs causing vasculitis

- Allopurinol
- Captopril
- Cimetidine
- Hydralazine
- Leukotriene antagonists
- Penicillin
- Quinidine
- Sulphonamides
- Thiazides

4.10 Acute pancreatitis

Acute pancreatitis is a recognised adverse effect of a number of drugs.

Drugs causing acute pancreatitis

- Anti-retrovirals (ritonavir, didanosine, zalcitabine, stavudine, lamivudine)
- Azathioprine
- Corticosteroids
- Fibrates
- HMG CoA reductase inhibitors
- Omega-3 fish oils
- Thiazide diuretics

4.11 Syndrome of inappropriate ADH (SIADH)

SIADH is characterised by hyponatraemia, concentrated urine and low plasma osmolality, all occurring in the absence of oedema, diuretic use or hypovolaemia.

Drugs causing SIADH

- Carbamazepine
- Chlorpropamide
- Cytotoxic agents
- Opiates
- Oxytocin
- Psychotropic agents
- Rifampicin

In addition there are a number of non-pharmacological causes, which include malignancy, central nervous system disorders, suppurative pulmonary disease and porphyria (*see* Chapter 4, Endocrinology, Section 4).

5. POISONING

5.1 Paracetamol overdose

Overdose with paracetamol is one of the most common causes of self-poisoning. Early features are minor (nausea and vomiting) but hepatic or renal failure occur later; and liver damage peaks at 1–2 days after ingestion. Paracetamol is normally metabolised by glucuronidation in the liver. Toxicity arises because excess oxidation products are formed in overdose; these overwhelm the capacity for endogenous detoxification (glutathione) and the active metabolite binds to liver cell macromolecules, causing necrosis.

- The international normalised ratio (INR), or prothrombin ratio, is the most sensitive indicator of liver damage. Hypoglycaemia is a feature of advanced liver damage.
- Poor prognosis is indicated by an INR above 3.0, raised serum creatinine or plasma pH <7.3 more than 24 hours after overdose.
- Patients taking enzyme inducers such as phenytoin have an increased risk of hepatic necrosis after paracetamol poisoning.
- Renal failure may sometimes develop before liver necrosis due to mixed-function oxidases generating the same dangerous metabolites within the renal parenchyma.
- *N*-Acetyl cysteine binds the hepatotoxic metabolites; it improves prognosis in paracetamol poisoning even after hepatic encephalopathy has developed. It is now administered continuously until the INR has returned to normal.

5.2 Tricyclic antidepressant overdose

Tricyclic antidepressants have anti-cholinergic (pupillary dilatation, confusion and tachycardia) and alpha-blocking (hypotension) side-effects. Sympathomimetic overactivity results.

- Prolonged QT interval on the ECG may predispose to ventricular arrhythmias; the QRS complex is widened in severe toxicity. Intravenous bicarbonate may reduce the risk of arrhythmias and seizures in these situations. In markedly widened QRS complex, it may be a prelude to cardiogenic shock and such patients require cardiac pacing.
- The seizure threshold is also reduced and status epilepticus may ensue; abnormalities of thermoregulation can also occur.
- Treatment is supportive, with emesis, gastric lavage and use of activated charcoal. Fluid and electrolyte balance should be maintained; diazepam is used for convulsions.

5.3 Theophylline toxicity

Theophylline causes tachycardia and may trigger arrhythmias in overdose due to phosphodiesterase inhibition. These are more likely in the presence of severe acidosis or hypokalaemia, the latter due to intractable vomiting. Seizures and confusion can occur.

- Treatment is with activated charcoal (which significantly reduces theophylline absorption) and correction of fluid and electrolyte depletion. Upper gastrointestinal endoscopy may be useful to remove tablet residuum that can remain within the stomach for many hours.
- Haemodialysis or, preferably, charcoal haemoperfusion is indicated for patients with severe toxicity (plasma theophylline >60 mg/l).

5.4 Carbon monoxide poisoning

Carbon monoxide binds to haemoglobin with high affinity (>200 times that of oxygen); poisoning leads to decreased haemoglobin oxygen-carrying ability, and consequent tissue anoxia. Normal carboxyhaemoglobin levels are <3% in non-smokers and 5–6% in smokers; at 10–30% exposed patients usually only complain of headaches and mild exertional dyspnoea.

Signs of marked toxicity (carboxyhaemoglobin 30–60%)

- Acute renal failure
- Agitation and confusion
- Bullous lesions
- ECG changes and arrhythmias
- Hyperpyrexia
- Hypertonia and hyperreflexia
- Muscle necrosis
- Pink mucosae
- Vomiting

- Severe toxicity is associated with coma, convulsions and cardio-respiratory arrest.
- Treatment is with 100% oxygen by mask; hyperbaric oxygen (2.5 atmospheres pressure) will decrease the elimination half-life of carbon monoxide (from 4 hours to 22 minutes), but this is not often available on site and hence patient transfer to a specialist centre may be required.
- Neuropsychiatric changes may develop over several weeks after recovery from poisoning and these include intellectual deterioration, personality change, cerebral and cerebellar damage, and midbrain damage (Parkinson's disease).

5.5 Quinidine and quinine toxicity

Quinidine and quinine poisoning may result in blurred vision and abdominal pain due to anticholinergic effects. Other features are:

- **arrhythmias**: because these drugs prolong the QT interval on the ECG
- **hypotension**: which may occur due to alpha-adrenoceptor blockade
- **tinnitus** and **irreversible blindness**.

5.6 Iron poisoning

The key features of iron poisoning are shown in the box below. Gastric lavage should be contemplated if the patient presents within 1 hour of ingestion. Desferrioxamine chelates iron and improves clinical outcome. It is given by intravenous infusion and the treatment is based upon the serum iron concentration; however, in severe cases, treatment should be commenced before iron levels are available.

Clinical features of iron poisoning

- Abdominal pain
- Diarrhoea
- Haematemesis
- Lower gastrointestinal blood loss
- Nausea and vomiting

Severe poisoning

- Coma
- Death
- Delayed hepatocellular necrosis
- Hypotension

5.7 Salicylate overdose

The adverse effects of salicylate poisoning are due to direct stimulation of the respiratory centre in the CNS (respiratory alkalosis) and to the acidic properties of the drug as well as the accumulation of organic acids (metabolic acidosis).

Early features of poisoning

- Hypokalaemia
- Respiratory centre stimulation in the CNS, and hence alkalosis
- Sweating
- Tinnitus

Later features of poisoning

- Acute renal failure
- Hypoglycaemia
- Hypoprothrombinaemia
- Metabolic acidosis
- Pulmonary oedema

Key aspects of management of salicylate poisoning involve:

- activated charcoal
- correction of electrolyte and metabolic abnormalities
- intravenous fluids to ensure adequate hydration (forced alkaline diuresis is now regarded as unsafe and is not recommended)
- **haemodialysis**: for very severe salicylism (blood salicylate >750 mg/l).

5.8 Ethylene glycol poisoning

Poisoning with ethylene glycol has the clinical appearance of alcohol intoxication with cerebellar symptoms and signs in the first 12 hours, but without any smell of alcohol. Subsequent breakdown of ethylene glycol to oxalate causes metabolic acidosis; there is a raised anion gap due to the presence of exogenous organic acid, as well as a raised osmolar gap. Within 2–3 days acute tubular necrosis results due to cellular damage by calcium oxalate crystals. Cardiac failure with pulmonary oedema may ensue.

Treatment for ethylene glycol poisoning

- **Sodium bicarbonate**
  To reduce acidosis
- **Intravenous ethanol**
  Can inhibit ethylene glycol metabolism
- **Fomepizole**
  This blocks the conversion of ethylene glycol to glycolate and it may be administered after the overdose
- **Calcium**
  To correct hypocalcaemia
- **Haemodialysis**
  Active elimination of ethylene glycol is by haemodialysis

5.9 Haemodialysis for overdose or poisoning

Drugs or poisons which are poorly removed by haemodialysis are those with a large volume of distribution (eg amiodarone and Paraquat) or those which are highly protein-bound (eg digoxin and phenytoin). Repeated or continuous dialysis treatment may be required for drugs which are widely distributed throughout the body, eg lithium, as there will be rebound increases in plasma concentration.

Removal of drugs or toxins by haemodialysis/haemoperfusion

- **Haemodialysis effective**
  Alcohol
  Barbiturates
  Ethylene glycol
  Lithium
  Methanol
  Salicylate
- **Charcoal haemoperfusion**
  Paracetamol metabolites
  Theophylline

Chapter 3
Dermatology

CONTENTS

8. Disorders of pigmentation

9. Drug eruptions

10. Skin tumours
- 10.1 Malignant melanoma
- 10.2 Basal cell carcinoma
- 10.3 Squamous cell carcinoma
- 10.4 Other skin tumours

11. Hair and nails
- 11.1 Disorders of hair
- 11.2 Disorders of nails

Dermatology

1. STRUCTURE AND FUNCTION OF SKIN AND TERMINOLOGY OF SKIN LESIONS

1.1 Structure

The skin consists of three distinctive layers: the epidermis, dermis and the subcutis.

- **Epidermis**: this forms the outermost layer and is the largest organ in the body. The principal cell is the keratinocyte. The epidermis has four layers which are the basal cell layer, stratum spinosum, stratum granulosum and the stratum corneum.
- **Dermis**: this lies beneath the epidermis and is a support structurally and nutritionally, and contributes 15–20% of total body weight. The principal cell is the fibroblast which makes collagen (giving the skin its strength), elastin (providing elasticity) and proteoglycans. It also contains adnexal structures including hair follicles, sebaceous glands, apocrine glands and eccrine glands.
- **Dermo-epidermal junction**: separates the epidermis from the dermis. Anomalies of this can give rise to some of the blistering disorders.
- **Subcutis**: contains adipose tissue, loose connective tissue, blood vessels and nerves.

1.2 Function

The skin has numerous functions, all of which are designed to protect the rest of the body.

- **Barrier properties**: the skin acts as a two-way barrier, preventing the inward or outward passage of fluid and electrolytes.
- **Mechanical properties**: the skin is highly elastic and so can be stretched or compressed.
- **Immunological function**: the skin provides defence against foreign agents. In the epidermis, antigen presentation is carried out by Langerhan's cells.
- **Sensory function**: the skin perceives the sensations of touch, pressure, cold, warmth and pain.
- **Endocrine properties**: as a result of exposure to ultraviolet B radiation, vitamin D3 is synthesised from previtamin D3.
- **Temperature regulation**: the rich blood supply of the dermis plays an important role in thermoregulation.
- **Respiration**: the skin plays a minor role in gaseous exchange with the environment.

1.3 Terminology of skin lesions

- **Macule**: a flat lesion due to a localised colour change; when >1 cm in diameter, this is termed a patch.
- **Papule**: a small solid elevation of skin <1 cm diameter.
- **Plaque**: a raised flat-topped lesion >1 cm diameter.
- **Nodule**: a raised lesion with a rounded surface >1 cm diameter.
- **Bulla**: a fluid-filled lesion (blister) >1 cm diameter.
- **Vesicle**: a fluid-filled skin lesion <1 cm diameter.
- **Pustule**: a pus-filled lesion.
- **Wheal**: a raised compressible area of dermal oedema.
- **Scale**: flakes arising from abnormal stratum corneum.
- **Crust**: dried serum, pus or blood.

2. SPECIFIC DERMATOSES AND INFECTIONS OF THE SKIN

2.1 Psoriasis

This is a genetically determined, inflammatory and proliferative disorder of the skin, occurring in 1–2% of the UK population. Its aetiology is unknown but there is an association with HLA Cw6, B13 and B17 in skin disease and HLA B27 in psoriatic arthropathy. The disease is more common in the second and sixth decades, with females generally developing psoriasis at an earlier age than males.

Psoriasis tends to affect the extensor surfaces and demonstrates the Köbner phenomenon. Other affected areas include the scalp, nails, genitalia and flexures.

Clinical presentation

- **Chronic plaque**: well-defined, red, disc-like plaques covered by white scale, which classically affect elbows, knees and scalp.
- **Pustular (generalised pustular)**: sheets of small, sterile yellow pustules on a red background. This presentation may be accompanied by systemic symptoms and progression to erythroderma.
- **Pustular (palmo-plantar pustulosis)**: yellow/brown sterile pustules and erythema on palms or soles. Strongly associated with smoking. This is most often seen in middle-aged women.
- **Guttate**: an acute eruption of drop-like lesions often following a streptococcal sore throat.
- **Erythrodermic**: confluent areas affecting most of the skin surface.
- **Nail psoriasis**: onycholysis, pitting and subungal hyperkeratosis.
- **Flexural**: affects axillae, submammary areas and the natal cleft. Lesions are often smooth, red and glazed in appearance.

Associations with psoriasis

- **Arthropathy**: arthritis occurs in about 8% of patients with psoriasis. There are several different forms (see Chapter 20, Rheumatology) – distal inter-phalangeal joint disease, large single joint oligoarthritis, arthritis mutilans, sacroiliitis and psoriatic spondylitis have all been described.
- **Gout**: this is due to deposits of urate crystals.
- **Malabsorption**: Crohn's and ulcerative colitis are associated with psoriasis.

Factors which can exacerbate psoriasis

- **Trauma**: the Köbner phenomenon.
- **Infection**: eg streptococci (guttate psoriasis as above) and HIV.
- **Endocrine**: psoriasis generally tends to improve during pregnancy and deteriorate in the post-partum period.
- **Drugs**: beta-blockers, lithium, antimalarials and the withdrawal of oral steroids can exacerbate psoriasis.
- **Alcohol**.
- **Stress**: severe physical or psychological stress.

Causes of the Köbner phenomenon

- Psoriasis
- Lichen planus
- Vitiligo
- Viral warts
- Molluscum contagiosum

Causes of erythroderma

- Psoriasis
- Eczema
- Mycosis fungoides
- Adverse drug reactions
- Underlying malignancy
- Pityriasis rubra pilaris

Management of psoriasis

A careful explanation of the disease process and the likely necessity for long-term treatment should always be given. The type and severity of psoriasis influence the choice of treatment. However, it is usual to prescribe topical agents as the first-line treatment.

- **Topical therapy**: emollients, tar preparations, dithranol, vitamin D analogues, weak topical steroids (for face, genitalia and flexures).

For widespread or severe disease further treatment options are **ultraviolet radiation**, **systemic treatment**, or newer **biological agents**.

Ultraviolet radiation

- PUVA (oral/topical psoralen and UVA).
- UVB narrowband (311–313 nm) is now replacing broadband UVB (290–320 nm).

Systemic treatment

The benefits must be weighed against side-effects of the drugs. Treatments include retinoids, methotrexate, ciclosporin, azathioprine, hydroxyurea, mycophenolate mofetil.

Biological agents

These are promising new treatments but not all are licensed for use in psoriasis. Etanercept has been recently approved by NICE for patients unresponsive or intolerant to other systemic agents. Efalizumab has been also approved for patients unresponsive to, intolerant of, or with contraindications to Etanercept.

- **Efalizumab**: this is a humanised monoclonal antibody which blocks T-cell activation/migration.
- **Alefacept**: a recombinant fusion protein which interferes with activation/proliferation of T-cells.
- **Etanercept**: human fusion protein of the tumour necrosis factor (TNF) receptor which acts as a TNFα inhibitor.
- **Infliximab**: a monoclonal antibody which binds to TNFα.

2.2 Eczema (dermatitis)

Eczema is an inflammatory skin disorder with characteristic histology and clinical features, that include itching, redness, scaling and a papulovesicular rash. Eczema can be divided into two broad groups, exogenous or endogenous:

- exogenous eczema – irritant dermatitis, allergic contact dermatitis
- endogenous eczema – atopic dermatitis, seborrhoeic dermatitis, pompholyx.

Seborrhoeic dermatitis is a red, scaly rash caused by *Pityrosporum ovale*. The eruption occurs on the scalp, face and upper trunk and is more common in young adults and HIV patients.

Pompholyx is characterised by itchy vesicles occurring on the palms and soles.

Atopic dermatitis is a characteristic dermatitic eruption associated with a personal or family history of atopy. The age of onset is usually between two and six months, with males being more affected than females. The disease is chronic but tends to improve during childhood. The flexural sites are commonly affected and features include itching, exudative papules or vesicles, dryness and lichenification. There is an increased risk of bacterial (staphylococcal or streptococcal) and viral (Herpes simplex) infection.

Management of atopic eczema

Initial treatment consists of avoidance of irritants and exacerbating factors. Thereafter:

- **Topical therapy**: regular emollients, topical steroids, tar bandages, wet wraps and antibiotic ointment (for minor infections). Topical tacrolimus and pimecrolimus may also have a place in treatment.

- **Ultraviolet radiation**: UVB or PUVA (*see* psoriasis Section 2.1).
- **Systemic treatment**: this can be with ciclosporin, azathioprine, antihistamines, as well as antibiotics for any infective episodes.

2.3 Lichen planus

This presents as an itchy, shiny, violaceous, flat-topped, polygonal, papular rash with white lines on the surface known as Wickham's striae. Other affected sites include mucous membranes, genitalia, palms, soles, scalp and nails. Lichen planus causes a white lace-like pattern on the buccal mucosa.

Causes of white lesions in the oral mucosa

- Lichen planus
- Leukoplakia
- Chronic candidiasis
- Chemical burns.

2.4 Erythema multiforme

This is usually a maculo-papular, targetoid rash, which can occur anywhere, including the palms, soles and oral mucosa. The aetiology is unknown but thought to be associated with infections, mainly viral. Stevens–Johnson syndrome, on the other hand, is more likely to affect mucosal surfaces and is thought to be associated with drug reactions.

Causes of erythema multiforme

- **Infections**
  Herpes simplex virus
  Mycoplasma
  Psittacosis
  Rickettsiae
  HIV
  Hepatitis B virus
  Orf
  Infectious mononucleosis
  Mumps
- **Drug reactions**
  Barbiturates
  Penicillin
  Sulphonamides
- **Others**
  Lupus erythematosus
  Polyarteritis nodosa
  Wegener's granulomatosis
  Underlying malignancy
  Sarcoidosis

2.5 Erythema nodosum

This is a hot, tender, nodular, erythematous eruption lasting three to six weeks, which is more common in the third decade and in females.

Causes of erythema nodosum

- **Bacterial infection**
  Streptococcal throat infection
- **Mycoses**
- **Sarcoidosis**
- **Tuberculosis**
- **Malignancy**
- **Viral/chlamydial infection**
- **Other infections**
  Salmonella gastroenteritis
  Campylobacter colitis
- **Inflammatory bowel disease**
- **Drugs**
  Penicillin
  Tetracyclines
  Oral contraceptive pill
  Sulphonamides
  Sulphonylureas

2.6 Specific skin infections

These can be sub-divided into bacterial, fungal and viral infections as well as infestations.

Specific infections of the skin

- **Bacterial infections**
  Streptococcal: cellulitis, erysipelas, impetigo, necrotising fasciitis, rheumatic fever (erythema marginatum), scarlet fever
  Staphylococcal: folliculitis, impetigo, staphylococcal scalded-skin syndrome, toxic-shock syndrome
  Mycobacterial: TB (lupus vulgaris, scrofuloderma), fish tank granuloma, Buruli ulcer, leprosy
  Spirochaetal: syphilis, Lyme disease (erythema chronicum migrans)
- **Fungal**
  Dermatophytes: *Trichophyton rubrum*, *Trichophyton interdigitale*, *Epidermophyton floccosum* (tinea pedis, tinea corporis, tinea cruris, tinea unguium)
  Yeasts: *Candida* (intertrigo, oral, genital or systemic)
  Pityrosporum orbiculare: pityriasis versicolor
- **Viral**
  Human papilloma virus: warts
  Herpes virus: varicella (chickenpox), zoster (shingles), simplex I (face and lips), simplex II (genital)
  Pox virus: molluscum contagiosum, parapox virus (orf)
  Parvovirus B19: erythema infectiosum (fifth disease)
  RNA virus: measles, rubella
  Coxsackie A16: hand, foot and mouth disease
  HIV/AIDS: skin disease is common, affecting 75% of patients who can be at any stage of HIV disease (see Chapter 8, Genito-urinary Medicine and AIDS)
- **Infestations**
  Sarcoptes scabiei: scabies mite infestation
  Lice infestation (pediculosis): head lice, pubic lice

3. BULLOUS ERUPTIONS

This is a rare group of disorders characterised by the formation of bullae. The development of blisters can be due to congenital, immunological or other causes. The level of split within the epidermis or within the dermo-epidermal junction determines the type of bullous disorder.

Causes of bullous eruptions

- **Congenital**
  Epidermolysis bullosa
- **Others**
  Staphylococcal scalded skin syndrome
  Toxic epidermal necrolysis
  Diabetic bullae
  Chronic renal failure
  Haemodialysis
- **Immunological**
  Pemphigus
  Bullous pemphigoid
  Cicatricial pemphigoid
  Herpes gestationis
  Dermatitis herpetiformis
- **Drug overdose**
  Barbiturates

Epidermolysis bullosa is the term used for a group of genetically determined disorders characterised by blistering of the skin, palms, soles and mucosae, especially the mouth and oesophagus.

Pemphigus is a rare group of disorders characterised by blistering of the skin and mucous membranes.

Bullous pemphigoid is more common than pemphigus. It is a disorder characterised by large tense blisters found on limbs, trunk and flexures in the elderly. Oral mucosal involvement is rare.

Cicatricial pemphigoid is a rare, chronic blistering disease of the mucous membranes and skin, which results in permanent scarring, particularly of the conjunctivae.

Dermatitis herpetiformis is an itchy, vesiculo-bullous eruption mainly occurring on the extensor areas. The majority of patients have asymptomatic gluten-sensitive enteropathy.

4. THE SKIN IN CONNECTIVE TISSUE DISORDERS

4.1 Systemic sclerosis

This is a rare, multisystem, connective tissue disease of unknown aetiology, characterised by fibrosis of the skin and visceral organs and accompanied by the presence of relatively specific antinuclear antibodies. The incidence peaks in the fifth and sixth decades and females are more affected than males.

Morphoea (localised scleroderma) consists of indurated plaques of sclerosis in the skin; systemic features are not found.

Skin changes in systemic sclerosis

- Facial telangiectasia
- Restricted mouth opening
- Peri-oral puckering
- Smooth shiny pigmented indurated skin
- Raynaud's phenomenon with gangrene
- Sclerodactyly
- Pulp atrophy
- Dilated nail fold capillaries
- Ragged cuticles
- Calcinosis cutis
- Livedo reticularis
- Leg ulcers

4.2 Rheumatoid arthritis

Specific skin changes in rheumatoid arthritis

- Rheumatoid nodules
- Nail fold infarcts
- Vasculitis with gangrene
- Pyoderma gangrenosum.

4.3 Dermatomyositis

Specific skin changes in dermatomyositis

- Heliotrope rash around eyes
- Gottron's papules: red plaques on extensor surfaces of finger joints
- Gottron's sign: erythema over knees and elbows
- Dilated nail fold capillaries and prominent, ragged cuticles
- Nail fold infarct.

4.4 Lupus erythematosus

Discoid lupus erythematosus is associated with scaly erythematous plaques with follicular plugging, on sun-exposed sites. These tend to heal with scarring.

Systemic lupus erythematosus (**SLE**) is commonly associated with dermatological manifestations. These include malar rash, photosensitivity, vasculitis, Raynaud's phenomenon, alopecia and oropharyngeal ulceration.

5. THE SKIN IN OTHER SYSTEMIC DISEASES

5.1 Sarcoidosis

Skin lesions are found in approximately 25% of patients with systemic sarcoid and can occur in the absence of systemic disease:

- erythema nodosum
- scar sarcoid
- lupus pernio
- scarring alopecia.

5.2 The porphyrias

- **Porphyria cutanea tarda** is the commonest of the porphyrias. Skin signs develop in sun-exposed areas. Patients have decreased levels of uroporphyrinogen decarboxylase. Eighty per cent of cases are acquired, in which case the condition is provoked by a hepatotoxic factor such as alcohol, oestrogens, hepatitis C, iron, lead and certain aromatic hydrocarbon hepatotoxins.
- **Acute intermittent porphyria**: skin signs are not seen.
- **Congenital erythropoietic porphyria**: patients have brown teeth which fluoresce red under Wood's light, giving the 'werewolf' appearance.

The typical skin signs of the porphyrias are:

- photosensitivity
- blister formation
- scarring with milia
- hypertrichosis.

5.3 Pyoderma gangrenosum

This is a painful ulcerating disease that typically occurs on the legs.

Causes of pyoderma gangrenosum

- **Gastrointestinal**
  Ulcerative colitis
  Crohn's colitis
- **Rheumatological**
  Rheumatoid arthritis
  Ankylosing spondylitis
- **Liver**
  Chronic active hepatitis
  Primary biliary cirrhosis
  Sclerosing cholangitis
- **Haematological**
  Leukaemia
  Lymphoma
  Myeloproliferative disorders
- **Others**
  Diabetes mellitus
  Thyroid disease
  Sarcoidosis
  Wegener's disease
- **Other malignancies**

5.4 Diabetes

Skin signs in diabetes mellitus

- Necrobiosis lipoidica
- Disseminated granuloma annulare
- Diabetic rubeosis
- Candidiasis and infection
- Vitiligo
- Neuropathic foot ulcers.

Diabetic rubeosis is an odd redness of the face, hands and feet thought to be due to diabetic microangiopathy.

6. GENERALISED PRURITUS

Pruritus is an important skin symptom and occurs in dermatological diseases such as atopic eczema. In the absence of localised skin disease or skin signs, patients should be fully investigated to exclude an underlying cause.

Causes of generalised pruritus

- **Obstructive liver disease**
- **Haematological**
  Iron deficiency anaemia
  Polycythaemia
- **Endocrine**
  Hyperthyroidism
  Hypothyroidism
  Diabetes mellitus
- **Chronic renal failure**
- **Malignancy**
  Internal malignancies
  Lymphoma
- **Drugs**
  Morphine
- **Other**
  Pregnancy
  Senility

7. CUTANEOUS MARKERS OF INTERNAL MALIGNANCY

There are numerous skin changes associated with internal malignancy. These can be either genetically determined syndromes with cutaneous manifestations, where there is a recognised predisposition to internal malignancy, or paraneoplastic syndromes, where the cutaneous signs are significantly associated with malignancy of various organs.

7.1 Genetically determined syndromes with skin manifestations

Most of these diseases have an autosomal dominant inheritance.

- **Gardner's syndrome**: epidermal cysts, lipomas and fibromas are associated with colonic carcinoma.
- **Peutz–Jeghers syndrome**: mucocutaneous pigmentation is associated with mainly gastrointestinal malignancy.
- **Howel–Evans syndrome**: tylosis (palmo-plantar keratoderma) has been reported with oesophageal carcinoma.
- **Torre–Muir syndrome**: sebaceous tumours are associated with gastrointestinal malignancy.
- **Cowden's disease**: tricholemmomas (facial nodules) and warty hyperplasia of the mucosal surface is associated with breast and thyroid carcinoma.
- **Neurofibromatosis**: the presence of six or more café-au-lait macules, axillary freckling and neurofibromas is associated with malignant schwannomas and astrocytomas.
- **Tuberous sclerosis**: angiofibromas, together with periungual fibromas, shagreen patches and ash-leaf macules are associated with sarcomas and rhabdomyomas.
- **Multiple endocrine neoplasia type 2b**: mucosal neuromas are associated with medullary thyroid carcinoma and phaeochromocytoma.
- **Gorlin's syndrome (basal cell naevus syndrome)**: multiple basal cell carcinomata associated with medulloblastoma, meningioma, astrocytoma and ovarian tumours.

- **von-Hippel Lindau syndrome**: café-au-lait macules and haemangiomas are associated with vascular tumours of the central nervous system, phaeochromocytoma, renal and pancreatic carcinoma.
- **Sturge–Weber syndrome**: port wine stain associated with ipsilateral vascular meningeal malformation and epilepsy.
- **Wiskott–Aldrich syndrome**: a sex-linked recessive disease characterised by eczema, immunodeficiency and an increased risk of lymphoma and leukaemia.
- **Chediak–Higashi syndrome**: a fatal autosomal recessive disease with recurrent bacterial infections and widespread infiltration with lymphocytes suggesting a lymphoma.
- **Ataxia telangiectasia**: an autosomal recessive disease characterised by mucocutaneous telangiectasia and an increased risk of lymphoma and leukaemia.
- **Xeroderma pigmentosum**: an autosomal recessive group of conditions characterised by multiple melanomas and non-melanoma skin malignancies which start developing from childhood in sun-exposed skin.

7.2 Skin disease as paraneoplastic features

Dermatological features can be seen in all types of malignant disease but some are more common in certain types of neoplasia.

Specific dermatological features and the common types of malignancy with which they are associated

- **Acanthosis nigricans**: gastrointestinal adenocarcinoma
- **Acanthosis palmaris (tripe palms)**: bronchial carcinoma
- **Acanthosis palmaris with nigricans**: gastrointestinal adenocarcinoma
- **Generalised pruritus**: lymphoma
- **Dermatomyositis (in adults)**: bronchial, breast and ovarian tumours
- **Erythema gyratum repens**: bronchial carcinoma
- **Acquired hypertrichosis lanuginosa**: gastrointestinal and bronchial tumours
- **Necrolytic migratory erythema**: glucagonoma
- **Migratory thrombophlebitis**: pancreatic carcinoma
- **Acquired ichthyosis**: lymphoma
- **Pyoderma gangrenosum**: myeloproliferative tumours
- **Erythroderma**: lymphoma and leukaemia
- **Clubbing**: bronchial carcinoma
- **Herpes zoster**: myeloproliferative tumours.

Other causes of acanthosis nigricans

- Internal malignancy
- Insulin-resistant diabetes mellitus
- Familial
- Acromegaly
- Cushing's disease
- Obesity
- Oral contraceptive pill
- Nicotinic acid
- Hypothyroidism

8. DISORDERS OF PIGMENTATION

The major colour determinant of the skin is melanin. This is produced by melanocytes, which are found in the basal layer of the epidermis. Pigmentary disorders usually present with either hypopigmentation or hyperpigmentation.

Causes of hypopigmentation

- **Genetic**
  Albinism
  Phenylketonuria
  Tuberous sclerosis
- **Chemical**
  Chloroquine
- **Infections**
  Pityriasis versicolor
- **Endocrine**
  Hypopituitarism
- **Autoimmune**
  Vitiligo
- **Post-inflammatory**
  Eczema
  Psoriasis
  Lupus erythematosus

Causes of hyperpigmentation

- **Genetic**
  Peutz–Jeghers syndrome
  Xeroderma pigmentosum
  Albright's syndrome
- **Metabolic**
  Cirrhosis
  Haemochromatosis
  Porphyria
  Renal failure
- **Drugs**
  Oral contraceptive pill
  Minocycline
  Amiodarone
- **Endocrine**
  Addison's disease
  Cushing's syndrome
  Nelson's syndrome
  Pregnancy
- **Nutritional**
  Malabsorption
  Carcinomatosis
  Kwashiorkor
  Pellagra
- **Post-inflammatory**
  Lichen planus
  Eczema
  Secondary syphilis
  Cutaneous amyloid

9. DRUG ERUPTIONS

The incidence of drug eruptions is approximately 2%.

The most common drug eruptions are:

- **Toxic erythema**: the commonest type of eruption. It is usually characterised by a morbilliform or maculopapular eruption which may become confluent. Causes include antibiotics (including sulphonamides), carbamazepine, allopurinol, gold, thiazides and anti-tuberculous drugs.
- **Fixed drug eruption**: this occurs in a localised site each time the drug is administered (see later).
- **Toxic epidermal necrolysis**: a life-threatening eruption due to extensive skin loss. This can be associated with allopurinol, sulphonamides, penicillin, carbamazepine, phenytoin, NSAIDS, gold, salicylates and barbiturates.
- **Urticaria**: (see below).
- **Photosensitivity** (see Chapter 2, Clinical Pharmacology, Toxicology and Poisoning).
- **Lupus erythematosus-like syndrome**: a number of drugs have been implicated to cause this relatively rare disorder (see Chapter 2, Clinical Pharmacology, Toxicology and Poisoning).
- **Vasculitis** (see Chapter 2, Clinical Pharmacology, Toxicology and Poisoning).
- **Erythema multiforme**: this is associated with penicillins, sulphonamides, phenytoin, carbamazepine, ACE inhibitors, NSAIDS, gold, barbiturates, thiazides.
- **Contact dermatitis**.
- **Hyperpigmentation** (see preceding page): associated with amiodarone, minocycline, bleomycin, chlorpromazine, antimalarials.

Urticaria is a transient, itchy, erythematous rash characterised by the presence of weals. It is thought to occur due to histamine release from mast cells, but other agents such as prostaglandins and leukotrienes have also been implicated. **Angio-oedema** is similar to urticaria, but histologically there is greater swelling of the subcutaneous tissue and mucosal sites are often affected. Ninety-five per cent of cases are idiopathic.

Drugs causing urticaria

- Penicillin
- Salicylates
- Quinidine
- Cephalosporin
- Angiotensin converting enzyme inhibitors
- Hydralazine
- Opiates

Drugs causing a fixed drug eruption

- Tetracyclines
- Barbiturates
- Dapsone
- Chlordiazepoxide
- Phenolphthalein
- Sulphonamides
- Benzodiazepines
- Non-steroidal anti-inflammatory drugs
- Quinine
- Paracetamol

Diseases aggravated by sunlight

- Lupus erythematosus
- Dermatomyositis
- Xeroderma pigmentosum
- Herpes simplex infection
- Porphyrias (except acute intermittent)
- Pellagra
- Carcinoid syndrome

10. SKIN TUMOURS

10.1 Malignant melanoma

This has an incidence of around 10 per 100, 000 per year; and this is doubling every decade. The prognosis is related to tumour thickness. Early lesions are often curable by surgical excision. Any changing mole (bleeding, increase in size, itching, etc) should be viewed suspiciously.

The different types of melanoma are:

- Superficial spreading: this is the most common. An irregularly pigmented macule or plaque which may have an irregular edge and colour variation.
- Nodular: a pigmented nodule, often rapidly growing and aggressive.
- Lentigo maligna melanoma: occurs in the elderly in a long-standing lentigo maligna (a slowly expanding, irregularly pigmented macule).
- Acral lentiginous melanoma: occurs on the palms, soles and nail beds. This is the commonest type of melanoma in Chinese and Japanese people.

10.2 Basal cell carcinoma

These are the commonest skin cancer and are seen most commonly on the face of elderly or middle-aged patients. They only very rarely metastasise. Predisposing factors for basal cell carcinoma are:

- prolonged sun exposure (most common)
- radiation treatment
- chronic scarring
- ingestion of arsenic (tonics)
- basal cell naevus syndrome (Gorlin's syndrome).

Basal cell carcinomas are classified as:

- nodular/cystic
- morphoeic
- pigmented.

10.3 Squamous cell carcinoma

There are several predisposing factors for squamous cell carcinoma:

- **actinic damage**: squamous carcinomas can also develop in just sun-damaged skin (in the absence of actinic keratosis)
- **X-irradiation**
- **chronic scarring or inflammation**
- **smoking (particularly lesions of the lip)**
- **arsenic ingestion**
- **organic hydrocarbons**
- **immunosuppression**
- **human papilloma virus.**

10.4 Other skin tumours

Keratoacanthoma

A rapidly growing tumour arising in sun-exposed skin. This is normally thought of as benign but histologically it is similar to squamous cell carcinoma.

Cutaneous T-cell lymphoma (mycosis fungoides)

A lymphoma that evolves in the skin, usually over a protracted course of many years. The clinical pattern may be varied.

11. HAIR AND NAILS

11.1 Disorders of hair

The first signs of hair follicles appear in the region of the eyebrows, upper lip and chin at about nine weeks' gestation. By 22 weeks the full complement of follicles is established. Hair abnormalities comprise either excessive hair growth or hair loss.

Excessive hair growth can be androgen-independent 'hypertrichosis' or androgen-dependent 'hirsutism'.

Causes of hypertrichosis

- **Congenital/hereditary**
  Congenital hypertrichosis lanuginosa
  Porphyrias
  Epidermolysis bullosa
  Hurler's syndrome
- **Acquired**
  Acquired hypertrichosis lanuginosa
- **Endocrine**
  Hypothyroidism
  Hyperthyroidism
- **Drugs**
  Diazoxide
  Minoxidil
  Ciclosporin
  Streptomycin
- **Other**
  Malnutrition
  Anorexia nervosa

Causes of hirsutism

- **Ovarian**
  Polycystic ovary syndrome
  Ovarian tumours
- **Androgen therapy**
- **Adrenal**
  Congenital adrenal hyperplasia
  Cushing's disease
  Prolactinoma

Loss of hair is called alopecia and can be scarring or non-scarring. Scarring alopecia is loss of hair with destruction of the hair follicles. Non-scarring alopecia is when the hair follicles are preserved. A good example of this is the 'exclamation mark' hair seen in alopecia areata.

Causes of scarring alopecia

- **Hereditary**
  Ichthyosis
- **Bacterial**
  Tuberculosis
  Syphilis
- **Physical injury**
  Burns
  Radiotherapy
- **Fungal**
  Kerion
- **Others**
  Lichen planus
  Lupus erythematosus
  Morphea
  Sarcoidosis
  Cicatricial pemphigoid

Causes of non-scarring alopecia

- **Male pattern/androgenetic alopecia**
  (the most common in men and women)
- **Alopecia areata**
- **Endocrine**
  Hypopituitary state
  Hypothyroidism
  Hyperthyroidism
  Hypoparathyroidism
  Pregnancy
- **Drugs**
  Retinoids
  Anticoagulants
  Antimitotic agents
  Oral contraceptive pill
  Carbimazole
  Thiouracil
  Lithium
- **Iron deficiency**
- **Chronic illness**

Alopecia areata is associated with nail dystrophy, cataracts, vitiligo, autoimmune thyroid disease, pernicious anaemia and Addison's disease.

11.2 Disorders of nails

Nails are derived from keratin. This is a protein complex, which gives the nail its hard property. The nail can be affected in a variety of skin and systemic disorders.

Causes of nail changes associated with skin disorders

- **Psoriasis**: nail changes include onycholysis, nail pitting, hyperkeratosis, pustule and occasional loss of nail.
- **Fungal**: signs include discoloration, onycholysis and thickening of the nail.
- **Bacterial**: usually due to staphylococcal infections. Pseudomonas infections give a green discoloration to the nail.
- **Lichen planus**: nail changes occur in 10% of cases, with thinning of the nail plate and longitudinal linear depressions. Occasionally there is destruction of the nail (pterygium).

- **Alopecia areata**: pitting, thickening and ridging of the nail (sandpaper nail) is seen.
- **Dermatitis**: coarse pits, cross-ridging and onycholysis may be seen.

Causes of nail changes associated with systemic disease

- **Koilonychia**: the nails are thin, brittle and concave. There is an association with iron deficiency anaemia.
- **Yellow nail syndrome**: the nails are yellow and excessively curved. Associations include recurrent pleural effusions, chronic bronchitis, bronchiectasis, nephrotic syndrome and hypothyroidism.
- **Nail–patella syndrome**: loss of ulnar half of the nails, usually the thumbnail, is seen. Associations include small patellae, bony spines over posterior iliac crests, renal abnormalities, over-extension of joints and laxity of the skin.
- **Beau's lines**: these are transverse depressions in the nail due to temporary arrest in growth. They usually occur after a period of illness or infection.
- **Half and half nails**: the proximal nail bed is white and distal, pink or brown. They are associated with chronic renal failure and rheumatoid arthritis.

Causes of onycholysis

- **Idiopathic**: excessive manicuring or wetting.
- **Dermatological disease**: psoriasis, fungal infection, dermatitis.
- **Systemic disease**: impaired peripheral circulation, hypothyroidism, hyperthyroidism.
- **Trauma**.

Chapter 4
Endocrinology

CONTENTS

Endocrinology

1. HORMONE ACTION

There are three main types of hormone:

- amine
- steroid
- peptide.

Knowing which category a particular hormone fits into makes it possible to guess much of its physiology. Thyroxine is an exception to this as shown below.

1.1 Types of hormone

- **Amine**: catecholamines, serotonin, **thyroxine**
- **Steroid**: cortisol, aldosterone, androgens, oestrogens and progestogens and **vitamin D**
- **Peptide**: everything else! (made up of a series of amino-acids).

Thyroxine is chemically an amine but it acts like a steroid. Vitamin D has the structure of a steroid hormone and it acts like one.

Amines/peptides

- Short half-life (minutes)
- Secretion may be pulsatile
- Act on a cell surface receptor
- Often act via a second messenger

Steroids

- Longer biological half-life (hours)
- Act on an intracellular receptor
- Act on DNA to alter gene expression

This information can be used to predict hormone action. For example, aldosterone is a steroid hormone so it must have a biological half-life of several hours, bind to an intracellular receptor and affect gene transcription. Glucagon is not a steroid or an amine so it must be a polypeptide hormone which has a short circulation half-life, acts via a cell-surface receptor and probably utilises a second messenger (cAMP in fact).

1.2 Hormones that act at the cell surface

Peptide and amine hormones act at the cell surface via specific membrane receptors. The signal is transmitted intracellularly by one of three mechanisms:

- via cAMP
- via a rise in intracellular Ca^{2+} levels
- via receptor tyrosine kinases.

If in doubt, assume the action of a peptide or amine hormone (excluding thyroxine) is via cAMP unless it is insulin or has the word 'growth' in its name, in which case it is likely to act via a receptor tyrosine kinase.

Via cAMP	Via Ca^{2+}	Via receptor tyrosine kinases
Adrenaline (α receptors)	GnRH	Insulin
All pituitary hormones except GH, PRL	TRH	GH, PRL
Glucagon	Adrenaline (α receptors)	'Growth factors': IGF-1, EGF
Somatostatin		

cAMP = cyclic adenosine monophosphate; GnRH = Gonadotrophin releasing hormone; GH = Growth hormone; PRL = Prolactin; TRH = Thyrotrophin releasing hormone; IGF-1 = Insulin-like growth factor 1; EGF = Epidermal growth factor

cAMP and G-proteins

Hormone receptors linked to cAMP (eg TSH receptor) typically have seven trans-membrane domains. The receptor does not directly generate cAMP but acts via separate 'G-protein' on the cell surface which, in turn, interact with the cAMP generating enzyme, adenylate cyclase, on the cell surface. (See figure 3 in Chapter 14, Molecular Medicine.)

Hormones that raise the level of cAMP intracellularly (all hormones in this category except somatostatin) act via a stimulatory G-protein, 'G_s'. Hormones that lower the level of cAMP (somatostatin) act via an inhibitory G-protein, 'G_i'.

G-proteins are important in endocrinology because mutations in G_s have been found to be associated with certain diseases:

- **Acromegaly**: 40% of patients with acromegaly have an activating somatic mutation of G_s in their pituitary tumour. As a result, the cells are always 'switched on' and continuously make GH (resulting in acromegaly).

- **McCune–Albright syndrome**: an activating mutation of G_s early in embryonic development causes hyperfunction of one or more endocrine glands, eg gonads (precocious puberty), GH (acromegaly), adrenal gland (Cushing's), thyrotoxicosis or hyperparathyroidism. The syndrome is associated with café-au-lait spots and polyostotic fibrous dysplasia. Because the mutation occurs after the zygote stage, affected individuals are a mosaic and different patterns of tissue involvement may be seen between individuals.
- **Pseudohypoparathyroidism**: inactivating germ-line mutations in G_s result in pseudohypoparathyroidism type 1A **if maternally inherited**, with dysmorphic features (including short 4th or 5th metacarpal) and resistance to a variety of hormones that act via cAMP (including parathyroid hormone, TSH and gonadotrophins). Spontaneously occurring or paternally inherited mutations cause the dysmorphic features alone (**pseudopseudohypoparathyroidism**). The dysmorphic bone features are sometimes referred to as '**Albright's Hereditary Osteodystrophy**' and they can be present in either the maternally or paternally inherited form.

Intracellular Ca^{2+}

Some hormones release intracellular Ca^{2+} as a second messenger (see box on previous page for examples). The receptors for these hormones activate different G proteins (eg G_q) which in turn activate the cytoplasmic enzyme phospholipase C (PLC). PLC releases the small molecule inositol 1,4,5-trisphosphate (IP_3) from membrane phospholipids. IP_3 in turn binds to the IP_3-sensitive receptor on the endoplasmic reticulum within the cell causing Ca^{2+} to be released from stores in the endoplasmic reticulum into the cytoplasm. The Ca^{2+} subsequently affects cell metabolism by binding to the protein calmodulin.

Receptor tyrosine kinases

The insulin, GH, prolactin and growth factor receptors do not use second messengers. The receptors themselves can act as enzymes which phosphorylate ('kinase activity') other proteins when hormone is bound at the cell surface. This is followed by a cascade of proteins phosphorylating other proteins until gene transcription in the nucleus is modulated.

1.3 Hormones that act intracellularly

Steroids, vitamin D and thyroxine are sufficiently lipid soluble that they do not need cell surface receptors but can diffuse directly through the cell membrane. They then bind to receptors in the cytoplasm which results in shedding of heat shock proteins that protect the empty receptor. The hormone–receptor complex migrates into the nucleus where the complex alters the transcription of a large number of genes (see diagram in Chapter 14, Molecular Medicine).

1.4 Hormone resistance syndromes

The following are conditions of hormone resistance with the site of the defect shown.

Receptor defect (hormone involved)	Second messenger defect
Laron dwarfism (GH)	Pseudohypoparathyroidism
Leprechaunism (Donahue syndrome, Rabson–Mendenhall syndrome (insulin))	**Defect unknown**
Nephrogenic DI (antidiuretic hormone (ADH))	Type 2 diabetes
Androgen resistance (testicular feminisation syndrome (testosterone))	
Vitamin-D-dependent rickets type 2 = hereditary vitamin D resistance rickets (vitamin D)*	

* Vitamin-D-dependent rickets type 1 is due to a failure of 1-hydroxylation of vitamin D

2. SPECIFIC HORMONE PHYSIOLOGY

2.1 Hormones in illness

During illness/stress, the body closes all unnecessary systems down 'from the top', eg the thyroid axis closes down by a fall in thyrotrophin releasing hormone (TRH), thyroid-stimulating hormone (TSH) and L-thyroxine/L-thyronine (T_4/T_3). It is orchestrated by the hypothalamus, not by the end organs. Hormones involved in the stress response may rise.

Hormones which fall	May rise (stress hormones)
TSH, T_4/T_3*	GH (though IGF-1 falls)
LH, FSH	ACTH, glucocorticoids
Testosterone, oestrogen	Adrenaline
Insulin (starvation)	Glucagon (starvation)
	Prolactin

* In this case conversion of T_4 to T_3 is inhibited so T_3 falls more than T_4

TSH = Thyroid-stimulating hormone; GH = growth hormone; IGF-1 = insulin-like growth factor 1; LH = luteinising hormone; FSH = follicle-stimulating hormone; ACTH = adrenocorticotrophic hormone; T_3 = L-thyronine; T_4 = L-thyroxine

In starvation alone, without illness, all hormones fall except glucagon. In anorexia nervosa there is also stress: all hormones fall except glucagon, GH and glucocorticoids.

2.2 Hormone changes in obesity and the physiology of leptin

In the absence of other diseases (eg type 2 diabetes) which might develop in obese patients, the following changes are seen in obesity.

- Hyperinsulinaemia
- Increased cortisol turnover but not hypercortisolism
- Increased androgen levels in women
- Reduced GH
- Conversion of androgens to oestrogens
- All bad lipid changes (low HDL, high LDL and triglyceride)

Leptin, adipokines and other hormones involved with appetite and weight

Leptin was identified as a product of the *ob* gene in 1994. *Ob/ob* mice make no leptin owing to a homozygous *ob* gene mutation and are grossly obese.

- Leptin is a polypeptide hormone, released from fat cells, that acts on specific receptors in the hypothalamus to reduce appetite.
- Circulating leptin levels are directly proportional to fat mass, and hence they tell the brain how fat an individual is.
- Leptin appears to have stimulatory effects on metabolic rate and levels fall in starvation (appropriate change for weight homeostasis).
- Adequate leptin levels are required for the onset of puberty.
- Persistently obese individuals appear relatively resistant to leptin.
- Hereditary leptin deficiency (very rare) results in grossly obese children due to a voracious appetite.

Several other hormones have recently been shown to affect appetite and weight:

- **Ghrelin**: this was first identified as a growth hormone releasing hormone. It is released from the stomach when subjects are fasting and triggers hunger. Ghrelin levels fall after gastric by-pass surgery which may help weight loss (by reducing appetite).
- **Peptide YY** (a member of the neuropeptide Y family): released from the small and large bowel. Levels rise after meals and reduce appetite. This may be the main regulator of day-to-day appetite.
- **Glucagon-like-peptide-1** (GLP-1): released from the intestine after meals and powerfully stimulates insulin secretion as well as possibly reducing appetite.
- In the hypothalamus itself, **neuropeptide Y (NPY)** and **Agouti-related protein (AgRP)** increase appetite while **α-MSH** (a melanocortin) reduces appetite.

In addition to leptin a number of other hormones have recently been identified as being released from fat cells. These 'adipokines' include **adiponectin**, which reduces insulin resistance, and **resistin** and **acylation stimulating protein (ASP)**, which both increase insulin resistance. Their role in the association between obesity and insulin resistance remains uncertain.

2.3 Hormones in pregnancy

As a general rule, most hormone levels rise in pregnancy. Insulin resistance develops, causing a rise in circulating insulin levels. Insulin requirements are highest in the last trimester but fall slightly in the last four weeks of pregnancy.

Other key features of hormone metabolism in pregnancy are as follows:

- **Prolactin** levels rise steadily throughout pregnancy and in combination with oestrogen prepare the breast for lactation. Post-partum surges of prolactin and oxytocin are generated by the nipple stimulation of breast-feeding. However, after several weeks prolactin levels fall almost to normal even if breast-feeding continues.
- **LH/FSH** from the pituitary are no longer necessary after conception for continued pregnancy (although the pituitary does double in size) – the placenta takes over.
- **Thyroid axis**. Thyroid binding globulin (TBG) levels rise in the first trimester causing a rise in total T_4 and total T_3. However, human chorionic gonadotrophin (HCG) from the placenta shares its alpha-subunit with TSH and very high levels in the first trimester can cause true mild thyrotoxicosis (not just a binding protein rise), especially associated with hyperemesis gravidarum. Note that T_4 and T_3 do not cross the placenta very efficiently but sufficient T_4 does cross to prevent a fetus with congenital hypothyroidism becoming hypothyroid until after birth.

2.4 Investigations in endocrinology

The plasma level of almost all hormones varies through the day (because of pulsatile secretion, environmental stress or circadian rhythms) and is influenced by the prevailing values of the substrates they control. This makes it hard to define a 'normal range'. For example, insulin values depend on the glucose level, GH levels depend on whether a pulse of GH has just been released or the blood sample is taken in the trough between pulses.

Dynamic testing is therefore frequently used, ie suppression or stimulation tests. The principle is, 'If you think a hormone level may be high, suppress it; if you think it may be low, stimulate it'.

- **Suppression tests** are used to test for hormone EXCESS – eg dexamethasone suppression for Cushing's syndrome, glucose tolerance for GH in acromegaly.
- **Stimulation tests** are used to test for hormone DEFICIENCY – eg synacthen tests for hypoadrenalism, insulin-induced hypoglycaemia for GH deficiency and/or hypoadrenalism.

2.5 Growth hormone

This is secreted in pulses lasting 30–45 minutes separated by periods when secretion is undetectable. The majority of GH pulses occur at night ('children grow at night'). In response to GH pulses, the liver makes insulin-like growth factor-1 (IGF-1, previously called somatomedin C), the plasma level of which is constant and which mediates almost all the actions of GH, ie GH does not act directly. The effective levels of IGF-1 are influenced by changes in the level of its six binding proteins (IGF-BP I–6).

2.6 Prolactin

Prolactin causes galactorrhoea but not gynaecomastia (oestrogen does this). Raised prolactin levels are essentially the only cause of galactorrhoea, although occasionally prolactin levels in the normal range can cause milk production in a sensitised breast. Raised prolactin levels also 'shut down' the gonadal axis 'from the top' (hypothalamic level) resulting in low GnRH, LH and oestrogen/testosterone levels. Surprisingly, prolactin is a stress hormone and levels rise after an epileptic fit.

Prolactin release from the pituitary is under **negative** control by dopamine from the hypothalamus. Oestrogens (the pill, pregnancy) and nipple stimulation raise prolactin.

Prolactin is raised by

- Phenothiazines (*not* tricyclics)*
- Anti-emetics (eg metoclopramide)
- Damage to hypothalamus (eg radiation)
- Pregnancy
- Nipple stimulation
- Damage to pituitary stalk (eg pressure from a pituitary tumour)
- Oestrogens
- Polycystic ovary syndrome

Prolactin is suppressed by

- Bromocriptine (dopamine agonist) and related drugs

* Female psychiatric patients may complain of galactorrhoea – doctors often do not believe them but the patients are right and it is due to the doctor's treatment!

Gynaecomastia

This is due to a decreased androgen:oestrogen ratio in men. Gynaecomastia is unrelated to galactorrhoea (which is always due to prolactin). Breast enlargement is not necessary to make milk.

Causes of gynaecomastia:

- pubertal (normal)
- obesity – not true gynaecomastia
- hypogonadism (eg Klinefelter's, testicular failure)

- cirrhosis, alcohol
- hyperthyroidism
- drugs: including spironolactone, digoxin, oestrogens, cimetidine, anabolic steroids, marijuana
- tumours, including adrenal or testicular making oestrogen; lung, pancreatic, gastric making HCG; hepatomas converting androgens to oestrogens.

2.7 Adrenal steroids

These act intracellularly to alter the transcription of DNA to mRNA (see Section 1, Hormone Action). Surprisingly, the mineralocorticoid (aldosterone) and glucocorticoid receptors have an equal affinity for cortisol. However, the cellular enzyme **11-beta hydroxysteroid dehydrogenase** 'protects' the mineralocorticoid receptor by chemically modifying any cortisol that comes near the receptor to an inactive form while having no effect on aldosterone itself. Inactivating mutations of this enzyme or inhibition of it by liquorice causes 'apparent mineralocorticoid excess' since cortisol (which circulates at much higher concentrations than aldosterone) is able to stimulate the mineralocorticoid receptor.

	Relative glucocorticoid effect	**Relative mineralocorticoid effect**	**Duration of action**
Cortisol = hydrocortisone	1	+	Short
Prednisolone	4	±	Medium
Dexamethasone	30	–	Long
Fludrocortisone	10	+++	

2.8 Thyroid hormone metabolism

More than 95% of thyroid hormones are bound to plasma proteins in the circulation, predominantly thyroid binding globulin (TBG) and thyroid binding prealbumin (TBPA). T_4 (L-thyroxine, four iodine atoms per molecule) has a half-life of seven days (so if a patient is in a confused state it is possible to administer his/her total weekly dose of thyroxine once a week). It is converted partly in the thyroid and partly in the circulation to T_3 (L-thyronine, three iodine atoms per molecule), which is the active form and has a half-life of one day.

There are three deiodinase enzymes that act on thyroid hormones (termed D_1–D_3). D_1 and D_2 promote the generation of active hormone (T_3) by converting T_4 to T_3, (see accompanying figure). D_3 opposes this by promoting conversion of T_4 to rT_3 and destroying T_3 by conversion to T_2 (inactive). The D_1 and D_2 enzymes are inhibited by illness, propranolol, propylthiouracil, amiodarone and ipodate (formerly used as X-ray contrast medium for study of gall bladder disease). This reduces the level of active hormone, T_3, with little change or a rise in T_4. rT_3 levels rise (T_4 spontaneously converts to rT_3 if the monodeiodinase is not available) but rT_3 is *not* detected in laboratory tests of T_3 levels.

Figure 1 Metabolism of thyroid hormones. $D_1 - D_3$ – different deidinase enzymes that act on thyroid hormone

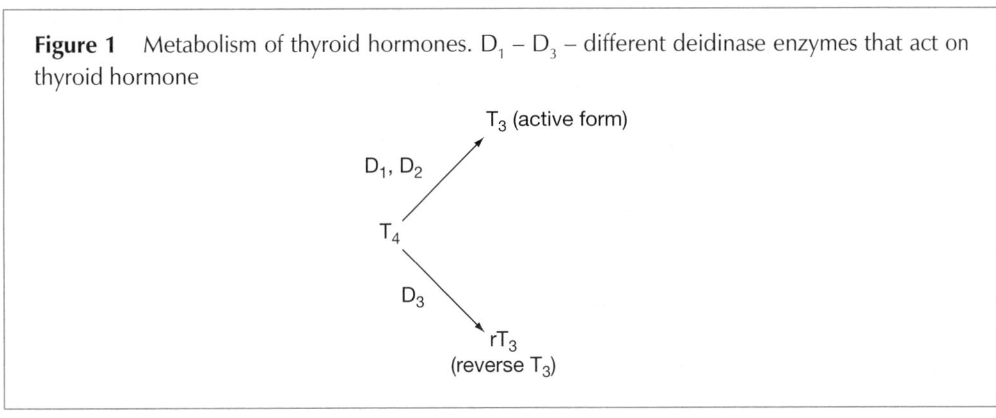

It is said that you should, 'Never measure thyroid function tests on ITU as you will not be able to interpret them'. In illness TSH and free T_3 levels fall ('sick euthyroidism'). The only interpretable finding in sick patients is a raised free T_3 – this would almost definitely indicate thyrotoxicosis.

2.9 Renin–angiotensin–aldosterone

Aldosterone secretion is controlled almost completely by the renin–angiotensin system, not by ACTH. The initial letters of the zones of the adrenal cortex from outside inwards spell 'GFR', like glomerular filtration rate: glomerularis, fasciculata, reticularis. Aldosterone is the 'outsider hormone' and is made on the 'outside' (zona glomerulosa).

Figure 2 The renin–angiotensin system

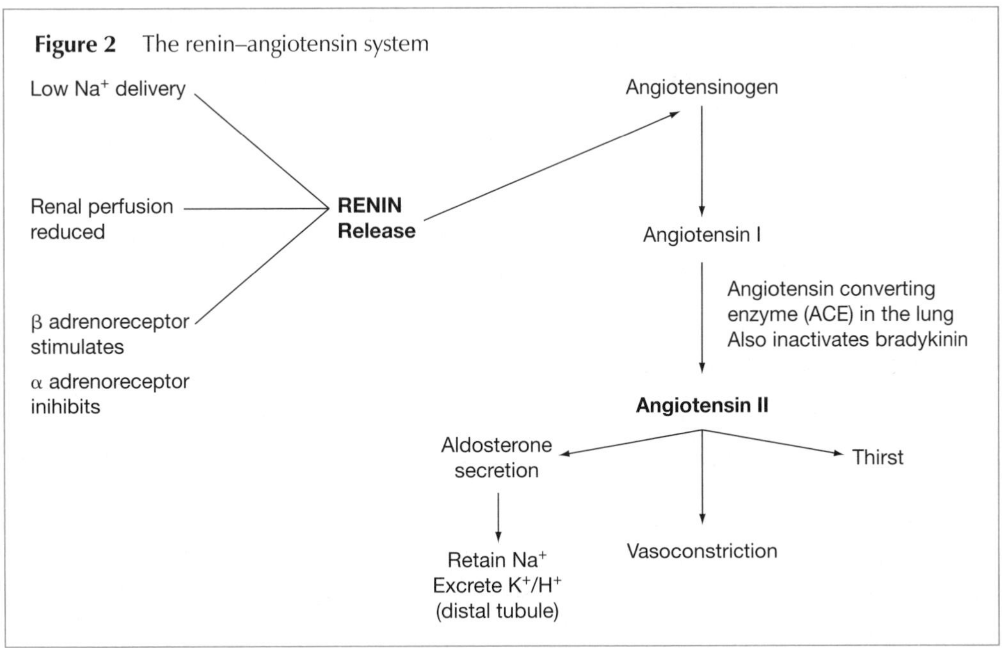

Renin is released from the JGA (juxtaglomerular apparatus) of the kidney in response to low Na^+ delivery or reduced renal perfusion. Renin is an enzyme which converts angiotensinogen to angiotensin I (10 amino acids). ACE (angiotensin converting enzyme) in the lung converts angiotensin I to angiotensin II, which is the active form. ACE also breaks down bradykinin: ACE inhibitors (eg captopril) are believed to cause cough by causing a build up of bradykinin in the lung. The renin–angiotensin system is designed to restore circulating volume. It is therefore activated by hypovolaemia (see above) and its end product, angiotensin II, has three actions which restore volume:

- releasing aldosterone from the adrenal (retains Na^+, excretes K^+ in the distal tubule)
- vasoconstriction (powerful)
- induction of thirst (powerful).

2.10 Calcium, PTH and vitamin D

(*See also* Chapter 13, Metabolic Diseases.)

Plasma calcium is tightly regulated by parathyroid hormone (PTH) and vitamin D, acting on the kidney (PTH), bone (PTH) and the gut (vitamin D).

PTH controls Ca^{2+} levels minute to minute by mobilising Ca^{2+} from bone and inhibiting Ca^{2+} excretion from the kidney. Vitamin D has a more long-term role, predominantly by promoting Ca^{2+} absorption from the gut. Its actions on the kidney and bone are of lesser importance. Ca^{2+} levels are sensed by a specific calcium-sensing receptor on the parathyroid glands. Mutations that reduce the activity of this enzyme result in a resetting of calcium and PTH to higher levels (**familial hypocalciuric hypercalcaemia, FHH**). Activating mutations can also occur which result in a picture almost indistinguishable from hypoparathyroidism, with a low Ca^{2+} (**autosomal dominant hypocalcaemia with hypercalciuria**). It is important to identify these conditions as they run a benign course and only attempted treatment causes problems (eg raising the serum Ca^{2+} in autosomal dominant hypocalcaemia will predispose to renal stone formation).

Precursor vitamin D, obtained from the diet or synthesised by the action of sunlight on the skin, requires activation by two steps:

- 25-hydroxylation in the liver
- 1-hydroxylation in the kidney.

PTH can promote 1-hydroxylation of vitamin D in the kidney, ie it can activate vitamin D thereby indirectly stimulating Ca^{2+} absorption from the gut.

Calcitonin (from the C-cells of the thyroid) behaves almost exactly as a counter-hormone to PTH (secreted by high Ca^{2+}, acts to lower serum Ca^{2+} by inhibiting Ca^{2+} release from bone) but its physiological importance is in doubt (thyroidectomy does not affect Ca^{2+} levels).

2.11 Atrial natriuretic peptide (ANP)

ANP physiology can be predicted from its name.

- **Atrial**: it is synthesised by the myocytes of the right atrium and ventricle.
- **Natriuretic**: it causes a natriuresis (urinary excretion of sodium). It thereby *reduces* circulating volume (opposite of renin–angiotensin). As you would predict therefore, it is secreted in conditions of *hyper*volaemia – via stretch of the right atrial and ventricular walls. It also antagonises the other actions of angiotensin II by causing vasodilatation and reduced thirst/salt craving.
- **Peptide**: it is a peptide hormone (which acts via cAMP).

There are two other natriuretic peptides, B-type and C-type natriuretic peptides (BNP and CNP). BNP is similar to ANP, and is produced from the heart especially in heart failure. Serum levels are more stable than ANP, and BNP is proving to be a useful test of heart failure. CNP is produced by the vascular endothelium rather than by cardiac myocytes.

3. THE PITUITARY GLAND

3.1 Anatomy

The anatomical relations of the pituitary are important as enlarging pituitary tumours may press on surrounding structures.

Figure 3 Schematic sagittal section through the pituitary to show its relation to surrounding structures

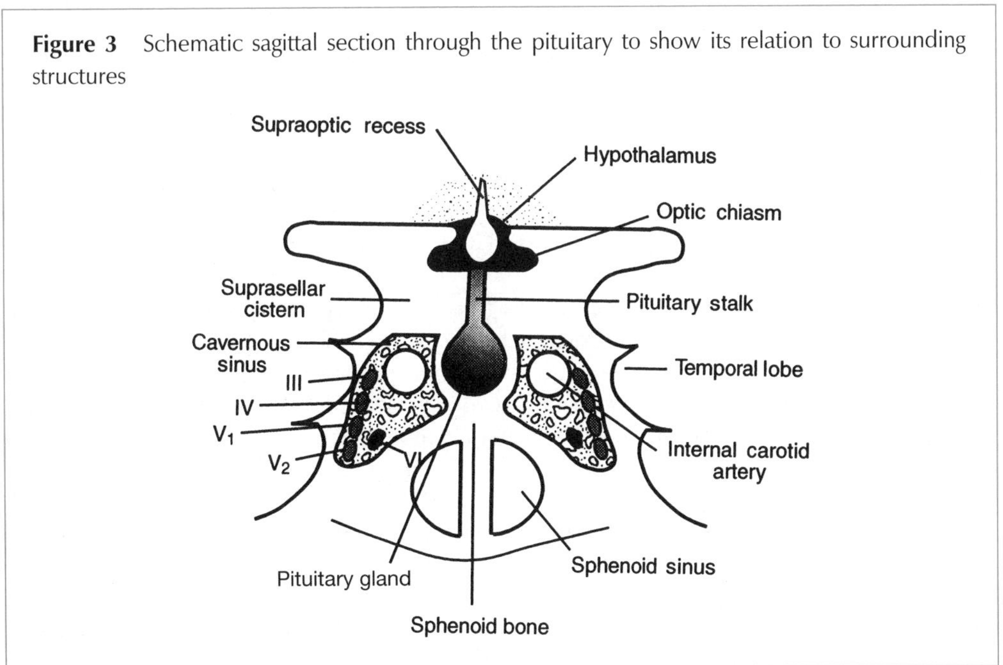

- **Above**: optic chiasm (causing bitemporal hemianopia if compressed), pituitary stalk, hypothalamus, temporal lobes.
- **Below**: sphenoid sinus (in front and below to allow transphenoidal surgery), nasopharynx.
- **Lateral**: cavernous sinus, internal carotid arteries, III, IV, V_1, V_2 and VI cranial nerves.

Expanding pituitary tumours may also compromise remaining anterior pituitary function but very rarely affect posterior pituitary hormones.

3.2 Pituitary tumours

A microadenoma is a pituitary tumour less than 1 cm in size. The size and frequency of pituitary tumours are related.

Pituitary tumours

Large – non-secreting (typically chromophobe)	50% of all tumours
Large – prolactinomas in men	25% of all tumours
Medium – acromegaly (typically 'acidophil', 70% are >1 cm)	12% of all tumours
Small – Cushing's disease (often undetectable on CT/MRI, typically basophil)	5–10% of all tumours
Small – TSH-secreting	1% – very rare

The commonest tumours are small, non-functioning microadenomas which have been reported to occur in up to 20% of people at post-mortem. Note that **prolactinomas** in women are usually picked up at the microadenoma size due to their effects upon menstrual disturbance.

Nelson's syndrome arises after adrenalectomy for pituitary-dependent Cushing's syndrome (Cushing's disease). The small tumour is no longer suppressed by high steroid levels and can become very invasive. Local tumour effects and hyperpigmentation result.

Pituitary apoplexy is sudden enlargement of the pituitary by haemorrhage into a tumour, typically causing the combination of headache, neck stiffness and sudden blindness associated with cardiovascular collapse due to hypopituitarism. Treatment is with steroid replacement and urgent surgery for visual loss (to decompress the optic chiasm). In **pituitary failure** the only two hormones that **must** be replaced for survival are thyroxine and hydrocortisone.

Forty per cent of cases of **acromegaly** (GH tumours) arise because of a G-protein mutation (see Section 1.2).

Craniopharyngiomas are benign tumours that arise from remnants of Rathke's pouch. Two-thirds arise in the hypothalamus itself (suprasellar), one-third in the sella. They are usually cystic, frequently calcify, often recur after aspiration and, although they represent an embryonic remnant, they not infrequently present in adulthood.

3.3 Diabetes insipidus

Antidiuretic hormone (ADH, also called vasopressin or arginine-vasopressin, AVP) is synthesised in the hypothalamus and transported to the posterior pituitary, along with oxytocin, for storage and release. Diabetes insipidus (DI) is caused either by a failure to secrete vasopressin from the posterior pituitary (**central or cranial DI**) or resistance to **the action of vasopressin in the kidney** (nephrogenic DI). To cause **cranial DI**, the hypothalamic nuclei (supraoptic and paraventricular) need to be damaged – it is not sufficient simply to compress the posterior pituitary as vasopressin can be secreted directly from the hypothalamus itself. Pituitary tumours therefore rarely cause DI.

Major causes of cranial diabetes insipidus

- Idiopathic
- Craniopharyngiomas
- Infiltrative processes of the hypothalamus (eg sarcoid, histiocytosis X)
- Trauma
- Pituitary surgery
- Lymphocytic hypophysitis
- Dysgerminomas

Causes of nephrogenic diabetes insipidus

Reduced action of ADH on the kidney may be due to several causes

- **Primary**
  Childhood onset: X-linked/dominant abnormality in tubular ADH receptor
- **Secondary (common)**
  Hypercalcaemia
  Hypokalaemia
  Renal disease (particularly if it involves the medullary interstitium)
  Lithium
  Demeclocycline

Water deprivation test

A water deprivation test is used to identify the cause of polydipsia and/or polyuria. Major metabolic causes should first be excluded (eg hyperglycaemia (diabetes mellitus), hypercalcaemia, hypokalaemia, chronic renal failure). The patient is then deprived of water (from the night before if polyuria is not excessive) and hourly urine and plasma osmolality are measured until 3% of the body weight is lost. The patient is then given an injection of DDAVP (a synthetic analogue of ADH).

Interpretation of the water deprivation test

	Initial plasma osmolality	Final urine osmolality (mosmol/kg)	Urine osmolality post-DDAVP (mosmol/kg)	Final plasma ADH
Normal	Normal	>600	>600	High
Cranial DI	High	<300	>600	Low
Nephrogenic DI	High	<300	<300	High
Primary polydipsia	Low	300–400 (approx.)	400 (approx.)	Moderate
Partial cranial DI	High	300–400	400–600	Relatively low

- **Primary polydipsia (compulsive water drinking)**: in this condition the patient is not dehydrated but water-overloaded in the resting state (Na <140 mmol/l). Chronic polydipsia in this condition can result in washout of the renal medullary concentrating gradient so that even if the patient does become dehydrated, with a rise in ADH, urine cannot be concentrated.
- **Partial cranial DI**: in this condition there is weak ADH production. There is a similar effect upon the renal medullary concentrating gradient to that seen in primary polydipsia, and hence the two conditions may not be differentiated unless a post-hydration serum ADH level is obtained.

3.4 Acromegaly

The common features of acromegaly are well known (hand and foot enlargement, coarse facial features, overbite of the lower jaw, splaying of teeth) but the following also occur:

Features of acromegaly

Diabetes
Sleep apnoea
Multinodular goitre
Hypertension
Twofold increase in death from cardiovascular disease
Enlarged testes
Raised phosphate
Raised triglycerides
Arthropathy – often pseudogout
Carpal tunnel syndrome
Increase in malignancies, especially colonic polyps
Cardiomyopathy
Left ventricular hypertrophy
Renal stones (hypercalciuria)
Raised prolactin, galactorrhoea, menstrual change

Acromegaly is almost always due to a GH-secreting pituitary tumour. Rarely the condition is due to ectopic GH-releasing hormone (GHRH) secretion from a tumour (typically carcinoid) which stimulates the normal pituitary (no discrete tumour seen on MRI scan). Acromegaly is diagnosed by failure of GH to suppress to less than 2 mU/l at any time in a standard 75 g glucose tolerance test (GTT). This may produce a double diagnosis as the GTT may diagnose acromegaly-induced diabetes at the same time.

First-line treatment is **transphenoidal surgery** to the pituitary tumour (or transcranial surgery if there is a large suprasellar extension of tumour). The cure rate (40–70%) depends on the initial tumour size. Alternative therapies are **octreotide** (long-acting analogue of somatostatin), **pituitary radiotherapy** (may take years to take effect and result in hypopituitarism), **pegvisomont** (GH antagonist derived from the GH receptor) or **bromocriptine** (effective in less than 20% of cases). After successful treatment of acromegaly (GH <5 mU/l, IGF-1 in the normal range), most physical features do not regress. Features of active disease are increased sweating and oedema of hands and feet which can regress after therapy.

3.5 Hypopituitarism and growth hormone deficiency in adults

Hypopituitarism

Pan-hypopituitarism can be caused by enlarging pituitary tumours, cranial irradiation (including specific pituitary radiotherapy), pituitary apoplexy, Sheehan's syndrome (infarction following post-partum haemorrhage), and then by any of the conditions which can cause cranial diabetes insipidus (see box on p. 129). Important features include the following:

- Patients present with a soft, smooth 'baby' skin, 'crows' feet' lines around the eyes and possibly features of other specific hormone loss (eg hypotension associated with hypoadrenalism, hypothyroidism).
- Only replacement therapy with steroids and thyroxine is essential for life.
- In suspected hypopituitarism, the steroids should be given first and certainly before thyroid replacement therapy. This is because correction of hypothyroidism will accelerate cortisol metabolism and would precipitate a hypo-adrenal crisis (if thyroxine is given before exogenous steroids).
- If the pituitary is damaged, GH production is lost early so that most patients are growth hormone deficient (see below).
- Despite conventional hormone replacement therapy (thyroxine, glucocorticoid and sex steroids), mortality rates are increased in hypopituitarism owing to either an increase in cardiovascular events or malignancy. The potential for GH therapy to reverse this trend is currently under research.

GH is required for growth in children. It was thought to have little function in adults but recently the following have been ascribed to **adult GH deficiency**:

- reduced muscle, increased fat
- low mood (some patients improve markedly with GH therapy)
- raised lipids
- reduced left ventricular function

- osteoporosis
- impaired endothelial function.

Treatment of adult GH deficiency with daily GH injections is now recommended in patients whose quality of life is shown to improve significantly after a three-month trial of GH therapy.

4. HYPONATRAEMIA AND SIADH

Antidiuretic hormone (ADH or vasopressin) is synthesised in magnocellular neurones in the supraoptic and paraventricular nuclei of the hypothalamus and stored in the posterior pituitary. ADH is released in response to rising plasma osmolality and acts on the distal tubule and renal collecting ducts to increase water permeability. Water is reabsorbed and the urine becomes more concentrated. When the ADH system is working normally, 'the urine should reflect the blood', that is, concentrated urine should occur when the plasma osmolality is high and vice versa.

However, hypovolaemia is also a strong signal for ADH release and in the presence of hypovolaemia ADH will be secreted even if the osmolality is low. This explains the hyponatraemia seen in renal, cardiac and liver failure as well as following excessive sodium loss (eg diarrhoea). Other stimuli can also commonly override control of ADH secretion by osmolarity (see SIADH below).

Syndrome of inappropriate ADH secretion (SIADH)

Many common stimuli override the control of osmolality and cause inappropriate amounts of ADH to be secreted, causing hyponatraemia. Sodium concentration should be high in the urine (excluding hypovolaemia), renal, adrenal and thyroid function should be normal and diuretic therapy needs to be excluded before SIADH is diagnosed. Treatment is by fluid restriction or, if necessary, oral demeclocycline.

Causes of inappropriate secretion of ADH include:

- Nausea
- Fits
- Other CNS/lung insults
- Chlorpropamide
- Head injury
- Tumours making ectopic ADH (eg bronchus)
- Pain
- Pneumonia
- Smoking
- Carbamazepine
- Cerebrovascular accidents (CVAs)

If a tumour is the cause, it is usually obvious: a search for malignancy beyond a chest X-ray is not required in SIADH. Smoking makes you pass less urine (releases ADH), drinking (alcohol) makes you pass more (inhibits ADH secretion).

Causes of hyponatraemia

Hyponatraemia can be divided into three categories.

- 'real' (low serum osmolality)
- pseudohyponatraemia: high triglycerides, high protein (eg myeloma), (normal serum osmolality)
- dilutional: high glucose, ethanol, mannitol.

If hyponatraemia is confirmed to be 'real' (low plasma osmolality, glucose not raised and no suggestion of ethanol or mannitol in blood) then the following clinical and laboratory pointers must be considered:

- careful history for drug use (especially diuretics) and of fluid loss (eg diarrhoea)
- examination for circulatory volume status (oedema, postural hypotension and skin turgor)
- measurement of urinary sodium concentration (see box below).

Hypoadrenalism is the most important diagnosis not to be missed, since untreated it can result in death.

Causes of hyponatraemia

Urine sodium (mmol/l)	Hypovolaemia present	Eu/Hypervolaemia ± oedema
>20	Diuretics	SIADH
	Hypoadrenalism	Hypothyroidism
	Salt-losing nephropathy	Renal failure
<10	Vomiting, diarrhoea	CCF, cirrhosis, nephrotic syndrome
	Loss of other fluid	

5. THE THYROID GLAND

5.1 Hyperthyroidism and hypothyroidism

The common features of hyperthyroidism (eg weight loss, tremor, palpitations) and hypothyroidism (eg weight gain, dry skin, slowing up) are well-known but questions are often asked on the more unusual features. The following are 'recognised' features of the two major thyroid syndromes.

Features of hyper and hypothyroidism

Features	Hyperthyroidism	Hypothyroidism
General	Weight gain (rarely)	Weight gain
	Gynaecomastia	Serous effusions (pleural, pericardial, ascites, joint)
	Occult in elderly	Hair loss
	Hair loss	
Gynae	Amenorrhoea	Menorrhagia
	Raised sex hormone binding globulin (SHBG)	Infertility
GI	Diarrhoea	Constipation
	Raised alkaline phosphatase (derived from liver and bone)	
	Vomiting	
Muscle	Proximal myopathy	Raised creatine kinase
	Periodic paralysis (especially Chinese)	Chest pain (muscular)
		Muscle cramps
CVS	Dyspnoea	Hypercholesterolaemia
	Atrial fibrillation with high stroke rate	Ischaemic heart disease
	High output cardiac failure	
Bone	Osteoporosis	
	Hypercalcaemia	
Neuro	'Apathetic thyrotoxicosis'	Deafness
		Ataxia, confusion, coma
Eyes	Eye signs (see Section 5.5)	Periorbital oedema
Blood	Leukopaenia	Macrocytic anaemia
	Microcytic anaemia	Microcytic if menorrhagia
Skin	Urticaria	Dry, orange (caroteinaemia)

Amenorrhoea is predictable in hyperthyroidism because of associated weight loss. In hypothyroidism, everything slows down except the periods! The menorrhagia can cause a microcytic anaemia in contrast to the more usual macrocytosis. In both conditions there may be subfertility. In the GI tract, the symptoms of hyperthyroidism are almost indistinguishable from those of anxiety. The diarrhoea is actually more like the increased bowel frequency before an examination.

- A patient with hypothyroidism could present in A&E with chest pain and have raised CKs like a myocardial infarct. The chest pain may be muscular, but it may also be myocardial ischaemia – the raised cholesterol of hypothyroidism accelerates atheroma.
- Both hyperthyroidism (if Graves' disease) and hypothyroidism can cause periorbital oedema. See note in Section 5.5 on eye signs in thyrotoxicosis.
- The leukopoenia of thyrotoxicosis often causes confusion: thionamide drugs (eg carbimazole) used as treatment also commonly cause a lymphopenia. Both of these are separate from the agranulocytosis that rarely occurs with thionamide drugs.
- In hyperthyroidism the urticaria due to the disease itself can cause confusion with the maculopapular rash which develops in 10% of patients treated with thionamide drugs.

Side-effects of anti-thyroid drugs (carbimazole, propylthiouracil)

- **Common**
  Rash
  Leukopoenia
- **Rare**
  Agranulocytosis
  Aplastic anaemia
  Hepatitis
  Fever
  Arthralgia
  Vasculitis (propylthiouracil)

(See *also* Chapter 2, Clinical Pharmacology, Toxicology and Poisoning)

5.2 Causes of thyrotoxicosis

The three common causes of thyrotoxicosis are:

- Graves' disease
- toxic multinodular goitre
- toxic (hot) nodule.

In all these conditions all or part of the gland is overactive and the gland takes up a normal or increased amount of radioiodine.

In the following conditions, there is thyrotoxicosis without increased production of new hormone by the thyroid gland itself, ie radioiodine uptake is suppressed:

- excess thyroxine ingestion
- thyroiditis: post-viral (De Quervain's), post-partum or silent thyroiditis

- ectopic thyroid tissue, eg lingual thyroid or ovary (struma ovarii)
- iodine administration: gland is actually still active but cold iodine competes with radioioodine during scanning.

5.3 Thyroid cancer and nodules

Only 5–10% of thyroid nodules are malignant (the rest are adenomas). Thyroid cancer virtually never causes hyperthyroidism so 'hot nodules' can usually be presumed to be benign. In order of increasing malignancy and decreasing frequency the thyroid epithelial cancers are:

- papillary
- follicular
- anaplastic.

Lymphomas occur in Hashimoto's disease. Medullary thyroid cancer is from the C-cells (calcitonin), not from the thyroid epithelium. Serum calcitonin is a tumour marker for this cancer which often occurs in families, sometimes as part of the multiple endocrine neoplasia type 2 syndrome (*see* Section 7).

5.4 Drugs and the thyroid

- **Lithium**
  Inhibits T_4 release from the gland causing hypothyroidism
- **Oestrogens**
  Raised thyroid binding globulin (TBG) and hence 'total' T_4/T_3
- **Frusemide**
  Displaces T_4/T_3 from TBG (reducing total T_4/T_3)
- **Interferon**
  Induces anti-thyroid autoantibodies and hypothyroidism
- **Amiodarone**
  Inhibits T_4 to T_3 conversion, increasing reverse T_3
  High iodine content can cause hyper- or hypothyroidism
- **Aspirin**
  Displaces T_4/T_3 from TBG (reducing total T_4/T_3)
- **Phenytoin**
  Displaces T_4/T_3 from TBG and increases T_4 metabolism

5.5 Autoimmunity and eye signs in thyroid disease

In areas such as the UK where there is no iodine deficiency, more than 90% of spontaneous hypothyroidism is due to autoimmunity. Anti-thyroglobulin autoantibodies are present in 60% of cases and antimicrosomal antibodies (now identified as anti-thyroid peroxidase antibodies) are present in up to 90%. Antibodies that block the TSH receptor may also be present. Similar antibodies are present in Graves' disease but the anti-TSH receptor antibodies are stimulatory, causing the thyrotoxicosis. The term LATS (long-acting thyroid stimulator) referring to this stimulatory antibody is no longer used.

The eye signs in thyroid disease are shown in the box below (*see also* Chapter 17, Ophthalmology). Retro-orbital inflammation and swelling of the extra-ocular muscles is only seen in Graves' disease. The target of the antibody or T-cell reaction causing this inflammation is not known for certain and eye disease activity can occur in the absence of thyrotoxicosis.

Thyrotoxicosis from any cause	Graves' disease only
Lid retraction	Soft tissue signs: periorbital oedema, conjunctival injection, chemosis
Lid lag	Proptosis/exophthalmos
	Diplopia/ophthalmoplegia
	Optic nerve compression causing visual failure

5.6 Thyroid function tests

TSH is the most sensitive measure of thyroid status in patients with an intact pituitary. T_4 and T_3 are over 95% protein bound, predominantly to TBG. The following alter TBG levels and hence total but not free hormone levels.

Conditions which alter thyroid binding globulin (TBG)

- **Raised TBG**
  Pregnancy
  Oestrogen
  Hepatitis
  Congenital TBG abnormality
- **Low TBG**
  Nephrotic syndrome
  Congenital TBG abnormality

6. ADRENAL DISEASE AND HIRSUTISM

6.1 Cushing's syndrome

Cushing's syndrome refers to the sustained over-production of cortisol (hypercortisolism) which causes:

- centripetal obesity with moon face
- 'buffalo hump'
- hirsutism
- recurrent infections
- osteoporosis
- oligomenorrhoea
- hypokalaemia
- striae
- acne
- proximal muscle weakness
- hyperglycaemia
- psychiatric disturbances
- hypertension.

If untreated, death is usually due to infection. Other than due to steroid treatment, Cushing's syndrome is rare. In the first instance, it needs to be distinguished from simple obesity. Once Cushing's syndrome is confirmed, the cause needs to be identified.

The diagnosis is made in two phases.

Tests to confirm hypercortisolism (Cushing's syndrome)

- Loss of diurnal variation (midnight cortisol not lower than morning cortisol)
- Overnight dexamethasone suppression test (1 mg at midnight then 9 am cortisol)
- Low-dose dexamethasone suppression test (0.5 mg qds for 48 hours)
- Urinary free cortisol (24-hour collection).

If one or more of these are positive then one can proceed to localisation. NB: Depression or alcoholism can both cause cortisol over-production ('pseudo-Cushing's'). If these conditions are present, further investigation is very difficult.

Tests to localise the cause of Cushing's syndrome

Possible causes of Cushing's syndrome are:

- adrenal tumour
- pituitary tumour (Cushing's disease)
- ectopic production of ACTH – either from cancer (eg small cell cancer of lung) or from a bronchial adenoma (often very small)
- ectopic production of corticotrophin releasing hormone (CRH) (very rare).

MRI scanning of the adrenal or pituitary alone cannot be relied on to localise the cause. Firstly, the tumours of the pituitary causing Cushing's disease are often too small to see, and secondly, incidental tumours of both the pituitary and adrenal are common and may not be functional. Tests used to identify the causes of Cushing's syndrome are shown in the following box.

Tests used to identify causes of Cushing's syndrome

	Adrenal	Pituitary	Ectopic
ACTH	Suppressed	Mid-range	High
High-dose dexamethasone suppression	No change in cortisol	Suppression of cortisol*	No change
CRH stimulation test	No change	Rise in ACTH and cortisol*	No change
Metyrapone	Rise in 11-deoxycortisol <220-fold	Rise in 11-deoxycortisol >220-fold*	Rise in 11-deoxycortisol <220-fold
Petrosal sinus ACTH**	Equals peripheral level	Higher than peripheral level	Equals peripheral level

* 'Under pressure' (ie at high doses), pituitary adenomas behave like a normal pituitary in dynamic endocrine testing, whereas adrenal or ectopic sources do not. A positive response to high-dose suppression (2 mg qds for 48 hours) is >10% suppression of plasma cortisol or 24-hour-urine free cortisol

** In a petrosal sinus sampling a catheter is placed in the draining sinus of the pituitary gland, via a femoral or jugular venous approach. The ACTH level is compared to that in the peripheral blood before and after CRH injection

- With modern assays, an undetectable ACTH level with confirmed hypercortisolism is sufficient for a diagnosis of an adrenal source.

Nelson's syndrome: bilateral adrenalectomy will cure the hypercortisolism of pituitary-dependent Cushing's syndrome but loss of suppression (provided by the previously high cortisol levels) may allow a pre-existing pituitary adenoma to grow very rapidly, years later causing local damage and generalised pigmentation.

Endocrine causes of obesity

- Steroid excess (Cushing's syndrome)
- Hypothyroidism
- Hypothalamic tumours (hyperphagia)
- Prader–Willi syndrome
- GH deficiency.

6.2 Primary hyperaldosteronism

Primary hyperaldosteronism comprises hypertension, hypokalaemia (80% of cases), hypomagnesaemia and metabolic alkalosis. Patients can, however, have a serum potassium within the normal range. Primary hyperaldosteronism is now thought to account for 1–3% of all cases of hypertension.

- **Symptoms (if present) relate to hypokalaemia**: weakness, muscle cramps, paraesthesiae, polyuria and polydipsia. Patients rarely develop peripheral oedema ('sodium escape' mechanism).
- **Causes**: aldosterone-secreting adenoma (**Conn's syndrome** is almost never caused by a malignancy), idiopathic bilateral adrenal hyperplasia, unilateral hyperplasia (rare).
- **Investigations** (not standardised): the **renin:aldosterone** ratio should be assessed to confirm high aldosterone levels in the presence of low renin. Ideally, the ratio should be assessed after the patient has ceased antihypertensive drugs (β-blockers lower renin and aldosterone levels, spironolactone, diuretics and vasodilators raise renin and aldosterone levels, whereas ACE inhibitors and calcium channel blockers raise renin but lower aldosterone levels, ie they may all lead to a false-negative result). α-blockers (eg doxazosin) have the least effect. However, discontinuing antihypertensive therapy for two to six weeks is often impractical and measurement of the ratio after the patient has been upright (sitting or standing) for two hours (to stimulate renin levels) is now considered to be a useful screening test for primary hyperaldosteronism, even in the presence of one or two drugs. If hyperaldosteronism is confirmed, a CT or MRI scan of the abdomen may identify a unilateral adrenal adenoma. However, the tumours are usually < 2 cm diameter and hence if imaging is negative, adrenal vein sampling may be required in order to distinguish unilateral hypoplasia or a tiny adenoma from idiopathic bilateral hyperplasia.
- **Treatment**: spironolactone or amiloride are often successful treatments when the cause is bilateral hyperplasia. An adenoma or unilateral adrenal hyperplasia may be surgically removed; hypertension may persist if this was previously longstanding.

(*See* Chapter 1, Cardiology, Section 9.3 systemic hypertension. *See also* Chapter 15, Nephrology, Section 3.4 for differential diagnoses of hypokalaemia.)

6.3 Congenital adrenal hyperplasia (CAH)

Two enzyme defects account for 95% of all CAH:

- 21-hydroxylase (90%)
- 11-hydroxylase (5%).

The block caused by these enzyme defects leads to reduced production of cortisol, but increased production of other intermediates in steroid metabolism, including androgenic steroids. 17-Hydroxylase, 3-β-hydroxysteroid dehydrogenase and cholesterol side-chain cleavage enzyme defects are very rare causes of CAH and have differing effects (see the following box).

Features of congenital adrenal hyperplasia

- Autosomal recessive
- Plasma ACTH is high (renin is high if salt-losing)
- Can cause ambiguous genitalia in females (not 17-hydroxylase or side-chain enzyme)
- Can have a minor, late-onset form resembling polycystic ovarian syndrome
- Antenatal steroid therapy to the mother has been used
- Both gene deletions and point mutations can occur
- Can cause male precocious puberty (not 17-hydroxylase or side-chain enzyme)
- Treat with glucocorticoids ± mineralocorticoids at night
- Surgery may be required to correct ambiguous genitalia/ cliteromegaly

It is possible to distinguish between the different enzyme defects in CAH (see following table).

Differentiating features in congenital adrenal hyperplasia

	21-Hydroxylase	11-Hydroxylase	17-Hydroxylase/side-chain enzyme
Frequency	90% cases	5% cases	Very rare
Presentation in female	Virilising, intersex 70% salt-losing*	Virilising hypertension low K^+	Non-virilising (intersex in boys)
Biochemistry	Raised 17-hydroxylase, progesterone	Raised 11-dehydroxycortisol	

* Salt-losing individuals can have Addisonian crises soon after birth

6.4 Hypoadrenalism

In the UK, spontaneous hypoadrenalism is most commonly due to autoimmune destruction of the adrenal glands (Addison's disease – adrenal autoantibodies present in 70% of cases). Vitiligo is present in 10–20% of cases. Other causes include TB, HIV or haemorrhage into the adrenal glands and anterior pituitary disease (secondary hypoadrenalism). Hypoadrenalism after withdrawal of long-standing steroid therapy is similar to secondary hypoadrenalism.

The following are 'recognised' features of hypoadrenalism:

- **Biochemical**: raised urea, hypoglycaemia, hyponatraemia, hyperkalaemia, raised TSH, hypercalcaemia.

- **Haematological**: eosinophilia, lymphocytosis, normocytic anaemia.
- **Clinical features**: weight loss, abdominal pain, psychosis, loss of pubic hair in women, hypotension, auricular cartilage calcification, increased pigmentation.

Hyperkalaemia and increased pigmentation are absent in secondary hypoadrenalism since there are low levels of circulating ACTH and mineralocorticoid continues to be secreted via the renin–angiotensin–aldosterone system. Hypoadrenalism is diagnosed by failure of plasma cortisol to rise above 550 nmol/l at 30 or 60 minutes following IM or IV injection of 250 μg of synthetic ACTH (short SYNACTHEN test).

Acute adrenal failure (Addisonian crisis)

Addisonian crisis presents with hypovolaemia, hyponatraemia, hyperkalaemia (if primary adrenal failure), hypoglycaemia and cardiovascular collapse, which can be fatal. A mildly raised TSH may also be seen even in the absence of thyroid disease. Urgent treatment is necessary and this includes intravenous fluid and electrolyte replacement as well as steroid replacement.

6.5 Polycystic ovarian syndrome (PCOS) and hirsutism

Hirsutism is the increased growth of terminal (dark) hairs in androgen-dependent areas. Virilisation is temporal hair recession (male pattern), breast atrophy, voice change, male physique and (most important) cliteromegaly. Hirsutism and acne are invariably also present.

Causes of hirsutism

Ovarian	Adrenal	Drugs
PCOS (>90% of cases)	CAH (may be late-onset)	Minoxidil
Virilising tumour	Cushing's/adrenal carcinoma	Phenytoin
		Diazoxide
		Ciclosporin
		Androgens

A serum testosterone >4.5 nmol/l (normal <1.8), recent onset of hirsutism and signs of virilisation in women should prompt a search for other causes (eg a tumour). Dehydroepiandrostenedione (DHEA) is a weak androgen produced in the adrenal only.

- Measure the 17-hydroxyprogesterone level after stimulation with ACTH to check for late-onset 21-hydroxylase deficiency (partial enzyme deficiency).
- Other than androgens, the drugs listed strictly cause hypertrichosis, an increase in vellus hair, rather than an increase in androgen-sensitive terminal hairs (see Chapter 3, Dermatology).

Polycystic ovarian syndrome

There is no widely recognised definition and up to 20% of women have a degree of hirsutism. In practice, the three main presenting complaints in PCOS are **hirsutism/acne**, **oligo/amenorrhoea** and **subfertility**. The following are recognised associations of PCOS:

- **Clinical features**: obesity, acanthosis nigricans, oligomenorrhoea, polycystic ovaries, subfertility, hypertension, premature balding in male relatives, hirsutism.
- **Biochemical**: insulin resistance and hyperinsulinaemia, raised testosterone, raised LH/FSH ratio, raised prolactin low HDL.
- **Treatment**: metformin will lower insulin resistance and it has been shown to promote ovulation, improve conception rates and reduce hirsutism.

7. PHAEOCHROMOCYTOMA AND MULTIPLE ENDOCRINE NEOPLASIA (MEN) SYNDROMES

Phaeochromocytomas are rare tumours of the adrenal medulla or ganglia of the sympathetic nervous system. They are the 'tumour of 10%':

- 10% are outside the adrenal glands – paragangliomas (including organ of Zuckerkandl)
- 10% are multiple (eg bilateral)
- 10% are malignant
- 10% are familial.

Diagnosis of phaeochromocytoma is by measurement of urinary catecholamines (this has now replaced measurement of urinary catecholamine metabolites – 3-methoxy-4-hydroxy-mandelic acid (VMAs)). As is the case with most endocrine tumours, the histology is not a reliable guide to the malignant potential in phaeochromocytomas. The diagnosis of malignancy is made by the presence of metastases.

Familial phaeochromocytomas occur in

- Multiple endocrine neoplasia type II (see below)
- Von Hippel–Lindau syndrome (retinal and cerebral haemangioblastomas and renal cystic carcinomas)
- Spontaneously in some families (not associated with a syndrome)
- von Recklinghausen's disease (neurofibromatosis) – 1–2%
- Carney's Triad: gastric leiomyosarcoma, pulmonary chondroma, Leydig testicular tumour

Important features of phaeochromocytomas

- 70% have persistent rather than episodic hypertension
- Extra-adrenal tumours do not make adrenaline (they secrete noradrenaline/dopamine)
- They give characteristically a 'bright' (white) signal on T_2-weighted MRI scan
- Phaeochromocytomas may produce chromogranin A
- The triad of headache, sweating and palpitations is said to be >90% predictive
- Hypotension or postural hypotension may occur particularly if adrenaline is produced
- MIBG (meta-iodobenzylguanidine) scanning may help localisation
- Pre-operative preparation is with alpha adrenergic blockade (eg phenoxybenzamine) *before* beta blockade

Causes of episodic sweating and/or flushing

- Oestrogen/testosterone deficiency (eg menopause, castration)
- Carcinoid syndrome (flushing, diarrhoea, wheeze)
- Phaeochromocytoma (sweat but do not flush)
- Hypoglycaemia (in diabetes)
- Thyrotoxicosis (not usually episodic)
- Systemic mastocytosis (histamine release)
- Allergy.

Multiple endocrine neoplasia (MEN) syndromes are syndromes with multiple benign or malignant endocrine neoplasms. They should not be confused with polyglandular autoimmune syndromes which relate to autoimmune endocrine diseases.

Classification of multiple endocrine neoplasia

	MEN-1	MEN-2A	MEN-2B
Genetics	*menin gene* Chromosome 11	*ret gene* Chromosome 10	*ret gene* Chromosome 10
Tumours	Parathyroid Pituitary Pancreas (Carcinoid) (Adrenal adenomas)	Parathyroid Phaeochromo Medullary thyroid cancer	Parathyroid Phaeochromo Medullary thyroid cancer Marfanoid Mucosal neuromas

- MEN-1 was formerly known as Werner's syndrome. MEN-2A was known as Sipple's syndrome. All MEN syndromes are autosomal dominant. Genetic (DNA-based) screening is being introduced for MEN-2 and may follow for MEN-1. The MEN-2 mutation in *ret* activates the protein. Inactivating mutations of *ret* are seen in Hirschsprung's disease.
- All MEN syndromes can be associated with hypercalcaemia. This is usually due to hyperplasia of all four parathyroids, not a single parathyroid adenoma as with sporadic hyperparathyroidism. Hypercalcaemia is often the first manifestation in MEN-1.
- Gastrinomas and insulinomas are the most common pancreatic tumours in MEN-1. Of the pituitary tumours, prolactinomas are the most common, followed by acromegaly and Cushing's disease.

Medullary thyroid cancer (MTC) is always malignant, secretes calcitonin and is preceded by C-cell hyperplasia. Prophylactic thyroidectomy in patients with confirmed MEN-2 should be performed to prevent this most serious manifestation. Medullary thyroid cancer in MEN-2 is less aggressive than sporadic MTC.

8. PUBERTY/GROWTH/INTERSEX

8.1 Normal puberty

In 95% of children, puberty begins between the ages of 8 and 13 in females and between 9 and 14 in males. The mean age of menarche is 12.8 years. The events of puberty occur in a particular order, although the later stages then overlap with the earlier ones.

Order of events in normal puberty (Earliest events listed first)

- **Male**
  Scrotal thickening (age 9–14)
  Testicular enlargement (>2 ml)
  Pubic hair
  Phallus growth
  Growth spurt (age 10–16)
  + increasing bone age
- **Female**
  Breast development (age 8–13)
  Growth spurt
  Pubic hair
  Menstruation (age 10–16)
  + increasing bone age

8.2 Precocious puberty

True precocious puberty is rare. It is diagnosed if multiple signs of puberty develop before age 8 in females and age 9 in males accompanied by increased growth rate, accelerated bone age and raised sex steroid levels. Isolated premature breast development (thelarche) or the appearance of pubic hair alone (from adrenal androgens – adrenarche) are both benign conditions if no other stages of puberty are entered.

Causes of precocious puberty

- **True 'central' gonadotrophin-dependent precocious puberty**
  Idiopathic
  Other CNS disease
  (eg hydrocephalus, encephalitis, trauma)
  CNS hamartoma (eg pineal)
- **Other causes (gonadotrophin-independent)**
  Adrenal, ovarian tumour
  CAH (males)
  Testotoxicosis (males)
  Exogenous oestrogen (females)
  McCune–Albright syndrome
  Follicular cysts (females)
  Profound hypothyroidism

McCune–Albright syndrome is more common in girls (*see* Section 1.2 on activating G-protein mutations).

8.3 Delayed puberty/short stature

Short stature in children is often due to delayed puberty and hence the two problems are usually grouped together. Three per cent of children are 'statistically delayed', ie for girls no breast development by age 13 or menses by age 15 and for boys no testicular enlargement by age 14. The majority will have 'constitutional delay' and will later enter puberty spontaneously. However, there is no endocrine test that can reliably distinguish constitutional delay from other organic causes of delayed puberty.

In investigation, systemic diseases or syndromes that can cause delayed puberty should be excluded before considering pituitary testing. A karyotype (for Turner's syndrome) should always be requested in girls (see following text).

Causes of delayed puberty/short stature

General causes	Occult systemic disease
Overt systemic disease	Renal failure/renal tubular acidosis
Social deprivation	Crohn's /coeliac disease
Anorexia, excess exercise	Hypothyroidism
Chemotherapy/gonadal irradiation	Asthma
Cranial irradiation	Anterior pituitary disease
	Hyperprolactinaemia
	Isolated GH deficiency

Syndromes causing delayed puberty/short stature	Syndromes causing delayed puberty but normal stature
Turner's (XO)	Androgen insensitivity (testicular feminisation – XY female)
Noonan's ('Male Turner')	Polycystic ovarian syndrome (delayed menarche only)
Prader-Willi	Kallman's (XY) anosmia
	Klinefelter's (XXY) – males

In Turner's syndrome, Noonan's syndrome, androgen insensitivity and Klinefelter's syndrome raised LH and FSH are present. **Kallman's syndrome** is due to failure of GnRH-secreting neurones to migrate to the hypothalamus. LH and FSH levels, as well as sex steroids, are low and patients typically have associated anosmia. More than one gene mutation can cause the syndrome; the X-linked locus (*KAL-1* also known as *anosmin-1*) has been cloned. There is no biochemical test that can currently distinguish Kallman's syndrome from constitutional delay of puberty, and hence a clinical diagnosis is made when delayed puberty is associated with anosmia.

Turner's syndrome (XO) (*see* Chapter 7, Genetics) occurs in 1 in 2500 live births. The typical features (abnormal nails, neonatal lymphoedema, web neck, widely spaced nipples, wide carrying angle) may be absent. A karyotype should always be requested in girls with short stature/delayed puberty since the final height can be increased by early treatment with high doses of growth hormone. Other important complications which may occur in Turner's syndrome include aortic root dilatation (often the cause of death) or coarctation, renal abnormalities, abnormal liver function tests and deafness. Women with Turner's syndrome are generally infertile but in some cases who have relatively minor X deletions and/or chimaerism with cells of a normal karyotype, both menstruation and pregnancy can occur.

Klinefelter's syndrome (XXY) (*see* Chapter 7, Genetics) occurs in 1 in 1000 live births (by meiotic non-disjunction) but is usually undiagnosed until adulthood. Testosterone production is around 50% of normal, but is sufficient to allow secondary sexual characteristics and normal height to develop. Patients usually come to attention because of small testes, gynaecomastia or infertility.

8.4 Intersex

(*See also* Chapter 7, Genetics.) Ambiguous genitalia at birth require urgent diagnosis with steroid profile and karyotype to assign the appropriate sex of rearing and identify the risk of a salt-losing crisis (CAH). Causes can be grouped as follows:

Causes of intersex

Virilised female (XX)	Non-masculinised male (XY)
CAH (21-OH or 11-OH)	Unusual CAH (17-hydroxylase/side-chain/3-beta-OH)
Maternal androgen ingestion	Androgen resistance: receptor defect ('testicular feminisation') 5-alpha-reductase deficiency

Mothers who have a virilised daughter with CAH can be treated antenatally with steroids in subsequent pregnancies in order to suppress androgen production by the fetus. Steroids are continued until the sex of the baby can be established by chorionic villous sampling.

9. DIABETES MELLITUS

Diabetes may be defined as chronic hyperglycaemia at levels sufficient to cause microvascular complications:

- 85% of cases are due to insulin resistance of unknown origin (type 2, maturity-onset, non-insulin dependent)
- 10% of cases are due to autoimmune destruction of the pancreatic islets causing insulin deficiency (type 1, juvenile-onset, insulin-dependent)
- around 5% of cases are due to miscellaneous secondary causes (*see* Section 9.3).

9.1 Risk factors and clinical features of type 1 and type 2 diabetes mellitus

The following table summarises the differences between type 1 and type 2 diabetes mellitus. Note that type 2 diabetes mellitus is more common in non-Caucasian races and that despite being 'late-onset', it is more strongly inherited than the juvenile-onset form.

In addition to insulin resistance, there is relative failure of the beta cells in type 2 diabetes: they are unable to maintain the very high insulin levels required.

Comparison between type 1 and type 2 diabetes mellitus

	Type 1	Type 2
Genetics	Both parents affected: 10–20% risk for child	Both parents affected: 70–100% risk for child
	Identical twins: 50% concordance	Identical twins: up to 90% concordance
	Caucasians	Asian, Black, Pima Indians, other indigenous peoples
	Increased risk: HLA DR3/4, DQ8, CTLA-4	No HLA association
	Protective: HLA-DR2, DQasp57	Increased risk alleles: potassium channel subunit KCNJ11
Autoantibodies	60-90% Islet Cell Ab (ICA) positive at diagnosis	No association with antibodies
	70–90% positive for anti-GAD and/or anti-IA2 antibodies Abs*	
	35% risk of diabetes in 5 years if ICA-positive	
	3% of sibs ICA-positive	
Other risk factors		Impaired glucose tolerance
		Gestational diabetes (50% diabetic in 10 years)
Incidence	Approx 1/10,000 per year	Approx 1–2/1000 per year
Prevalence	Approx 1/1000	Approx 2–3/100

continued overleaf

Comparison between type 1 and type 2 diabetes mellitus *(continued)*

	Type 1	Type 2
Clinical features (at diagnosis and pathology)	Age <40	Age>40 (except MODY – see below) often asymptomatic
	Weight loss	Overweight
	Ketosis prone	Ketone negative
	Insulin-deficient	Insulin-resistant
	Autoimmune aetiology (associated with other autoimmune disorders)	Acanthosis nigricans
		Associated with 'syndrome X': (hypertension, IHD, hyperinsulinaemia, glucose intolerance)
		Amyloid deposition in islet

*GAD = glutamic acid decarboxylase; IA2 = Islet-associated antigen 2 (a protein tyrophosphatase). These are both proteins largely confined to the islet

Rule of 10s (approximate)

- Incidence of type 1 – 0.01%
- Prevalence of type 1 = incidence of type 2 – 0.1%
- Prevalence of type 2 (10 times type 1) – 1% (actually closer to 2–3%).

Maturity-onset diabetes of the young (MODY) is the term used to describe type 2 diabetes occurring in patients under the age of 25 with a strong family history. Single gene defects with an autosomal dominant mode of inheritance have been found in the majority of cases (see following table).

Classification of MODY disorders

Gene	% of MODY cases	Classification
Glucokinase	20	MODY 2 – 'mild'; complications are rare
HNF-1α	60	MODY 3 – diagnosed later (around 35 years of age) Progressive beta cell failure but very sensitive to sulphonylureas
HNF-4α	1	MODY 1
HNF-1β	1	MODY 5
IPF-1	1	MODY 4
Unknown	15	'MODY X'
SUR1	< 1%??	Hyperinsulinism in infancy and beta cell failure in adulthood

9.2 Diagnostic criteria for diabetes

This remains a controversial area. The key criterion is a plasma glucose of >11.1 mmol/l two hours after 75 g of glucose, but this is an inconvenient test to perform in routine practice. The original 1985 WHO definition equated this to a fasting level of >7.8 mmol/l; but this was later improved to 7.0 mmol/l, a fasting figure that was used to replace the glucose tolerance test (GTT) in the new American Diabetes Association (ADA) 1997 criteria. However, some individuals can have fasting glucose levels as low as 5.8 mmol/l and yet are diabetic as their two-hour GTT level is >11.1 mmol/l. It is therefore recommended that a GTT be performed when the fasting glucose is between 6.0 and 7.0 mmol/l.

ADA 1997 diagnosis of diabetes*

*Values are based on venous plasma. Glucose values are lower with capillary samples or whole blood.

- **With symptoms**: fasting glucose >7.0 mmol/l or random glucose >11.1 mmol/l or a glucose of >11.1 mmol/l two hours after 75 g GTT (GTT to be performed when fasting glucose 6 mmol/l and, if diabetes suspected, when random blood glucose is >11.1 mmol/l).
- **Without symptoms**: either fasting glucose >7 mmol/l or random glucose >11.1 mmol/l, present on two occasions.
- **Impaired glucose tolerance**: two-hour GTT glucose 7.8–11.1 mmol/l.
- **Impaired fasting glucose**: fasting glucose >6.0 but <7.0 mmol/l (approximately equivalent to impaired glucose tolerance, above).

In impaired glucose tolerance (IGT) glucose levels are insufficient to cause microvascular complications but there is still an increased macrovascular risk (see p. 154). Twenty per cent or more of individuals with IGT will progress to type 2 diabetes within 10 years.

Note that most people with normal glucose tolerance will have fasting glucose <6.0 mmol/l.

9.3 Secondary diabetes

A variety of conditions can lead secondarily to chronic hyperglycaemia fulfilling the criteria of diabetes either by reducing insulin secretion (type 1-like) or by increasing insulin resistance (type 2-like). A pigmented rash in the axillae, neck and groin (acanthosis nigricans) is seen in many conditions associated with insulin resistance.

Causes of secondary diabetes

- **Insulin deficiency**
  Pancreatitis
  Haemochromatosis
  Pancreatic cancer/surgery
  Cystic fibrosis
  Somatostatin
- **Insulin resistance**
  Polycystic ovarian syndrome
  Cushing's, steroid use
  Acromegaly
  Glucagonoma
  Phaeochromocytoma
  Insulin-*receptor* (see Section 1.4) or signalling defect
  Anti-insulin *receptor* antibodies
  Partial lipodystrophy

9.4 Treatment of type 2 diabetes mellitus

Five categories of drug are used to lower glucose levels in type 2 diabetes mellitus. A gradual decline in insulin reserve leads to an increasing requirement for medication over time and around 30% of type 2 diabetes patients ultimately require insulin therapy to achieve satisfactory glycaemic targets. **Weight loss** (diet and exercise, orlistat and other weight loss drugs), **antihypertensive agents** and drugs to **reduce cardiovascular risk** (aspirin, statins, and other lipid-lowering drugs) are also equally important in the management of type 2 diabetes mellitus.

Drugs used in treatment of type 2 diabetes mellitus

Drug	Action/comments
Sulphonylureas	Increase insulin secretion
Biguanides (eg metformin)	Reduce insulin resistance (less hepatic glucose production) Do not cause hypoglycaemia but risk of lactic acidosis
Alpha-glucosidase inhibitor (acarbose)	Slows carbohydrate absorption, not complicated by hypoglycaemia
Glitazones (eg rosiglitazone and pioglitazone). Troglitazone has been withdrawn in the UK because of cases of liver failure	Activate intracellular peroxisome proliferator activated receptors (PPAR-gamma) so reducing insulin resistance
Insulin	Often used in combination with other drugs (eg metformin). Leads to weight gain

Insulin analogues: these have now been introduced for the treatment of both type 1 and type 2 diabetes mellitus. Examples are lispro (a lysine to proline substitution) and insulin-aspart (an asparagine substitution) both of which are designed to replace soluble (regular) insulin. They have an ultra-fast absorption and elimination so reducing late hypoglycaemia. Newer intermediate-acting insulin analogues have also been developed with a smoother 24-hour profile ('peakless') and these include insulin glargine (which is soluble in the vial at pH 4 but precipitates under the skin at pH 7) and insulin detemir (whose action is prolonged by binding to albumin due to a fatty acid side-chain). These analogues also reduce the likelihood of hypoglycaemia.

9.5 Glycated haemoglobin (HbA1, HbA1c)

Red cell haemoglobin is non-enzymically glycated at a low rate according to the prevailing level of glucose. The percentage of glycated haemoglobin provides an accurate estimate of mean glucose levels over the preceding six weeks and correlates well with the risk of microvascular complications. HbA1c is a more specific fraction of glycosylated haemoglobin than HbA1 and values are 1–2% lower. Optimal control equates to an HbA1c of 7% in most assays. Modern assays for glycated haemoglobin are rarely misleading but the following conditions should be considered if the results do not correlate with home glucose monitoring results.

Abnormally low HbA1c	**Abnormally high HbA1c**
Haemolysis	Persistent HbF (fetal haemoglobin)
Increased red cell turnover	Thalassaemia
Blood loss	Uraemia (carbamylated Hb)
HbS or HbC	

9.6 Microvascular and macrovascular complications of diabetes

Long-term diabetic complications are due to vascular damage. Damage to the microvasculature and its consequences (see box below) correlate well with levels of glycaemic control and can be delayed or prevented by maintaining near-normal glucose levels. Microvascular complications take a minimum of five years to develop even with poor glycaemic control. However, they may be apparently present 'at diagnosis' in type 2 diabetes as hyperglycaemia has often been present for many years prior to diagnosis. Neuropathy (70–90%) and retinopathy (90%) occur in virtually all patients if control is not perfect and diabetes is present for long enough. Thirty to forty per cent of patients will develop diabetic nephropathy, usually within 20 years of onset of the diabetes (*see* Chapter 15, Nephrology, Section 12.4).

The incidence of microvascular complications was reduced by around 50% in the 'Diabetes Control and Complications Trial' (DCCT) by tight glycaemic control.

In contrast, macrovascular disease, which is responsible for most of the increased mortality in diabetes, does not appear to be related to the level of glycaemic control. However, the increased risk of macrovascular disease in diabetes is at least partly explained by a combination of higher blood pressure, lower HDL and higher triglyceride levels, although absolute cholesterol levels are not raised. Macrovascular complications are markedly reduced by hypertension treatment (which also reduces microvascular complications) and treatment of dyslipidaemia. Proteinuria is a strong risk factor for ischaemic heart disease in diabetes, presumably as it is a marker for endothelial dysfunction.

Micro- and macrovascular complications of diabetes

Microvascular	**Macrovascular**
Retinopathy (90%)*	Ischaemic heart disease (accounts for up to 70% of deaths in diabetes)
Neuropathy (70–90%)*	Peripheral vascular disease
Nephropathy (30–40%)*	CVA, hypertension
HbA1c dependent	HbA1c independent
	(Also present in IGT)

* Approximate percentages of diabetics who will have this complication to some degree during their lifetime (data from retrospective studies)

9.7 Autonomic neuropathy

Autonomic complications of diabetes mellitus occur in very long-standing disease and include the following:

Manifestations of diabetic autonomic neuropathy

- Postural hypotension
- Gustatory sweating
- Cardiac arrhythmia ('dead-in-bed')
- Gastroparesis
- Generalised sweating
- Diarrhoea
- Reduced appreciation of cardiac pain

10. HYPOGLYCAEMIA

10.1 Hypoglycaemia in diabetes mellitus

Hypoglycaemia can occur in diabetic patients taking either insulin or sulphonylurea drugs. Autonomic symptoms (sweating, tremor) appear when the blood glucose is <3.5 mmol/l and cerebral function becomes progressively impaired at glucose levels <2.5 mmol/l. In patients on insulin, failure of the normal counter-regulatory responses (sympathetic nervous system activation, adrenaline and glucagon release) may develop in long-standing insulin-treated diabetes, particularly in the presence of frequent hypoglycaemic episodes. This results in **hypoglycaemia unawareness**. The patient has no warning of impending neurological impairment and cannot take appropriate action (glucose ingestion). More frequent hypoglycaemic episodes result, exacerbating the problem – 'hypos beget hypos'. Hypoglycaemia awareness can be restored by relaxing control to allow a prolonged (3-month) hypoglycaemia-free period. There is no proof that hypoglycaemia unawareness is more common with human as compared with animal insulin.

10.2 Hypoglycaemia unrelated to diabetes

True hypoglycaemic episodes unrelated to diabetes therapy are rare. A blood sugar of 2.5 mmol/l or less should be documented, associated with appropriate symptoms which resolve after treatment (eg food – 'Whipples' triad'). A supervised 72-hour fast can be used to precipitate and document an episode, particularly to diagnose an insulinoma.

Causes of hypoglycaemia

- **Fasting**
  Insulinoma*
  Tumour (IGF-2)
  Hypoadrenalism
  Alcohol
  Severe liver failure
  Factitious (insulin or sulphonylurea)*
  Drugs (pentamidine, quinidine)
  Anti-insulin antibodies (delayed post-prandial release of insulins)*
- **Post-prandial**
  Post-gastrectomy
  Idiopathic (rare)

* Associated with detectable insulin levels and low β-hydroxybutyrate levels at the time of hypoglycaemia.

Chapter 5
Epidemiology

CONTENTS

Epidemiology

1. COMPARING DISEASE RATES

In clinical textbooks, the term 'epidemiology' is commonly used to describe which groups of people are most likely to present with a specific disease. This usage of the word 'epidemiology' hints at one of epidemiology's defining characteristics: the comparison of disease rates between different groups of people. As well as providing a general guide to clinical practice, comparing disease rates between different groups of people can:

- suggest **causes** of a disease (the usual goal of observational epidemiological studies, such as cohort studies and case control studies)
- identify effective **treatments** of a disease (the usual goal of experimental epidemiological studies, ie randomised trials).

A fundamental strategy of epidemiological research is to investigate **associations** between **variables** in large populations, while taking proper account of extraneous factors.

1.1 Variables

Five key types of variable are important in comparing disease rates between different groups of people:

- exposure variables (**exposures**)
- outcome variables (**outcomes**)
- confounding variables (**confounders**)
- intermediate variables (**intermediate factors**)
- risk-modifying variables (**effect modifiers**).

Exposure

An exposure is the variable that is used to define the comparison groups. It is often a risk factor for, or a cause or a treatment of, the outcome. For example, in an observational study of the causes of high blood pressure, possible exposures of interest could include salt intake or physical activity; whilst in a randomised trial of blood pressure lowering, the exposure would be the intervention intended to lower blood pressure.

Outcome

The outcome is the disease (or other health-related endpoint) under investigation. Assuming all else is equal, if the exposure causes the outcome then outcome occurrence can be expected to vary between exposure groups. Measures of outcome occurrence include:

- **Incidence rate**: the number of new cases divided by the total person-years at risk of becoming a case (where the person-years is the number of people multiplied by the average number of years of follow-up).
- **Incidence proportion** (or '**average risk**'): the proportion of people who became new cases during a specified period of follow-up.
- **Survival time**: for each person, the length of time from the start of follow-up until the person became a case or, if they did not become a case, until the end of follow-up.
- **Prevalence**: the proportion of people in a given population, at a given point in time, who had the disease. (Prevalence can provide useful information for clinical practice and public health planning, but it is less useful for indicating the effects of an exposure, as it is determined not only by the incidence of new cases, but also by how long people have the disease before they either die or recover.)

Confounders

A confounder is an extraneous variable whose own effects on the outcome are mixed in with those of the exposure. To be a confounder, a variable must be related independently to both the exposure and the outcome, while not being an intermediate factor that causally links the two. For example, any attempt to estimate the relationship between alcohol intake (as an exposure) and lung cancer (as an outcome) will be susceptible to confounding by smoking, because smoking is related both to alcohol intake (smoking and heavier drinking tend to go together) and – causally, as it happens – to lung cancer, while not being an intermediate factor that somehow causally links alcohol intake with lung cancer.

Intermediate factors

As with confounders, intermediate factors are related to both the exposure and the outcome, but, in contrast to confounders, they are simultaneously effects of the exposure *and* causes of the outcome. To take a common example, higher blood pressure is an intermediate factor in the relationship between obesity and coronary heart disease.

Effect modifiers

An effect modifier is a variable that can be used to define two or more categories in which the strength of the relationship between the exposure and the outcome differs. The presence of effect modification is sometimes called statistical interaction. For example, if the relationship between the exposure and the outcome is stronger at one age than another, then the relationship is said to be modified by age, or alternatively, that there is an interaction between age and the exposure. Quite commonly, relationships are stronger* in middle age than old age. For example, this is true for blood pressure and blood total cholesterol in relation to coronary heart disease and stroke.

*When indicated by relative risks (the opposite may apply with absolute risk).

Figure 1 Relationships between key types of epidemiological variable

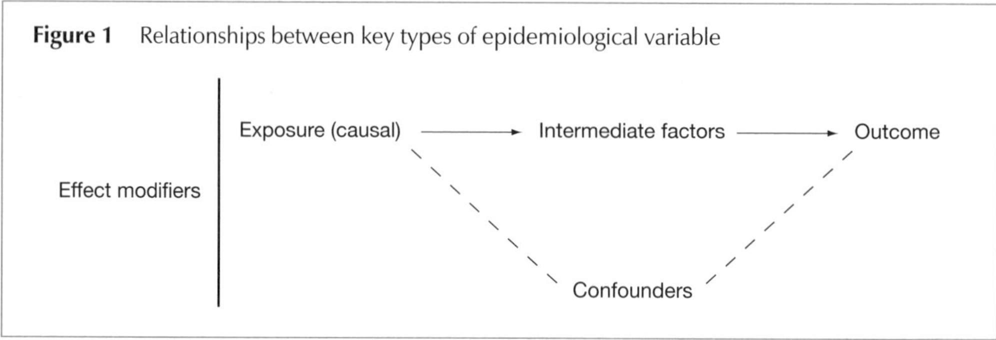

1.2 Associations

Investigating associations (termed 'relationships' above) between exposures and outcomes is a cornerstone of epidemiology. An exposure is said to be associated with the outcome if the outcome occurs more frequently in one exposure group than another, and the difference is greater than would reasonably be expected by the play of chance alone. Associations often need to be controlled for **confounding** (otherwise the effects of extraneous variables might remain mixed in with the estimated effects of the exposure), but they should not be controlled for intermediate factors (otherwise some or all of the effects of the exposure will be masked).

Measures of association compare outcome occurrence in different exposure groups. These measures fall into two categories: relative risks (which are ratios) and absolute risks (which are differences).

Relative risks

Commonly used measures of relative risk include:

- **Incidence rate ratio**: the ratio of incidence rates in different exposure groups; this ratio is often considered the basic building block of aetiological epidemiology.
- **Risk ratio**: the ratio of the average risk (incidence proportion) in different exposure groups; this ratio is nearly always a good approximation to the incidence rate ratio.
- **Hazard ratio**: the usual measure of relative risk in a study with information on survival time; this ratio is potentially even more informative than the incidence rate ratio.
- **Odds ratio**: the ratio of the odds of exposure in the cases to the odds of exposure in the controls; in a case control study, this is usually a reasonable approximation to the incidence rate ratio if the control selection was appropriate. (The odds of an event is the ratio of its probability to one minus its probability; eg if the probability is 0.20, then the odds will be 0.25).

Relative risks provide a better measure of the 'aetiological force' of an exposure than do absolute risks; they therefore also tend to be more generalisable between populations.

Example

During a specified period of time, people with a body mass index (BMI) of 30 kg/m^2 or more are on average twice as likely to develop coronary heart disease as people with a BMI of 20–24 kg/m^2: the relative risk of coronary heart disease in the more obese group, compared with the leaner group, is therefore about 2. If obesity were a weaker cause of coronary heart disease, then the relative risk would tend to be less extreme, and if it was not a cause at all, then the real relative risk would be 1.

Absolute risks

The main measures of absolute risk are:

- **Rate difference**: the difference between the incidence rates in different exposure groups.
- **Risk difference**: the difference between the average risks (incidence proportions) in different exposure groups.

Absolute risks generally give a better estimate of the public health and clinical burden of disease associated with an exposure than do relative risks.

Example

Again comparing people with a BMI of 30 kg/m^2 or more to people with a BMI of 20–24 kg/m^2, if in a western European population the annual incidence rate of coronary heart disease was 100 per 10, 000 people in the more obese group and 50 per 10, 000 people in the leaner group, while in an eastern Asian population it was 10 and 5 per 10, 000 people in these two groups, respectively, then while the relative risk would still be 2 in both populations, the annual absolute risk would be 50 per 10, 000 people in the European population but only 5 per 10, 000 people in the Asian population. Thus while obesity would be as strong a *cause* of coronary heart disease in the two populations (as indicated by the relative risks), the importance of the association to *population health* would be much greater in the European population (as indicated by the absolute risks).

1.3 Causation

The existence of an association between an exposure and an outcome does not imply that the exposure necessarily caused the outcome. Other mechanisms that can account for an observed association include:

- **Chance**: even if the association is greater than 'would reasonably be expected by the play of chance alone', chance can occasionally be unreasonable.
- **Bias**: measurement error or misclassification (of exposures, outcomes or confounders) – note that random errors in exposure measurement tend to attenuate associations (this is sometimes called regression dilution bias, eg blood pressure in relation to vascular risk – see Section 2.2 on cohort studies page 168); selection biases (eg inappropriate control selection in a case control study, or losses to follow-up in a cohort study); and confounding.

- **Statistical artefact**: these may result from violation of assumptions involved in statistical modelling (eg if in a multiple linear regression model, the level of the outcome does not vary linearly with the level of the exposure).
- **Reverse causation**: the outcome causing the exposure (eg in a study of the association between BMI and ovarian cancer, an inverse association might be accounted for by the tendency of ovarian cancer itself to cause weight loss).

Factors that lend support to the interpretation that an exposure caused the outcome are:

- **Random** allocation to the exposure (ie the study is a randomised trial).
- A **stronger** association (ie a more extreme relative risk).
- A **dose response** association (ie outcome occurrence either only increases, or only decreases, as exposure levels increase; this might be indicated by a *p*-value for trend).
- **Low plausibility** of competing explanations: chance (this is less likely if there are a larger number of outcome events, tighter confidence intervals and lower *p*-values), bias (eg confounding is well controlled, and there is little exposure or outcome measurement error), statistical artefact (eg modelling assumptions are not violated) and reverse causation (eg in a cohort study, people with the outcome at the start of the study are excluded from the analysis).
- **High plausibility** of possible biological mechanisms.
- **Consistency** of the total body of epidemiological, clinical and biomedical evidence.

Example

The evidence that smoking causes lung cancer does not include direct evidence from randomised trials in humans (long-term trials of smoking in humans would clearly be unethical), but the other strands of evidence together make the case conclusive:

- Studies sufficiently large to rule out the play of chance have consistently reported that the association between smoking and lung cancer is strong, with relative risks of 10–20 when comparing long-term smokers with lifelong non-smokers.
- The association is stronger among heavy smokers than light smokers.
- No known bias or statistical error could plausibly account for associations of such strength.
- Additionally, tobacco smoke contains a large number of known carcinogens, and observational studies have shown that smoking cessation is associated with lower lung cancer risk.

1.4 Attributable fractions

Attributable fractions estimate both the proportion of cases attributable to the exposure and the proportion of cases that could theoretically be avoided if the exposure were eliminated. The two most commonly used measures of attributable fraction, which each assume that the exposure caused the outcome, are the **aetiological** and **population attributable fractions**.

- **Aetiological fraction**: the proportion of exposed cases that is attributable to the exposure
- **Population attributable fraction**: the proportion of cases in a particular population that is attributable to the exposure

Example

If the relative risk of lung cancer in smokers compared with lifelong never-smokers is 15, then 14 out of every 15 lung cancer cases that occur among *smokers* in that population would be attributable to smoking (ie the aetiological fraction would be 14/15ths, or about 93%). If the prevalence of smoking was 25% in this population, then 78% of *all* lung cancer cases in that population would be attributable to smoking; or if the prevalence was 50%, then the population attributable fraction would be 88% instead. (The formulas for attributable fractions can be found in epidemiological textbooks.)

1.5 Generalisability

If an association is similar in a wide range of populations, then it is said to be generalisable. Purely descriptive associations (eg the prevalence of smoking in various communities) tend not to be generalisable, whereas aetiological associations tend to be so (eg smoking is about as likely to cause lung cancer in doctors, or in bricklayers, as in the general population). Being representative of the general population is therefore usually more important for descriptive studies than for aetiological studies.

2. STUDY DESIGNS

There are several study designs that allow direct or indirect comparisons of disease rates between different exposure groups. The most important are:

- randomised trials
- cohort studies (which can be prospective or retrospective)
- case control studies
- cross-sectional studies
- ecological studies.

Figure 2 Some shared and distinguishing characteristics of common epidemiological study designs

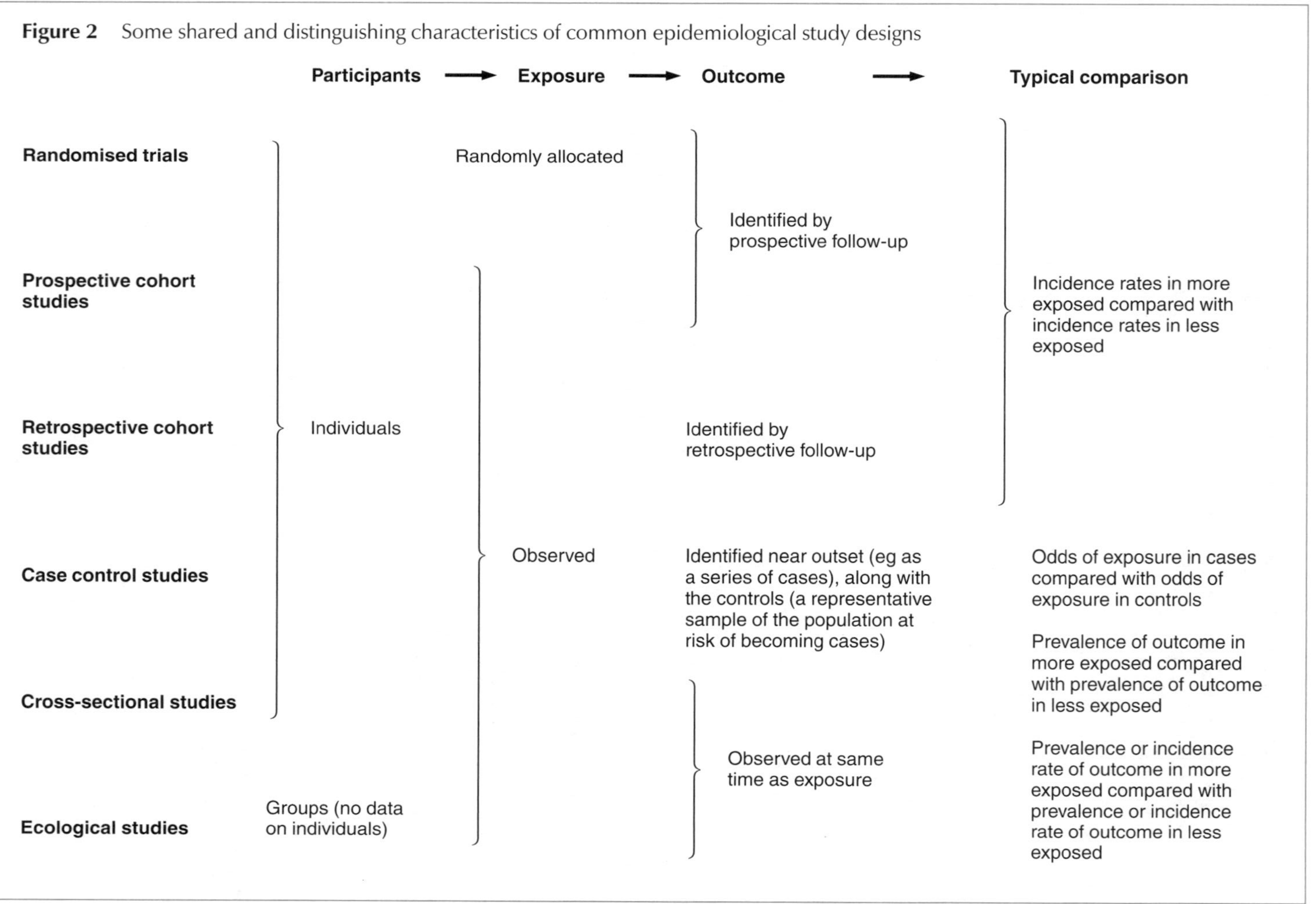

The value of the evidence from an epidemiological study depends not only on the characteristics of the study itself, but on the nature of the question being asked. For example, if a study is trying to determine whether a treatment is effective, and the real effect is not large, then anything other than a large randomised trial (or perhaps a meta-analysis of smaller ones) is unlikely to provide a clear and reliable answer. If, however, the question is whether smoking causes pancreatic cancer, a randomised trial would certainly be unethical (a cohort study or a case control study would be indicated); alternatively, if the question is what proportion of people in a given country regularly eat fish, then a randomised trial would probably be unhelpful (a representative cross-sectional study would be better).

2.1 Randomised trials

The hallmark of a randomised trial is random allocation of participants to exposures. Usually, each participant is randomly allocated to either the treatment under investigation or an established alternative (or possibly, if there is no such alternative, to a placebo). Participants are then followed up for a certain period of time, and at the end of follow-up, the disease rates (often called event rates) in the different treatment groups are compared.

A large, well-designed and appropriately analysed randomised trial can provide the highest standard of epidemiological evidence possible. Proper randomisation blocks confounding by preventing associations from forming between the treatment and factors related to prognosis. *Non*-randomised studies of treatments are generally susceptible to confounding (eg by age) because those with a poorer prognosis (eg older people) often are more – or less – likely to be allocated the treatment.

- Randomised trials avoid this possibility because all levels of the prognostic factor (eg age) are, by design, equally likely to be allocated the treatment.
- Randomised trials consequently provide a reliable way to identify treatment effects. Indeed, if the real effects are only small or moderate, large randomised trials (or, potentially, meta-analyses of smaller ones) are the only reliable way to identify them.

Randomised trials

Major advantages

Greatly reduced potential for bias, particularly:

- Confounding (eg confounding by indication)
- Observer or investigator recall bias (if there is blinding)

Major disadvantages

- Expensive
- For some exposures/treatments, randomisation is not feasible
- Special ethical issues (cf the **uncertainty principle**: a patient should be randomised only if there is substantial uncertainty about which trial treatment is appropriate for that patient)

The features of a randomised trial that can influence the trustworthiness of its findings include the:

- quality of randomistion
- number of outcome of events
- compliance with treatment allocation
- losses to follow-up
- presence of participant or investigative blinding
- use of appropriate analyses.

The quality of randomisation

Even slight deviations from true randomisation potentially create cracks through which confounding can leak. Proper randomisation requires that foreknowledge of a participant's treatment allocation must be impossible, and that once the allocation has been made, it is irreversible. Any scheme which allows an investigator or participant to know, or guess, the next allocation – for example, by holding an envelope up to the light – can influence the treatment allocation, whether consciously or subconsciously, according to factors that might be related to prognosis.

The number of outcome events

The smaller the real effect, the larger the number of events needed to reliably detect the effect's existence. Additionally, a study with a small number of events typically cannot rule out the existence of a potentially important real effect. Insufficient events are more likely if a study has too few participants, they are followed up too briefly, or they are at low risk of the outcome. Randomised trials (and other epidemiological studies) need to be sufficiently large to have a reasonably high probability (eg 80%) of detecting an association, or treatment effect, if one really exists. This probability is called a study's statistical **power**. Methods are available for estimating a planned study's statistical power based on the expected effect size, the expected number of events, and a specified level of 'statistical significance' (often 0.05 or less, ie $P < 0.05$).

Compliance with treatment allocation

Compliance with (or equivalently, adherence to) treatment allocation is the extent to which participants keep to their allocated treatment during the follow-up period. Non-compliance occurs when participants allocated the treatment stop taking it ('treatment drop-out'), or when participants not allocated the treatment start taking it ('treatment drop-in'). Non-compliance generally makes estimated treatment effects smaller, and therefore harder to detect, but it can also mimic or exaggerate real effects, particularly if the non-compliance is substantial or unevenly balanced between treatment groups.

Losses to follow-up

If a participant's health (or vital status) is not determined up to the end of the follow-up period, then the participant is lost to follow-up. As with non-compliance, losses to follow-up generally attenuate estimated treatment effects, but they can also mimic or exaggerate real effects, especially if the losses are substantial or unequal between treatment groups.

Presence of participant or investigator blinding

In a double-blind study, neither the investigators nor participants know any of the individual treatment allocations, while in a single-blind study, one of these parties (usually the investigators) does. Blinding adds further protection against biases, such as the tendency for participants or investigators to misreport or misrecord data if they have prior beliefs about what to expect with any given treatment.

Use of appropriate analyses

Potential pitfalls in the analysis of randomised trials include inadequate emphasis on **intention-to-treat analyses**, and undue emphasis on analyses of subgroups.

- **Intention-to-treat analyses** compare the event rates in different treatment groups by analysing each participant in their originally allocated group, regardless of any dropping in or out from that allocation, or of any losses to follow-up, during the course of the study. This approach provides the greatest assurance that deviations from true randomisation (and therefore potential for confounding) are minimised.
- Alternative approaches, such as so-called **on-treatment analyses**, can be appropriate for investigating adverse effects.
- **Subgroup analyses** are particularly susceptible to the play of chance because they necessarily involve smaller numbers of events. As a consequence they often suggest differences between subgroups (ie effect modification) that tend to be refuted by larger (and therefore generally more reliable) studies. The results of subgroup analyses are less likely to be misleading if the study has a larger total number of events, and if subgroup analyses were specified at the time that the study was designed, rather than, for example, after the study data had been collected and explored.

The usual ethical principle guiding modern randomised trials is the uncertainty principle, in which a person is regarded as eligible for randomisation if there is substantial uncertainty about which trial treatment is more appropriate for that individual (ie none of the possible treatment allocations is definitely indicated or contraindicated in that person).

Variants of the basic randomised trial design include:

- **Factorial trials**: trials in which participants are randomly allocated to each of two active treatments, or to their respective comparison treatments.
- **Crossover trials**: trials in which participants are switched to another treatment part way through the study.

Randomised trials have contributed enormously to the armory of effective treatments now available to physicians for combatting cancer, communicable diseases and vascular diseases. For example, the **Heart Protection Study** (2002) randomised about 20, 000 patients to either 40 mg simvastatin daily or a matching placebo, and showed that treatment with the statin substantially lowered risks of coronary heart disease and stroke at all ages, and in both sexes, irrespective of initial blood cholesterol concentration.

2.2 Cohort studies

A **prospective** cohort study can be viewed, in a sense, as a randomised trial in which the exposure is merely observed at the start of the study ('baseline') rather than randomly allocated. As in a randomised trial, participants are then followed up, and at the end of follow-up, disease rates in the different exposure groups are compared. **Retrospective** cohort studies differ from prospective cohort studies in that follow-up had already ended when the investigators started the study (ie the follow-up was retrospective rather than prospective).

Prospective cohort studies

Major advantages

- Less susceptible to reverse causation or exposure recall bias
- Can investigate multiple outcomes

Major disadvantages

- Relatively expensive (might involve a large number of participants followed up for many years)
- Potential bias due to losses to follow-up
- Might be more difficult to obtain rigorous outcome data

Cohort studies are most often used to identify causes of, or risk factors for, disease. Prospective cohort studies are often considered to provide the best observational (ie non-randomised) epidemiological evidence possible. The key factors that can affect the quality of the findings from a cohort study are the:

- **Kind of follow-up**: studies with prospective follow-up are generally less susceptible to reverse causation than studies in which the follow-up is retrospective (in a prospective study it is easier to determine disease status at the start of follow-up, and therefore to exclude participants with known disease at baseline).
- **Number of outcome events (and quality of ascertainment)**: as for randomised trials. Cohort studies vary greatly in the rigour with which they ascertain the outcome. Some actively follow up participants using regular health examinations and intensive scrutiny of personal health records, while others passively follow up participants by screening routinely collected data in national mortality or morbidity databases. The appropriateness of the method used will depend on the outcome in question. For instance, national mortality and morbidity databases might be adequate for investigating associations with total stroke, but less so for investigating associations with particular stroke subtypes.
- **Exposure measurement error**: snapshot assessment of exposure levels at the start of a study can provide a good estimate of usual exposure levels throughout the follow-up period if the exposure is more-or-less fixed (eg gender) or otherwise stable (eg height). But if the exposure fluctuates considerably (eg blood pressure), or tends to systematically increase (or, alternatively, to systematically decrease) with time, then steps need to

be taken to ensure that the estimated associations are not biased. The best strategy is usually to estimate the direction and extent of change in the exposure levels by measuring exposure levels at least once after baseline. For example, repeat measurements of blood pressure several months or years apart enable associations with *usual* blood pressure to be estimated; because of regression dilution bias, these associations are typically 50% to 100% stronger than associations with blood pressure if blood pressure is measured at a single survey only. Retrospective studies are usually more susceptible to exposure measurement error as they often have to estimate exposure levels many years previously.

- **Losses to follow-up**: as for randomised trials above.
- **Use of appropriate analyses**: because the exposure is not randomised, the exposure is often associated with extraneous variables that are themselves risk factors for the disease. Control for confounding – for example, by restricting the analysis to one level of the potential confounder, or by statistical adjustment – is therefore usually essential. For example, a cohort study of the association between parity and risk of breast cancer which fails to control for confounding by age could be heavily confounded by that variable, as both the exposure (parity) and the outcome (breast cancer) will be strongly associated with age. The potential hazards of subgroup analyses are much the same for cohort studies as for randomised trials.

Example

Among the most well known British cohort studies is the **British Doctors' Study**, which recruited and surveyed about 34,000 male British doctors in 1951, and then followed them up for the next 50 years using periodic resurveys and regular monitoring of national mortality records. The 50-year follow-up results showed that prolonged cigarette smoking tripled overall mortality rates (on average resulting in death 10 years earlier than lifelong non-smoking), but that cessation at age 50 halved this hazard, and that cessation at age 30 avoided nearly all of it.

2.3 Case control studies

As the name might suggest, a case control study recruits two types of participant: cases and controls. Exposure status is assessed in each participant, then the ratio of the odds of exposure in the cases to the odds of exposure in the controls (the odds ratio) is estimated.

- In a case control study, incidence rates in exposed and unexposed participants cannot be estimated directly because, in the absence of any follow-up, data on person-years at risk are unavailable.

Case control studies

Major advantages

- Relatively inexpensive
- Can investigate rare outcomes

Major disadvantages

More susceptible to:

- Selection biases (eg if the controls are not representative of the population at risk of becoming cases)
- Exposure recall bias (eg cases might tend to overestimate their exposure levels if they are aware of the study hypothesis)

As with cohort studies, case control studies are most often used to investigate causes of, and risk factors for, disease. But because case control studies recruit cases directly (rather than waiting for them to arise during follow-up), and merely a sample of the population at risk (rather than an entire population at risk), they are usually much more cost-efficient than prospective cohort studies.

A good case control study can provide evidence that is as reliable as a good prospective cohort study, but it is perhaps easier for a case control study to go wrong. The major points to check in a case control study are:

- **The quality of control selection**: the purpose of the controls is to provide an estimate of the exposure distribution in the population at risk of becoming cases (eg in a case control study of asbestos in relation to laryngeal cancer, the controls should give a reliable estimate of asbestos exposure in the source population from which the laryngeal cancer cases arose); therefore, it is essential that the probability of control selection is not itself related to exposure status (eg if people who were exposed to asbestos were more likely to agree to take part in the study – as controls – then the distribution of asbestos exposure in the population at risk would be overestimated, and the odds ratio biased). Biases introduced by poor control selection can fatally invalidate the results of a case control study.
- **The number of cases**: as for randomised trials and cohort studies above.
- **The potential for recall bias**: cases and controls are usually asked to recall their exposure experience during some earlier, aetiologically relevant, period. In some situations, cases might be more likely than controls to over-report (or to under-report) exposure levels, particularly if they are aware of the hypothesised association. Such recall biases can be minimised by: ensuring that information is elicited from cases and controls in an identical manner; ensuring that no information about specific hypotheses is needlessly disclosed; and, if possible, by gathering corroborating objective data about early exposure levels.
- **The use of appropriate analyses**: as for cohort studies above.

Two notable case control studies published in 1950 – one British (a precursor to the British Doctors' Study mentioned above) and one American – provided the first strong evidence that smoking is associated with lung cancer. In both studies, the proportion of smokers was much higher among people who had lung cancer than among those who did not.

2.4 Cross-sectional studies

Cross-sectional studies assess both the exposure and the outcome at one point in time. The prevalence of the outcome can then be compared between different exposure groups. Cross-sectional studies can suggest possible causes of, or risk factors for, disease, but they are generally more useful for describing the distributions of disease, or of risk factors, in specific populations. When investigating aetiological hypotheses, the chief limitation of cross-sectional studies is the difficulty of ruling out the possibility that outcome status somehow influenced the measured exposure levels (whether by reverse causation, or as a result of recall bias).

Example

The World Health Organization's ongoing MONICA project monitors trends in vascular risk factors, such as blood pressure, blood lipids and BMI, through regular cross-sectional surveys of risk factor levels in representative samples of the adult populations in several different countries.

2.5 Ecological studies

In each of the above study designs, investigators gather data (eg on exposures, outcomes and confounders) for each individual participant. Ecological studies differ in that they involve no data on individuals – merely average values for one or more groups of people. Data of this kind sometimes permit the average incidence rate or prevalence of a given disease to be compared between different populations (eg comparing bowel cancer mortality rates between countries), or within a given population over time (eg bowel cancer mortality rates in a country over a period of decades). While potentially providing clues about causes of disease, ecological studies are not themselves adequate for testing aetiological hypotheses, primarily because the absence of data on confounders in individuals greatly hampers the ability to control for confounding.

Example

International ecological studies of dietary fat and salt intake were among the first to suggest that a high intake of saturated fat is associated with increased risk of coronary heart disease, and that high salt intake is associated with high blood pressure.

2.6 Meta-analyses

Epidemiological evidence can be most trusted when biases are small and the number of participants (or, more particularly, the number of cases) is large. Meta-analysis can help achieve this second criterion by quantitatively combining data from two or more relevant studies.

Meta-analysis has at least three potential goals

- To identify important gaps in existing knowledge
- To obtain overall precise estimates of associations ('lumping')
- To identify possible sources of heterogeneity in associations ('splitting')

If there are substantial differences in the relative risks obtained in different studies, then it makes more sense to explore the sources of this heterogeneity than to obtain some overall pooled estimate. But if there is only slight or modest heterogeneity, an overall pooled estimate can potentially be informative. Pooled estimates are likely to be biased if (i) the studies utilised are a biased sample of all of the available studies (it is therefore essential to try to include *all* relevant studies), or (ii) if the available studies misrepresent reality, for example because the studies themselves were biased, or because of the dual tendency for studies with more striking findings to be published even if the findings are spurious, and for studies with statistically non-significant findings to remain unpublished even if the findings are real (two aspects of publication bias).

- Publication bias can be explored using a funnel plot, in which an estimate of effect size is plotted against a measure of study size (deviation from a symmetrical funnel shape sometimes indicates publication bias).
- Meta-analyses that merely combine the published results of studies (literature-based meta-analyses) are much less able to control for confounding than are meta-analyses that combine data on all the individuals decided in several studies (individual participant data meta-analyses).

Until the late 1980s, the net benefits and risks of streptokinase in the treatment of acute myocardial infarction were controversial. The many small randomised trials to have investigated this question had produced inconsistent results; however, when the data were combined in meta-analyses, a moderate but clear net benefit (which was subsequently confirmed by large randomised trials) became evident.

3. INTEGRATING THE EVIDENCE

The results of a single randomised trial or observational study are seldom definitive. It is therefore essential for anyone wanting a good understanding of the evidence about a particular question to weigh the evidence from all relevant studies (or to consult a source that has already done this), rather than to focus on the results of a single study, or of just a few selected studies. In weighing the evidence from all sources, more weight should be assigned to studies that are likely to have tackled chance and bias more effectively. Thus, more weight should generally be assigned:

- to studies that are bigger, especially if they involve more cases or events, as these studies will generally be less susceptible to the play of **chance**
- to **randomised trials** than to observational studies,
  to **prospective studies** than to **retrospective studies**, and
  to studies that use **individual participant data** than
  to studies that use aggregated data

As the first type of study in each of these pairs is usually less vulnerable to **bias**.

- to studies with fewer evident flaws in their conduct or analysis, as these studies may generally also be less susceptible to bias.

However, these criteria should not be viewed as prescriptive: how much weight to assign to the evidence from a particular study will inevitably involve a degree of judgement. On occasion, the findings from a large case control study, for example, will be more important than those from a small randomised trial; yet on other occasions, the opposite may be true. The value of the evidence from any given study will frequently depend more on the nature of the question being asked than on the criteria listed above.

Chapter 6
Gastroenterology

CONTENTS

Gastroenterology

1. ANATOMY AND PHYSIOLOGY OF THE GI TRACT

1.1 Oesophagus

The oesophagus is 25 cm long, and is composed of outer longitudinal and inner circular muscle layers. In the upper part these are both striated muscle and in the lower part both are smooth muscle, with the myenteric plexus lying between the two layers. The mucosa is lined with squamous epithelium.

The oesophagus is protected from acid damage by a number of defences including the lower oesophageal sphincter pressure (10–30 mmHg), salivary bicarbonate, oesophageal *bicarbonate* secretion, gravity and the 'pinchcock' effect of the diaphragmatic crura.

1.2 Stomach

At the gastro-oesophageal junction the squamous epithelium of the oesophagus changes to columnar epithelium. Secretions total approximately 3 litres per day. In gastric pits there are chief cells producing pepsin, and parietal cells (fuelled by H^+ K^+ATPase) producing hydrochloric acid and intrinsic factor. Mucus and bicarbonate are secreted by surface cells.

Innervation is both parasympathetic via the vagus (motor and secretory supply) and sympathetic via Meissner's and Auerbach's plexi. Blood supply is derived from the coeliac trunk.

The control of gastric acid secretion is summarised in the diagram overleaf.

Figure 1 Control of gastric secretion

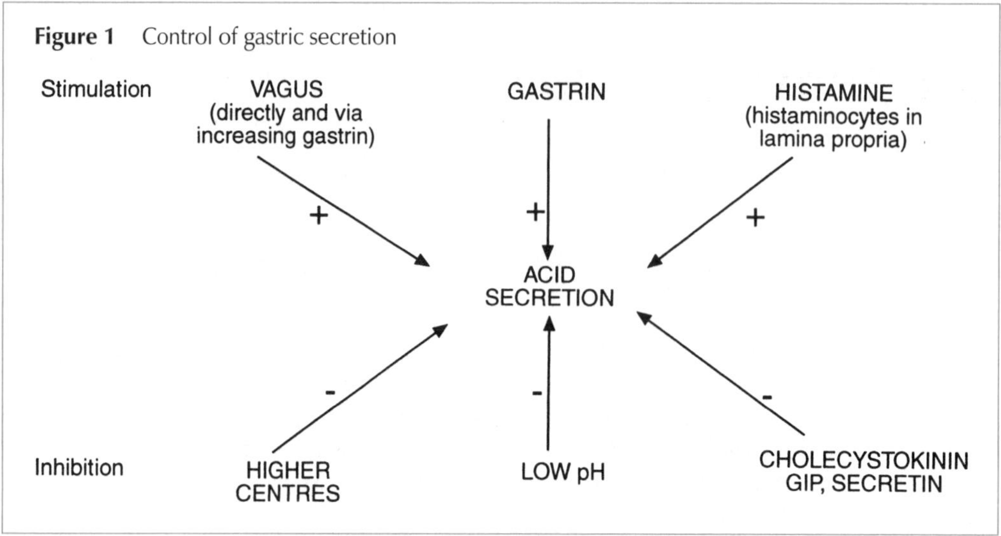

1.3 Pancreas

Between 1200 ml and 1500 ml of alkaline fluid, containing proteins and electrolytes, is secreted daily. Ninety-eight per cent of the pancreatic mass consists of exocrine acini of epithelial cells; the islets of Langerhans from which endocrine secretion occurs make up the remaining 2%. Innervation is via the coeliac plexus.

Pancreatic secretions

- **Exocrine (from acini of epithelial cells)**
  Trypsinogen
  Chymotrypsinogen
  Pancreatic amylase
  Lipase
- **Endocrine (from islets of Langerhans)**
  Glucagon from α cells
  Insulin from β cells
  Somatostatin from δ cells
  Pancreatic polypeptide

1.4 Liver

Blood supply is from the hepatic artery and portal vein (bringing blood from the gut and spleen); drainage is via the hepatic vein into the inferior vena cava. Between 250 and 1000 ml of bile is produced daily; stimulation of release from the gallbladder is by cholecystokinin.

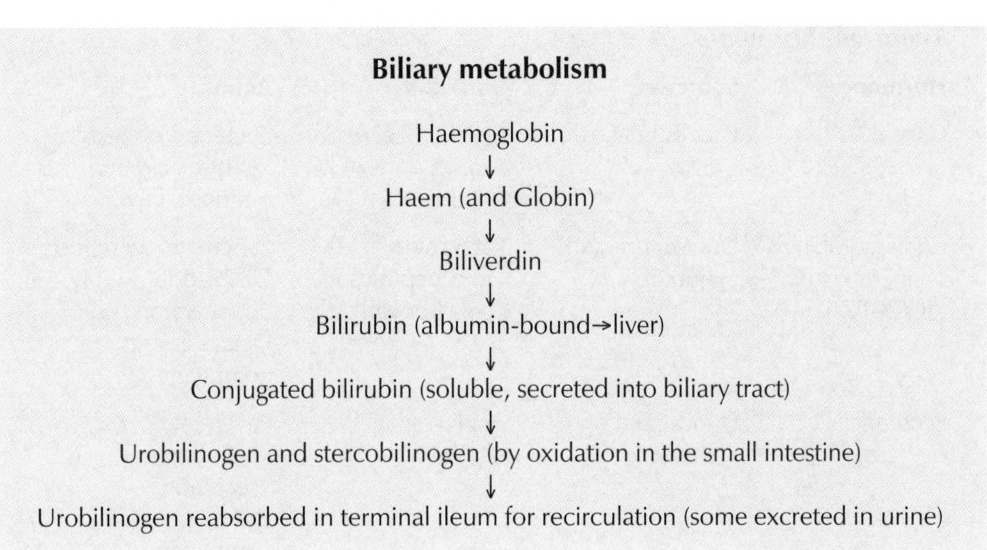

Biliary metabolism

Haemoglobin
↓
Haem (and Globin)
↓
Biliverdin
↓
Bilirubin (albumin-bound→liver)
↓
Conjugated bilirubin (soluble, secreted into biliary tract)
↓
Urobilinogen and stercobilinogen (by oxidation in the small intestine)
↓
Urobilinogen reabsorbed in terminal ileum for recirculation (some excreted in urine)

1.5 Small intestine

This is 2–3 metres in length with the villi and enterocytes providing a huge surface area which allows the absorption of up to 6 litres daily. The main function of the small intestine is absorption, with most taking place in the duodenum and jejunum. However, it also has an important immune role with lymphoid aggregates throughout, especially in the form of Peyer's patches in the ileum.

There is secretion of approximately 2 litres of alkaline fluid with mucus and digestive enzymes daily, from the enterocytes of the villi, Paneth cells at the bases of the crypts of Lieberkühn and Brunner's glands.

Blood supply from the mid-duodenum onwards is derived from the superior mesenteric artery.

1.6 Colon

This is 90–125 cm in length and its main function is the absorption of water, sodium and chloride. Typically 1–1.5 litres is absorbed daily but in some circumstances this can rise to 5 litres per day. Secretion of mucus, potassium and bicarbonate also takes place.

The blood supply is derived from the superior mesenteric artery up to the distal transverse colon; the inferior mesenteric artery supplies the remainder.

1.7 Gut hormones

The response to a meal is regulated by complex hormonal and neural mechanisms. Secretion of most hormones is determined by the composition of intestinal contents.

Major gut hormones

Hormone	Source	Stimulus	Action
Gastrin	G cells in antrum	Gastric distension Amino acids in antrum	Secretion of pepsin, gastric acid and intrinsic factor
Cholecystokinin-pancreozymin (CCK-PZ)	Duodenum and jejunum	Fat, amino acids and peptides in small bowel	Pancreatic secretion Gallbladder contraction Delays gastric emptying
Secretin	Duodenum and jejunum	Acid in small bowel	Pancreatic bicarbonate secretion Delays gastric emptying
Motilin	Duodenum and jejunum	Acid in small bowel	Increases motility
Vasoactive intestinal peptide (VIP)	Small intestine	Neural stimulation	Inhibits gastric acid and pepsin secretion Stimulates secretion by intestine and pancreas
Gastric inhibitory peptide	Duodenum and jejunum	Glucose, fats and amino acids	Inhibits gastric acid secretion Stimulates insulin secretion Reduces motility
Somatostatin	D cells in pancreas	Vagal and β-adrenergic stimulation	Inhibits gastric and pancreatic secretion
Pancreatic polypeptide	PP cells in pancreas	Protein-rich meal	Inhibition of pancreatic and biliary secretion

1.8 Metabolism of haematinics

Iron

Total body iron is between 4 and 5 g, with iron content being maintained by control of absorption in the upper small intestine. Most iron intake is in the Fe^{3+} form and approximately 5–10% of that consumed is absorbed. Iron is better absorbed from foods of animal than of plant origin.

Factors which affect iron absorption

- **Increased absorption**
  Increased erythropoiesis (eg pregnancy)
  Decreased body iron (eg GI blood loss)
  Vitamin C*
  Gastric acid*
- **Decreased absorption**
  Partial/total gastrectomy
  Achlorhydria
  Disease of small intestine (eg Crohn's disease, coeliac disease)
  Drugs (eg desferrioxamine)

*Gastric acid and vitamin C promote reduction of Fe^{3+} to Fe^{2+} which is more easily absorbed

For a more detailed account of iron metabolism *see* Chapter 9, Haematology.

Folate

The usual requirement for this nutrient is approximately 50–200 μg/day. It is present in green vegetables. Absorption takes place in the duodenum and jejunum, thus deficiency may occur with coeliac disease, Crohn's disease or any other small bowel pathology. Dietary folate is converted into 5-methyltetrahydrofolate which enters the portal blood. Deficiency may also develop if the demands of the body increase, for example in haemolysis, pregnancy and in patients being treated with antimetabolites such as methotrexate. Clinical deficiency results in a macrocytic anaemia, and in pregnancy this can be associated with neural tube defects in the fetus.

Vitamin B_{12}

Adults require 1–2 μg of dietary vitamin B_{12} daily. This is predominantly obtained from foods of animal origin. It is tightly protein bound and is released by peptic digestion. Oral B_{12} binds to intrinsic factor in the stomach and is then absorbed in the terminal ileum. Thus deficiency can occur for several reasons:

- dietary deficiency in vegetarians or vegans
- post-gastrectomy (lack of intrinsic factor)
- atrophic gastritis (pernicious anaemia)
- terminal ileal disease
- blind loops.

The Schilling test

The **Schilling test** determines whether deficiency is due to malabsorption in the terminal ileum or to lack of intrinsic factor (eg post-gastrectomy, pernicious anaemia)

1. Administer orally labelled B_{12}
2. Administer intramuscular unlabelled B_{12} to saturate body binding sites
3. Assay amount of labelled B_{12} excreted in urine (>10% in normal subjects)
4. Repeat above with concurrent administration of intrinsic factor: the amount excreted will rise if B_{12} deficiency was due to lack of intrinsic factor which is now corrected

In pernicious anaemia, autoantibodies to gastric parietal cells result in B_{12} deficiency, atrophic gastritis and achlorhydria. Approximately 1% of the population aged over 50 years is affected, with a female preponderance and a familial tendency.

Autoantibodies to gastric parietal cell are present in 90%, and autoantibodies to intrinsic factor are present in 50%. Pancytopenia may occur and other autoimmune disease may be present. The risk of gastric cancer is increased threefold.

2. DISORDERS OF THE OESOPHAGUS

2.1 Achalasia

Achalasia is a condition of unknown aetiology resulting in abnormal peristalsis and lack of relaxation of the lower oesophageal sphincter. The incidence is approximately 1/100, 000 per year, occurring at any age (usually 3rd to 5th decade) but rare in children.

It is demonstrable on manometry, endoscopy or barium studies where it is characterised by oesophageal dilation with a smooth distal 'bird's beak' stricture. Chest X-ray may show an air/fluid level behind the heart. Presentation is usually with dysphagia which, unlike other types of stricture, may affect solids and liquids from the outset.

Regurgitation, pain and weight loss may occur. There is a risk of recurrent aspiration. Squamous carcinoma is a late and rare complication.

Treatment is with endoscopic dilatation or surgical myotomy.

2.2 Reflux oesophagitis

Acid reflux is extremely common – *approximately 40% of Western populations experience 'heartburn' at least once per month*. The development of reflux oesophagitis depends on a number of factors.

Factors predisposing to reflux oesophagitis

- **GI factors**
  Acid content of refluxate
  Mucosal defences in oesophagus
  Gastric/oesophageal motility
  Hiatus hernia
- **Other factors**
  Obesity
  Smoking
  Alcohol and coffee intake
  Large meals (especially late at night)
  Drugs (most commonly theophyllines, nitrates, calcium antagonists and anticholinergics)

The correlation between symptoms and endoscopic appearances is poor; severe symptoms are compatible with a normal gastroscopy. The gold standard for diagnosis is oesophageal pH monitoring.

- The main symptom is heartburn but other symptoms include chest pain, odynophagia (painful swallowing) and dysphagia due to oesophageal dysmotility.
- Complications include strictures, haemorrhage, Barrett's oesophagus and carcinoma of the oesophagus (independent of Barrett's).

Treatment of reflux oesophagitis

Treatment is with lifestyle modifications (not evidence-based), antacids, H_2 antagonists or proton pump inhibitors with the addition of a pro-motility agent (metoclopramide, domperidone or erythromycin) for large volume reflux. Surgery is indicated for patients failing medical therapy, those with large volume reflux, bile reflux and those preferring to avoid long-term medical therapy. Most fundoplication procedures are now performed laparoscopically and endoscopic anti-reflux procedures are under evaluation.

2.3 Other causes of oesophagitis

Candidal oesophagitis may occur in patients who are immunosuppressed, on antibiotics or steroids (especially inhaled corticosteroids), or suffering from diabetes mellitus. Barium swallow shows irregular filling defects in the oesophagus and white patches can be seen on endoscopy – biopsy will confirm the diagnosis.

Chemical oesophagitis may be caused by drugs such as NSAIDs, tetracycline and potassium chloride tablets.

2.4 Barrett's oesophagus

This is found in 10–20% of patients with long-standing acid reflux. It consists of extension of the columnar gastric epithelium into the oesophagus to replace the normal squamous epithelium. It is usually caused by chronic acid exposure, and it is premalignant, although estimates of the rate of transformation to adenocarcinoma vary widely from 30 to 100 times greater than in the normal population. Treatment is of the underlying reflux disease; the benefits of regular endoscopic screening and biopsy to detect dysplastic change are controversial although most centres undertake periodic endoscopy with multiple biopsies to detect evidence of dysplastic change. Photodynamic therapy and argon beam ablation are being assessed as potential cures.

Hiatus hernia occurs when part of the upper stomach herniates through the diaphragm into the chest and is extremely common, especially with increasing age and obesity. The majority are asymptomatic and found incidentally during investigations. There are two types:

- sliding 80% – may cause aspiration and acid reflux
- rolling 20% – may obstruct or strangulate.

Hiatus hernia can be diagnosed at endoscopy, by CT scan or with barium studies and may be seen on a plain chest X-ray. Treatment is symptomatic with acid suppression where necessary. Surgical correction may sometimes be warranted.

2.5 Oesophageal carcinoma

Most oesophageal carcinomas are squamous carcinoma; adenocarcinoma is rare unless arising from ectopic gastric mucosa or Barrett's oesophagus. The incidence is rising and also increases with advancing age. The majority of tumours arise in the mid-thoracic portion of the oesophagus.

Risk factors and clinical features of oesophageal carcinoma

- **Risk factors**
  Smoking
  High alcohol intake
  Plummer–Vinson syndrome
  Achalasia
  Barrett's oesophagus
  Chronic reflux (independent of Barrett's oesophagus)
  Chinese or Russian ethnicity
  Tylosis (autosomal dominant palmar and plantar keratosis – very high risk)
- **Clinical features**
  Pain and dyspepsia
  Progressive dysphasia for liquids then solids
  Weight loss

Oesophageal carcinoma is often asymptomatic until a late stage, resulting in poor survival figures. Diagnosis is by endoscopy or barium swallow (this shows a stricture with irregular shouldering, unlike the smooth outline of a benign peptic stricture). CT scanning is used for staging, although the accuracy is very poor especially for lymph node spread; laparoscopy may be useful. Endoscopic ultrasound is especially useful for assessing transmural extension but is not yet generally available.

Treatment of oesophageal carcinoma

- Surgery
  Radical, high operative mortality (up to 10%)
  Only 1/3 lesions suitable for resection at presentation
  Improves five-year survival to approximately 10%
- Endoscopic dilatation and stenting
- Radiotherapy*
- Chemotherapy* (eg cisplatin, 5-fluorouracil)

*Used alone or in combination with surgery

Over 50% of patients have local or distant spread such that palliation is the only option. The overall five-year survival is less than 5%.

3. DISORDERS OF THE STOMACH

3.1 Peptic ulcer disease

Most epidemiological data are from studies pre-dating the re-discovery and treatment of *Helicobacter pylori*. The incidence rates of peptic ulcer are 0.1–0.3%; the ratio of duodenal to gastric ulceration is 4:1 and males are more susceptible than females. Incidence peaks at approximately 60 years of age. Most patients are treated medically with acid suppression and *H. pylori* eradication, and surgery is limited to those with complications unresponsive to medical or endoscopic therapy.

Recent NICE guidelines recommend a 'test and treat' strategy for the management of dyspepsia. This will heal underlying lesions and avoid the necessity for endoscopy in many cases. Patients with 'sinister' symptoms (weight loss, iron deficiency, dysphagia or an abdominal mass) require urgent endoscopy to exclude gastric and oesophageal malignancy.

Peptic ulcer disease

- **Risk factors**
  High alcohol intake
  NSAID use
  High-dose steroids
  Male sex
  Smoking (↑ acid, ↓ protective prostaglandins)
  H. pylori colonisation
  Zollinger–Ellison syndrome

- **Clinical symptoms**
  Epigastric pain (sometimes radiating to back if posterior duodenal ulcer)
  Vomiting
  Symptoms often relapsing/remitting
  Weight loss
  Iron deficiency anaemia
  Acute haemorrhage*

*Duodenal ulcers are the most common cause of upper GI haemorrhage

- **Treatment**
  Remove precipitating factors
  Acid-suppressing drugs
  Eradication of *H. pylori*
  Surgery if perforation, pyloric stenosis, or resistant haemorrhage

Causes of upper gastrointestinal haemorrhage

- **Common**
  Duodenal ulcer – 35%
  Gastric ulcer – 20%
  Gastric erosions – 18%
  Mallory–Weiss tear – 10%

- **5% or less**
  Duodenitis
  Oesophageal varices
  Oesophagitis
  Upper GI neoplasia

- **Rare (1% or less)**
  Angiodysplasia
  Hereditary haemorrhagic telangiectasia
  Portal hypertensive gastropathy
  Aorto-duodenal fistula

Helicobacter pylori

This Gram-negative spiral bacillus is the primary cause of most peptic ulcer disease. Infection rates increase with age – more than half of those over 50 years of age are colonised by *H. pylori* in the gastric antral mucosa. *H. pylori* has been detected in 70% of patients with gastric ulcer and over 90% of patients with duodenal ulcer compared with 50% of control subjects.

Detection of *Helicobacter pylori*

- Antral biopsy at endoscopy with haematoxylin/eosin or Giemsa stain
- Urease testing – the bacillus secretes a urease enzyme which splits urea to release ammonia. A biopsy sample is put into a jelly containing urea and a pH indicator; this will thus change colour if *H. pylori* is present
- ^{14}C breath testing – the patient ingests urea labelled with ^{14}C; CO_2, produced by urease, is detected in the exhaled breath
- Serology (stays positive after treatment and NOT useful for confirming eradication)

H. pylori causes chronic gastritis and is associated with gastric carcinoma. All patients with peptic ulceration or gastritis found to be positive should undergo eradication therapy. Effective eradication should be assessed by either repeat biopsies or breath testing in patients with complications (perforation or haemorrhage) and those with persistent symptoms.

Relapse of peptic ulcer disease after *H. pylori* eradication is less than 5% per year, compared with more than 60% in patients without eradication therapy. Evidence to support eradication of *H. pylori* in patients with non-ulcer dyspeptic symptoms is mixed, although a recent meta-analysis suggested that the number needed to be treated to cure one patient is 20. Eradication regimes vary but usually involve triple therapy of a proton pump inhibitor and two antibiotics (eg amoxicillin and clarithromycin); metronidazole resistance is a problem in some areas.

3.2 Zollinger–Ellison syndrome

This is a rare condition with an incidence of one per million population. Gastrin-secreting adenomas cause severe gastric and/or duodenal ulceration – the tumour is usually pancreatic in origin, although it may arise in the stomach, duodenum or adjacent tissues. Fifty to sixty per cent are malignant, 10% are multiple neoplasms. It may occur as part of the syndrome of multiple endocrine neoplasia type I in which case malignancy is more likely.

Clinical signs of Zollinger–Ellison syndrome

- **Pain and dyspepsia**
  From multiple ulcers
- **Steatorrhoea**
  From acid-related inactivation of digestive enzymes and mucosal damage in the upper small bowel
- **Diarrhoea**
  Due to copious acid secretion

Diagnosis is suggested by very high serum fasting gastrin levels, with little further increase with pentagastrin, and elevated basal gastric acid output. There is a rise in gastrin with secretin (unlike raised gastrin secondary to achlorhydria or proton pump inhibitor (PPI) therapy). CT scanning may be useful to locate the adenoma and assess for hepatic metastases, although 40% of adenomata are smaller than 1 cm and thus difficult to detect on CT.

Treatment of Zollinger–Ellison syndrome

- **High-dose acid suppression**
  (eg omeprazole 80–120 mg o.d.)
- **Surgical resection of adenoma**
  (May be possible)
- **Somatostatin analogues**
  To reduce gastric secretion and diarrhoea
- **Chemotherapy**
  (Although poor response) and embolisation may be used for hepatic metastases

The five-year survival rate is 80% for a single resectable lesion but falls to 20% if hepatic metastases present.

3.3 Gastric carcinoma

The incidence of gastric carcinoma is decreasing in the Western world but it still remains one of the commonest causes of cancer deaths. It usually takes the form of an adenocarcinoma, most commonly in the pyloric region; however, the incidence of carcinoma occurring in the cardia is rising. There is very little early detection in the UK, unlike Japan where the extremely high incidence of the disease merits an intensive screening programme. Most patients have local spread at the time of diagnosis, making curative resection unusual.

Gastric carcinoma

- **Risk factors**
  Japanese
  Hypo/achlorhydria (pernicious anaemia, chronic atrophic gastritis, partial gastrectomy)
  Male sex
  Dietary factors (high salt, nitrites)
  Gastric polyps (rare)
- **Clinical presentation**
  Dyspepsia (often only symptom)
  Epigastric pain
  Anorexia and weight loss
  Early satiety
  Iron deficiency anaemia
  Haematemesis/melaena

Very few tumours are confined to the mucosa at diagnosis, when cure rates are above 90%. Overall survival is below 10%. Diagnosis is by endoscopy and biopsy; endoscopic ultrasound and CT scan of the abdomen and thorax are used to determine resectability. Adjuvant chemotherapy before and after surgery may improve prognosis, although patients are often too unwell post-operatively to receive the second course.

Other gastric tumours include lymphoma (about 5%), which has a good prognosis, and leiomyosarcoma (<1%), which has a 50% five-year survival.

3.4 Other gastric pathology

Gastroparesis

Reduced gastric motility results in vomiting, bloating and weight loss. Some cases are idiopathic, others are due to diabetes, autonomic neuropathy or following vagotomy. Gastric distension and delayed emptying can be demonstrated using a barium meal (which is useful to exclude obstructing lesions) or isotope emptying studies (which are more useful for quantifying the amount of delay). Treatment is with pro-motility agents such as metoclopramide, domperidone or erythromycin but if symptoms are severe or if aspiration pneumonia occurs a feeding jejunostomy may be required.

Ménétrière's disease

This is a very rare condition associated with mucus cell hypertrophy and parietal cell atrophy, mediated by epidermal growth factor. This results in gross thickening of the gastric mucosa, hypochlorhydria and protein-losing enteropathy.

Gastric polyps

Unlike colonic polyps, most gastric polyps are rare and usually benign, occurring in about 2% of the population.

- Multiple hamartomatous polyps are occasionally found in Peutz–Jeghers syndrome and adenomata in polyposis coli, but over 90% are hyperplastic (usually arising from Brunner's glands).
- Adenomatous polyps should be removed in view of their pre-malignant potential.

3.5 Complications of gastric surgery – dumping syndrome

Gastric surgery is much less common since the advent of H_2 antagonists and PPIs, but long-term complications of previous gastric surgery are frequently encountered. **Dumping syndrome** results from an inappropriate metabolic response to eating and can occur within half an hour of eating (early dumping) or between 1 and 3 hours (late dumping).

- Symptoms include palpitations, sweating, hypotension and light-headedness.
- Early dumping is a vagally mediated response to rapid gastric emptying.

- Late dumping is due to hypoglycaemia – a rebound insulin-mediated phenomenon following transient hyperglycaemia due to a heavy carbohydrate load to the duodenum.
- Diagnosis is usually clinical, but may be confirmed by glucose, electrolyte or blood pressure monitoring during an attack.

4. DISORDERS OF THE PANCREAS

4.1 Acute pancreatitis

Acute pancreatitis is a common and potentially fatal disease. Mortality in hospital remains at 7–10%, usually due to multi-organ failure or peripancreatic sepsis. Scoring systems, such as the APACHE II or the Glasgow score, aim to identify those patients at high risk by assessing factors such as age, urea, hypoxia and white cell count but are unreliable within the first 48 hours. Obstruction of the pancreatic duct by gallstones accounts for over 50% of cases, most of the rest being alcohol-related. Four per cent are thought to have a viral aetiology; all other causes are rare. Oxygen free radicals are thought to mediate tissue injury.

Acute pancreatitis

- **Causes**
  Gallstones
  Alcohol
  Viral (eg mumps, Coxsackie B)
  Trauma
  Drugs (eg azathioprine, oral contraceptive pill, frusemide, steroids)
  Hypercalcaemia
  Hyperlipidaemia
  Post-surgery to bile duct/ endoscopic retrograde cholangiopancreatography (ERCP)

- **Early complications**
  Adult respiratory distress syndrome
  Acute renal failure
  Disseminated intravascular coagulation

- **Poor prognostic indicators**
  Age >55 years
  WCC >15 × 10^9/l
  Urea >16 mmol/l
  pO_2 <60 mmHg (<8 kPa)
  Calcium <2 mmol/l
  Albumin <32 g/l
  Glucose >10 mmol/l
  LDH >600 IU/l
  (Severe attack if more than three factors are present)

- **Late complications**
  Abscess
  Pseudocyst
  Splenic or portal vein thrombosis

Clinical presentation is usually with abdominal pain and vomiting with tachycardia and hypotension in more severe cases. Amylase (in blood, urine or peritoneal fluid) is raised, usually to at least four times normal values. A plain abdominal X-ray may show a sentinel loop of adynamic small bowel adjacent to the pancreas.

Treatment is supportive with fluids and analgesia; the presence of three or more poor prognostic indicators suggests that referral to ITU should be considered. Prophylactic antibiotics reduce morbidity. In severe pancreatitis due to gallstones (where jaundice and cholangitis are present), early ERCP to achieve duct decompression is of proven value. Any patient with a biliary aetiology should have cholecystectomy during the same admission once the acute symptoms have settled.

4.2 Chronic pancreatitis

Chronic pancreatitis is an inflammatory condition characterised by irreversible damage to the exocrine and later to the endocrine tissue of the pancreas. Most cases are secondary to alcohol but it is occasionally due to cystic fibrosis or haemochromatosis. There is a male predominance, often with a long history of alcohol abuse.

Chronic pancreatitis

- **Clinical signs**
  Malabsorption and steatorrhoea
  Abdominal pain radiating to the back, often severe and relapsing
  Diabetes mellitus

- **Diagnosis**
  X-ray may show speckled calcification, present in 50–60% of advanced cases
  CT is the most sensitive for detection of pancreatic calcification
  ERCP shows irregular dilation and stricturing of the pancreatic ducts although MRCP is the modality of choice for diagnostic pancreatography
  Pancrealauryl and PABA (*p*-aminobenzoic acid) testing are of use to assess exocrine function – both these involve ingestion of an oral substrate which is cleaved by pancreatic enzymes and can then be assayed in the urine

Treatment is with pancreatic enzyme supplementation, analgesia and abstention from alcohol. Antioxidants (vitamins A, C and E) are of unproven value and coeliac axis block for pain relief is now rarely performed because of poor results and surgical complications. Sixty per cent survive for 20 years – death is usually from complications of diabetes or alcohol.

4.3 Pancreatic carcinoma

Carcinoma of the exocrine pancreas is responsible for more than 6000 deaths per year in the UK, with an incidence of 110–120 per million, rising to 800–1000 per million over the age of 75 years. Seventy to eighty per cent arise in the head of the pancreas where there is maximal pancreatic tissue; those in the tail are often silent in the early stages and present at an advanced stage. Pancreatic carcinoma may invade into the duodenum and this can lead to small bowel obstruction.

- The risk is increased 2- to 3-fold in smokers, and also possibly in those with diabetes, although it has been suggested this is an early symptom of carcinoma rather than a risk factor. Alcohol does not increase the risk.
- Clinical signs include abdominal pain radiating through to back, weight loss and obstructive jaundice in 80–90%. The exocrine and endocrine functions are usually maintained.
- Ultrasound and CT are both useful diagnostic tools, although ERCP is probably of most use, enabling stenting to relieve jaundice and pruritus.

Between 10 and 20% of patients are suitable for surgery but perioperative mortality is high. Radiotherapy and chemotherapy are under evaluation but so far have been shown to confer little survival benefit. Median survival remains 2–3 months from diagnosis, with one- and five-year survival rates of 10% and 3%, respectively.

4.4 Endocrine tumours

These are very rare with an annual incidence of 4 per million but they are incidentally detected at post mortem. They can occur independently, or as part of multiple endocrine neoplasia (MEN I) syndrome.

The more important lesions include:

- **insulinoma**
- **gastrinoma** (**Zollinger–Ellison syndrome**, *see* Section 3.2)
- **glucagonoma**
- **VIPoma**
- **somatostatinoma.**

Insulinoma

These arise from the Islets of Langerhans and often present with unusual symptoms (visual disturbances, irritability, abnormal behaviour, confusion, amnesia, paraesthesia and drowsiness) after overnight fast or before meals as a result of hypoglycaemia. Patients often discover that glucose is helpful and may go for years without diagnosis.

Glucagonoma

These tumours arise from alpha cells of the pancreas and present clinically with a characteristic rash (migratory necrolytic erythema), weight loss, glucose intolerance or frank diabetes, and anaemia. Tumours are often very large at diagnosis and are usually malignant.

VIPoma

Excessive VIP (vasoactive intestinal polypeptide) produces an extreme secretory diarrhoea (usually >3 litres per day) resulting in hypochlorhydria and hypokalaemia.

Somatostatinoma

This rare tumour was only described 27 years ago. It produces a syndrome of diabetes mellitus, diarrhoea, gallbladder disease, weight loss, steatorrhoea and hypochlorhydria due to inhibition of insulin and pancreatic enzymes.

5. SMALL BOWEL DISORDERS

The small bowel is the main site of absorption of nutrients for the body. Thus small bowel diseases such as coeliac or Crohn's disease often result in malabsorption and malnutrition.

Small bowel pathology can be difficult to diagnose because of the inaccessibility of this part of the GI tract. Special investigations, such as enteroscopy or white cell scanning, may be of use in addition to more routine tests such as gastroduodenoscopy or barium studies.

5.1 Coeliac disease

Also known as gluten-sensitive enteropathy, this common and under-diagnosed condition is caused by an immunological reaction to the gliadin fraction of wheat and other cereals. Some 0.1–0.2% of the population are affected and the onset may be at any age, although peaks occur in babies and in the third decade. The incidence is greatly increased in western Ireland and it has been postulated that this is due to increased reliance on potatoes rather than wheat products as a source of carbohydrate. Thus those affected with gluten intolerance continued to thrive and reproduce.

HLA B8 DRW3 is present in 90%. Pathologically, gliadin provokes an inflammatory response which results in partial or total villous atrophy in the proximal small bowel; this reverses on a gluten-free diet but recurs on re-challenge.

Coeliac disease

- **Clinical picture**
  Diarrhoea
  Oral aphthous ulcers
  Weight loss
  Growth retardation
  General malaise
  Neurological symptoms – ataxia, weakness and paraesthesiae
  Amenorrhoea

- **Complications**
  Anaemia – folate, B_{12} or iron deficiency
  Increased malignancy*
  Hyposplenism
  Dermatitis herpetiformis – itchy rash, improves with dapsone
  Osteomalacia

- **Diagnosis**
  Upper GI endoscopy with jejunal biopsy
  Antiendomyseal antibody
  Antigliadin antibody – may become negative after treatment

*There is an increased risk of all GI malignancies but especially small bowel lymphoma, occurring in approximately 6% of cases. This risk returns to almost normal with treatment of the disease

Treatment is by strict avoidance of wheat, rye and barley. The role of oats is debatable and many patients can eat oats without significant pathological or clinical effects. Patients require folate, iron and calcium supplements in the early stages of treatment. Failure to respond to treatment is usually due to non-compliance (often unwittingly) with diet. However, supervening pathology, such as lymphoma, should always be excluded and a small number of patients may require steroids to control their symptoms.

Although 10% of first-degree relatives will develop coeliac disease routine screening is not advocated unless they have symptoms to suggest the diagnosis.

Other causes of villous atrophy:

- Whipple's disease
- hypogammaglobulinaemia
- lymphoma
- tropical sprue: aetiology unknown, but likely to be infective as it responds to long-term tetracycline therapy.

5.2 Carcinoid tumours

These are relatively common; it is estimated that carcinoid tumours are an incidental finding in up to 1% of post-mortems. **Carcinoid syndrome**, however, is extremely rare. Carcinoid tumours arise from the enterochromaffin cells of intestinal mucosa (neuroendocrine cells found in the lamina propria) throughout the gut. The most common GI sites are the appendix (from which site metastasis is rare) and the ileum.

- The tumours secrete serotonin and therefore can be detected by assay of the metabolite 5-hydroxyindoleacetic acid (5-HIAA) in the urine.
- Serotonin causes bronchoconstriction and increased gut motility, resulting in the symptoms documented below.
- Histamine and adrenocorticotrophin may also be synthesised.
- Carcinoid syndrome occurs only when secondaries in the liver release serotonin into the systemic circulation; any hormone from non-metastatic gut carcinoids will be metabolised in the liver.

Clinical features of carcinoid syndrome

- Diarrhoea
- Bronchospasm
- Local effect of the primary (eg obstruction, intussusception)
- Flushing
- Right heart valvular stenosis (left heart may be affected in bronchial carcinoid or if an atrial septal defect (ASD) is present)

- **Treatment** depends on the site of the primary and presence of metastases. Many carcinoids are very slow growing, with patient survival of more than 20 years. With widespread metastases five-year survival varies from zero to 25%, the better figures reflecting the less aggressive nature of appendiceal primaries.

Treatment of carcinoid tumours and syndromes

- **Surgical resection**
  Good prognosis if no metastases
- **Resection or embolisation**
  Of hepatic metastases
- **Octreotide, methysergide and cyproheptadine**
  For diarrhoea
- **Phenoxybenzamine**
  For flushing

Carcinoid tumours may occasionally cause pellagra due to tumour uptake of tryptophan (the precursor of nicotinic acid).

5.3 Whipple's disease

This is an uncommon condition usually affecting middle-aged men (occasionally women and children) caused by infection with *Tropheryma whippeli*. Jejunal biopsy shows deposition of macrophages containing PAS-positive granules within villi. There is a clinical syndrome of diarrhoea, malabsorption, arthropathy and lymphadenopathy. Whipple's disease remains poorly understood but symptoms respond to extended courses of tetracycline or penicillin.

5.4 Angiodysplasia

Although most commonly occurring in the caecum and ascending colon, angiodysplasia is included here because of the diagnostic challenge it may present when present in the small intestine. Angiodysplasia may be found throughout the GI tract and its frequency in the population is unknown. It is a rare but significant cause of acute gastrointestinal haemorrhage, but presents more frequently as occult iron-deficiency anaemia.

Diagnosis of angiodysplasia

This can be difficult, but useful investigations include:

- **Gastroscopy/colonoscopy**: may detect gastric and large bowel lesions.
- **Mesenteric angiography**: only of use if currently bleeding; if so, will localise source in approximately 40%.
- **Small bowel enteroscopy**: intubation of the upper small bowel is possible using an elongated endoscope with an overtube to provide rigidity.
- **Capsule enteroscopy**: this is the most effective method of detecting small bowel angiodysplasia and other sources of small bowel bleeding. A small (11 × 27 mm) capsule is swallowed which transmits thousands of images from the gut as it transits. Images are analysed manually and with computer assistance. The technique is not yet widely available.

Treatment of angiodysplasia

Treatment is by heat or laser coagulation at endoscopy or by embolisation of the bleeding point during angiography. Surgery may be indicated if the lesions are very numerous or if there is severe bleeding. Drug therapy with danazol is thought to reduce the risk of bleeding but is poorly tolerated by many patients.

6. NUTRITION

The maintenance of adequate nutrition requires three main criteria to be fulfilled.

1. **Intact GI tract**
   This may be compromised by resections resulting in a short bowel syndrome, or by fistulas such that segments of bowel are bypassed. As different nutrients are absorbed from different parts of the gut a variety of clinical sequelae may occur depending upon the segment of bowel affected (eg B_{12} deficiency after terminal ileal resection, iron deficiency after partial gastrectomy).

2. **Ability to absorb nutrients**
   Impairment of absorptive function may be caused by mucosal damage such as occurs in Crohn's or coeliac disease, or after radiation damage. Motility problems resulting in accelerated transit times may reduce absorption.

3. **Adequate intake**
   This is dependent both on the motivation to maintain an adequate oral intake, often lacking in sick or elderly patients, and on the composition of the diet.

Inability to maintain nutrition is an indication to provide supplementation by one of the three routes listed below. The underlying disease will determine which is appropriate.

- **Oral**: obviously the most simple form but relies on a conscious patient with an intact swallowing mechanism. High protein or carbohydrate drinks may be used to provide good nutritional intake in a small volume.
- **Enteral**: useful when swallowing impaired (eg in neurological disease) or when high volume intake is needed. May take the form of a simple nasogastric tube, or a percutaneous gastrostomy (PEG) or jejunostomy which can be inserted endoscopically or surgically. Can be for short- or long-term supplementation.
- **Parenteral**: this is intravenous feeding, either to supplement enteral nutrition or to provide total support in the case of complete intestinal failure.

Problems with parenteral nutrition

- Central venous access needed
- Patient/carer must be sufficiently motivated and competent to master aseptic techniques and care for venous line
- Electrolyte abnormalities may occur – need for careful monitoring; also need to monitor trace elements such as zinc and selenium
- Risk of sepsis – line infections, right heart endocarditis

Examples of specific nutritional deficiencies are covered in Chapter 13, Metabolic Diseases.

6.1 Diarrhoea

Diarrhoea means different things to different people but medically is defined as >200 ml of stool per day. In lay terms, diarrhoea is used to describe increased frequency and/or decreased consistency of motions. There are multiple causes (as illustrated below), and these result in diarrhoea by differing mechanisms.

Various classifications can be used:

- acute or chronic
- large bowel (often smaller amounts, may contain blood or mucus)
- small bowel (often voluminous, pale and fatty).

Causes of diarrhoea

- **Osmotic** (osmotic agents draw water into gut)
  Osmotic laxatives (lactulose, polyethylene glycol)
  Magnesium sulphate
  Lactase deficiency* (poorly absorbed lactose acts as a laxative)
  Stops with fasting

- **Altered motility** (altered peristalsis or damage to autonomic nervous system)
  Irritable bowel syndrome
  Thyrotoxicosis
  Post-vagotomy
  Diabetic autonomic neuropathy
  Stops with fasting

- **Secretory** (failure of active ion absorption ± active ion secretion)
  Infection (eg *E. coli*, cholera)
  Malabsorption
  Bile salts (↑ deposition into bowel after cholecystectomy)
  Continues with fasting

*Lactase deficiency may be congenital (possibly severe) or acquired, and often occurs in the setting of viral gastroenteritis or coeliac disease. Complete exclusion of lactose from diet usually not necessary – there is often a threshold below which symptoms are absent

Causes of bloody diarrhoea

- Crohn's disease
- Ulcerative colitis
- Colorectal cancer
- Ischaemic colitis
- Pseudomembranous colitis
- Schistosomiasis
- *Salmonella*
- *Shigella*
- Amoebiasis
- *Campylobacter*
- *Strongyloides stercoralis*
- Haemolytic uraemic syndrome (which can be caused by *E. coli* type O157, *Campylobacter*, *Shigella*, etc)

Investigations for diarrhoea

- **History and examination vital, including rectal examination**
  History may be suggestive of large or small bowel cause; examination per rectum to exclude overflow or rectal tumour
- **Sigmoidoscopy/colonoscopy**
  If large bowel cause suspected
- **Folate and iron assay**
  If small bowel cause suspected
- **Gastroscopy**
  With duodenal biopsy if small bowel cause suspected
- **Biochemistry**
  Electrolyte disturbance; include thyroid function tests
- **Stool examination**
  Including examination for ova, cysts and parasites and laxative screen
- **Three-day faecal fat assay**
  If small bowel cause suspected
- **Small bowel radiology**
  If small bowel cause suspected
- **Gut hormone assay**
- **Urine analysis**
  Laxative screen
- **Hydrogen breath test**
  Bacterial overgrowth in the small bowel can be identified by detection of exhaled hydrogen from ingested glucose or lactulose. False positives occur with rapid small bowel transit that results in prolonged hydrogen release

Treatment of diarrhoea

Depends on the underlying disease process, which should be treated if possible. Loperamide or codeine increase gut transit time thus may control symptoms. **Octreotide** may be useful for chronic secretory diarrhoea, short bowel symptoms and diarrhoea secondary to endocrine tumours.

6.2 Malabsorption

Malabsorption may be defined as a failure to absorb sufficient exogenous nutrients or reabsorb endogenous substances such as bile salts. It may be caused by several factors since normal absorption depends on gut structure, motility and secretion of hormones and enzymes. Malabsorption usually results in diarrhoea. Clinical presentation depends on the type and site of defect, and includes weight loss and general ill health, osteomalacia, or specific nutritional deficiencies such as of B_{12} and folate.

Investigation of malabsorption

Investigation is as for diarrhoea. In addition, specific tests for malabsorption include:

- **Schilling test**: see earlier.
- **Xylose absorption test**: 25 g of xylose is given orally. Urinary excretion of xylose is quantified. More than 20% should appear in the urine if small bowel absorption is normal.
- **Pancreatic function testing.**
- **^{14}C breath testing**: to detect overgrowth (although the most accurate test remains quantitative bacteriological assay of jejunal aspirates).

Causes of malabsorption

- **Structural abnormalities**
  Coeliac disease*
  Crohn's disease*
  Post-surgical resections*
  Bacterial overgrowth due to blind loops or anatomical abnormalities
  Whipple's disease
  Tropical sprue
- **Motility abnormalities**
  Thyrotoxicosis
  Drugs (eg neomycin)
  Diabetes
- **Secretory abnormalities**
  GI tract infection (eg *Giardia*, amoebiasis)
  Chronic pancreatitis*
  Cystic fibrosis

*Common causes in the UK

Bacterial overgrowth of the small bowel

This is common in patients who have undergone small bowel resections or in those with jejunal diverticulae or systemic sclerosis. These bacteria are able to metabolise vitamin B_{12} and carbohydrate but the serum folate usually remains normal or elevated. Patients usually have diarrhoea, and malabsorption may ensue. Treatment is with antibiotics such as metronidazole, tetracycline or ciprofloxacin, and recurrent courses of these antibiotics may be necessary.

7. LARGE BOWEL DISORDERS

7.1 Crohn's disease and ulcerative colitis

Crohn's disease and ulcerative colitis are both chronic relapsing inflammatory diseases of the gastrointestinal tract.

Aetiology of inflammatory bowel disease

There is an undoubted genetic predisposition based on the identification of at least five susceptibility loci in family studies, and the recent discovery of the NOD2/CARD15 gene on chromosome 16 which is clearly associated with the development of Crohn's disease. This gene codes for a protein which facilitates opsonisation of gut bacteria, and animal studies have conformed that colitis does not develop in animals raised in a sterile environment. Putative infectious agents including *Mycobacterium paratuberculosis* have not been confirmed, and recent speculation about the role of measles or the measles vaccination in Crohn's disease has no epidemiological basis. The use of NSAIDs and the oral contraceptive pill have also been implicated but mechanisms remain unclear.

The major similarities and differences between the two diseases are detailed below.

Clinico-pathology of Crohn's disease and ulcerative colitis

Crohn's disease	**Ulcerative colitis**
Affects any part of the GI tract from mouth to anus. Commonly terminal ileum (70%), colon (30%), anorectum (30%). May be 'skip lesions' of normal mucosa between affected areas	Always involves rectum and extends confluently into the colon. Terminal ileum may be affected by 'backwash ileitis' but remainder of gut unaffected
Pathology	
Transmural inflammation	Mucosa and submucosa only involved
Non-caseating granulomata (in 30% only)	Mucosal ulcers
Fissuring ulcers	Inflammatory cell infiltrate
Lymphoid aggregates	Crypt abscesses
Neutrophil infiltrates	
Clinical	
Abdominal pain prominent and frequent fever	Diarrhoea, often with blood and mucus
Diarrhoea ± blood p.r.	Fever
Anal/perianal/oral lesions	Abdominal pain less prominent
Stricturing common, resulting in obstructive symptoms	

Continues ...

... Continued

Crohn's disease	Ulcerative colitis
Associations	
Increased incidence in smokers (50–60% smokers)	Decreased incidence in smokers (70–80% non-smokers)
Skin disorders: erythema nodosum (5–10%) pyoderma gangrenosum (0.5%) iritis/uveitis (3–10%)	Increased incidence of: primary biliary cirrhosis chronic active hepatitis sclerosing cholangitis
Joint pain/arthritis (6–12%) Cholelithiasis (common) Clubbing Depression	Other systemic manifestations occur but less common than in Crohn's disease
Diagnosis	
Barium studies: cobblestoning of mucosa rosethorn ulcers strictures skip lesions	Barium studies: pseudopolyps between ulcers loss of haustral pattern featureless shortened colon
Endoscopy with biopsy	Sigmoidoscopy with biopsy may be sufficient
Isotope leukocyte scans useful to diagnose active small bowel disease	
Complications	
Fistulae: entero-enteral entero-vesical entero-vaginal perianal	Fistulae do not develop Toxic megacolon (uncommon – usually an indication for urgent colectomy) Increased risk of carcinoma* (risk increases with time since diagnosis, extent of disease and early age of onset)
Carcinoma – slightly increased risk of colonic malignancy (see later)*	Iron deficiency anaemia
B_{12} deficiency common (decreased absorption in terminal ileal disease)	
Iron deficiency anaemia	
Abscess formation	

*See section 'Carcinoma complicating inflammatory bowel disease'

Treatment of inflammatory bowel disease

Treatment is similar for both Crohn's disease and ulcerative colitis, although the latter may be more amenable to topical drug therapy. The major treatment strategies are:

- **5-ASA compounds** (sulfasalazine, mesalazine, olsalazine, balsalazide): these are used to treat mild–moderate relapses of colitis and are taken long-term to maintain remission. Oral 5-ASAs are targeted to the colon using pH-dependent or bacterial cleavage systems to release active 5-ASA from carrier molecules. Side-effects are common with sulfasalazine, and these include rash, infertility, agranulocytosis, headache, diarrhoea and renal failure. Interstitial nephritis is a rare side-effect of all 5-ASA drugs.
- **Steroids**: this is the main treatment for active disease, and is available for topical, oral and intravenous administration. Terminal ileal Crohn's disease may be treated with topically acting oral budesonide, which is metabolised in the liver and has far fewer systemic side-effects.
- **Immunosuppressants**: **azathioprine** is very effective as a steroid-sparing agent and in some patients who are steroid unresponsive. Its use is limited by gastrointestinal and systemic side-effects and close monitoring for evidence of marrow suppression and hepatotoxicity is necessary. Pancreatitis is an uncommon but potentially serious idiosyncratic side-effect. **Methotrexate** is useful in patients with Crohn's disease but does not appear to be effective in patients with ulcerative colitis. **Intravenous ciclosporin** is sometimes effective in the treatment of acute, steroid-resistant colitis, but long-term benefit has not been established.
- **Metronidazole and ciprofloxacin**, used in treatment of perianal disease.
- **Anti-tumour necrosis factor alpha (infliximab)**: this chimeric (mouse/human) monoclonal antibody is very effective in the treatment of active Crohn's disease and many patients benefit from long-term maintenance therapy. The cost (up to £15,000/year) has to be balanced against the reduced costs of hospital admission, surgery, lost productivity and improved quality of life. In the UK its use is restricted to patients who are unresponsive to immunosuppressant therapy, have severe symptoms and who are unsuitable for surgery. Newer immunological therapies are currently under evaluation.
- **Nutritional support and treatment**: patients with inflammatory bowel disease are often malnourished and require nutritional supplementation (enteral or parenteral), especially if surgery is planned. An elemental diet may be as effective as steroids in inducing remission in Crohn's disease.
- **Surgery**: surgical resection is very effective for symptom relief in obstructive Crohn's disease, and colectomy offers a cure to patients with ulcerative colitis. The recurrence rate for Crohn's disease after surgery is approximately 50%, although this can be reduced with post-operative azathioprine. Ileo-anal pouch surgery restores continence to patients undergoing colectomy.

Carcinoma complicating inflammatory bowel disease

The risk of carcinoma associated with inflammatory bowel disease is increased if:

- onset occurs at less than 15 years of age
- disease duration has been longer than 10 years
- there is widespread disease (eg total colitis)
- the disease takes an unremitting course
- compliance with treatment and follow-up is poor.

The value of screening for colonic carcinoma in ulcerative colitis and Crohn's disease is controversial. Some units advise a screening colonoscopy every 3 years for patients who have had extensive disease for more than 10 years. This is certainly indicated if one or more adenomatous colonic polyps are present at sigmoidoscopy, if there is long-standing extensive ulcerative colitis, or if the patient has a family history of colonic carcinoma at a young age. In patients with long-standing and extensive colitis, prophylactic colectomy may be recommended for persistent moderate/severe dysplasia.

7.2 Pseudomembranous colitis

This is acute colitis due to the enterotoxin of *Clostridium difficile*, usually precipitated by broad-spectrum antibiotics (particularly clindamycin). It is common in the elderly or chronically ill, and mortality may be as high as 20%. Patient-to-patient spread in hospital is common. Diagnosis is by demonstration of the toxin in stools or by endoscopy (which shows inflamed mucosa with yellow pseudomembranes). Treatment is with oral vancomycin or metronidazole.

7.3 Familial polyposis coli

This is an autosomal dominant condition, caused by mutation in the APC tumour suppressor gene which is located on the long arm of chromosome 5. Estimates of the incidence vary from 1 in 7000–30, 000 of the population in the UK.

Multiple adenomata occur throughout the colon; if untreated, malignancy is inevitable, often when patients are aged only 30 or 40 years. Surveillance colonoscopy begins in adolescence and prophylactic colectomy usually follows at around age 20 years in view of the high risk of malignant change. Many patients opt for an ileo-anal pouch. Screening of family members is essential.

7.4 Peutz–Jeghers syndrome

This is an autosomal dominant condition in which multiple hamartomatous polyps occur throughout the GI tract (particularly in the small bowel). Patients may have mucocutaneous pigmentation and perioral freckles. Lesions may lead to GI haemorrhage and may undergo malignant change (carcinoma is increased 12-fold in patients with this condition).

7.5 Hereditary non-polyposis colorectal cancer (HNPCC)

This is a dominantly inherited disorder of DNA mismatch repair genes located on chromosomes 2 and 3. Malignancies such as those affecting the colon, breast, ovary and endometrium occur at a young age. Relatives of affected patients require genetic counselling and cancer screening.

7.6 Colorectal cancer

This is the second most common cause of cancer death in the UK, with an incidence of approximately 30/100, 000 in the UK. Because of its frequency, screening of the asymptomatic population by faecal occult blood testing has been evaluated but not found to be worthwhile, partly due to poor patient compliance. It is likely that a national screening programme based on fibre-optic sigmoidoscopy will be introduced in the UK within the next year or two. Colorectal cancer is common from the sixth decade onwards and the incidence increases with advancing age. Recent studies have suggested that non-steroidal anti-inflammatory agents (NSAIDs) may have a protective effect.

Pathologically, it is an adenocarcinoma usually arising from tubular and villous adenomatous polyps (although in inflammatory bowel disease, malignant change arises directly from the mucosa). The commonest sites are the rectum and sigmoid colon.

Risk factors and clinical features of colorectal cancer

- **Increased incidence**
  Male sex
  Inflammatory bowel disease, especially ulcerative colitis
  Familial polyposis coli
  Diet low in fibre, fruit and vegetables
  Diet high in fat and red meat
  Cholecystectomy (bile salts 'dumped' in colon)

- **Genetics**
  Sporadic mutations may occur in the p53, Ras and APC genes. p53 regulates the cell cycle and causes apoptosis in the event of DNA damage – its loss therefore leads to uncontrolled proliferation of cells

- **Clinical signs**
  These depend on the site of the lesion; all can cause weight loss and obstructive symptoms.

Right-sided	*Left-sided*	*Rectum*
Iron deficiency anaemia	Blood p.r.	Blood p.r.
Abdominal pain	Altered bowel habit	Tenesmus
Abdominal mass	Abdominal mass	

- **Complications**
  Local spread to organs and lymph nodes
  Metastasis to liver, lung, brain and bone
  Obstruction ± perforation

Treatment of colorectal cancer

This consists of surgery (for cure) or symptomatic relief depending, on **Duke's staging**.

Duke's classification and prognosis of colorectal cancer

Stage	Five-year survival
A – confined to mucosa and submucosa	80% +
B – extends through muscularis propria	60–70%
C – regional lymph nodes involved	30–40%
D – distant spread	0%

- **Radiotherapy** may be used as an adjuvant, particularly to reduce tumour bulk before surgery.
- Adjuvant chemotherapy (eg 5-fluorouracil post-operatively) has been shown to improve prognosis for patients at Duke's stages B and C, toxicity is low so quality of life tends to be good.
- Serial monitoring of carcinoembryonic antigen (CEA), a glycoprotein from gastrointestinal epithelia, may be of use in detecting recurrence.
- Some surgeons are now resecting hepatic metastases isolated to a single lobe of liver.

Carcinoma complicating inflammatory bowel disease: this is discussed in Section 7.1, Crohn's disease and ulcerative colitis.

7.7 Irritable bowel syndrome (IBS)

This is a chronic, relapsing functional gut disorder with no recognisable pathological abnormality. In most cases the diagnosis is based on clinical presentation although symptoms presenting in older patients require investigation to exclude other pathologies. IBS affects up to 10% of the population with a ratio of 5:1 female dominance. Strict diagnosis is based on Rome II criteria requiring abdominal pain provoked by eating or relieved by defecation and a change in bowel habit occurring for at least 3 months in a year.

Full blood count, ESR, CRP, thyroid function tests (TFTs) and stool culture are useful screening investigations to exclude common diagnoses, and sigmoidoscopy provides reassurance for patients and clinicians that there is no underlying pathology.

- Bloating, borborygmi, excessive flatus, belching and mucorrhoea are common gastrointestinal symptoms.
- IBS is often associated with alternating bowel habit but may also present with 'diarrhoea-dominant' or 'constipation-dominant' symptoms.
- Patients with IBS often complain of other 'functional' symptoms and have a higher prevalence of fibromyalgia, non-cardiac chest pain, tension headache, sterile cystitis, dyspareunia, back pain, anxiety and depression.

- There is a clear association with a history of childhood abuse.
- In about a quarter of cases IBS is preceded by gastrointestinal infection, raising the possibility of damage to the neuroenteric innervation in some cases.

Treatment of irritable bowel syndrome

Treatment is usually symptomatic and includes antispasmodics, increased dietary fibre, laxatives, constipating agents, antidepressants, hypnotherapy and psychotherapy. The latter are particularly useful for patients whose symptoms occur on a background of significant psychological morbidity.

8. GASTROINTESTINAL INFECTIONS

AIDS and the gut is covered in Chapter 8, Genito-urinary Medicine and AIDS.

8.1 Gastroenteritis

Most gastrointestinal infections in the UK are viral or self-limiting bacterial infections such as *Staphylococcus aureus* or *Campylobacter*. Most patients require no treatment but antidiarrhoeals (such as loperamide) and oral rehydration therapy (ORT) may be required in patients who are at risk of dehydration. ORT utilises the capacity of the small bowel to absorb chloride, sodium and water via a glucose-dependent active transport channel that is not disrupted by infections. More intensive therapy is confined to those systemically unwell or immunosuppressed.

The following are some of the more important gastrointestinal infections. (*See also* Chapter 11, Infectious Diseases.)

Amoebiasis

- Infection is due to *Entamoeba histolytica* with faecal–oral spread.
- The clinical spectrum ranges from mild diarrhoea to dysentery with profuse bloody stool; a chronic illness with irritable-bowel-type symptoms may also occur. Colonic or hepatic abscesses occur, the latter commonly in the setting of a severe amoebic colitis.
- Treatment is with metronidazole.

Campylobacter

This is due to a Gram-negative bacillus; spread is faecal–oral.

- Gram-negative rods.
- Clinically, patients are often systemically unwell with headache and malaise prior to the onset of diarrhoeal illness. Abdominal pain may be severe, mimicking an acute abdomen.
- Erythromycin may be indicated if symptoms are prolonged.

Cholera

- Infection is due to *Vibrio cholerae* (Gram-negative rods) which colonise the small bowel; spread is faecal–oral. A high infecting dose is needed as the bacteria are susceptible to gastric acid.
- A severe toxin-mediated diarrhoea occurs with 'rice-water' stool which may exceed 20 litres per day. Dehydration is the main cause of death especially in young or elderly, and mortality is high without rehydration treatment.
- Tetracycline may reduce transmission.

Giardiasis

- Infection is due to *Giardia lamblia* (a flagellate protozoan) which colonises the duodenum and jejunum; spread is faecal–oral.
- Bloating and diarrhoea (not bloody) occur and may be chronic. Malabsorption may occur with small intestinal colonisation. Asymptomatic carriage is common and duodenal biopsy may be necessary to make the diagnosis in patients with chronic diarrhoea or malabsorption symptoms.
- Treatment is with metronidazole.

Salmonella

- A Gram-negative bacillus with multiple serotypes divided into two main groups: those causing typhoid and paratyphoid (enteric fever), and those causing gastroenteritis. Spread is faecal–oral.
- Diarrhoea (may be bloody) occurs, with or without vomiting and abdominal pain.
- Treatment is supportive but occasionally ciprofloxacin or trimethoprim may be required for chronic symptoms or severe illness in the very young or elderly. Chronic asymptomatic carriage is rare (less than 1% compared with 3–4% in typhoid/paratyphoid).

Shigella

- Gram-negative rods. Spread is faecal–oral with a very low infecting dose of organisms needed owing to its high virulence.
- The clinical spectrum ranges from diarrhoeal illness to severe dysentery depending on the infecting type: *S. sonnei*, *S. flexneri*, *S. boydi*, *S. dysenteriae*.
- Diarrhoea (may be bloody), vomiting, abdominal pain.
- Treat if severe with ampicillin or tetracycline although there is widespread resistance.

8.2 Gastrointestinal tuberculosis

This is common in developing countries, and causes ileo–caecal TB (mimicking Crohn's disease) or occasionally spontaneous TB peritonitis. There has been a recent increase in abdominal TB particularly in patients with AIDS. The infection may occur secondary to pulmonary TB as a result of swallowing infected sputum or by haematogenous spread; it may also result from drinking unpasteurised milk.

- Clinical features are often non-specific such as malaise, fever and weight loss, as well as diarrhoea and abdominal pain.
- Ultrasound, barium studies or CT may suggest the diagnosis but biopsy, either by laparoscopy or endoscopy, is confirmative.
- Treatment is with conventional anti-tuberculous therapy.

9. HEPATOLOGY

9.1 Jaundice

Jaundice is one of the most common symptoms of liver disease, caused by the accumulation of bilirubin in the tissues. Bilirubin is formed as the end product of catabolism of haem-containing compounds and is clinically detectable at a level of >40 μmol/l. The formation and excretion of bilirubin is shown in the following figure.

The most common causes of jaundice in the UK are alcoholic liver disease, gallstones and tumours of the liver and pancreas.

Hyperbilirubinaemia may occur because of excess production or decreased elimination of bilirubin. Jaundice can thus be broadly divided into three categories depending on the site of the pathology.

Prehepatic

Figure 2 Enterohepatic circulation of bile

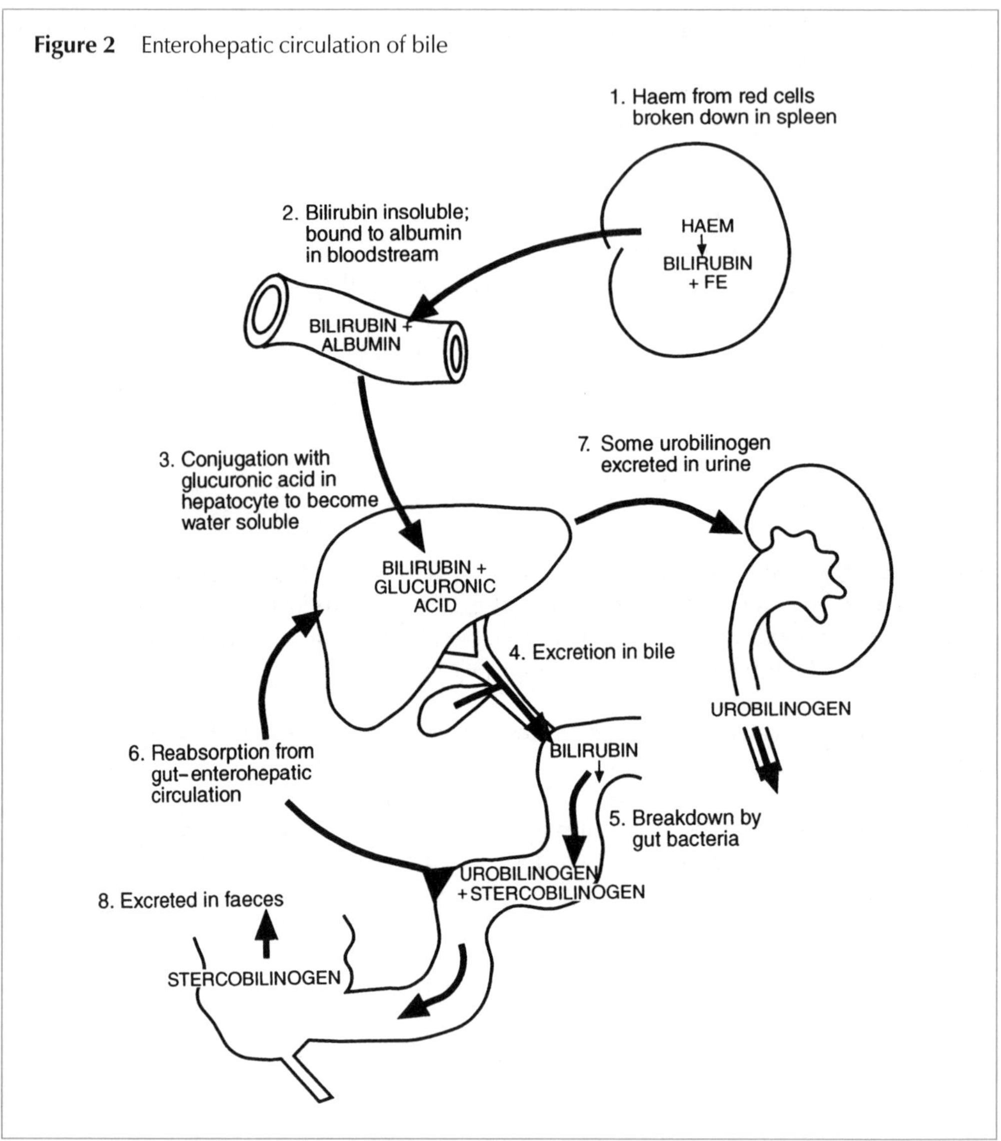

Causes of jaundice

The following classification is used:

- **Pre-hepatic**: excess production of bilirubin or failure of uptake into the liver. Bilirubin is unconjugated and insoluble thus it does not appear in the urine – acholuric jaundice.
- **Hepatic**: defect is at the level of hepatocyte. There is diminished hepatocyte function, and thus both conjugated and unconjugated bilirubin appear in the urine.
- **Post-hepatic**: there is impaired excretion of bile from liver into the gut. Conjugated bilirubin is therefore reabsorbed which increases serum and urine levels and produces dark urine. The stools become pale due to lack of stercobilinogen; urobilinogen (produced in the gut – see figure on previous page) becomes undetectable in urine.

Causes of jaundice	
Pre-hepatic	• Haemolysis causing excess haem production • Congenital hyperbilirubinaemia (eg Gilbert's syndrome, Crigler–Najjar syndrome (see following box)
Hepatic	• Viral infection (eg hepatitis A, B, EBV) • Drugs (eg phenothiazines) • Wilson's disease • Rotor and Dubin–Johnson syndromes (see following box) • Cirrhosis • Multiple hepatic metastases • Hepatic congestion in cardiac failure
Post-hepatic	• Gallstones • Carcinoma of pancreas or bile ducts • Lymph nodes at porta hepatis (eg metastatic, lymphomatous) • Primary biliary cirrhosis – small bile duct obliteration • Sclerosing cholangitis • Structural abnormality of the biliary tree – post-surgery, congenital (eg biliary atresia)

Classification of congenital hyperbilirubinaemia

Syndrome	Genetics	Defect	Clinical features	Treatment
Gilbert's	Aut Dom	Defect in conjugation	↑ Unconjugated bilirubin Asymptomatic ± jaundice, increases with fasting	Nil as benign condition
Crigler–Najjar	Type 1 – Aut Rec	Both due to defective conjugation	Neonatal kernicterus and death	None; fatal
	Type 2 – Aut Dom		Jaundice as neonate/child; survive to adulthood	Phenobarbitone to ↓ jaundice
Dubin–Johnson	Aut Rec	Defect in hepatic excretion	Jaundice with right upper quadrant pain and malaise	Nil as benign condition
Rotor	Aut Rec	Defect in uptake and storage of bilirubin	↑ Conjugated bilirubin	Nil as benign condition

Aut Dom = autosomal dominant; Aut Rec = autosomal recessive

Investigation of jaundice

The following would be a typical systematic approach.

Blood tests

- **Liver function tests** may indicate if jaundice is obstructive (elevated alkaline phosphatase from cells lining canaliculi) or hepatocellular (elevated transaminases). Patients with chronic liver disease may have normal enzyme levels but poor synthetic function (low albumin, prolonged prothrombin time) will indicate a hepatic aetiology. Full blood count, reticulocyte count and blood film are useful if haemolysis is suspected.
- **Viral serology** (hepatitis A, B and C), **autoantibody titres** (antimitochondrial M2 for primary biliary cirrhosis and anti-smooth muscle for chronic autoimmune hepatitis), α1-antitrypsin, alpha fetoprotein (AFP), ferritin and copper studies are essential when investigating unexplained jaundice or chronic liver disease.

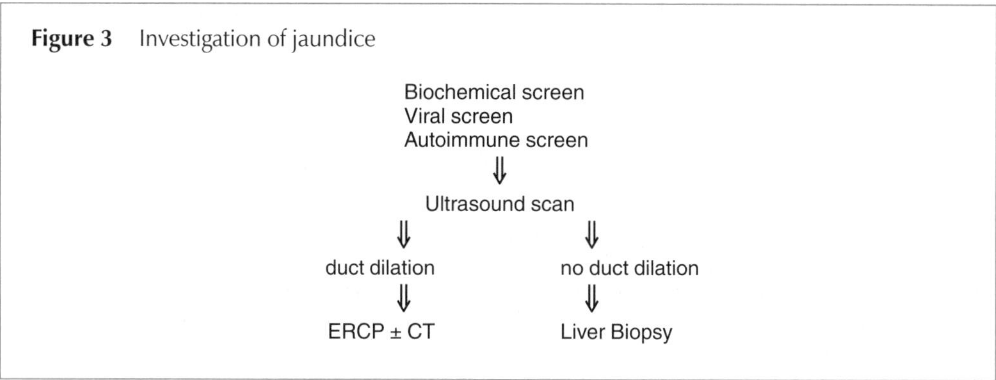

Figure 3 Investigation of jaundice

Imaging and biopsy

- **Liver ultrasound**: is the single most useful radiological test and will identify obstruction, metastases, cirrhosis and hepatoma.
- **CT scanning**: is frequently used to complement ultrasound images, to define lesions more clearly and to diagnose lesions not seen on ultrasound.
- **ERCP**: is used to investigate obstructive jaundice and to stent obstructing tumours or remove obstructing gallstones.
- **Liver biopsy**: may be helpful in non-obstructive jaundice, but is contraindicated in the presence of uncorrected coagulation disorders and is technically difficult if ascites is present.

Liver function tests in jaundice

	Unconjugated bilirubin	Conjugated bilirubin	ALT/AST	Alk phos	Gamma GT
Pre-hepatic	↑↑	Normal	Normal	Normal/↑	Normal/↑
Hepatic	Normal	↑↑	↑↑	Mod ↑	Mod ↑
Post-hepatic	Normal	↑	Mod ↑	↑↑↑	↑↑

9.2 Gallstone disease

Gallstones are one of the commonest causes of jaundice, usually presenting with colicky upper abdominal pain and cholestatic liver function tests. Approximately 1 litre of bile is secreted by the hepatocytes each day. Half of this drains directly into the duodenum whilst the remainder is stored and concentrated in the gallbladder by removal of sodium, chloride, bicarbonate and water. Cholecystokinin (CCK) then stimulates its release.

- Stones are found in 10–20% of the population (with a female preponderance) but are asymptomatic in the majority.
- 70–90% gallstones are a mixture of cholesterol and bile pigment and 10% are pure cholesterol. Pure pigment stones are rare except with chronic haemolysis (eg sickle cell disease, spherocytosis).

Risk factors for and clinical presentation of gallstones

- **Risk factors for stone formation**
  Female sex
  Increasing age
  Drugs (eg oral contraceptive pill, clofibrate)
  Crohn's disease (terminal ileum)
  Short bowel syndrome
  Haemolysis (pigment stones)
- **Clinical presentation**
  Acute/chronic cholecystitis
  Biliary colic
  Cholestatic jaundice if duct obstruction
  Pancreatitis
  Cholangitis
  Gallstone ileus

NB Stones may form in the common bile duct even after cholecystectomy

- **Diagnosis** in most cases may be established by ultrasound with/without ERCP. **MRCP** is replacing ERCP as a useful, non-invasive investigation but it does not allow therapeutic intervention during the procedure.
- Definitive treatment is by cholecystectomy. ERCP with sphincterotomy and balloon clearance of the common bile duct may be indicated for duct stones. Medical treatment with ursodeoxycholic acid can be used to dissolve cholesterol stones; however, this is extremely slow and should be reserved only for patients who are unfit for other treatment.

9.3 Ascites

Ascites is defined as the accumulation of free fluid within the peritoneal cavity. It can be subdivided into transudate or exudate depending on whether the protein content is less or greater than 30 g/l, respectively. The most common causes in the UK are cirrhosis and malignant disease.

Causes of ascites

- **Transudate**
  Portal hypertension
  Nephrotic syndrome
  Malnutrition
  Cardiac failure
  Budd–Chiari syndrome
  Myxoedema
- **Exudate**
  Hepatic or peritoneal malignancy
  Intra-abdominal TB
  Pancreatitis

The **treatment** of ascites depends on the aetiology.

- **Transudates** respond to fluid restriction, low sodium intake and diuretic therapy, to promote sodium and water excretion via the kidneys. Paracentesis may be used for tense ascites or ascites which is not responding to diuretics. However, paracentesis may result in a further shift of fluid from the intravascular space into the peritoneal cavity with the risk of circulatory collapse. This can be reduced by supporting the circulation using intravenous albumin.
- Exudates can be safely paracentesed without protein replacement.

9.4 Viral hepatitis

The six major hepatitis viruses are described below, but further types are already postulated. Hepatitis B and C in particular are major causes of morbidity and mortality worldwide, although recent advances in treatment with interferon and other antivirals have improved the outcome in certain groups.

Hepatitis A

Spread: faecal–oral
Virus: RNA
Clinical: anorexia, jaundice, nausea, joint pains, fever
Treatment: supportive
Chronicity: no chronic state
Vaccine: yes.

Hepatitis B

Spread: blood-borne (eg sexual, vertical, congenital transmission)
Virus: DNA
Clinical: acute fever, arteritis, glomerulo-nephritis, arthropathy
Treatment: supportive; chronic HBV may respond to interferon (the effectiveness of antiviral agents lamivudine and famciclovir are under evaluation)
Chronicity: 5% → chronic carriage (risk of cirrhosis and hepatocellular carcinoma)
Vaccine: yes.

Hepatitis C

Spread: blood-borne, sexual
Virus: RNA
Clinical: acute hepatitis – less severe than A or B, fulminant failure rate
Treatment: pegylated interferon alpha (interferon bound to polyethylene glycol) for chronic HCV. This may be more effective when used in combination with ribavirin
Chronicity: 60–80% develop chronic hepatitis and 20% of these progress to cirrhosis (of whom a third will develop hepatocellular carcinoma). IV-drug-related hepatitis C represents a major public health problem in the UK
Vaccine: no.

Hepatitis D (delta agent)

Spread: blood-borne (dependent on concurrent hepatitis B infection for replication)
Virus: incomplete
Clinical: exacerbates established hepatitis B infection and increases risk of hepatic failure and cirrhosis
Treatment: interferon of limited benefit
Chronicity: increases incidence of cirrhosis in chronic HBV
Vaccine: no.

Hepatitis E

Spread: faecal–oral
Virus: RNA
Clinical: acute self-limiting illness, but there is a 25% mortality (fetal and maternal) in pregnancy, which increases in later stages of gestation
Treatment: supportive
Chronicity: no chronic state
Vaccine: no.

Hepatitis G

Spread: blood-borne
Virus: RNA
Clinical: doubtful relevance; 20% of patients with chronic HCV are infected with hepatitis G
Treatment: viraemia may decline with interferon
Chronicity: unknown – may cause cirrhosis and hepatocellular carcinoma
Vaccine: no.

Interferon in viral hepatitis

Interferon is predominantly of benefit in patients suffering from chronic hepatitis B and C. In hepatitis B, there is a response in 40% of chronic carriers. The response is poorer in Asian patients. The response is likely to be very poor if the patient is also infected with HIV and thus treatment is not usually indicated in this group. In hepatitis C, there is a response in 50% of chronic carriers but 50% of these will relapse despite treatment.

Hepatitis B serology

Antigens/antibodies related to viral surface (**s**), envelope (**e**) and core (**c**) are useful for determining the stages, infectivity and chronicity of hepatitis B infection:

- **HBsAg**: present in acute infection; if present longer than 6 months = chronic hepatitis
- **HBeAg**: present in acute or chronic infection; signifies high infectivity
- **HBcAg**: present in acute or chronic infection; found only in liver tissue; present for life
- **AntiHBs**: signifies immunity after vaccination or acute infection
- **AntiHBe**: signifies declining infectivity and resolving infection
- **AntiHBe IgM**: signifies recent acute infection; lasts less than 6 months
- **AntiHBc IgG**: is a lifelong marker of past acute or chronic infection; does not signify immunity or previous vaccination

9.5 Drug-induced hepatitis

Many drugs can cause hepatitis. Toxicity may be due to overdose (eg paracetamol), idiosyncratic (eg flucloxacillin) or may be related to dosage or duration of therapy (eg azathioprine). Three patterns of damage can occur:

- **Cholestasis**: some drugs produce a functional obstruction to bile flow by causing bile duct inflammation and interfering with excretory transport mechanisms. The commonest examples are flucloxacillin, chlorpromazine, oral contraceptives and anabolic steroids.
- **True hepatitis**: some drugs produce direct hepatocellular damage which may be trivial or result in fulminant liver failure. Several mechanisms are responsible. Common examples include statins, antituberculous drugs, immunosuppressants, ketoconazole and halothane.
- **Hepatic necrosis**: if the ability of the liver to detoxify metabolites is overwhelmed, glutathione levels fall and toxic metabolites accumulate causing liver necrosis. This is the pattern of damage with carbon tetrachloride ingestion and paracetamol overdosage.

Other causes of acute hepatitis include:

- alcohol
- other viruses (eg Epstein–Barr, yellow fever, CMV, rubella, Herpes simplex)
- other infections (eg malaria, toxoplasmosis, leptospirosis, brucellosis).

9.6 Chronic hepatitis

Chronic hepatitis is defined as any hepatitis persisting for longer than 6 months. The main differentiation is between chronic persistent hepatitis, which is a benign condition with a good prognosis, and the more serious chronic active hepatitis.

Chronic persistent hepatitis

This is defined as a benign inflammatory reaction lasting longer than 6 months. It will remit spontaneously after several months or years. Biopsy (necessary to exclude chronic active hepatitis) shows portal fibrosis but no piecemeal necrosis. Patients are often asymptomatic; there may be hepatomegaly but signs of chronic liver disease are absent. Liver biochemistry is often normal except for elevated aspartate aminotransferase.

Causes of chronic hepatitis

- Viral hepatitis
- Drugs (eg methyldopa, isoniazid, cytotoxics)
- Alcohol

Because of its benign nature, treatment is not indicated.

Chronic active hepatitis (CAH)

This is an aggressive persistent hepatitis characterised by piecemeal necrosis on biopsy. Progression to cirrhosis with the associated risk of hepatocellular carcinoma is common.

Causes of chronic active hepatitis (CAH)

- Hepatitis B ± hepatitis D (20% of all CAH; not responsive to steroids but may respond to interferon – see earlier)
- Alpha-1 antitrypsin deficiency
- Hepatitis C (see earlier)
- Autoimmune (see below)
- Wilson's disease

Autoimmune 'lupoid' hepatitis

This condition occurs predominantly in female patients. Other autoimmune disease is often present and patients are usually ANF positive. It responds to steroids and azathioprine but the majority progress to cirrhosis, although 90% are alive at 5 years and may be candidates for transplantation.

9.7 Cirrhosis

Cirrhosis is characterised by the irreversible destruction and fibrosis of normal liver architecture with some regeneration into nodules.

There are four stages of pathological change:

- liver cell necrosis
- inflammatory infiltrate
- fibrosis
- nodular regeneration.

Regeneration may be macronodular (eg alcohol- or drug-induced), micronodular (eg viral hepatitis) or mixed, but a more useful categorisation is according to the aetiological agent.

Causes of cirrhosis

- Alcohol (most common in the UK, approximately 30% of all cases)
- Hepatitis B or C (most common worldwide)
- Cryptogenic
- Primary biliary cirrhosis
- Haemochromatosis
- Wilson's disease
- Alpha-1 antitrypsin deficiency

Evidence of chronic liver disease may or may not be present

Clinical features of cirrhosis

Clinical features are related to hepatic insufficiency:

- **Confusion/encephalopathy**: due to failure of liver to metabolise ammonium salts.
- **Haemorrhage**: bruising/bleeding/petechiae secondary to deficiency in factors II, VII, IX and X, and thrombocytopenia.
- **Oedema**: secondary to hypoalbuminaemia.
- **Ascites**: due to portal hypertension, hypoalbuminaemia and secondary hyperaldosteronism.
- **Jaundice**: failure to metabolise and/or excrete bilirubin.
- **Other clinic features include**: palmar erythema, spider naevi and splenomegaly (due to portal hypertension).

Diagnosis of cirrhosis

Cirrhosis may be suspected on ultrasound scanning but biopsy is required to confirm this and to help identify the aetiology. Ultrasound guided biopsy is mandatory as the liver is often very small. Rarely, a transjugular biopsy is attempted, particularly if clotting is markedly deranged.

Treatment of cirrhosis

Treatment is aimed at the removal of causal factors such as alcohol. Specific treatments include interferon for viral hepatitis and ursodeoxycholic acid for primary biliary cirrhosis. Transplantation is the best hope but many patients are not suitable.

Contraindications for liver transplantation include:

- poor cardiac reserve
- co-morbidity such as HIV infection or severe respiratory disease
- failure to abstain from alcohol.

There is no definitive cut-off regarding age but patients over 70 years are less likely to be suitable.

Conditions which may be amenable to hepatic transplantation

- **Fulminant hepatic failure**
  (eg due to hepatitis C or paracetamol toxicity)
- **Primary biliary cirrhosis**
- **Hepatitis B**
  Although frequent recurrence after transplant – reduce using pre-transplant treatment with interferon
- **Cholangiocarcinoma**
  If unresectable at presentation
- **Alcohol**
  Following psychological review and if abstained for more than 6 months
- **Wilson's disease**
- **Haemochromatosis**
- **Hepatocellular carcinoma**
  If not multifocal, <5 cm and no evidence of vascular invasion

9.8 Portal hypertension and varices

Portal hypertension occurs as a result of increased resistance to portal venous flow. Pressure in the portal vein rises and is said to be pathological when >12 mmHg, although pressures of up to 50 mmHg may occur. The spleen enlarges and anastomoses may open between the portal and systemic circulation. Some of the collaterals, which most commonly occur at the oesophago-gastric junction, umbilicus and rectum, may become very large with a risk of bleeding.

A variety of conditions may cause portal hypertension; in the UK the single most common is cirrhosis secondary to alcohol.

Causes of portal hypertension

- Cirrhosis due to any cause
- Portal vein thrombosis (congenital malformation, pancreatitis, tumour)
- Budd–Chiari syndrome (thrombosis or obstruction of hepatic vein due to tumour, haematological disease or the oral contraceptive pill)
- Intrahepatic tumours such as cholangiocarcinoma or hepatocellular carcinoma
- Constrictive pericarditis
- Right heart failure

Variceal haemorrhage

Thirty per cent of patients with varices will bleed at some point with a mortality of 50% for that episode. The majority of survivors will rebleed with a mortality of 30%. Bleeding is often catastrophic as many patients also have coagulopathy as a result of their underlying liver disease.

Primary prevention of haemorrhage

All patients with cirrhosis of the liver should have upper GI endoscopy to determine the presence or absence of varices. If there are none, or only very small varices, no treatment is required except regular endoscopic review every 2–3 years. Larger varices in patients with no history of variceal haemorrhage should be treated with prophylactic beta-blockade (or nitrates if beta-blockers are contraindicated). This reduces portal pressure and significantly reduces the risk of haemorrhage.

Treatment of variceal haemorrhage

After resuscitation and correction of any coagulopathy the treatment of choice is early gastroscopy with band ligation of the varices (now shown to be superior to injection sclerotherapy). Temporary balloon tamponade (Sengstaken–Blakemore tube) may be useful if endoscopy is not immediately available or if bleeding cannot be stopped endoscopically. Vasoactive drugs, such as terlipressin (Glypressin®), are widely used but should not be viewed as a substitute for endoscopy and banding. Bleeding which does not respond to these measures may be an indication for emergency transjugular intrahepatic porto-systemic shunting (TIPSS).

Secondary prevention of haemorrhage

Patients should undergo repeated band ligation until varices are eradicated. Beta-blockade should be given as this reduces the risk of rebleeding by up to 40%. Recurrent haemorrhage may be an indication for TIPSS.

Transjugular intrahepatic porto-systemic shunting (TIPSS)

This involves placement of a shunt under radiological screening which decompresses the portal venous system. As it is less invasive than surgery it may be a useful rescue procedure for patients with recurrent or resistant haemorrhage who are not fit for surgery. The major problems are that shunting may precipitate hepatic encephalopathy (this occurs in up to 24%, but seems more responsive to treatment than encephalopathy from other causes), and shunt blockage. In the latter case a second shunt may be 'piggy-backed' across the first. TIPSS may be particularly helpful as a palliative procedure in patients with recurrent haemorrhage due to malignancy.

9.9 Hepatic encephalopathy

Hepatic encephalopathy is a neuropsychiatric syndrome which may complicate acute or chronic liver disease from any cause. Symptoms include confusion, falling level of consciousness, vomiting, fits and hyperventilation. Renal failure may often supervene – the chance of recovery from hepato-renal failure is extremely poor. The underlying mechanisms are complex but the absorption of toxins such as ammonia from bacterial breakdown of proteins in the gut is thought to play a major part. Porto-systemic shunting of blood occurs – toxins thus bypass the liver and cross the blood–brain barrier.

The most common causes of **acute hepatic encephalopathy** are fulminant viral hepatitis and paracetamol toxicity which are potentially fully reversible. Indicators of poor prognosis are:

- worsening acidosis
- rising prothrombin time
- falling Glasgow Coma Scale.

These patients should be referred to a specialist centre as they may need transplantation.

Chronic hepatic encephalopathy may supervene in chronic liver disease of any type. It is often precipitated by:

- alcohol
- drugs
- GI haemorrhage
- infections
- constipation.

It is characterised by a flapping tremor, decreased consciousness level and constructional apraxia.

Treatment of hepatic encephalopathy

- Screen for and treat sepsis aggressively – if ascites is present consider bacterial peritonitis and perform a diagnostic ascitic tap. This should be a low threshold for prescribing ciprofloxacin
- Strict fluid and electrolyte balance
- Low protein diet
- Laxatives to clear the gut and thus reduce toxin absorption; neomycin is now rarely used
- Remove or treat precipitants

Mortality is high, especially if renal failure supervenes when the mortality exceeds 50%.

9.10 Primary biliary cirrhosis

Primary biliary cirrhosis accounts for approximately 5% of deaths due to cirrhosis. The cause is unknown although factors point to an autoimmune aetiology, especially the strong association with other autoimmune disease such as rheumatoid arthritis, Sjögren's syndrome and CREST syndrome. Histologically, progressive inflammation and destruction of small intrahepatic ducts leads to eventual cirrhosis. Ninety per cent of patients are female, often in middle age. There are four stages of primary biliary cirrhosis:

1. Destruction of interlobular ducts
2. Small duct proliferation
3. Fibrosis
4. Cirrhosis.

Primary biliary cirrhosis

- **Clinical features**
  Cholestatic jaundice
  Xanthelasmata due to hypercholesterolaemia
  Skin pigmentation
  Clubbing
  Hepatosplenomegaly
  Portal hypertension ± varices
  Osteoporosis and osteomalacia
- **Diagnosis**
  Antimitochondrial (M2) antibody present in 95%
  Predominantly raised alkaline phosphatase – often raised in advance of symptoms/signs
  Raised IgM
  Liver biopsy showing the features listed above

Treatment is symptomatic; cholestyramine relieves pruritus. Ursodeoxycholic acid is widely used but it is doubtful whether this agent either improves the prognosis or delays time to liver transplantation. Rising bilirubin levels are an indication that the disease is approaching end stage, and as liver transplantation remains the only hope of cure, patients should be assessed for this later treatment at an appropriate stage of their disease process.

9.11 Other causes of chronic liver disease

Haemochromatosis: this is an autosomal recessive disorder of iron metabolism leading to deposition in the liver, pancreas, pituitary and myocardium. (*See* Chapter 13, Metabolic Diseases.)

Wilson's disease: this is an autosomal recessive disorder of copper metabolism causing deposition in the liver, basal ganglia and cornea (Kayser–Fleischer ring). (*See* Chapter 13, Metabolic Diseases.)

9.12 Parasitic infections of the liver

Hydatid disease

This is caused by *Echinococcus granulosus* (a dog tapeworm), and is most common in areas of sheep and cattle farming. Ingestion results from eating contaminated vegetables or as a result of poor hand hygiene. The parasitic embryos hatch in the small intestine and enter the bloodstream via the portal venous circulation to the liver, but there may also be spread to lung or brain.

- Many cases are asymptomatic but right upper quadrant pain is the commonest symptom. Jaundice occurs if there is duct obstruction, and peritonitis will result from cyst rupture.
- Diagnosis is confirmed using a haemagglutination test, but eosinophilia or the presence of cystic lesions on liver ultrasound in an at-risk individual is strongly suggestive of the disease.
- Active infection is treated with albendazole followed by surgical resection of the intact cyst. Chronic calcified cysts can be left untreated.

Schistosomiasis

This affects about 250,000,000 people worldwide. It is caused by *Schistosoma mansoni* (Africa, South America) or *Schistosoma japonicum* (Asia). Infection occurs when the parasite penetrates the skin during swimming or bathing in infected water contaminated by the intermediate host – the freshwater snail. The parasite migrates to the liver via the portal venous system where it matures, migrates back along the portal (and mesenteric) veins and produces numerous eggs which penetrate the gut wall and are excreted to continue the cycle. A chronic granulomatous reaction occurs in the liver leading to periportal fibrosis and cirrhosis.

- Early symptoms are related to the site of entry of the organism (swimmer's itch) and systemic effects including malaise, fever, myalgia, nausea and vomiting.
- Diagnosis confirmed by detecting ova in stool or liver biopsy. Liver function tests show raised alkaline phosphatase, and there is an eosinophilia.
- Treatment is with praziquantel.

9.13 Hepatic abscesses

Pyogenic abscesses most commonly occur following intra-abdominal sepsis but they can occur spontaneously. The commonest organism isolated is *E. coli* but *Enterococcus*, *Proteus*, *Staphylococcus aureus* and anaerobes are recognised.

- Patients present with swinging pyrexia, weight loss, right upper quadrant pain and anorexia. Septic shock or jaundice may develop.
- Diagnosis is confirmed by liver ultrasound which is used to guide aspiration or insertion of a drain.
- Broad-spectrum antibiotics are given until sensitivities are available; occasionally surgical resection is required.

Amoebic abscesses are caused by *Entamoeba histolytica* which spreads from the gut (where it can cause an acute diarrhoeal illness) via the portal system to the liver. Single or multiple cysts may be found on ultrasound and treatment is with metronidazole.

9.14 Hepato-biliary tumours

There are a number of types of primary hepatic malignancy, all of which are rare. Secondary tumours, however, are common, typically metastasising from the stomach, colon, breast and lung.

Treatment of metastatic tumours is usually not indicated as the disease process is far advanced, although chemotherapy may slow progression in selected patients.

Hepatocellular carcinoma

This is rare in the UK (1–2/100, 000 population) but the incidence is increased 20–30 times in Africa, Asia and Japan.

Incidence is increased by:

- hepatitis B (commonest cause worldwide) and hepatitis C virus
- cirrhosis from any cause, particularly hepatitis B, C and haemochromatosis
- aflatoxin – a carcinogen from the mould *Aspergillus flavus* which may contaminate food
- long-term oral contraceptive use.

Raised serum AFP suggest the diagnosis and, in association with ultrasound, has been suggested as an appropriate annual screening for patients with cirrhosis.

Prognosis of hepatocellular carcinoma

Treatment	Prognosis
No treatment	Five-year survival <25%
Resection	Only 5–15% are suitable, with 20% operative mortality; five-year survival <30%
Transplant	Very few patients are suitable – they should have single tumours smaller than 5 cm with no vascular or metastatic spread; five-year survival 90%
Chemotherapy/ethanol injection into tumour/embolisation	Palliative with little survival benefit

Cholangiocarcinoma

This is an uncommon adenocarcinoma arising from the biliary epithelium.

Predisposing factors:

- sclerosing cholangitis
- choledochal cyst or other biliary tract abnormality
- liver fluke infection
- Carolli's disease (dilation of the intrahepatic bile ducts predisposing to infection and stone formation).

Treatment	Prognosis
No treatment	Average survival 2 months
Resection	Fewer than 20% of patients are suitable; average survival approximately 3 years
Transplant	Very few patients are suitable but this gives the best prognosis

Carcinoma of the gall bladder

This adenocarcinoma occurs in the elderly but is uncommon. It has usually invaded locally or metastasised by the time of diagnosis.

Benign hepatic adenoma

The incidence of this is increased in patients who have been taking oral contraceptives for longer than 5 years and also with the use of anabolic steroids. It is usually asymptomatic but may rarely cause intraperitoneal bleeding or right upper quadrant pain.

Hepatic haemangioma

This is common, and is often an incidental finding on ultrasound. It is benign but may occasionally rupture.

Chapter 7
Genetics

CONTENTS

Genetics

1. CHROMOSOMES

Within the nucleus of somatic cells there are 22 pairs of autosomes and one pair of sex chromosomes. Normal male and female karyotypes are 46,XY and 46,XX, respectively. The normal chromosome complement is known as **diploid**. Genomes with a single copy of each chromosome are known as **haploid**, and those with three copies of each chromosome are known as **triploid**. A karyotype with too many or too few chromosomes, in which the total is not a multiple of 23, is called **aneuploid**. Chromosomes are divided by the centromere into a short 'p' arm ('petit') and long 'q' arm. **Acrocentric** chromosomes (13, 14, 15, 21, 22) have the centromere at one end.

Lyonisation is the process whereby in a cell containing more than one X chromosome, only one is active. Selection of the active X is usually random and each inactivated X chromosome can be seen as a Barr body on microscopy. **Mitosis** occurs in somatic cells and results in two diploid daughter cells with nuclear chromosomes that are genetically identical both to each other and the original parent cell.

Meiosis occurs in the germ cells of the gonads and is also known as 'reduction division' because it results in four **haploid** daughter cells, each containing just one member (homologue) of each chromosome pair and all genetically different. Meiosis involves two divisions (**meiosis I and II**). The reduction in chromosome number occurs during meiosis I and is preceded by exchange of chromosome segments between homologous chromosomes called **crossing over**. In males the onset of meiosis and spermatogenesis is at puberty. In females, replication of the chromosomes and crossing over begins in fetal life but the oocytes remain suspended prior to the first cell division until just before ovulation.

Translocations

- **Reciprocal**: exchange of genetic material between non-homologous chromosomes
- **Robertsonian**: fusion of two acrocentric chromosomes at their centromeres (eg 14;21)
- **Unbalanced**: if chromosomal material has been lost or gained overall
- **Balanced**: if no chromosomal material has been lost or gained overall.

Figure 1 Mitosis

Chromosomes replicate forming
2 chromatids joined at the centromere,
and condense

Homologous chromosomes
align independently on the spindle

Chromatids move to opposite
poles and cell divides

2 diploid daughter cells, genetically
identical to each other and the
parent cell

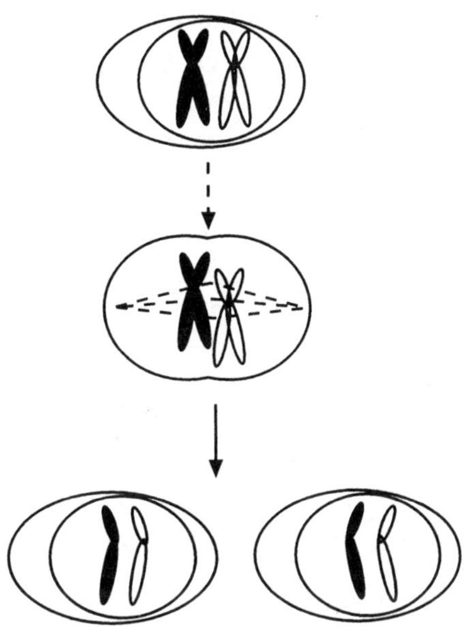

Figure 2 Meiosis

Chromosomes replicate, condense
and homologues pair up and cross-over

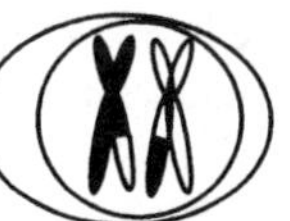

Meiosis I (reduction division)
Homologous chromosomes move to opposite
poles and the cell divides

chromosomes align on
spindle in pairs

Meiosis II
Chromatids move to opposite poles
and the cells divide

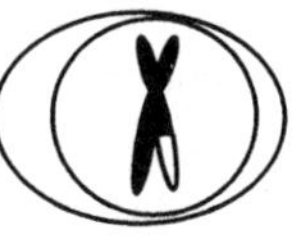

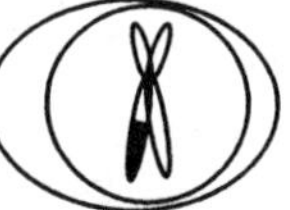

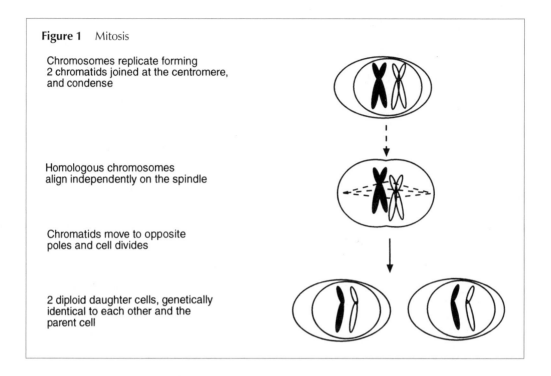

chromosomes align on
spindle

4 haploid daughter
cells, all genetically
different

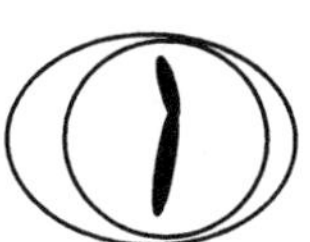

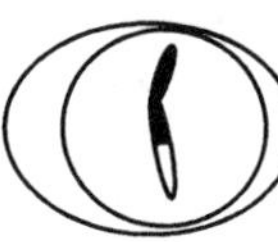

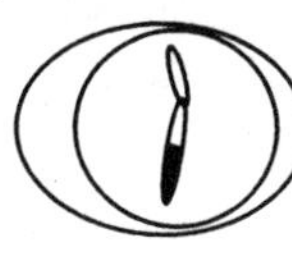

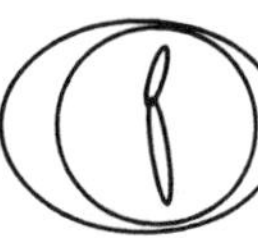

1.1 Common sex chromosome aneuploidies

Turner's syndrome (karyotype 45,X)

This affects one in 2500 live-born females but it is a frequent finding amongst early miscarriages. Patients are usually of normal intelligence. They have streak ovaries which result in failure of menstruation, low oestrogen with high gonadotrophins and infertility.

Normal secondary sexual characteristics may develop spontaneously or be induced with oestrogens. Short stature throughout childhood with failure of the pubertal growth spurt is typical. Final height can be increased by early treatment with growth hormone. Other features may include the following.

Features of Turner's syndrome

- Webbed or short neck
- Shield chest with widely spaced nipples
- Renal abnormalities (eg horseshoe kidney, duplicated ureters, renal aplasia) in approximately 30%
- Low hairline
- Cubitus valgus (wide carrying angle)
- Cardiovascular abnormalities, particularly aortic coarctation in 10–15%
- Non-pitting lymphoedema in approximately 30%

Triple X syndrome (karyotype 47,XXX)

These patients show little phenotypic abnormality but tend to be of tall stature. Intelligence is typically reduced compared with siblings but usually falls within normal or low–normal limits. Mild developmental and behavioural difficulties are more common. Fertility is normal but the incidence of early menopause is increased.

Klinefelter's syndrome (karyotype 47,XXY)

This affects 1 in 600 newborn males. Phenotypic abnormalities are rare prepubertally other than a tendency to tall stature. At puberty, spontaneous expression of secondary sexual characteristics is variable but poor growth of facial and body hair is common. The testes are small in association with azoospermia, testosterone production around 50% of normal and raised gonadotrophins. Gynaecomastia occurs in 30% and there is an increased risk of male breast cancer. Female distribution of fat and hair and a high-pitched voice may occur but are not typical. Intelligence is generally reduced compared with siblings but usually falls within normal or low–normal limits. Mild developmental delay (especially speech) and behavioural problems are more common.

47,XYY males

These males are phenotypically normal but tend to be tall. Intelligence is usually within normal limits but there is an increased incidence of behavioural abnormalities.

1.2 Common autosomal chromosome aneuploidies

Down's syndrome (trisomy 21)

Down's syndrome affects one in 700 live births overall and is usually secondary to meiotic non-disjunction during oogenesis, which is more common with increasing maternal age. Around 5% of patients have an underlying Robertsonian translocation, most commonly between chromosomes 14 and 21. Around 3% have detectable **mosaicism** (a mixture of trisomy 21 and karyotypically normal cells) usually resulting in a milder phenotype. Phenotypic features include the following.

Phenotypic features of Down's syndrome

- Brachycephaly
- Protruding tongue
- Single palmar crease, 5th finger clinodactyly, wide sandal gaps between 1st and 2nd toes
- Upslanting palpebral fissures, epicanthic folds, Brushfield spots on the iris
- Hypotonia and moderate mental retardation

The following are more common in patients with Down's syndrome.

Common features of Down's syndrome

- Cardiovascular malformations in 40%, particularly atrioventricular septal defects (AVSD)
- Haematological abnormalities, particularly acute lymphoblastic leukaemia (ALL), acute myeloblastic leukaemia (AML) and transient leukaemias
- Gastrointestinal abnormalities in 6%, particularly duodenal atresia and Hirschsprung's disease
- Hypothyroidism
- Cataracts in 3%
- Alzheimer's disease in the majority by 40 years of age

Edwards' syndrome (trisomy 18 [eighteen])

This typically causes intrauterine growth retardation, a characteristic facies, prominent occiput, overlapping fingers (2nd and 5th overlap 3rd and 4th), rockerbottom feet (vertical talus) and short dorsiflexed great toes. Malformations, particularly congenital heart disease, diaphragmatic hernias, renal abnormalities and dislocated hips, are more common. Survival beyond early infancy is rare but associated with profound mental handicap.

Patau syndrome (trisomy 13)

Affected infants usually have multiple malformations, including holoprosencephaly and other CNS abnormalities, scalp defects, microphthalmia, cleft lip and palate, post-axial polydactyly, rockerbottom feet, renal abnormalities and congenital heart disease. Survival beyond early infancy is rare and associated with profound mental handicap.

1.3 Microdeletion syndromes

These are caused by chromosomal deletions that are too small to be seen microscopically but involve two or more adjacent genes. They can be detected using specific fluorescent probes (**f**luorescent **i**n **s**itu **h**ybridisation (**FISH**)).

Examples of microdeletion syndromes are:

- **Di George syndrome** (parathyroid gland hypoplasia with hypocalcaemia, thymus hypoplasia with T-lymphocyte deficiency, congenital cardiac malformations particularly interrupted aortic arch and truncus arteriosus, cleft palate, learning disability) due to microdeletions at 22q11. There is an increased incidence of psychiatric disorders, particularly within the schizophrenic spectrum.
- **William's syndrome** (supravalvular aortic stenosis, hypercalcaemia, stellate irides, mental retardation, chatty, sociable behaviour known as a 'cocktail party manner') due to microdeletions involving the elastin gene on chromosome 7.

2. MENDELIAN INHERITANCE

2.1 Autosomal dominant (AD) conditions

These result from mutation of one copy (allele) of a gene carried on an autosome. All offspring of an affected person have a 50% chance of inheriting the mutation. Within a family the severity may vary (**variable expression**) and known mutation carriers may appear clinically normal (**reduced penetrance**). Some conditions, such as achondroplasia and neurofibromatosis (type 1), frequently begin de novo through new mutations arising in the egg or (more commonly) in the sperm.

Examples of autosomal dominant (AD) conditions*

Achondroplasia
Ehlers–Danlos syndrome (most)
Facioscapulohumeral dystrophy
Familial adenomatous polyposis coli
Familial hypercholesterolaemia
Gilbert's syndrome
Huntington's chorea
Marfan's syndrome
Neurofibromatosis types 1 and 2
Porphyrias (except congenital erythropoietic and erythropoietic protoporphyria which are autosomal recessive)
Tuberous sclerosis
von Willebrand's disease

An exception is hereditary haemochromatosis which is autosomal recessive (see Section 2.2).

* Conditions prefixed 'hereditary' or 'familial' are usually autosomal dominant

Noonan's syndrome

This is an autosomal dominant condition which is known to be heterogeneous (ie mutations at more than one gene locus can cause the Noonan phenotype). In around 40% of patients the condition is caused by mutations in the *PTPN11* gene (*Protein Tyrosine Phosphatase Non receptor type 11*) on chromosome 12. In the remainder, the gene is still unknown, and it is likely that there will be more than one gene locus involved. The karyotype is usually normal.

Clinical features of Noonan's syndrome

- **Cardiac**
  Pulmonary valve stenosis
  Hypertrophic cardiomyopathy
  Septal defects (ASD, VSD)
  Branch pulmonary artery stenosis
- **Other features**
  Ptosis
  Low-set and/or posteriorly rotated ears
  Small genitalia and undescended testes in boys
  Coagulation defects in 30% (particle factor XI:C, XIIC and VIIIC deficiencies)
  von Willebrand's disease
  Thrombocytopenia
  Mild mental retardation in 30%
- **Musculoskeletal**
  Webbed or short neck
  Pectus excavatum or carinatum
  Wide-spaced nipples
  Cubitus valgus
  Short stature in 80%

2.2 Autosomal recessive (AR) conditions

These result from mutations in both copies (alleles) of an autosomal gene. Where both parents are carriers each of their offspring has a one in four (25%) risk of being affected, and a 50% chance of being a carrier.

Examples of autosomal recessive (AR) conditions

Alkaptonuria	Homocystinuria
Ataxia telangiectasia	Haemochromatosis
β-thalassaemia	Mucopolysaccharidoses (all except Hunter's syndrome)
Congenital adrenal hyperplasia	Oculocutaneous albinism
Crigler–Najjar (severe form)	Phenylketonuria
Cystic fibrosis	Rotor (usually)
Dubin–Johnson	Sickle cell anaemia
Fanconi anaemia	Spinal muscular atrophy
Galactosaemia	Wilson's disease
Glucose-6-phosphatase deficiency (von Gierkes)*	Xeroderma pigmentosa
Glycogen storage diseases	

Most metabolic disorders are autosomal recessive – remember the exceptions

X-linked recessive exceptions: Hunter's syndrome (mucopolysaccharidosis type 2), glucose-6-phosphate dehydrogenase deficiency (Favism), childhood form of adrenoleukodystrophy.

Autosomal dominant exceptions: acute intermittent porphyria, variegate porphyria, familial hypercholesterolaemia.

* Do not confuse with glucose-6-phosphate dehydrogenase deficiency (favism) which is X-linked recessive

Hereditary haemochromatosis

As stated previously, 'hereditary' or 'familial' conditions are usually autosomal dominant. Although hereditary haemochromatosis is autosomal recessive, the carrier frequency is high (around 1 in 10 or greater) and so **pseudo dominant** inheritance has been observed. The latter occurs because the partner of an affected person is coincidently a carrier so that, on average, 50% of their offspring will have a genotype predisposing to clinical haemochromatosis. An apparent vertical (dominant) transmission is noted. Only a proportion of patients with mutations on both alleles will become symptomatic and the penetrance is higher in males than females. (*See also* Chapter 6, Gastroenterology and Chapter 13, Metabolic Diseases.)

2.3 X-linked recessive (XLR) conditions

These result from a mutation in a gene carried on the X chromosome and affect males because they have just one gene copy. Females are usually unaffected but may have mild manifestations as a result of lyonisation. This form of inheritance is characterised by the following:

- no male-to-male transmission (an affected father passes his Y chromosome to all his sons)
- all daughters of an affected male are carriers (an affected father passes his X chromosome to all his daughters)
- sons of a female carrier have a 50% chance of being affected and daughters have a 50% chance of being carriers.

Examples of X-linked recessive (XLR) conditions

Alport's syndrome (usually)
Becker muscular dystrophy
Duchenne muscular dystrophy
Fabry's disease
Fragile X syndrome
Glucose-6-phosphate dehydrogenase deficiency (favism)
Haemophilias A and B (Christmas disease)
Hunter's syndrome (MPS II)
Lesch–Nyhan syndrome
Ocular albinism
Red–green colour blindness
Testicular feminisation syndrome
Wiskott-Aldrich syndrome

2.4 X-linked dominant (XLD) conditions

These are caused by a mutation in one copy of a gene on the X chromosome but both male and female mutation carriers are affected. Because of lyonisation, females are usually more mildly affected and these disorders are frequently lethal in males, for the reasons outlined above.

- There is no male-to-male transmission.
- All daughters of an affected male are affected.
- All offspring of an affected female have a 50% chance of being affected.

Examples of X-linked dominant (XLD) conditions include:

- **Vitamin D-resistant rickets**: this results from mutations in the *PHEX* (phosphate regulating gene with homology to endopeptidases, X-linked) gene.
- **Incontinentia pigmenti**: a disorder of girls causing vesicular skin lesions in infancy with variable hypodontia (small teeth), alopecia, retinal and other abnormalities. This results from mutations in the *NEMO* (NF-κ-B essential modulator) gene.
- **Rett syndrome**: a disorder of girls associated with developmental regression, progressive microcephaly, stereotypic hand movements and irregular breathing patterns. This results from mutations in the *MECP2* (methyl CpG binding protein 2) gene.
- **Periventricular nodular heterotopia**: this is associated with epilepsy and occasional learning disability in females and with embryonic lethality in males. It results from certain mutations in the *FLNA* (filamin A) gene.

3. MOLECULAR GENETICS

3.1 DNA (deoxyribonucleic acid)

DNA is a **double-stranded** molecule composed of purine (adenine + guanine) and pyrimidine (cytosine and thymine) bases linked by a backbone of covalently bonded **deoxyribose sugar** phosphate residues. The two anti-parallel strands are held together by hydrogen bonds, which can be disrupted by heating, and re-form on cooling.

- **Adenine (A)** pairs with **thymine (T)** by two hydrogen bonds.
- **Guanine (G)** pairs with **cytosine (C)** by three hydrogen bonds.

3.2 RNA (ribonucleic acid)

DNA is **transcribed** in the nucleus into messenger RNA (mRNA) which is **translated** by ribosomes in the cytoplasm into a polypeptide chain. RNA differs from DNA in that:

- it is **single-stranded**
- thymine is replaced by **uracil**
- the sugar backbone is **ribose**.

3.3 Polymerase chain reaction (PCR)

This is a widely used method for generating large amounts of DNA from very small samples. PCR can be adapted for use with RNA providing the RNA is first converted to DNA. For a more detailed account *see* Chapter 14, Molecular Medicine.

4. TRINUCLEOTIDE REPEAT DISORDERS

(*See also* Chapter 14, Molecular Medicine.) These conditions are associated with genes containing stretches of repeating units of three nucleotides and include the following.

Trinucleotide repeat disorders

- Fragile X syndrome XLR
- Huntington's chorea AD
- Spinocerebellar ataxia AD
- Myotonic dystrophy AD
- Friedreich's ataxia AR

In normal individuals the number of repeats varies slightly but remains below a defined threshold. Affected patients have an increased number of repeats, called an **expansion**, above the disease-causing threshold. The expansions may be unstable and enlarge further in successive generations causing increased disease severity ('**anticipation**') and earlier onset, eg **myotonic dystrophy**, particularly congenital myotonic dystrophy following transmission by an affected mother.

4.1 Fragile X syndrome

This causes mental retardation, macro-orchidism and seizures and is often associated with a cytogenetically visible constriction on the X chromosome. The inheritance is X-linked but complex. Among controls there are between 6 and 55 stably inherited trinucleotide repeats in the *FMR1* gene. People with between 55 and 230 repeats are said to be premutation carriers but are unaffected. During oogenesis in female premutation carriers the triplet repeat is unstable and may expand into the disease causing a range (230 to >1000 repeats) known as a **full mutation**. All males and around 50% of females with the full mutation are affected.

5. MITOCHONDRIAL DISORDERS

(*See also* Chapter 14, Molecular Medicine.) Mitochondria are **exclusively maternally inherited**, deriving from those present in the cytoplasm of the ovum. They contain copies of their own **circular 16.5-kilobase chromosome** carrying genes for several respiratory chain enzyme subunits and transfer RNAs. Mitochondrial genes differ from nuclear genes in having no introns and using some different amino acid codons. Within a tissue or even a cell there may be a mixed population of normal and abnormal mitochondria known as **heteroplasmy**. Different proportions of abnormal mitochondria may be required to cause disease in different tissues, known as a **threshold effect**. Disorders caused by mitochondrial gene mutations include the following:

- **MELAS** (**m**itochondrial **e**ncephalopathy, **l**actic **a**cidosis, **s**troke-like episodes)
- **MERRF** (**m**yoclonic **e**pilepsy, **r**agged **r**ed **f**ibres)
- mitochondrially inherited diabetes mellitus and deafness
- Leber's hereditary optic neuropathy (NB other factors also contribute so that penetrance is much higher in males).

6. GENOMIC IMPRINTING

For most genes both copies are expressed but for some genes, either the maternally or paternally derived copy is preferentially used, a phenomenon known as genomic imprinting. The best examples are the **Prader–Willi** and **Angelman** syndromes, both caused by either cytogenetic deletions of the same region of chromosome 15q or by **uniparental disomy** of chromosome 15 (where both copies of chromosome 15 are derived from one parent with no copy of chromosome 15 from the other parent).

Other well recognised imprinting disorders include:

- Beckwith–Wiedemann syndrome
- Russell–Silver syndrome
- Albright's hereditary osteodystrophy.

Each of the above conditions is described below.

Genomic imprinting: comparison between Prader–Willi and Angelman syndromes

	Prader-Willi	Angelman
Clinical	Neonatal hypotonia and poor feeding Moderate mental handicap Hyperphagia + obesity in later childhood Small genitalia	'Happy puppet', unprovoked laughter/clapping Microcephaly, severe mental handicap Ataxia, broad-based gait Seizures, characteristic EEG
Genetics	70% deletion on **p**aternal chromosome 15 30% maternal uniparental disomy 15 (ie no paternal contribution)	80% deletion on maternal chromosome 15 2–3% paternal uniparental disomy 15 (ie no maternal contribution); remainder due to subtle mutations

Albright's hereditary osteodystrophy

Autosomal dominant.

This results from the deactivating mutations in the *GNAS* gene (alpha subunit of the adenylyl cyclase stimulating G-protein, Gs) on chromosome 20q13. Mutations on the maternally derived *GNAS* allele result in an associated pseudohypoparathyroidism. The typical clinical features are:

- short adult stature with a tendency to obesity
- round facies
- mild-moderate learning disabilities
- brachydactyly: short metacarpals, particularly 4 and 5, and short distal phalanges (particularly the thumb)
- ectopic ossifications.

Beckwith–Wiedemann syndrome

This is due to abnormal imprinting of the *IGF2/H19/p57^{KIP}/KvLqQT1* gene cluster on chromosome 11p15.

The clinical features are of:

- large birth weight
- neonatal hyperinsulinism causing hypoglycaemia
- omphalocele (exomphalos)
- hemihypertrophy
- facial nevus flammeus
- increased risk of childhood abdominal tumours (particularly Wilms' tumour and hepatoblastoma).

Russell–Silver syndrome

- This condition has a prenatal onset with small stature and relative macrocephaly
- Patients also have a triangular face, asymmetry and 5th finger clinodactyly
- Maternal uniparental disomy for chromosome 7 is seen in around 10% of cases.

7. OTHER IMPORTANT GENETICS TOPICS

This section includes short notes on conditions that form popular exam topics. See also homocystinuria (Chapter 13, Metabolic Diseases) and muscular dystrophy (Chapters 14, Molecular Medicine, and 16, Neurology).

7.1 Ambiguous genitalia

(*See also* 'intersex' in Chapter 4, Endocrinology.)

Figure 3 Outline of the normal development of the reproductive tract and external genitalia

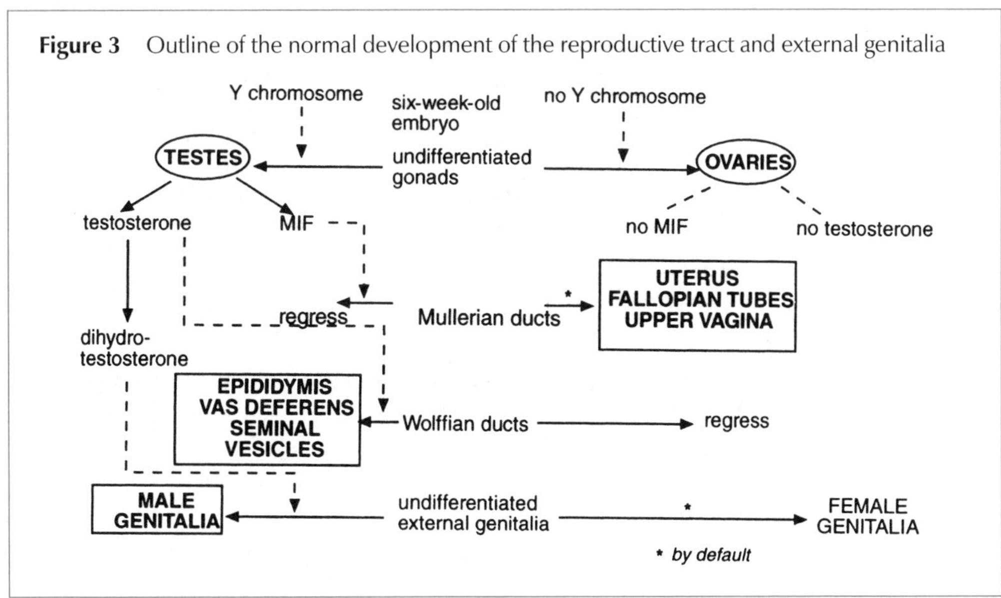

The six-week embryo has undifferentiated gonads, Mullerian ducts (capable of developing into the uterus, Fallopian tubes and upper vagina), Wolffian ducts (capable of forming the epididymis, vas deferens and seminal vesicles) and undifferentiated external genitalia.

In the presence of a Y chromosome the gonads become testes which produce testosterone and Mullerian inhibiting factor (MIF). Testosterone causes the Wolffian ducts to persist and differentiate and, after conversion to dihydrotestosterone (by 5α-reductase), masculinisation of the external genitalia. MIF causes the Mullerian ducts to regress.

In the absence of a Y chromosome the gonads become ovaries which secrete neither testosterone nor MIF. In the absence of testosterone the Wolffian ducts regress and the external genitalia feminise. In the absence of MIF, the Mullerian ducts persist and differentiate.

The causes of **ambiguous genitalia** divide broadly into those resulting in undermasculinisation of a male fetus, those causing masculinisation of a female fetus, and those resulting from mosaicism for a cell line containing a Y chromosome and another which does not. They are summarised in the diagram below.

Figure 4 Outline of causes of ambiguous genitalia

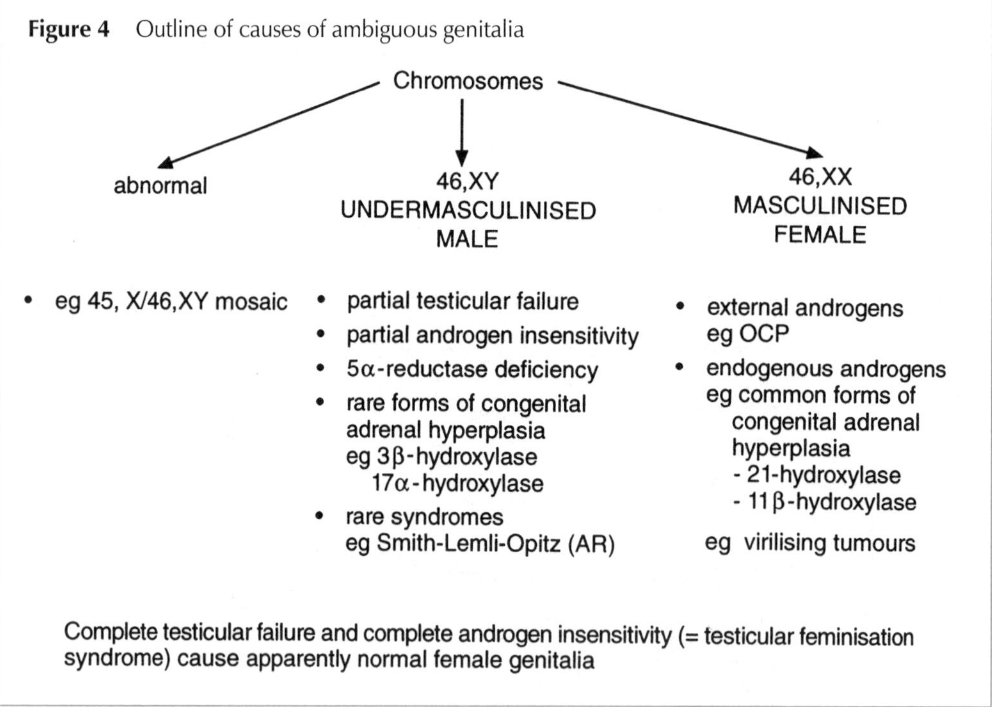

7.2 Cystic fibrosis

This results from mutations in the **CFTR** (cystic fibrosis transmembrane conductance regulator) gene and the **ΔF508** mutation (deletion of three nucleotides coding for a phenylalanine residue) accounts for 75% of mutations in Caucasians. Around 15% of cystic fibrosis mutations cannot be detected so that molecular testing cannot exclude a diagnosis of cystic fibrosis. (*See also* Chapter 19, Respiratory Medicine.)

7.3 Neurofibromatosis (NF)

There are two forms of NF which are clinically and genetically distinct.

Comparison of both forms of neurofibromatosis

	NF1	NF2
Major features	≥6 café-au-lait patches (CALs) Axillary/inguinal freckling Lisch nodules on the iris Peripheral neurofibromas	Bilateral acoustic neuromas (vestibular schwannomas) Other cranial and spinal tumours Lens opacities/cataracts Peripheral schwannomas
Minor features	Macrocephaly Short stature	CALs (usually < 6) Peripheral neurofibromas
Complications	Plexiform neuromas Optic glioma (2%) Other cranial and spinal tumours Pseudoarthrosis (especially tibial) Renal artery stenosis Phaeochromocytoma Learning difficulties Scoliosis Spinal cord and nerve compressions Malignant change/sarcomas	Deafness/tinnitus/vertigo Spinal cord and nerve compressions Malignant change/sarcomas
Gene	Chromosome 17	Chromosome 22

7.4 Tuberous sclerosis (TS)

There are at least two separate genes that cause TS, one on chromosome 9 (*TSC1*, hamartin) and the other on chromosome 16 (TSC2, tuberin).

Clinical features of tuberous sclerosis

- **Skin/nails**
  Ash-leaf macules
  Shagreen patches (especially over the lumbosacral area)
  Adenoma sebaceum (facial area)
  Subungual/periungual fibromas
- **Kidneys**
  Renal cysts
- **Neuro-imaging**
  Intracranial calcification (periventricular)
  Subependymal nodules
- **Eyes**
  Retinal hamartomas
- **Heart**
  Cardiac rhabdomyomas, detectable antenatally, usually regressing during childhood
- **Neurological**
  Seizures
  Mental handicap

7.5 Marfan's syndrome

This results from mutations in the fibrillin gene on chromosome 15. Intelligence is usually normal.

Clinical features of Marfan's syndrome

- **Musculoskeletal**
  Tall stature with disproportionately long limbs (dolichostenomelia)
  Arachnodactyly
  Pectus carinatum or excavatum
  Scoliosis
  High, narrow arched palate
  Joint laxity
  Pes planus
- **Heart**
  Aortic root dilatation and dissection
  Mitral valve prolapse
- **Eyes**
  Lens dislocation (typically up)
  Myopia
- **Skin**
  Striae
- **Pulmonary**
  Spontaneous pneumothorax
  Apical blebs on chest X-ray
- **Radiological**
  Protrussio acetabulae
  Dural ectasia on spinal MRI

The diagnosis of Marfan's syndrome is based upon the Ghent criteria (which are beyond the scope of this section) which divide clinical features into major and minor within each body system. For a definite diagnosis of Marfan's syndrome patients should have:

- a major criterion in at least two body systems and involvement of a third **or**
- a major criterion in one body system with involvement of a second system **and**
- a first-degree relative with confirmed Marfan's syndrome.

Chapter 8
Genito-urinary Medicine and AIDS

CONTENTS

Genito-urinary Medicine and AIDS

1. SEXUALLY TRANSMITTED INFECTIONS

The incidence of sexually transmitted infection (STI) has increased dramatically over the past 40 years both globally and in the UK. As well as the more 'traditional' diseases such as syphilis and gonorrhoea, a wider spectrum of diseases transmitted by sexual contact has increasingly been recognised (eg oro-anal transmission of enteric infections such as giardiasis and hepatitis A). HIV infection arrived on the scene in the late 1970s.

1.1 Gonorrhoea

Transmission is primarily sexual; there is a large asymptomatic reservoir, mainly pharyngeal, rectal and cervical. *Neisseria gonorrhoea* is a capsulated organism, and it therefore resists phagocytosis. In the UK penicillin is the most appropriate treatment for susceptible organisms. However, resistance is present in 10% of cases and quinolones or ceftriaxone can be used depending on anti-microbial sensitivities.

Disseminated (bacteraemic) infection is unusual but is more common in women. Responsible strains are nearly always highly susceptible to penicillin. Pharyngeal and rectal infection is often asymptomatic. Ophthalmia neonatorum is treated with systemic anti-microbials and appropriate eye drops.

1.2 Syphilis

Transmission is primarily sexual, congenital or, rarely, by blood transfusion. Penicillin is the drug of choice, or alternatively tetracycline. **Concurrent HIV infection may increase the risk of neurosyphilis**, and extended courses of treatment are required. Diagnosis is by:

- **Serology**: two treponemal tests, enzyme immunoassay (EIA) and *Treponema pallidum* haemagglutination assay (TPHA) (would use specific treponemal antigen) plus a quantitative non-treponemal test, rapid plasma reagin (RPR) or venereal disease reference laboratory (VDRL). The latter are non-specific (cardiolipin antigen) and biologically false-positive results can be obtained in other conditions.
- **Dark ground microscopy**: of **fresh** material from chancres or lesions of secondary syphilitic rash.

1.3 *Chlamydia* infections

Non-gonococcal urethritis (NGU) due to *Chlamydia trachomatis* is the most common bacterial STI in the Western world. Serovars D to K are responsible. It is also a major cause of pelvic inflammatory disease in women (frequently silent) and prostatitis/epididymitis in men. Neonatal conjunctivitis and, more rarely, diffuse interstitial pneumonia are both complications of serovars D to K; infection is acquired by passage through an infected birth canal.

- **Trachoma** (corneal scarring) is caused by serovars A, B and C.
- **Lymphogranuloma venereum (LGV)** is due to serovars L1, L2 and L3.

Both pneumonia and conjunctivitis need systemic treatment with erythromycin. Tetracycline or azithromycin is the drug of choice for adults.

2. BASIC EPIDEMIOLOGY AND VIROLOGY OF HIV/AIDS

2.1 Epidemiology

HIV/AIDS is a global disease. Of the estimated 42 million people infected with HIV, 30 million are from sub-Saharan Africa. In the UK the cumulative incidence of HIV (in 2002) is approximately 54, 000, and of AIDS 19, 000.

The following are the estimated routes of transmission in the current UK HIV population:

- sexual intercourse between men (30%)
- sexual intercourse between men and women (50%) – mainly acquired abroad
- injecting drug abuse (7%)
- blood and blood products (5%).

Risk factors facilitating sexual transmission include:

- seroconversion and advancing stage of disease
- concurrent STIs, particularly ulcerative disease of the genitalia.

Materno-fetal transmission occurs in 15–20% of non-breast-fed and 33% of breast-fed infants of patients with HIV/AIDS.

The risk of transmission from mother to baby can be reduced by:

- anti-retroviral therapy (this can reduce transmission to only 1–2% if therapy is started before the third trimester)
- avoidance of breast feeding
- delivery by Caesarean section.

2.2 The virus

Human retrovirus is a member of the lentivirus family. It contains RNA which is transcribed to DNA via a reverse transcriptase enzyme. The main target sites of action of anti-retroviral drugs are reverse transcriptases and proteases. There are two types of human immunodeficiency virus:

- **HIV-1**: (previously known as HTLV III) is prevalent world-wide.
- **HIV-2**: is common in West Africa.

Pathogenesis

The HIV virus has tropism for the following CD4 cells:

- T-helper lymphocytes
- B-lymphocytes
- macrophages
- CNS cells.

It causes progressive immune dysfunction, characterised by CD4 cell depletion. Impairment of immunity is primarily cell-mediated, but as the disease progresses there is general immune dysregulation.

The following laboratory markers are associated with disease progression:

- Decreased CD4 lymphocyte count (normal > $500/mm^3$ or $0.5 \times 10^9/l$). In the USA, a CD4 count of $<200/mm^3$ is regarded as acquired immune deficiency syndrome (AIDS), irrespective of the presence of clinical disease.
- High HIV viral load, using HIV PCR assay (note that CD4 and HIV viral load are the only markers monitored in clinical practice which help to predict progression as well as the response to treatment).

2.3 Seroconversion and the HIV antibody test

After inoculation the window or seroconversion period can be up to three months; HIV antibody may not be detectable during this time. The HIV p24 antigen becomes detectable during seroconversion. Current antibody tests detect HIV-1 and HIV-2. Approximately 60–90% of patients develop clinical seroconversion illnesses of variable severity, and which are often diagnosed retrospectively. HIV PCR and p24 antigen are used to diagnose HIV infection during this window period, and they are then confirmed by a positive antibody test. If the seroconversion illness is severe then anti-retroviral combination treatment should be used. Whether such early treatment improves long-term prognosis is unknown.

Seroconversion illnesses

- Fever
- Malaise
- Diarrhoea
- Meningo-encephalitis
- Rash
- Sore throat
- Lymphadenopathy
- Arthralgia

2.4 Center for Disease Control (CDC) classification of HIV/AIDS

The CDC classification is adopted in the USA and most developed countries. HIV infection is not synonymous with AIDS; the latter is a stage of severe immunodeficiency characterised by opportunistic infections and/or tumour.

CDC classification of HIV/AIDS

- **Stage 1**
  Primary seroconversion illness
- **Stage 2**
  Asymptomatic
- **Stage 3**
  Persistent generalised lymphadenopathy
- **Stage 4a**
  AIDS-related complex (ie advanced HIV disease, but having none of the features of stages 4b–d)
- **Stages 4b–d**
  AIDS: patient may have opportunistic infection or tumours, which are termed 'AIDS indicator' illnesses

3. RESPIRATORY DISEASES ASSOCIATED WITH HIV/AIDS

3.1 *Pneumocystis carinii* pneumonia (PCP)

Pneumonia is the most common opportunistic infection and clinical presentation of AIDS. *Pneumocystis carinii* pneumonia (PCP) constitutes 40% of all AIDS-defining illness.

The symptoms of PCP include dry cough, dyspnoea, fever and malaise. There are remarkably few abnormal signs on chest examination.

Investigations for PCP

- **Chest X-ray**: the typical appearance of PCP is bilateral mid- and lower-zone interstitial shadowing. Atypical chest X-ray findings are found in 10% of PCP cases and include: cavitation, upper zone opacities, pneumothorax or unilateral consolidation. The chest X-ray may be normal and effusions are rare.

- **Pulse oximetry**: hypoxia with low/normal pCO_2 is typically seen in moderate to severe infection. If O_2 saturation is normal then exercise-induced oxygen desaturation (O_2 saturation falling by ≥5% and/or to a saturation of ≤90%, with exercise) will support the diagnosis of PCP.
- **Identification of pneumocystis cysts**: samples obtained by inducing sputum or from broncho-alveolar lavage (BAL) can be stained with silver or immunofluorescent antibody.
- The combination of an HIV-positive person (usually with CD4 <200/mm^3) who is not taking PCP prophylaxis and who has a typical radiological appearance and hypoxia is sufficient for a confident diagnosis to be made. Empirical treatment with cotrimoxazole should be started. It is now unusual to have to result to lung biopsy for PCP diagnosis.

Poor prognostic features in PCP include poor response to treatment, co-infection, requirement for assisted ventilation and pneumothorax.

Treatment for PCP

- Treatment is with high-dose cotrimoxazole or intravenous pentamidine for severe cases. Clindamycin/primaquine, atovaquone and dapsone/trimethoprim are alternative treatments.
- Intolerance to cotrimoxazole is common, with nausea, vomiting, rash, leukopenia and thrombocytopenia.
- Steroids have been shown to improve prognosis in those with pO_2 <8 kPa (60 mmHg).

There is a 50% risk of recurrence within 12 months. **PCP prophylaxis** (cotrimoxazole, nebulised pentamidine, dapsone or atovaquone) is always given to patients with a CD4 count <200/mm^3 and to those who have already had an episode of PCP. Prophylaxis is continued until the CD4 count is increased above 200/mm^3 with the use of highly active anti-retroviral treatment (HAART).

3.2 Pulmonary tuberculosis

The incidence of infection depends upon the prevalence of TB in the rest of the general population and it is therefore much more common in African patients. In some areas of the UK up to a quarter of patients with TB are HIV positive.

Atypical features include:

- Extra-pulmonary involvement.
- Normal or atypical appearances on chest X-ray.
- Occurs at any stage of HIV disease, and at any level of CD4 count.
- Atypical mycobacterial infections (when CD4 count <50/mm^3) – usually *Mycobacterium avium intracellulare*. The usual presenting features are fever, anaemia, anorexia and the disease is commonly extra-pulmonary.

3.3 Other respiratory diseases in HIV/AIDS

Other causes of respiratory disease in HIV/AIDS

- **Viral**
  Cytomegalovirus (CMV) pneumonitis
- **Fungal**
  Candida
  Histoplasmosis
  Cryptococcus
  Nocardia
- **Bacterial**
  Streptococcus pneumoniae
  Staphylococcus aureus
  Mycobacterium tuberculosis
  Mycobacterium avium intracellulare
- **Protozoal**
  Toxoplasma
- **Tumour**
  Kaposi's sarcoma (see Section 6.1)
  Non-Hodgkin's lymphoma

Radiological appearance of other infections

- **Cavitation**: *M. tuberculosis*, *Nocardia*, *S. aureus*
- **Consolidation**: *Streptococcus pneumoniae*, Toxoplasma
- **Effusion**: TB (Kaposi's sarcoma may also cause effusion).

4. GASTROINTESTINAL DISEASES IN PATIENTS WITH HIV/AIDS

There are four main presentations:

- oral/oesophageal disease
- abdominal pain/diarrhoea
- biliary/pancreatic disease
- ano-rectal symptoms.

4.1 Oral/oesophageal conditions

Ninety per cent of patients will develop an oral/oesophageal condition:

- oral and oesophageal candidiasis
- periodontal disease (including gingivitis)
- herpes simplex
- lymphoma

- oral hairy leukoplakia (caused by EBV)
- aphthous ulcers
- kaposi's sarcoma
- cytomegalovirus.

These conditions may be asymptomatic, or patients may have dysphagia or odynophagia.

4.2 Diarrhoea/abdominal pain

Weight loss, diarrhoea and malnutrition are very common in patients with any stage of HIV infection, and can be due to specific infection or advanced disease. Approximately 50% of diarrhoeal illnesses are infective in origin (due to specific enteropathogens or opportunistic infections).

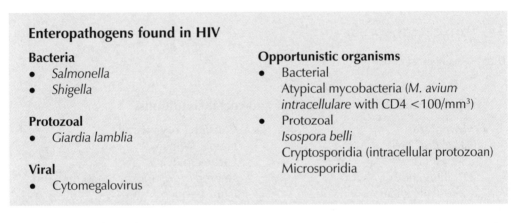

Enteropathogens found in HIV

Bacteria
- *Salmonella*
- *Shigella*

Protozoal
- *Giardia lamblia*

Viral
- Cytomegalovirus

Opportunistic organisms
- Bacterial
  Atypical mycobacteria (*M. avium intracellulare* with CD4 <100/mm^3)
- Protozoal
  Isospora belli
  Cryptosporidia (intracellular protozoan)
  Microsporidia

Clinical presentation can be with watery diffuse diarrhoea as exemplified by *Cryptosporidium*, or abdominal pain and bloody diarrhoea (eg cytomegalovirus procto-colitis).

- **Cryptosporidiosis**: this is a coccidian parasite of the gastrointestinal tract which is responsible for 10–15% of HIV-associated diarrhoeas, particularly occurring in patients with advanced HIV disease.
- **Salmonella**: much more frequent in HIV-infected patients than in the general population. More likely to cause bacteraemia and recurrence is common.

The investigation of infective diarrhoea includes the following:

- Identification of organisms in stool samples: microscopy and culture for pathogens, ovae and parasites.
- If stool specimen negative, stain with modified Ziehl–Neelsen for *Cryptosporidium*.
- Sigmoidoscopy/colonoscopy with biopsy: with culture of the specimen for viruses, mycobacteria, bacteriology and mycology. Histological appearances are often important.

Gastrointestinal tumours

These may also cause abdominal pain and diarrhoea.

- Kaposi's sarcoma.
- Intra-abdominal lymphoma (often high-grade non-Hodgkin's B cell lymphoma).

4.3 Biliary and pancreatic disease

The two most common presentations are **cholangiopathy** and **pancreatitis**.

- **Cholangiopathy**: due to *Cryptosporidium*, cytomegalovirus, or *Microsporidium*.
- **Pancreatitis**: this can be induced by drugs used in HIV treatment (eg DDI (didanosine), or DDC (zalcitabine) which are both reverse transcriptase inhibitors), or by the biliary organisms listed previously.

4.4 Ano-rectal conditions

These usually present with proctitis.

Symptoms and infective causes of ano-rectal conditions

- **Symptoms**
  Anal discharge
  Tenesmus
  Pruritus ani
  Rectal bleeding
  Diarrhoea
- **Causative organisms**
  Herpes simplex
  Cytomegalovirus
  Neisseria gonorrhoeae (gonorrhoea)
  Non-specific/*Chlamydia*
  Wart virus
  Treponema pallidum (syphilis)

5. HIV/AIDS-RELATED NEUROLOGICAL DISORDERS

Neurological disease is the first presentation of AIDS in 10% of HIV patients. An acute self-limiting lymphocytic meningitis may occur at the time of seroconversion. Chronic neurological syndromes or opportunistic infections occur later in the course of HIV infection. The most common cause is the neurotropic effect of the virus itself.

Clinical presentation may be:

- **focal**: hemiparesis, fits
- **generalised**: drowsiness, confusion, behavioural change
- **asymptomatic**: in early HIV disease.

Patients may also develop proximal myopathy, or drug-induced neuropathy (eg didanosine) and myopathy (eg zidovudine).

5.1 Direct neurotropic effects of HIV

These include:

- AIDS dementia complex (see below)
- vacuolar myelopathy
- neuropathy (see below).

Neurotropic disorders are diagnosed with the help of:

- **CSF analysis**: raised protein, and pleocytosis
- **MRI brain scan**: cerebral atrophy
- **nerve conduction studies**: distal symmetric sensory neuropathy.

AIDS dementia is the most frequent neurological condition of HIV infection, and is directly caused by the virus. Impairment of concentration and memory leads to progressive decline in widespread cognitive function. Occasionally psychiatric symptoms may be prominent. The EEG shows generalised slowing with no specific features, and imaging demonstrates cortical atrophy.

Sensorimotor neuropathy associated with HIV/AIDS usually has mild sensory symptoms and signs. Less commonly, a mononeuritis multiplex or a chronic painful myelopathy may develop.

5.2 Neurological infections

Opportunistic infections of the CNS are common.

Causes of focal neurological disease

- ***Toxoplasma gondii***
  Cerebral abscess
- ***Mycobacterium tuberculosis***
  Meningitis
  Tuberculosis abscess

Causes of generalised neurological disease

- ***Cryptococcus neoformans***
  Meningitis
- **Virus family (papovaviro)**
  Progressive multifocal leukoencephalopathy
- **Cytomegalovirus**
  Encephalitis/retinitis
  Peripheral neuropathy

Specific CNS infections

Cerebral toxoplasmosis is the most common CNS infection (90% of focal lesions) and occurs in 10% of AIDS patients. The organism is the crescentic trophozoite form of *Toxoplasma gondii*.

- **Investigations**: CT brain scan shows solitary or multiple ring-enhancing lesions. *Toxoplasma* IgG serology is positive in >90% of cases.
- First-line anti-toxoplasma therapy is pyrimethamine plus sulfadiazine (with folinic acid to prevent bone marrow suppression).
- **Prognosis**: 10% mortality with first episode; 25% of patients have residual neurological deficit.
- It is important to differentiate from primary CNS lymphoma causing a space-occupying lesion.

Cryptococcal meningitis is due to a 'budding' yeast; it occurs in 5–10% of AIDS patients. It presents with a sub-acute meningitic illness.

- Cryptococcal antigen is present in blood and CSF in most cases.
- **India ink stain**: positive in 70% of CSF samples.

Neurosyphilis: the co-existence of HIV and syphilis can result in aggressive and atypical neurosyphilis. Previous syphilis infection may re-activate. The following features are recognised:

- myelopathy
- retinitis
- meningitis
- meningovascular.

Diagnosis: from syphilis serology (rising VDRL and TPHA) and CSF, although serology may be modified by immune dysfunction.

Treatment

The first-line therapy is intramuscular procaine penicillin and probenecid for 14–21 days.

5.3 Ophthalmic disorders

AIDS may affect the lids or any layer of the eye.

Ophthalmic features of AIDS

- **Molluscum contagiosum of lids**
- **Episcleritis and keratitis**
- **Uveitis**
- **Choroidal granulomas**
- **Cytomegalovirus (CMV) retinitis**
- **Neuro-ophthalmic manifestations** (eg cranial nerve palsies, optic neuritis, sequelae to CNS infection or space-occupying lesion)
- **Kaposi's sarcoma of the eyelids or conjunctiva**
- **Retinal changes**: haemorrhages, cotton wool spots, oedema and vascular sheathing
- **Toxoplasmosis**: may develop acquired disease or reactivation of pre-existing disease
- **Candida endophthalmitis**

Retinitis is common and may be caused by HIV itself (non-specific micro-angiopathy which is present in 75% of HIV patients) or by CMV.

CMV retinitis usually occurs when the CD4 count is $<50/mm^3$. This is the most common AIDS-related opportunistic infection in the eye (occurring in 25% of patients).

- **Symptoms**: blurred or loss of vision; floaters.
- **Signs**: soft exudates, and retinal haemorrhages.
- **Prognosis**: initially unilateral eye involvement; ultimately both eyes are affected.

6. MALIGNANT DISEASE IN PATIENTS WITH HIV/AIDS

Despite the introduction of HAART, the incidence of malignant disease in patients with HIV/AIDS has increased in recent years. The most frequently occurring malignancies are:

- Kaposi's sarcoma (83%)
- non-Hodgkin's lymphoma (13%)
- primary CNS lymphoma (4%).

6.1 Kaposi's sarcoma (KS)

This occurs in 10–15% of HIV patients as the first AIDS-defining presentation. The tumour is derived from vascular or lymphatic endothelial cells and is due to infection with human herpes virus type 8 (HHV8). This virus is closely related to EB virus and is transmitted sexually, vertically and via organ transplantation.

- **Clinical presentation**: Kaposi's sarcoma (KS) can be cutaneous visceral involvement. Lesions appear as purple plaques or nodules. The most common systems involved are the gastro-intestinal tract (30% of patients with KS of the skin also have gastrointestinal involvement), lymph nodes and the respiratory system. Patients with pulmonary Kaposi's have cough, dyspnoea and infiltrates, lymphadenopathy or effusion on chest X-ray. KS is now quite uncommon owing to the effect of the new anti-retroviral combination therapies.
- **Diagnosis**: clinical appearance (or biopsy in difficult cases).

7. HIV/AIDS-RELATED SKIN DISEASE

Dermatological diseases are extremely common in HIV patients (affecting 75%), especially in those who have AIDS. During the acute HIV illness, patients may develop an asymptomatic maculo-papular eruption affecting the face and trunk. During seroconversion, they may also develop marked seborrhoeic dermatitis. As the disease progresses to AIDS, the development of tumours and atypical infections is seen.

Dermatological associations of HIV disease

- **General inflammatory dermatoses**
  Psoriasis
  Eczema
  Seborrhoeic dermatitis
  Folliculitis
- **Viral infections**
  Herpes zoster/Herpes simplex
  Human papilloma virus*
  Cytomegalovirus
  Molluscum contagiosum*
- **Fungal/yeast infections**
  *Pityrosporum ovale**
  Candidiasis*
  Cryptococcus neoformans
  Histoplasma capsulatum
- **Bacterial infections**
  Tuberculosis
  Syphilis
  Bacillary angiomatosis
  Staphylococcus aureus
- **Malignancy**
  Kaposi's sarcoma
  Lymphomas
  Cervical intra-epithelial neoplasia*

*Features common in HIV patients

Other skin diseases that are recognised include:

- **generalised maculo-papular rash** (due to drugs): cotrimoxazole (25%), nevirapine (14%), efavirenz (4%), abacavir (5%), dapsone (5%)
- **nail pigmentation**: zidovudine, indinavir.

8. DRUG THERAPIES IN HIV/AIDS PATIENTS

8.1 Specific therapy of common opportunistic infections

Infection	First-line drugs	Side-effects
Pneumocystis pneumonia	Cotrimoxazole (oral, or iv for moderate to severe infection)	Rash, bone marrow toxicity, nausea and fever
	Pentamidine (iv)	Hyper/hypoglycaemia, pancreatitis, hypotension
Cerebral toxoplasmosis	Pyrimethamine and sulfadiazine (in combination)	Bone marrow suppression, fever, gastrointestinal reactions, rash
Cryptococcal meningitis	Amphotericin and flucytosine (in combination)	Chills, fever, gastrointestinal reactions, renal impairment (amphotericin), bone marrow toxicity, liver toxicity
CMV retinitis	Ganciclovir or valganciclovir	Bone marrow suppression
	Foscarnet	Renal impairment
	Cidofovir	Nephrotoxicity

8.2 Anti-retroviral therapy

Anti-retroviral therapy is usually given as combination therapy with the following aims:

- suppression of viral replication
- reducing the risk of viral resistance emerging with three or more drugs
- improving patient immunity with reduction of morbidity and mortality.

Highly active anti-retroviral treatment (HAART)

This involves combinations of at least three drugs; for example, two different nucleoside/nucleotide reverse transcriptase inhibitors (NRTI) in addition to a protease inhibitor (PI), or a non-nucleoside reverse transcriptase inhibitor (NNRTI).

There are three main classes of anti-retroviral drugs currently licensed in the UK. Their modes of action are by inhibition of the viral reverse transcriptase enzyme or by inhibition of protease enzymes.

- Between 20% and 25% of ward admissions in patients with known HIV are due to drug toxicity.
- Patients who fail combination therapy switch to salvage regimens, which might include drugs from all classes (sometimes combinations of four to six drugs are used).

Reverse transcriptase inhibitors

- **Nucleoside/nucleotide analogues (NRTI)**: zidovudine, lamivudine, didanosine, stavudine, zalcitabine, abacavir, tenofovir
- **Non-nucleoside analogues (NNRTI)**: efavirenz, nevirapine, delavirdine.

Protease inhibitors (PI)

These act by inhibiting a protease which is needed to make the virus viable outside the cell. Particular PIs include saquinavir, ritonavir, indinavir, nelfinavir, amprenavir, lopinavir and atazanavir.

Other drugs used as anti-retrovirals

- **Interleukin-2**: this is used to boost CD4 counts in those patients who have had good HIV suppression with therapy, but who have failed to recover CD4 counts. The agent has little effect on HIV viral load.
- **Enfuvirtide (T-20)**: amino acid peptide (GP41) competes with the HIV viral envelope protein for fusion to the cell membrane (therefore, a fusion receptor inhibitor). This is used in conjunction with HAART salvage therapy.

Side-effects of anti-retroviral drugs

- **NRTI**
  Zidovudine: myopathy, anaemia, fatigue, bone marrow toxicity, nail changes
  Stavudine: peripheral neuropathy, lactic acidosis, lipoatrophy
  Lamivudine: peripheral neuropathy, fatigue
  Abacavir: hypersensitivity reaction (can be fatal on re-challenge)
  Didanosine: pancreatitis, peripheral neuropathy
  Zalcitabine (rarely used): peripheral neuropathy

- **NNRTI**
  All agents: potential for drug interactions via the CYP 450 cytochrome family; they can act as inhibitors or inducers
  Nevirapine: rash, hepatitis
  Efavirenz: rash, vivid dreams, hallucinations and depression
  Delavirdine (rarely used): rash

- **PI**
  All agents: diabetes, hypertriglyceridaemia and hypercholesterolaemia (except atazanavir), central adiposity, buffalo hump, peripheral fat loss (lipodystrophy syndrome); there is also great potential for drug interaction via the CYP 450 cytochrome family (ritonavir is the most potent inhibitor known)
  Indinavir: nephrolithiasis, asymptomatic hyperbilirubinaemia
  Nelfinavir: diarrhoea, nausea
  Atazanavir: a new PI which has no effect on lipids but hyperbilirubinaemia occurs in 5%

Monitoring of HIV patients on treatment

- **Clinical assessment**: examination of mouth (for ulcers and candidiasis), skin, lymph nodes, chest, fundoscopy and weight.
- Renal and hepatic function.
- CD4 lymphocyte count.
- HIV viral RNA load.
- Cholesterol, blood sugar, triglycerides.
- Lactate if symptoms of lactic acidosis (muscle pains, malaise, gastrointestinal symptoms, breathlessness) are present.
- **Adherence to treatment**: >90–95% of therapy must be taken to maintain adequate viral suppression and this will also reduce the chance of resistance developing to therapy. If there is evidence of virological failure (increased viral load on >2 tests) then HIV **resistance testing** is indicated. The latter involves viral genotype assay of point mutations associated with anti-retroviral resistance to specific drugs.

8.3 Prognosis of patients with HIV/AIDS

HIV was previously the leading cause of death in the USA in people aged 25–40 years (40 deaths/100, 000). The prognosis of HIV/AIDS patients has now been revolutionised by HAART (introduced 1997) and the death rate has reduced.

- Life expectancy may surpass 25 years after diagnosis.
- All opportunistic illnesses have been reduced dramatically; however, the incidence of **lymphoma** has increased steadily.
- The new anti-retroviral agents also significantly reduce mother-to-baby transmission of the virus from 20% to <2% (if breast-feeding is avoided).
- Individual prognosis depends on viral resistance (10% of new infections in Europe involve a resistant virus), side-effects and adherence to treatment; prognosis is worse if treatment is started when the CD4 count is below 200 cells/mm^3.
- Prognosis is worse in patients who present late with AIDS (mainly heterosexuals who may have no obvious risks); death is due to delay in diagnosis.
- Coronary heart disease, end-stage liver failure (due to co-infection with hepatitis B and C) and malignancy (lymphoma) are now common causes of death in patients with HIV/AIDS.

HIV has now become a treatable chronic illness rather than a fatal disease.

Chapter 9
Haematology

CONTENTS

6. Coagulation

6.1 The coagulation mechanism and detection of factor deficiencies
6.2 Haemophilia
6.3 von Willebrand's disease
6.4 Disseminated intravascular coagulation (DIC)
6.5 Vitamin K dependent coagulation factors (II, VII, IX, X)

7. Thrombosis

7.1 Thrombosis and the pill
7.2 Thrombophilia
7.3 Therapeutic fibrinolysis
7.4 Low molecular weight heparins (LMWH)

8. The spleen

8.1 Causes of splenomegaly
8.2 Splenectomy
8.3 Causes of hyposplenism

9. Blood transfusion

9.1 Transfusion-transmitted infection
9.2 Platelet transfusion in marrow failure
9.3 Indications for the transfusion of fresh frozen plasma

Haematology

1. ANAEMIAS

Anaemia is defined as a reduction in the concentration of circulating haemoglobin. The normal haemoglobin level varies with age and sex; neonates having a relative polycythaemia, infants having a lower haemoglobin level than adults, and women lower levels than men.

Common features of anaemias

- Pallor
- Decreased oxygen-carrying capacity (shortness of breath on exertion, tiredness)
- Increased cardiac output (palpitations, haemic ejection murmurs, cardiac failure in the elderly)

Examination of a bone marrow aspirate allows microscopic examination of the maturing erythroid cells. Normal maturation is termed **normoblastic erythropoiesis**. In conditions where there is interference with DNA synthesis, for example due to lack of vitamin B_{12} or folate, morphological abnormalities are seen. These include chromatin deficiency, premature haemoglobinisation, giant metamyelocytes and other morphological features which, put together, are termed **megaloblastic erythropoiesis**.

Anaemia may be classified by its cause, for example iron deficiency anaemia, but often the cause is not known at the start of investigations so the usual method of classification uses the red cell size (MCV) to classify the anaemias:

- **macrocytic**: anaemia with large red cells
- **microcytic**: anaemia with small red cells
- **normocytic**: anaemia with normal red cell size.

1.1 Causes of macrocytosis

Macrocytosis with a megaloblastic bone marrow

- **B_{12}** deficiency: pernicious anaemia most common
- **Folate deficiency**
- **Drugs**: methotrexate, hydroxyurea, cytosine, azathioprine.

Many other chronically administered cytotoxics also affect nucleic acid synthesis.

Macrocytosis with a normoblastic bone marrow

- **Reticulocytosis**: young cells are big cells
- **Liver disease**
- **Alcohol**
- **Myxoedema** (but check not the associated autoimmune disease pernicious anaemia!)
- **Pregnancy**: usually mild.

Liver disease is associated with anaemia because of interference with manufacture of the lipid envelope of red cells, associated with abnormal liver function tests and target cells on blood film. Alcohol has a direct toxic effect on the marrow and may cause liver disease or folate deficiency.

Macrocytosis associated with haematological diseases with their own special features

- **Myelodysplasia**: associated with cytopenias, monocytosis and dysplastic morphology (with blasts when transforming to acute myeloid leukaemia (AML))
- **Myeloma**: look for paraprotein, high erythrocyte sedimentation rate (ESR), leukoerythroblastic blood picture
- **Myeloproliferative disorders**: polycythaemia rubra vera, essential thrombocythaemia, myelofibrosis, chronic myeloid leukaemia (CML)
- **Aplastic anaemia**: look for pancytopenia with hypoplastic bone marrow.

1.2 Causes of microcytosis

- **Iron deficiency anaemia**: look for pencil cells, check Fe/total iron binding capacity (TIBC) or ferritin
- **Thalassaemia trait**: look for Mediterranean/Asian origin, check Hb A2 level (elevated)
- **Anaemia of chronic disease**: often normocytic, usually obvious disease
- **Sideroblastic anaemia**: the MCV in this disorder may be low, normal or high (see opposite)
- **Aluminium toxicity**: affecting some haemodialysis patients (now uncommon).

1.3 Red cell morphology

Sometimes morphological abnormalities of the red cells are sufficiently characteristic to suggest a diagnosis. These may be commented on in blood film reports. Abnormalities of red cell shape are termed **poikilocytosis**.

Type of poikilocytosis	Found in
Tear drops	Myelofibrosis
Helmet cells and fragmented cells	Microangiopathic haemolysis
Pencil cells	Iron deficiency (with hypochromic microcytes)
Elliptocytes	Hereditary elliptocytosis
Sickle cells	Sickle cell diseases (with target cells)

Other red cell morphological changes

- **Spherocytes**: found in any cause of haemolysis but particularly hereditary spherocytosis and autoimmune haemolytic anaemia.
- **Target cells**: found in liver disease, post-splenectomy, iron deficiency, thalassaemia and haemoglobinopathies.
- **Polychromasia**: young red cells, implies a high reticulocyte count if this is measured.
- **Dimorphic blood picture**: two populations of red cells. Easily spotted using modern blood counters which can provide a graph of cell size and/or haemoglobin content. It is caused by treatment of a haematinic deficiency (the new normal red cells contrast with the persisting cells characteristic of the anaemia); it may also be seen after transfusion of normal red cells to a patient with macro- or microcytosis and occasionally in combined deficiency when separated in time (eg patient with folate deficiency then becomes iron deficient). In primary sideroblastic anaemia the clone of abnormal erythroblasts produces abnormal red cells which contrast with those being produced by residual normal erythropoiesis.

1.4 Sickle cell disease

The sickle cell diseases consist of homozygous sickle cell anaemia (Hb SS), haemoglobin SC disease (Hb SC) and haemoglobin S beta thalassaemia trait (Hb S Thal). The clinical manifestations of sickle cell disease are mainly due to occlusion of small blood vessels by log-jams of sickled red cells. Precipitating causes may be hypoxaemia, infection and dehydration, but often no cause is identified for a vaso-occlusive crisis.

Clinical syndromes recognised in sickle cell disease

- **Simple pain crisis**: due to infarction of red bone marrow, a common problem in sickle cell disease. Deep-seated bone pain often requires opiate analgesia. Vigorous hydration may shorten the duration of the crisis. Hypoxaemia should be corrected and infection treated with antibiotics.

- **Sickle dactylitis**: infarction of the small bones of the hands or feet may be the earliest manifestation of sickle cell disease. Local pain and swelling result, with possible long-term deformity.
- **Splenic sequestration crisis**: in adults the spleen has usually atrophied by repeated infarction but children may have enlarged spleens and sometimes the spleen may rapidly enlarge (over hours) and be painful. This is associated with massive retention of sickled red cells in the spleen resulting in severe anaemia with requirement for urgent transfusion.
- **Localised areas of splenic infarction**: results in pleuritic pain in the left hypochondrium radiating to the left shoulder, sometimes associated with rubs.
- **Thrombotic stroke**: fortunately this is relatively rare but it may be catastrophic and is an indication for urgent exchange transfusion.
- **Pulmonary infarction–chest syndrome**: may be associated with infection. It is another serious complication of sickle cell disease, often requiring exchange transfusion.
- **Priapism**: painful sustained penile erection due to sickling of red cells in the corpora cavernosa. It may require surgical intervention and lead to impotence.
- **Other areas of sickle infarction**: the retina may be affected, particularly in haemoglobin SC disease leading to retinal detachment and blindness. Infarction of the placenta may lead to fetal loss and small-for-weight babies. Intractable leg ulcers are common in countries where the ankles are not protected by shoes and socks. Avascular necrosis of the head of femur may be seen in adults.

Aplastic crisis

This is a syndrome of severe anaemia with a lower reticulocyte count and bilirubin level than usual for the patient. It is usually due to parvovirus B19 infection. In normal people this infection results in a mild febrile illness with infection of red cell precursors in the bone marrow causing shutdown of marrow red cell production for a few days. In patients with increased red cell turnover, such as sickle cell disease, a precipitous drop in haemoglobin level may result from a short shutdown in red cell production. Aplastic crisis may be found in other patients with sickle cell disease and those with other congenital haemolytic anaemias associated with a high red cell turnover.

Transfusion in sickle cell disease

Because the oxygen dissociation curve of sickle haemoglobin is shifted to the right, oxygen is more easily released from haemoglobin to the tissues. Anaemia is therefore well tolerated and blood transfusion for the correction of anaemia is rarely required except in aplastic or sequestration crisis. For severe sickle problems exchange transfusion with non-sickling HbA-containing red cells is required. To be effective the percentage of haemoglobin A needs to be raised to 80–90% and care needs to be taken not to increase the haematocrit, which may lead to stagnation and increased sickling.

1.5 Thalassaemia

In contrast to the true haemoglobinopathies, such as sickle cell disease (which are associated with abnormal substitutions of amino acids in the globin chains), in thalassaemia the globin chains are normal in structure but not enough of the globin chains can be manufactured. The disorder may affect alpha chains (**alpha thalassaemia**) or beta chains (**beta thalassaemia**). Both types of thalassaemia may be severe (homozygous, **major**) or mild (heterozygous, **minor**).

- In the first year of life adult haemoglobin (Hb A) gradually replaces fetal haemoglobin (Hb F) as the major circulating haemoglobin.
- About 4% of haemoglobin is the second adult haemoglobin (HbA2).
- These normal haemoglobins differ from each other by the nature of the polypeptide chains which make up the globin part of the molecule.

Haemoglobin type	**Globin chain content**
Hb F	$2\,\alpha + 2\,\gamma$
Hb A	$2\,\alpha + 2\,\beta$
HbA2	$2\,\alpha + 2\,\delta$

Thalassaemia major

It may be seen that alpha chains are required in all the normal haemoglobins. It follows that in **alpha thalassaemia major**, where there is major failure of alpha chain manufacture, none of the haemoglobins are made and death in utero results. In **beta thalassaemia major** the blood is normal at birth, since beta chains are not required for the production of fetal haemoglobin. During the first year of life there is failure to switch over from fetal to adult haemoglobin and the syndrome of anaemia, stunting of growth and hepatosplenomegaly arises.

Treatment of beta thalassaemia major

- Effective treatment depends on regular transfusions, which leads to iron overload.
- Iron overload results in cardiomyopathy, endocrine failure and cirrhosis, and can be prevented by iron chelation therapy with desferrioxamine.
- **Desferrioxamine**: is given by overnight subcutaneous infusion (using a syringe driver or balloon infuser) on two to five nights of the week, depending on the degree of iron overload. The aim of therapy is to maintain the ferritin level at about 1000 mg/l. Overtreatment may lead to toxic effects on eyes or ears.

In women with beta thalassaemia trait, intra-uterine diagnosis is possible allowing the option of therapeutic abortion of a fetus with thalassaemia major.

Thalassaemia trait

Beta thalassaemia trait is associated with minor suppression of beta chain manufacture and a mild microcytic hypochromic anaemia difficult to distinguish from iron deficiency, although the MCV is often surprisingly low for the level of haemoglobin (which is usually over 9 g/dl). Besides assessing iron status (Section 2.1) an elevated Hb A2 is also a useful marker of this trait.

In **alpha thalassaemia trait** the clinical picture is more complex as four genes control alpha chain production compared to the two genes that control beta chain production.

- The mildest varieties of alpha thalassaemia trait are manifested by a microcytosis without anaemia.
- More severe cases have a microcytic anaemia with splenomegaly and **Hb H** in the red cells.

In **haemoglobin H** a tetramer of beta chains (that are unable to pair with alpha chains) replaces the $\alpha2\beta2$ chains of Hb A. Haemoglobin H may be detected by haemoglobin electrophoresis or by the presence of characteristic inclusion bodies in red cells (Hb H inclusions) seen on an incubated reticulocyte stain.

1.6 Aplastic anaemia

This is a pancytopenia secondary to marrow hypoplasia.

Aplastic anaemia

Causes:

- **idiopathic**: most cases are in fact autoimmune
- **drugs**: an idiosyncratic reaction to drugs such as gold, phenylbutazone and chloramphenicol
- **post-hepatitis**: viruses that are toxic to hepatocytes may also kill bone marrow stem cells
- as a predictable reaction to chemotherapy or radiation.

Treatment:

- **supportive**: red cell transfusion for correction of anaemia, antibiotics for infections, platelet transfusion for thrombocytopenic bleeding
- **immunosuppression**: high-dose steroids, anti-lymphocyte globulin, ciclosporin
- **stimulation of residual marrow activity**: anabolic steroids
- **bone marrow transplantation**: only in severe cases, particularly in children with an HLA-matched sibling.

2. IRON METABOLISM

A representation of the body's iron economy is shown in the figure below.

Figure 1 Iron economy in the body

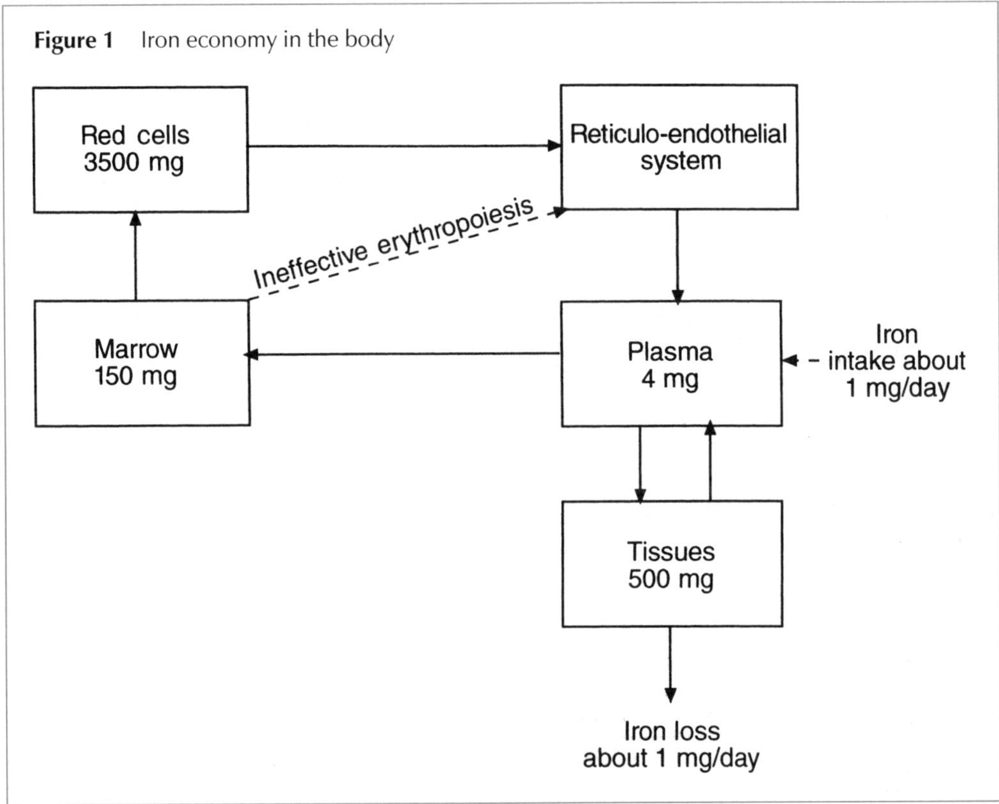

Iron absorption may be greatly increased in iron deficiency, but iron excretion cannot be increased in the case of iron overload. Most iron in the body lies within red cells, so chronic bleeding is a potent cause of iron deficiency.

The marrow normally contains stainable iron but it is possible to have no stainable iron in the bone marrow but a normal haemoglobin level. The converse is not true; however, in iron deficiency anaemia the marrow will not contain stainable iron. In megaloblastic anaemias, haemoglobinopathies and myelodysplasia, red cells may die and enter the reticulo-endothelial system without leaving the bone marrow – this is termed **ineffective erythropoiesis**.

2.1 Assessment of iron status

- **Serum iron**: on its own, not very useful. Serum iron is reduced in patients with inflammatory disease. False elevations may be found if the patient is taking iron at the time of the test (stop the day before). Serum iron should always be measured with total iron binding capacity (TIBC).
- **Total iron binding capacity (TIBC), transferrin**: always measure with serum iron. In iron deficiency the TIBC is increased, reflecting the body's desire to mop up and conserve all free iron molecules. False elevation of the TIBC may be found in pregnancy and oestrogen administration.
- **Transferrin saturation**: may be calculated by dividing the TIBC by the serum iron. Low in iron deficiency, high in iron overload. More useful than serum iron or TIBC assessed on their own.
- **Serum ferritin**: a major transport and storage form of iron which is high in iron overload states and low in iron depletion. It is one of the acute phase proteins, so like C-reactive protein (CRP), fibrinogen and immunoglobulins it is increased in inflammatory illness. If the ESR is increased then the serum ferritin may not be an accurate reflection of iron stores. It is also released from damaged liver cells, so if the patient has a transaminitis then it will be falsely elevated.
- **Iron stain**: on particles from bone marrow aspirate. This is the gold standard, but it is invasive!
- **Serum soluble transferrin receptor**: the latest index for measuring iron status, being high in iron deficiency and low in iron overload. It is still a research tool but shows promise.

2.2 Sideroblastic anaemia

In this disorder there is a failure to incorporate iron into the haemoglobin molecule, due to a biochemical block, and it accumulates in the mitochondria. These become poisoned and are visible as iron granules lying in a ring around the erythroblast nucleus. Hence the diagnostic feature is **ring sideroblasts** in the bone marrow.

Causes of sideroblastic anaemia:

- **congenital**: rare, pyridoxine responsive
- **acquired – primary**: one of the myelodysplastic disorders
- **acquired – secondary**: alcohol, malignancy in the body, drugs (eg antituberculous), connective tissue disorders, heavy metal poisoning.

3. HAEMOLYSIS

Destruction of red cells may occur in the:

- circulation (*intravascular*)
- reticulo-endothelial system (*extravascular*).

If haemolysis is intravascular then the haemoglobin liberated from red cells will be conserved in the body by binding to plasma proteins. Initially this will be haptoglobin so haptoglobin levels will be reduced. Then albumin will bind free haemoglobin, forming methaemalbumin, which may be detected by a positive Schumm's test. Without a protein to bind to, the haemoglobin will pass through the glomerulus to appear in the urine – **haemoglobinuria**.

3.1 General features and causes of haemolysis

The anaemia is commonly macrocytic and associated with:

- **Elevated reticulocyte count**: > 2%.
- **Jaundice**: pre-hepatic, unconjugated, water-insoluble bilirubin. Therefore NOT found in urine, but **urobilinogen** may be found in urine – due to increased breakdown products of porphyrins secreted into the bile and reabsorbed from the bowel. Detected by simple stick test.
- **Abnormal red cell morphology**: particularly spherocytes (see above).

Causes of haemolysis

Mainly intravascular

Immediate haemolytic transfusion reaction
Paroxysmal cold haemoglobinuria
Micro-angiopathic haemolytic anaemia
Glucose-6-phosphate dehydrogenase deficiency
Infections – malaria
Phosphokinase deficiency
Paroxysmal nocturnal haemoglobinuria

Mainly extravascular

Warm autoimmune haemolytic anaemia
Cold haemagglutination disease
Haemolytic disease of the newborn
Hereditary spherocytosis
Haemoglobinopathies (eg sickle cell disease)

3.2 The antiglobulin (Coombs') test

The direct antiglobulin test detects antibody on the patient's red cells. The antibody coating on the red cells may be:

- **opsonising**: making the red cells attractive to the phagocytes of the reticulo-endothelial system
- **complement fixing**: causing a local enzymatic explosion blowing a hole in the red cell envelope
- **agglutinating**: in which case the red cell clumping may be visible in the test tube without resorting to a Coombs' test to discover the antibody.

The indirect antiglobulin test detects antibody in the patient's serum. This involves incubation of serum with test red cells bearing various surface antigens. This test is most frequently used as part of the 'cross-match' or compatibility test. The donor's red cells are mixed with the recipient's serum and if there is incompatibility a positive indirect antiglobulin test will result.

3.3 Microangiopathic haemolytic anaemia (MAHA)

Fibrin strands are laid down in small blood vessels and these chop up red cells (like a wire cheese cutter). The red cells reseal themselves if not too badly damaged and circulate as helmet cells or, if multiply chopped, as fragmented cells. All the features of haemolysis will be present, as well as reticulocytosis due to increased marrow activity.

Haematological features of microangiopathic haemolytic anaemia:

- anaemia
- Helmet cell
- fragmented cells
- polychromasia
- reticulocytosis.

Sometimes thrombocytopenia and consumption coagulopathy may be associated, depending on diagnosis.

Causes:

- disseminated intravascular coagulation (DIC) (*see* Section 6.4)
- haemolytic uraemic syndrome (HUS)
- thrombotic thrombocytopenic purpura (TTP)
- malignant (accelerated-phase) hypertension
- severe pre-eclampsia.

Thrombotic thrombocytopenic purpura (TTP) and haemolytic uraemic syndrome (HUS)

The general features of microangiopathic haemolytic anaemia, as described above, are present in these overlapping syndromes. However, in addition there is often fever, renal impairment and cerebral dysfunction (*see also* Chapter 15, Nephrology).

- In TTP neurological symptoms dominate the clinical picture and adults are frequently affected.
- In HUS renal failure and fever are the predominant clinical problems and children are usually affected. Infection with verotoxin-producing strains of *E. coli* due to faecal contamination of food (in particular, meat) is a well-recognised cause (diarrhoea-associated HUS), but many cases are idiopathic or familial.

Pathogenesis of TTP and HUS

The essential problem is an excess of sticky high-molecular-weight von Willebrand factor (vWF) in the plasma, which causes the platelets to adhere to vascular endothelium. This results in thrombocytopenia and the blockage of small capillaries in the brain and kidney by platelet thrombi. Activation of the coagulation system causes fibrin strands to be laid down and these shred passing red cells, causing the classic features of microangiopathic haemolysis.

- In normal plasma high-molecular-weight vWF is cleaved to less sticky vWF by a plasma protease.
- Low levels of this protease have been found in many cases of TTP and, in some cases, antibody directed against the protease has been found.
- In contrast to DIC, the screening tests of coagulation (but not the platelet count) are normal.
- In sporadic HUS (not associated with diarrhoea), 20% of patients are shown to have a genetic defect for the complement regulatory protein Factor H.

Treatment of TTP and HUS

The mainstay of treatment is large volume infusion of fresh frozen plasma (FFP) which contains the vWF-cleaving protease, coupled with **plasma exchange**. The latter has the advantage of removing any antibodies and toxins involved in the pathogenesis of disease. Cryo-poor FFP (from which cryoprecipitate and hence vWF has been removed) may be used for the plasma exchange.

- High-dose steroids may be of benefit in cases with an autoimmune aetiology and are often given (eg non-epidemic forms of HUS, or in TPP).
- **Vincristine** causes premature release of platelets from developing marrow megakaryocytes (in addition to its immunosuppressive properties) and is useful in cases with marked thrombocytopenia and it may be useful in cases of TPP with marked thrombocytopenia.
- Once the platelet count has exceeded 50×10^9/l, aspirin may be used to inhibit further adhesion of platelets to vascular endothelium.
- Other specific therapies may be indicated for particular disease sequelae (eg haemodialysis for acute renal failure).

3.4 Paroxysmal nocturnal haemoglobinuria (PNH)

This is a rare acquired disorder that may affect all haematological cells. There is increased sensitivity of the cell membranes to the action of the patient's own complement which damages red cells, white cells, platelets and stem cells. This results in intravascular haemolysis with haemoglobinuria, leukopenia, thrombocytopenia and (sometimes) pancytopenia with an 'empty bone marrow' – aplastic anaemia. Other clinical features:

- In addition to episodes of haemoglobinuria, the release of tissue thromboplastin from damaged cells leads to an **acquired thrombophilia** when thrombosis may present in unusual sites such as the hepatic or portal veins.
- There is an increased incidence of **acute myeloid leukaemia**.

Pathogenesis and diagnosis of PNH

A trans-membrane glycoprotein is missing from the blood cell surface in PNH, and this 'fence post' would carry molecules that inactivate local complement.

- The glycoprotein would normally carry various CD antigens (eg CD55 and CD59) and so these are missing from the cell surface in PNH. This allows diagnosis by **immunophenotyping** of red cells, white cells or platelets.
- The classic diagnostic test is the **Ham acid serum haemolysis test** in which the patient's red cells are placed in hydrochloric acid with fresh complement. The red cells will haemolyse, but normal control red cells do not.
- The Ham acid lysis test will be negative if the patient has recently been transfused.

Treatment of PNH

This consists of:

- **red cell transfusion**: the correction of anaemia often requires use of washed red cells as the transfusion of complement in the donor plasma may exacerbate haemolysis
- **anticoagulation**: thrombosis is a frequent cause of death so anticoagulation with warfarin is usual if the platelet count permits
- **other therapies**: erythropoietin, steroids and danazol are of unproven value, although folate supplements should be given.

4. DISORDERS OF LEUKOCYTES

4.1 Leukocytosis

An elevated white cell count may be due to an increase in any of the individual types of white cell in the blood and should prompt examination to determine if there is a neutrophilia, lymphocytosis or, more rarely, an increase in other types of white cell to give a leukocytosis.

Neutrophilia (>7.5 × 10^9/l)

This is by far the commonest cause of a leukocytosis. If acute it may be associated with young neutrophils (band cells) in the blood or 'left shift'.

Causes of neutrophilia

- **Bacterial infections**
  Localised or generalised
- **Metabolic disorders**
  (eg uraemia, acidosis, gout, eclampsia, poisoning)
- **Malignant neoplasms**
  Particularly when associated with tissue necrosis
- **Inflammation or necrosis**
  (eg myocardial infarction, trauma, vasculitis)
- **Corticosteroid therapy**
- **Myeloproliferative disorders**
  (eg chronic granulocytic leukaemia, myelofibrosis, essential thrombocythaemia, polycythaemia rubra vera)

Lymphocytosis (>3.5 × 10^9/l)

The morphology of the lymphocytes may give valuable clues. For example, in acute viral infections the lymphocytes may show morphological abnormalities termed 'reactive changes' and in chronic lymphocytic leukaemia the mature-looking small lymphocytes characteristic of the disease are fragile and become crushed during the spreading of the blood film – 'smear cells'.

Causes of lymphocytosis

- **Acute viral infections**
  (eg influenza, glandular fever, rubella, mumps, acute HIV)
- **Chronic lymphocytic leukaemia**
- **Thyrotoxicosis**
- **Chronic infections**
  (eg TB, brucella, hepatitis, syphilis)
- **Other chronic leukaemias and lymphomas**

A lymphocytosis is normal in infancy

Eosinophilia (>0.5 × 10^9/l)

In the developed world allergic disorders are the main cause of eosinophilia.

Causes of eosinophilia

- **Allergies**
  (eg asthma, hay fever, drugs)
- **Skin diseases**
  (eg eczema, psoriasis, dermatitis herpetiformis)
- **Tropical eosinophilia**
- **Hypereosinophilic syndrome**
  (See below)
- **Eosinophilic leukaemia**
  (Very rare)
- **Parasites**
  (eg ankylostomiasis, ascariasis, filariasis, trichinosis, toxocariasis)
- **Neoplasms**
  (eg Hodgkin's disease)
- **Miscellaneous conditions**
  (eg sarcoidosis, polyarteritis nodosa, eosinophilic granuloma)

Hypereosinophilic syndrome

This condition is associated with a high eosinophil count, up to 100×10^9/l. The aetiology is obscure. Some cases are myeloproliferative disorders equivalent to eosinophilic variants of chronic myeloid leukaemia, some are T-cell lymphomas which produce large amounts of cytokines such as interleukin-5 (IL-5), which stimulate eosinophil proliferation. Treatment is with steroids and hydroxyurea.

Hypereosinophilic syndrome

Clinical features	**Pathological features**
Weight loss	Acute arteritis
Rashes	Pericarditis
Fever	Cardiac mural thrombus
Peripheral neuropathy	Chronic endocardial fibrosis
Oedema	Pulmonary abnormalities
Cardiac disturbances	Splenomegaly

Monocytosis (>0.8×10^9/l)

Monocytes are tissue phagocytes ('dustbin lorries') en route to the tissues to phagocytose and digest dead cells and other debris.

Causes of monocytosis

- **Recovery**
  (from chemotherapy or radiotherapy)
- **Chronic inflammatory disease**
  (eg sarcoidosis, Crohn's, ulcerative colitis, rheumatoid arthritis, systemic lupus erythematosus (SLE))
- **Myelodysplastic syndromes**
  (and chronic myelomonocytic leukaemia)
- **Infections**
  (eg TB, brucella, kala-azar, typhus, bacterial endocarditis, malaria, trypanosomiasis)
- **Hodgkin's disease**
  (and other neoplasms)
- **Acute myelomonocytic leukaemias**
  (when associated with increased blast cells)

4.2 Leukoerythroblastic change

This is defined as the presence of nucleated red cells and primitive white cells of any type in the peripheral blood. There are two major causes: either the normal cells inhabiting the bone marrow are being evicted by a marrow infiltration, or the patient has acute severe illness.

Causes of a leukoerythroblastic blood picture

Invasion of marrow space
Tumour (metastatic carcinoma), leukaemia, myeloma, lymphoma, myelofibrosis, osteopetrosis, storage disease (eg Gaucher's disease)

Severe illness
(eg severe haemolysis, massive trauma, septicaemia)

4.3 Neutropenia

This is defined as a neutrophil count less than 2×10^9/l. Below 1×10^9/l, some risk of infection exists; below 0.5×10^9/l this may be severe and such patients, if in hospital, will usually be isolated and subject to a regimen of care including prophylactic antiseptic mouth-washes and anti-fungal agents and avoidance of foods with a high bacterial load. In the event of significant fever a broad-spectrum antibiotic regimen reserved for 'febrile neutropenia' is instituted.

Causes of neutropenia

- **Associated with intercurrent viral infections**
- **Idiosyncratic drug reactions** (eg carbimazole)
- **Collagen diseases** (eg SLE, rheumatoid)
- **Myelodysplasia**
- **After chemotherapy or radiotherapy**
- **Racial** (eg in Blacks or Arabs)
- **Hypersplenism** Often low platelet count and haemoglobin as well
- **Marrow infiltration** May be associated with leukoerythroblastic change

5. HAEMATOLOGICAL MALIGNANCIES

These may be broadly divided into:

- leukaemias
- lymphomas
- myelodysplasias
- myeloproliferative disorders.

Acute leukaemias are characterised by primitive blast cells in the bone marrow and blood; chronic leukaemias with an excess of mature cells in the marrow and blood. In leukaemias the malignant cells lie mainly in marrow and blood, whereas in the lymphomas they lie mostly in lymph nodes. There is an overlap, however, so many cases of lymphoblastic lymphoma have marrow involvement by cells of the disease in addition to enlargement of thymus and lymph nodes.

5.1 Acute leukaemias

Acute	Chronic
Myeloid (AML)	Myeloid (CML (CGL))
Lymphoid (ALL)	Lymphoid (CLL)

Acute lymphoblastic leukaemia:

- predominantly affects children
- remission may be induced with non-myelosuppressive chemotherapy
- CNS involvement common
- >60% cure rate with chemotherapy
- further classified by immunological surface markers.

Acute myeloid leukaemia:

- predominantly affects adults
- marrow hypoplasia required to induce remission
- CNS involvement unusual
- >30% cure rate with chemotherapy
- further classified by morphological appearance (see opposite).

How to identify the leukaemic blast cell

- **Morphology**: often this is not helpful as myeloblasts look similar to lymphoblasts. One give-away is the presence of Auer rods which are diagnostic of AML.
- **Cytochemistry**: the leukaemic cells are tested for their biochemical activities. Important cytochemistry tests in acute leukaemia: Sudan black (stains lipid material in AML); Periodic Acid Schiff (PAS) (stains carbohydrate material in ALL); esterase (stains monocytic variants of AML).
- **Immunological surface markers**: these are particularly useful in ALL when they allow classification into T-cell, B-cell and other immunological types.

Treatment strategies in acute leukaemia

Bone marrow transplantation is a powerful treatment for acute leukaemia, as it also harnesses the power of graft-versus-leukaemia effect. It is a risky treatment, however, and this risk increases with age. The total body irradiation also results in sterility. Chemotherapy also carries major risks and so patients with acute leukaemia are stratified by **risk of relapse**. This allows the selective application of stronger, and hence riskier, chemotherapeutic regimes for those cases that require them, and less stringent chemotherapy in cases with better prognosis (see below).

Prognostic factors in acute leukaemia

Acute lymphoblastic leukaemia

- Age (< 1 year or over 10 years worsens prognosis; adults do particularly badly)*.
- Height of highest pre-treatment white cell (blast) count (a higher count = a higher tumour load and worse prognosis).
- Cytogenetics (see below).
- Sex (males do worse).
- Immunophenotype (T-cell ALL usually has a high presenting white cell count – see below).
- **Response to treatment** is measured by blast cell count in the marrow, one or two weeks into chemotherapy treatment, or by assessment of minimal residual disease. The latter uses the polymerase chain reaction (PCR) to amplify clonal rearrangements of T-cell receptor genes, or immunoglobulin genes, characteristic of that patient's disease. The persistence of $> 1 \times 10^4$ malignant cells in the marrow at one month into chemotherapy mandates use of more intensive MRC childhood leukaemia protocols.

Acute myeloid leukaemia

- Cytogenetics (see below).
- Age (over 60s do worse).
- Response to first course of chemotherapy.

5.2 Specific chromosome abnormalities in leukaemia/lymphoma

Cytogenetic techniques

Morphological examination of the chromosomes of malignant haematological cells is possible by culturing them in tissue culture medium and then 'freezing' the cell in division with the chromosomes spread out (metaphase arrest) by adding colchicine or vincristine which poison the spindle apparatus. The cells are then swollen in hypotonic salt solution and the cell suspension is dripped onto glass microscope slides so that the cells split open releasing a cloud of contained chromosomes. This is examined under the microscope and usually analysed with the aid of a computerised image analysis system. The chromosomes are arranged in order of their length to form a karyotype (see Chapter 7, Genetics). Cytogenetic abnormalities are found in two-thirds of cases of AML and three-quarters of cases of ALL.

*Highest presenting white cell count, age and sex may be combined in the Medical Research Council's risk algorithm.

Chromosome abnormalities in leukaemia and lymphoma are important for the following reasons:

- They act as a marker of the disease, indicating remission or relapse.
- Some have a prognostic significance. If the prognosis is especially bad (eg Philadelphia chromosome in childhood ALL) then a high-risk treatment such as bone marrow transplantation may be employed early in treatment. If the prognosis is especially good (eg t(8;21) in adult AML) then conventional chemotherapy may be employed without a transplant unless the patient relapses.
- Some of the abnormal DNA sequences that result from chromosomal translocation can be amplified by the polymerase chain reaction to allow the detection of incredibly small amounts of residual leukaemia. The prognostic significance of this minimal residual disease is now being investigated in international trials.

Many of the chromosomal abnormalities in leukaemia and lymphoma are translocations, involving the exchange of material between chromosomes. For example, t(9;22) involves a reciprocal translocation between chromosomes 9 and 22. Chromosome 22 comes off worst in this exchange, gaining only a small amount of extra material. The abnormally shortened long arms of this chromosome are visible morphologically as the Philadelphia chromosome (*see* Section 5.4).

Cytogenetic abnormality	**Found in**
t(9;22)	Philadelphia chromosome in CML
t(15;17)	Acute promyelocytic leukaemia (M3) – *see* Section 5.3 opposite
t(8;21)	AML with differentiation (M2) – better prognosis
inv(16)	(inversion of the long arm of chromosome 16) Acute myelomonocytic leukaemia (AML M4) with marrow eosinophilia (M4Eo)
Hyperdiploidy	(More than 47 chromosomes) Childhood ALL – better prognosis
t(1;19)	Childhood pre-B ALL
t(8;14)	ALL L3 Burkitt type
5q-	Myelodysplastic syndrome (refractory anaemia) with abnormal megakaryocytes particularly in women (loss of part of the long arm of chromosome 5)
t(14;18)	Follicular NHL – found in 3/4 of cases

5.3 The French–American–British (FAB) classification of acute leukaemia

This morphological classification is widely used for AML but in ALL has been largely supplanted by the immunophenotype. It depends on the degree of differentiation of the leukaemic cells and whether a recognisable tendency to differentiate along one of the myeloid pathways (eg monocytic) is present. As with any morphological classification it is rather subjective and there will be some cases which would be best classified between grades, eg M2½!

FAB type	Description
M0	Acute myeloid leukaemia undifferentiated – no morphological feature to distinguish it from ALL
M1	Acute myeloid leukaemia with recognisable myeloid features such as Auer rods
M2	Acute myeloid leukaemia with a few cells differentiating to the promyelocyte stage
M3	Acute promyelocytic leukaemia – see below
M4	Myelomonocytic leukaemia
M5	Pure monocytic leukaemia
M6	Acute erythroleukaemia
M7	Acute megakaryoblastic leukaemia

Acute promyelocytic leukaemia (AML M3)

- Majority of leukaemic cells are abnormal hypergranular promyelocytes
- Auer rods and collections of Auer rods (Faggots) common
- Strongly Sudan black/peroxidase positive
- Characteristic chromosome abnormality t(15;17), involving retinoic acid receptor gene alpha (RARA)
- Variant M3 (M3v) is **hypo**granular but otherwise the same.

The disease and its treatment are associated with acute fibrinolysis/DIC – tranexamic acid is used to block fibrinolysis and heavy platelet and fresh frozen plasma support are needed. Remission can be induced with all-*trans* retinoic acid (ATRA) – a differentiating agent which also helps with the coagulopathy. Prognosis is good providing death from DIC does not occur during induction.

5.4 Chronic myeloid leukaemia (CML)

CML is a disease of middle age, the majority of patients presenting with tiredness, weight loss and sweating. Splenomegaly is found in 90% of cases. If the white cell count is very high (over 500 × 10^9/l) then problems associated with hyperleukocytosis may be found: visual disturbance, priapism, deafness. Eventually almost all patients transform to blast crisis in 1–10 years. This may be myeloid, lymphoid or mixed transformation. At this stage it is very difficult to treat.

Blood and marrow features of CML

- High white cell counts (100–500) × 10^9/l
- Absolute basophilia and eosinophilia
- Platelet count high, normal or low
- Low neutrophil alkaline phosphatase (NAP) score
- Increased blood colony-forming cells (stem cells)
- High serum B_{12} due to production of a B_{12} binding protein by white cells
- Massive neutrophilia with left shift
- Anaemia in relation to height of WBC
- Philadelphia chromosome (see following text)
- Marrow hyperplasia sometimes with increased reticulin (fibrosis)

Philadelphia chromosome (Ph)

This is a balanced translocation between chromosomes 9 and 22, termed t(9;22). Ninety per cent of cases of CML have Ph chromosome; the breakpoints are at the *bcr* gene on 22 and *abl* gene on 9. The majority of Ph-negative CML cases have a translocation at the *molecular* level.

Ph is also found in:

- 5% childhood ALL
- 25% adult ALL
- 1% adult AML.

It carries a bad prognosis if found in these diseases. The protein product of the hybrid gene has protein tyrosine kinase activity.

Treatment of CML

The aims of treatment of CML include normalisation of the blood count, reduction of hypercatabolic symptoms and reduction of splenomegaly. Drugs such as **hydroxyurea** and **busulfan** do this effectively but they do not modify the underlying cytogenetic abnormality or prevent transformation into acute blast crisis. **Interferon** and **imatinib** can inhibit the proliferation of Philadelphia-positive marrow precursors, allowing return of normal haematopoiesis:

- **Interferon** is associated with a high incidence of systemic side-effects including malaise, myalgia and arthralgia, and it has to be given by injection.
- **Imatinib** has been created to specifically inhibit the abnormal tyrosine kinase produced by the leukaemic cells as a result of the *bcr/abl* new gene. It has proved spectacularly effective in inducing Philadelphia-negative haematopoiesis and this is likely to be reflected in improved survival, although it is an expensive treatment.

Bone marrow transplantation remains a curative option for young and fit patients who are not fully responsive to imatinib, but who have a suitable donor. Low levels of marrow disease can be monitored by PCR for the *bcr/abl* translocation.

5.5 Chronic lymphocytic leukaemia (CLL)

This is the most indolent of the chronic leukaemias. Many cases are discovered as an incidental finding when blood counts are done for some other reason, such as health screening.

- Commonest cause of a lymphocytosis in the elderly.
- 95% of cases are of B-cell lineage.
- Mature-looking lymphocytes and smear cells on the blood film.
- Progression through lymphocytosis to lymphadenopathy, hepatosplenomegaly, marrow failure though patients may skip stages in this progression.
- Increased incidence of certain antibody-mediated autoimmune disorders such as warm autoimmune haemolytic anaemia and immune thrombocytopenia (in B-cell CLL).

Treatment of CLL

Many patients with CLL require no treatment, living at peace with their lymphocytosis to die of an unrelated complaint. Early antibiotic treatment of intercurrent infection is indicated because of the associated immunoglobulin deficiency, and some patients with recurrent infections may benefit from immunoglobulin administration, particularly during the winter months.

Chemotherapy is indicated for:

- patients with bulky disease
- cytopenias due to marrow failure
- a short lymphocyte doubling time.

The most commonly used chemotherapy is single-agent oral **chlorambucil** or **fludarabine**. The latter is highly immunosuppressive, and *Pneumocystis* prophylaxis with cotrimoxazole should accompany its use.

The antibody-mediated autoimmune disorders are treated along conventional lines when they occur.

5.6 Hodgkin's disease (HD)

Prognosis of Hodgkin's disease is related to clinical stage, bulk of tumour and histopathological type.

Ann Arbor clinical staging	
Stage I	One involved lymph node group
Stage II	Two nodal areas on one side of the diaphragm
Stage III	Lymph nodes on both sides of the diaphragm
Stage IV	Involvement of extra-nodal tissues, such as liver or bone marrow

The spleen is an 'honorary' lymph node, ie if involved this is not necessarily stage IV.

The clinical stage may be given the letter suffix A or B, to reflect presence or absence of symptoms:

- **A**: no 'B' symptoms
- **B**: B symptoms consist of significant fever (>38°C), night sweats (drenching) or weight loss of more than 10% in the last six months.

Pruritus and alcohol-induced pain are not B symptoms, although they are useful indicators of relapse.

Investigation

- Many patients have neutrophilia, thrombocytosis and anaemia of chronic disease; some patients have eosinophilia
- The ESR and other inflammatory markers are elevated
- Lactate dehydrogenase (LDH) is elevated and provides a useful guide to bulk of disease; 'bulky disease' is a node mass more than 10 cm in diameter
- Clinical examination and CT scanning are used to establish clinical stage; there is almost no role for staging laparotomy if suitable imaging facilities are available
- Residual masses are common after treatment and it is often difficult to decide whether or not they represent active disease. Positron emission tomography (PET) scanning uses a form of radioactive glucose that helps distinguish tissue that is metabolically active. The place of this investigation remains uncertain.

Histological types of Hodgkin's disease

The Reed–Sternberg (RS) cell is the most useful diagnostic feature. This is a giant cell, often with twin mirror-image nuclei and prominent 'owls-eye' nucleoli. Histological typing depends on the other cells within the involved tissue:

- **lymphocyte predominant**: there is an infiltration with reactive T-lymphocytes
- **nodular sclerosing (NS)**: bands of fibrous tissue separate nodules of the Hodgkin tissue
- **mixed picture**
- **lymphocyte depleted**: no infiltrating lymphocytes.

The prognosis worsens through the histological types from lymphocyte predominant (best) to lymphocyte depleted (worst). With the benefit of modern immunophenotyping methodology (which uses monoclonal antibodies) many cases of Hodgkin's disease that were historically classified as lymphocyte-predominant Hodgkin's disease are now recognised to be non-Hodgkin's lymphomas. More than two-thirds of cases of Hodgkin's disease are of the nodular sclerosing type; this category can be subdivided into Grade I and Grade II NS Hodgkin's disease, depending on the number of RS cells and other histological features.

Treatment

Early clinical stages of Hodgkin's disease are treated with radiotherapy, and later stages with combination chemotherapy. The dividing line depends on national and institutional preferences. The classical (and some would say gold standard) chemotherapy is MOPP which contains Mustine, Oncovin (vincristine), Procarbazine and Prednisolone. As mustine is associated with severe vomiting it has been replaced by an alternative alkylating agent, chlorambucil, in many countries.

- Alkylating agents are associated with sterility and secondary leukaemogenesis. Hence, attempts have been made to dispense with them in regimens such as ABVD (Adriamycin, Bleomycin, Vinblastine and Dacarbazine) which is the current most popular regimen in the USA.
- Many relapsed patients may be salvaged with second-line chemotherapy and stem cell autografts, particularly if the relapse occurs more than one year after completion of initial treatment.

5.7 Non-Hodgkin's lymphoma (NHL)

Despite the general acceptance of the REAL (Revised European American Lymphoma) histological classification, the categorisation of non-Hodgkin's lymphoma (NHL) remains in a state of flux. For clinical purposes the NHLs are divided into three groups:

Low-grade NHL

- The cells are relatively mature and the disease pursues an indolent course without treatment. In many cases it is acceptable to watch and wait for symptoms or critical organ failure.
- Local radiotherapy to involved nodal regions is effective and should always be given in stage I disease (infrequent) as some patients can be cured by this treatment.
- Single agent chemotherapy (eg chlorambucil) is usually used for diffuse disease.
- Interferon may prolong remission duration.

High-grade NHL

- The cells are immature and the disease is rapidly progressive without treatment
- Combination chemotherapy is usual from the outset (eg CHOP regime: Cyclophosphamide, adriamycin (Hydroxydaunorubicin), vincristine, (Oncovin) Prednisolone)
- Usual to give six (monthly) courses
- No benefit of maintenance therapy
- Multi-agent, alternating and hybrid regimes may be advantageous.

Lymphoblastic NHL

- The cells of the disease are very immature and have a propensity to involve the CNS
- Treat as for ALL with CNS prophylaxis.

High-dose therapy with haemopoietic stem cell rescue may salvage some younger patients with aggressive chemotherapy-responsive lymphomas.

Prognosis

Low-grade (indolent) lymphomas are readily controllable initially but relapse usually occurs even after many years of remission. Approximately 40% of high-grade lymphomas are cured.

5.8 Myeloma

In myeloma there is a clonal proliferation of plasma cells and the clinical manifestations of disease are related to substances secreted by the plasma cells as much as to the effects of marrow infiltration. **Clonality** (all diseased cells originating from one parent plasma cell) may be confirmed by:

- the presence of a paraprotein (monoclonal) band on serum electrophoresis, or by
- immunophenotyping the increased numbers of plasma cells in the bone marrow, and finding that they all express either kappa or lambda light chains rather than a mixture of the two.

Paraprotein sub-types

The normal immunoglobulin concentrations in serum parallel the relative frequency of the three main sub-classes of myeloma paraprotein. Hence, IgG is the most common form of myeloma, followed by IgA, with IgM being the least common type.

Plasma hyperviscosity syndrome may be found when plasma viscosity exceeds 4 CpA. This consists of confusion, capillary bleeding, oedema and renal impairment. The incidence of hyperviscosity syndrome relates to the size of the immunoglobulin molecule as well as its concentration. As IgM is the largest molecule (750, 000 daltons) this syndrome is seen relatively frequently in IgM myeloma, less frequently in IgA myeloma and rarely in IgG myeloma. Transfusion should be avoided in patients with plasma hyperviscosity syndrome, as it will cause a big increase in whole blood viscosity.

- **Cryoglobulin**: rarely, the paraprotein may be a cryoglobulin, so that the protein precipitates from plasma in the cold. This may be a cause of vasculitis.
- Some myeloma paraproteins precipitate within tissue to form amyloid.

Bence–Jones protein

Sometimes, the malignant plasma cells are so defective that they cannot make a complete immunoglobulin molecule and are only able to make light chains. The latter are small enough to be filtered within the glomerulus and to appear in the urine as Bence–Jones proteinuria. They may obstruct the renal tubules and contribute to the renal failure which is often found in myeloma (see Chapter 15, Nephrology).

Role of cytokines in myeloma

Osteoclast-activating factors stimulate the normal osteoclasts to dissolve bone and lead to bone pain, hypercalcaemia and pathological fractures in myeloma. In other myeloma cases, IL-6 may be produced in excess by bone marrow stromal cells infected with human herpes virus (HHV8).

Treatment of myeloma

In younger patients, most centres are moving away from single-agent melphalan therapy towards continuous low-dose combination chemotherapy such as VAD (Vincristine, Adriamycin and Dexamethasone) or ZDex (oral idarubicin and dexamethasone). Malignant cells are most sensitive to the action of chemotherapy when they are dividing; as plasma cells divide relatively infrequently, it is necessary to administer the chemotherapy over several days in order to maximise the chances of treating dividing cells.

- **Thalidomide** has a proven role in myeloma treatment although its mechanism of action remains uncertain. It is likely to inhibit cytokine release, but an anti-angiogenesis activity has not been ruled out.
- **Bisphosphonates**, such as monthly intravenous pamidronate, have an important role in the prevention of pathological fractures and in the treatment of myeloma-associated hypercalcaemia.

Monoclonal gammopathy of undetermined significance (MGUS)

A common clinical problem is the differentiation between myeloma and MGUS (benign monoclonal gammopathy) in patients found to have a paraprotein. Ten per cent of patients with MGUS develop myeloma at 5 years, and 50% at 15 years. It is probable that most patients would eventually develop myeloma but many die of other causes before this occurs.

Differentiation of myeloma from MGUS

- **MGUS**
  Low level of paraprotein (< 20 g/l for an IgG paraprotein)
  Paraprotein level remains stable over a period of observation (months or years)
  Other immunoglobulin levels are normal
  No clinical evidence of myeloma (bone disease, renal disease)
- **Myeloma**
  High level of paraprotein
  Level rises
  Other immunoglobulin levels are depressed
  Clinical evidence of myeloma

5.9 Monoclonal antibodies in the treatment of haematological diseases

Monoclonal antibodies that are directed against various antigens on haemopoietic cells are now established in the treatment of a variety of haematological diseases. In many cases these are being used on a trial basis. Such antibodies may be administered in their native state or after conjugation to cell poisons or radioactive isotopes.

Monoclonal antibodies after haematology treatment

Antibody	Disease treated	Antibody specificity	Comments
Rituximab	B-cell non-Hodgkin's lymphoma	CD20	In routine use
Campath	Immunosuppression in bone marrow transplantation	CD56	In routine use
	Lymphoproliferative disorders		CD 56 is present on both T and B cells
Gemtuzumab	Acute myeloid leukaemia	CD33	Coupled to an anthracycline cell poison
Anti-D	Prevention of rhesus sensitisation in pregnancy	Anti-D	In trial – no risk of infectious disease transfer

5.10 Polycythaemia

Polycythaemia refers to an increase in red cell count, haematocrit and (usually) haemoglobin. There are two main types of polycythaemia, the classification depending on the results of measurement of red cell mass and plasma volume:

- **relative (pseudo) polycythaemia**: due to a decrease in plasma volume
- **true polycythaemia**: the red cell mass is increased.

True polycythaemia may be either a primary or secondary.

Primary true polycythaemia

In the myeloproliferative disorder polycythaemia rubra vera (PRV), there is uncontrolled production of red cells by the bone marrow, even though erythropoietin is switched off.

- **Clinical features**: hypertension, splenomegaly, arterial and venous thrombosis, pruritus, plethoric features, peptic ulceration, gout.
- **Laboratory features**: there is high red cell count, haemoglobin, haematocrit, whole blood viscosity and uric acid. The white cell count, platelet count and neutrophil alkaline phosphatase are also increased, and the latter three parameters help to distinguish PRV from secondary polycythaemia.

Secondary true polycythaemia

This condition is associated with increased levels of erythropoietin, which is produced by either the kidney or an ectopic tumour.

Causes of secondary polycythaemia

Increased renal erythropoietin production due to hypoxia

- **Physiological**
  Adaptation to altitude
  In neonates
- **Congenital cyanotic heart disease**
  (eg Fallot's tetralogy, Eisenmenger's complex)
- **Respiratory-related**
  Smoking*
  COPD
- **High-affinity haemoglobins**
  (eg Haemoglobin M**)

Inappropriate erythropoietin production

- **From the kidney**
  (eg pyonephrosis, renal cysts, renal artery stenosis after renal transplantation***)
- **From a tumour (ectopic erythropoietin secreted in an uncontrolled fashion)**
  (eg carcinoma of the kidney, giant uterine fibroids, hepatoma, cerebellar haemangioma)

* Inhaled carbon monoxide combines irreversibly with haemoglobin, forming carboxyhaemoglobin, which is unavailable for oxygen transport

** An abnormal structure of the globin chains decreases the ability of the haemoglobin to release oxygen to hypoxic tissues (including the kidney), so more erythropoietin is released

*** All these pathologies result in decreased oxygen delivery to the juxtaglomerular apparatus, either by increasing the pressure within the renal capsule or by reducing blood supply to the whole kidney

Relative polycythaemia

A reduction in circulating plasma volume can be due to pyrexia, diarrhoea, vomiting and diuretic therapy.

Gaisböck's polycythaemia refers to a form of 'stress polycythaemia'; this has been noticed in middle-aged men who have stressful occupations, a chronically reduced plasma volume of uncertain cause.

Treatment of polycythaemia

Treatment is indicated for polycythaemia as high blood viscosity leads to an increased incidence of thrombosis, hypertension, stroke and atheromatous vascular disease.

The main treatment options are:

- **Venesection to a target haematocrit**: the packed cell volume is more closely related to the blood viscosity than is the haemoglobin (as repeated venesection may result in iron-deficient red cells with a low haemoglobin content). Venesection may be traditional or **isovolaemic** (with saline replacement). The latter is used in patients with cardiovascular risk factors (eg angina or hypertension), in those who are taking drugs that may impair physiological response to venesection (ACE inhibitors, beta-blockers), or in patients with relative polycythaemia.
- **Cytotoxic agent** (particularly hydroxyurea): this presupposes erythropoiesis and causes a macrocytosis which is not related to vitamin B_{12} or folate deficiency. Unlike other cytotoxic agents (eg busulfan) it is unlikely to be leukaemogenic.
- **Aspirin and anticoagulants**: if the patient presents with thrombosis.

5.11 Thrombocytosis (platelets > 500 × 10^9/l)

Primary (essential) thrombocythaemia

In practice it is often difficult to distinguish between essential thrombocythaemia and reactive causes of thrombocytosis unless other markers of either a myeloproliferative disorder (polycythaemia, splenomegaly, basophilia, increased bone marrow reticulin cytogenetic abnormality) or hyposplenism (due to multiple splenic infarcts) are present.

It is often necessary to treat any potential cause of secondary thrombocytosis that may be present and see what happens to the platelet count over months.

Causes of secondary (reactive) thrombocytosis

- Bleeding
- Infection
- Trauma
- Thrombosis
- Infarction
- Iron deficiency (even if not due to bleeding)

5.12 Myelodysplasias (myelodysplastic syndromes – MDS)

This group of haematological malignancies is being seen with increasing frequency as the mean age of the population rises and general practitioners perform screening blood counts more frequently on their patients. As a group, they hang together less well than other haematological malignancies, but they do have the following features in common.

- Increased frequency in the elderly, but no age is exempt.
- Cytopenias – anaemia most common, also leukopenia and thrombocytopenia or combinations of these.
- Dysplastic changes seen in blood and bone marrow. These include hypogranular neutrophils, abnormal neutrophil nuclear lobulation, changes in red cell precursors mimicking megaloblastic change ('megaloblastoid') with vacuolated erythroblasts and mononuclear megakaryocytes.
- A monocytosis in the blood. This may be found in all the myelodysplastic disorders but is most marked ($>1 \times 10^9$/l) in chronic myelomonocytic leukaemia (CMML).
- Propensity to transform into acute myeloid leukaemia. This may be an acute transformation but usually takes a number of years.
- Cytogenetic abnormalities as seen in AML may be seen in MDS. A rare variant of MDS with a relatively good prognosis is 5q minus syndrome found mainly in women with a normal or even high platelet count and deletion of part of the long arm of chromosome 5.
- Mainstay of treatment is support – transfusion for anaemia, antibiotics for infection, platelet transfusion for bleeding.

Classification of myelodysplastic syndromes

MDS	Special features
Refractory anaemia (RA)	Dysplastic morphological features seen as above but difficult to diagnose in early stages
Refractory anaemia with excess of blasts (RAEB)	As above plus increased number of blast cells in marrow (5–20%)
Refractory anaemia with excess of blasts in transformation to AML (RAEB-t)	As above but 20–30% blasts in marrow
Chronic myelomonocytic leukaemia (CMML)	Monocytosis in marrow and blood leukaemia
Primary acquired sideroblastic anaemia	Ring sideroblasts in marrow

5.13 Bone marrow transplantation

Bone marrow or stem cell transplantation works by using a strong (myelo-ablative) treatment such as high-dose cyclophosphamide with total body irradiation to wipe out residual malignant disease. In addition, the donor's transplanted immune system may recognise malignant cells and destroy them – graft-versus-leukaemia (GVL) effect. The down side of GVL is that the donor immune system may attack the recipient's tissues, particularly liver, intestine and skin, causing graft-versus-host disease (GVHD).

Peripheral blood stem cells

In the rebound after marrow recovery from chemotherapy, stem cells appear in the peripheral blood. They can be made to appear in larger numbers by using growth factors such as granulocyte colony-stimulating factor (G-CSF). They can then be harvested using a cell separator and frozen. Peripheral blood stem cells are further down the differentiation pathway to mature cells than marrow stem cells, so their use is associated with quicker haematological recovery than seen when bone marrow is used.

Types of donor and stem cells used

Type	Advantages	Disadvantages
Autologous	Donor available!	Poor GVL, possibility of residual marrow disease being harvested and returned to patient
Syngeneic (identical twin)	Full house HLA match – no GVHD	Reduced GVL effect
HLA-matched sibling	Controllable GVHD but some GVL	GVHD unpredictable
Matched volunteer unrelated donor	Available if no family match	GVHD unpredictable

GVHD = Graft-versus-host disease, GVL = graft-versus-leukaemia effect

The following are conditions in which a bone marrow allograft is a useful treatment if a matched sibling is available and the recipient is fit enough for the procedure:

- **Acute myeloid leukaemia**: in first or subsequent remission. However, if good prognosis, cytogenetics are present (see Section 5.2) and the patient is in remission after the first course of chemotherapy, then bone marrow transplant (BMT) may not be necessary.
- **Acute lymphoblastic leukaemia**: in second or later remission unless adverse prognostic features (such as age beyond childhood) are present, in which case BMT should be performed in first remission.

- **Chronic myeloid leukaemia**: in first chronic phase if imatinib does not induce complete cytogenetic response. BMT is also indicated when a patient who has undergone CML disease transformation is in remission.
- **Other indications**: BMT for thalassaemia major and sickle cell disease remains controversial.
- **Others**: storage disease, thalassaemia major, sickle cell disease.

6. COAGULATION

6.1 The coagulation mechanism and detection of factor deficiencies

A representation of the coagulation cascades is shown in the following figure. It consists of an extrinsic pathway (in which tissue thromboplastin plays an important part) and an intrinsic pathway (intrinsic to the blood itself – what happens when blood clots away from the body in a tube). These two pathways share a final common pathway resulting in the production of a fibrin clot.

Figure 2 Representation of the coagulation cascades

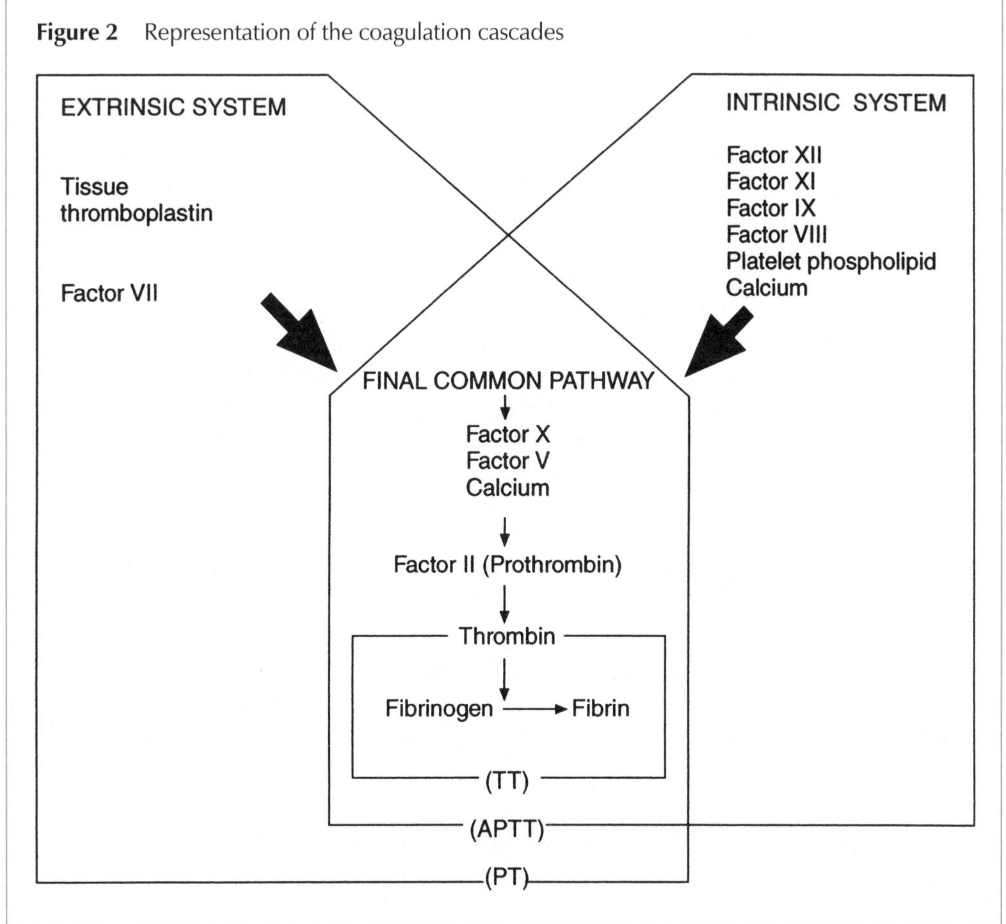

The system can be divided into boxes, each box representing one of the following three basic screening tests of coagulation.

- **Prothrombin time** (PT) measures the extrinsic system and final common pathway.
- **Activated partial thromboplastin time** (APTT) measures the intrinsic system and final common pathway. It is also known as the kaolin cephalin clotting time (KCCT) and the partial thromboplastin time (PTT), which are technical variations of the same test.
- **Thrombin time** (TT) measures the final part of the final common pathway. It is prolonged by lack of fibrinogen to convert to fibrin, and by inhibitors of this conversion, including heparin and high levels of fibrin degradation products.

If one of these screening tests of coagulation is significantly prolonged then it should be repeated using a mixture of 50% patient plasma and 50% normal plasma. If the cause of the prolonged time is factor deficiency then the abnormal time should correct more than halfway back to the control value. If it does not, this suggests the presence of an inhibitor such as the lupus anticoagulant. The diagram shows which factors should be assayed after finding a prolonged, correctable coagulation time. For example, an isolated prolonged APTT should prompt assay of the coagulation factors XII, XI, IX and VIII in the intrinsic system.

6.2 Haemophilia

This disease is characterised by deep muscular haematomas and haemarthroses with prolonged bleeding after trauma or operation. It is caused by a deficiency of clotting factor VIII (classical haemophilia A) or factor IX (Christmas disease) and is classed as severe if the factor VIII level is less than 1% of normal (<1 unit/dl).

There is a sex-linked inheritance but one-third of cases have no family history, which are due to spontaneous mutation. Carriers may be detected as they have half the amount of clotting factor measured by a coagulation assay than they have measured by an immunological assay. Also, restriction fragment length polymorphisms (RFLP) can track the affected chromosome. Diagnosis is by prolonged APTT, with low factor VIII or IX. The range of treatments is shown below.

Treatment	Rationale
Viral inactivated coagulation factor concentrate	Should be given early in course of a bleed, ideally home treatment
DDAVP (a synthetic ADH analogue)	Releases factor VIII from storage sites in endothelial cells, so can temporarily boost blood level in mild haemophilia A
Fibrinolytic inhibitors (eg tranexamic acid)	Useful for bleeding wounds and tooth sockets but avoid in haemarthrosis, muscle haematomas and urinary bleeding as may lead to resolution by local fibrosis
Ancillary treatments (part of 'total haemophilia care')	Physiotherapy, hydrotherapy, immunisation against hepatitis B, dental and orthopaedic advice

Complications of treatment include hepatitis, HIV, factor VIII antibodies and opiate addiction.

6.3 von Willebrand's disease

This is the commonest inherited coagulopathy in the UK. It is coded for on chromosome 12 – hence it shows an autosomal dominant inheritance pattern. It is caused by a quantitative or qualitative abnormality of von Willebrand factor (vWF) production. vWF is made in endothelial cells and forms variable-size polymers in plasma.

vWF acts as a protective carrier for factor VIII in the circulation and is responsible for gluing the platelets to exposed vascular subendothelium. Hence, the factor VIII coagulation factor level in vWD is often reduced but (in contrast to the haemophilias) the disease manifests as a platelet-type bleeding disorder, with bruising, superficial purpura, menorrhagia, nosebleeds and bleeding from cuts and mucous membranes.

Diagnosis

- Low factor VIIIC (C for 'clotting' activity, measured by a coagulation test)
- Low vWF Ag (von Willebrand factor antigen, measured in an immunological assay)
- Prolonged template bleeding time
- Deficient ristocetin-induced platelet aggregation.

Ristocetin is an antibiotic that clumps platelets in normal plasma but fails to clump them in vWF-deficient plasma. The disease may be divided into types according to the size of vWF multimers present.

Treatment is with DDAVP if mild, and with vWF concentrate. Many intermediate-purity factor VIII concentrates contain enough vWF for treatment, otherwise cryoprecipitate is used.

6.4 Disseminated intravascular coagulation (DIC)

This disorder is caused by the release into the circulation of a pro-coagulant – something that makes the blood clot. There is massive activation of coagulation factors and platelets, with laying down of fibrin. This fibrin clot is immediately removed as the fibrinolytic system is also put into overdrive, worsening the haemorrhagic tendency.

The treatment is to remove the cause if possible, and transfuse with blood, platelets, fresh frozen plasma or cryoprecipitate.

Features and causes of disseminated intravascular coagulation (DIC)

- **Laboratory features of DIC**
  Prolongation of all coagulation times (prothrombin, APTT and thrombin)
  Activation of the fibrinolytic system leading to high fibrin degradation products
  Thrombocytopenia
  Microangiopathic blood film with fragmented red cells and helmet cells
- **Obstetric causes**
  Retroplacental haemorrhage
  Retained dead fetus
  Amniotic fluid embolus
  Severe pre-eclampsia
- **Other causes**
  Crush injury
  Septicaemia
  Haemolytic transfusion reaction
  Malignancy

6.5 Vitamin K dependent coagulation factors (II, VII, IX, X)

Vitamin K is a fat-soluble vitamin essential for the carboxylation of inactive coagulation factors into their active functional form. These coagulation factors are manufactured in the liver, consequently levels are low in liver disease, obstructive jaundice and when there is fat malabsorption (loss of vitamin K). Levels are also low in the neonate due to liver immaturity – this can lead to haemorrhagic disease of the newborn, particularly when breast-fed. These coagulation factors are also reduced by warfarin anticoagulation. Deficiency causes prolonged prothrombin time and APTT.

7. THROMBOSIS

There are many well-recognised risk factors associated with venous thromboembolism, and in these situations it may be appropriate to take prophylactic measures.

Therapeutic ranges for warfarin anticoagulation

The necessary degree of anticoagulation will vary depending on the indication and whether the causes (eg bed rest, fracture) can be removed.

Indication	INR
Treatment of deep vein thrombosis (DVT), pulmonary embolism (PE), systemic embolism, post myocardial infarction (MI), mitral stenosis with embolism, transient ischaemic attacks, atrial fibrillation	2.0–3.0
Recurrent DVT and PE, arterial disease, including MI, mechanical prosthetic valves	3.0–4.5

Clinical risk factors for venous thrombosis

- Increasing age
- Immobility
- Varicose veins
- Major abdominal and hip operations
- Oestrogen/contraceptive pill therapy
- Increased blood viscosity
- Nephrotic syndrome
- Cigarette smoking
- Paroxysmal nocturnal haemoglobinuria
- Protein S or C or antithrombic III deficiency
- Obesity
- Previous family history of thrombosis
- Cancer
- Trauma to the lower limbs
- Pregnancy and puerperium
- Post-myocardial infarction or CVA
- Diabetic hyperosmolar state
- Homocystinuria
- Presence of Leiden factor V mutation

7.1 Thrombosis and the pill

Administration of oestrogen-containing pills:

- increases fibrinogen and vitamin K dependent coagulation factors
- decreases antithrombin III levels
- gives a four times greater risk of thromboembolism.

The risk of thromboembolism is increased by eight times if factor V Leiden is present – it is important to screen all women with a history of thrombosis if starting on the combined oral contraceptive pill.

Hormone replacement therapy is also associated with a small risk of thrombosis and patients with a previous history of thromboembolism should be screened for thrombophilia.

7.2 Thrombophilia

This may be defined as recurrent venous thromboembolism without any of the usual predisposing causes outlined above.

Groups for investigation of thrombophilia

- Venous thrombosis age < 40 years without cause
- Recurrent venous thrombosis
- Arterial thrombosis age < 30 years without cause
- Family history
- Unusual anatomical site

Congenital causes of thrombophilia

The blood contains clotting factors that promote the formation of thrombus when activated. The blood also contains natural *anticoagulant* factors that inhibit the formation of clot. These factors are:

- antithrombin
- protein C
- protein S.

A congenital deficiency of these factors results in a tendency to thrombosis, so they should be tested for when screening for congenital thrombophilia.

Normally, activated clotting factor V is inhibited by the anticoagulant protein C. Approximately 3–5% of Europeans have an abnormal structure to their clotting factor V caused by a single point mutation in the factor V gene. This means that protein C cannot bind to it and inactivate it. This abnormal factor V is called **V Leiden**, after its place of discovery, and it is found in 30% of patients with recurrent venous thrombosis. Screening for V Leiden may be done by PCR (looking for the abnormal gene) but this is expensive, so it is usual to screen using the **activated protein C resistance test**. In this test, protein C is added to the patient's plasma and an APTT is performed. In normal subjects the added protein C has an anticoagulant action resulting in prolongation of the APPT. In a patient with factor V Leiden the added protein C cannot bind to activated factor V so the APTT coagulation time will not be prolonged by protein C.

Other causes of inherited thrombophilia include:

- abnormal prothrombin molecule
- dysfibrinogenaemia
- fibrinolytic defects.

Acquired causes of thrombophilia

- Polycythaemia and essential thrombocythaemia
- Lupus anticoagulant/anti-phospholipid antibodies.

Anti-phospholipid antibodies and lupus anticoagulant, which are not always the same molecules, have a strong association with each other and with immune thrombocytopenia. Paradoxically, lupus anticoagulant, causing venous thrombosis, is detected by a prolonged coagulation test such as the APTT (or the more sensitive DRVT - dilute Russell viper venom time). The coagulation times are prolonged because anti-phospholipid antibodies neutralise phospholipids that are essential for the coagulation reaction. Although it may be found in patients with systemic lupus erythematosus (SLE), most patients with lupus anticoagulant do not have SLE. The disorder may present with recurrent venous thromboembolism or recurrent miscarriages. (See *also* Chapter 12, Maternal Medicine.)

7.3 Therapeutic fibrinolysis

Therapeutic fibrinolysis

- **Action**
  Conversion of plasminogen to plasmin, which dissolves fibrin to fibrin degradation products

- **Indications**
  Early stage of myocardial infarction, young patient with proximal DVT (eg ilio-femoral), survivors of massive pulmonary embolism, peripheral arterial thrombosis

- **Drugs**
  Streptokinase, urokinase, tissue plasminogen activator (TPA), anisoylated plasminogen streptokinase activator complex (APSAC)

- **Unwanted effects**
  Bleeding

- **Reversal**
  Administration of tranexamic acid, cryoprecipitate

7.4 Low molecular weight heparins (LMWH)

Conventional heparin is a mixture of different sized polymers. Low molecular weight fractions can be separated by various chemical and physical methods. Low molecular weight heparin (LMWH) has a molecular weight of 5000, compared with 15, 000 for unfractionated heparin. LMWH has a strong anti-Xa and relatively weak antithrombin action compared with conventional heparin. It is claimed that this gives it more antithrombotic effect with less risk of bleeding. It certainly means that no significant prolongation of APTT is found, so this test is not used for monitoring therapy. Measurement of its anti-Xa effect is possible, though this is only necessary if prolonged treatment is required.

Advantages

- Long half-life – once or at most twice a day administration
- Laboratory assays are not required for short-term administration
- Less heparin-induced thrombocytopenia and osteopenia than conventional heparin.

Disadvantages

- Expensive
- Different doses for different brands
- When given for more than a few weeks require (relatively) complicated anti-Xa assay for monitoring.

8. THE SPLEEN

8.1 Causes of splenomegaly

- **Myeloproliferative disorders**
  Myelofibrosis
  Chronic myeloid leukaemia
  Polycythaemia rubra vera
  Essential thrombocythaemia
  (splenic atrophy also common)
- **Portal hypertension**
  Cirrhosis
  Congestive cardiac failure
- **Infection**
- **Bacterial**
  (eg typhoid, brucella, TB)
- **Collagen diseases**
- **Chronic haemolytic anaemias**
  Autoimmune haemolytic anaemia
  Cold haemagglutinin disease
  Hereditary spherocytosis
  Haemoglobinopathies
- **Lymphoproliferative disorders**
  Most lymphomas
  Chronic lymphocytic leukaemia
  Hairy cell leukaemia
- **Viral**
  (eg glandular fever, hepatitis)
- **Tropical**
  (eg malaria, kala-azar)
- **Storage diseases**

8.2 Splenectomy

Often performed because of traumatic injury or haematological disease, this operation results in a characteristic blood film appearance and a well-recognised predisposition to sudden overwhelming bacterial infection with capsulated organisms such as *Pneumococcus* or *Haemophilus*.

Clinical indications for splenectomy

- **Traumatic rupture**: but surgeons may preserve splenic function by surgical repair of capsular tears, omental patches, and sometimes implantation of some splenic tissue in the retroperitoneum.
- **Autoimmune destruction of blood cells**: immune thrombocytopenic purpura and warm autoimmune haemolytic anaemia after failure of steroid treatment.
- **Haematological malignancies**: low-grade lymphoproliferative disorders associated with painful splenomegaly, hypersplenism and not much disease outside the spleen. Also sometimes performed in the myeloproliferative disorders, particularly in myelofibrosis when the enlarged or painful spleen is destroying more blood cells than it is producing.
- **Congenital haemolytic anaemias**: such as hereditary spherocytosis and elliptocytosis and some cases of hypersplenic thalassaemia major.
- **Staging of Hodgkin's disease and NHL**: this is no longer performed where adequate imaging is available (CT or MRI).

Haematological and immune changes after splenectomy

- **Howell–Jolly bodies** (Nuclear remnants in the red cells – the spleen is responsible for removing particulate material from red cell cytoplasm – pitting function)
- **Enhanced neutrophilia** in response to infection
- **Target cells**, increased platelet count and occasionally spherocytes with increased aniso- and poikilocytosis
- **Decreased IgM level**

8.3 Causes of hyposplenism

- Splenectomy (see above)
- Sickle cell disease
- Coeliac disease
- Myeloproliferative diseases, particularly essential thrombocythaemia
- Congenital asplenism (rare)

Infection prophylaxis necessary in hyposplenism (recent UK working party report).

Pneumococcal vaccine and one dose of Haemophilus influenzae vaccine (Hib) are required at least two weeks before planned splenectomy; if the operation is unplanned then these should be given as soon as possible afterwards.

Post-operatively, prophylactic life-long penicillin V 250 mg b.d. is necessary (or erythromycin if the patient is penicillin allergic). Meticulous malaria prophylaxis is vital including insect repellent and mosquito nets. Meningococcal vaccine is necessary if the patient is going to equatorial Africa – the meningitis belt. A warning card is now available from the Department of Health.

The above applies to hyposplenic patients (eg adult sickle cell disease) as well as previously splenectomised patients (recognised by the film comment 'Howell–Jolly bodies' on routine blood count) who have not been taking prophylaxis. If penicillin prophylaxis is refused then they should keep a supply of amoxicillin at home.

9. BLOOD TRANSFUSION

9.1 Transfusion-transmitted infection

Periodically, transfusion-transmitted infections hit the headlines, resulting in patient's reluctance to accept blood products. The infection which is of most concern currently is **variant Creutzfeldt-Jakob disease** (vCJD or 'mad cow disease'), the prion protein of which is not destroyed by conventional heat-detergent viral inactivation processes. A screening test for carriers of this disease is being developed, although it is feared that introducing such a test may shrink the donor pool, as potential donors would not wish to have a test for a disease for which no treatment is currently available.

All cellular blood products issued by the UK blood service have been **leukodepleted at source** for some years so as to reduce the possibility of transmitting vCJD.

Leukocyte depletion at source will:

- make bedside leukodepletion blood filters obsolete
- reduce the incidence of non-haemolytic febrile blood transfusion reactions due to HLA antigen sensitisation in recipients
- decrease transmission of CMV to CMV-negative blood transfusion recipients
- reduce the risk of third-party graft-versus-host disease caused by the transfusion of immunocompetent lymphocytes to immunodeficient recipients.

Testing donations for transfusion-transmitted infection in the UK

- HIV antibodies – small risk of viral transmission from infected donors in the period up to 8 weeks before antibody production
- Hepatitis B surface antigen
- Hepatitis C antibody
- Syphilis screen
- CMV antibody – some donations only, to ensure enough CMV-negative products for transfusion to premature neonates and immunosuppressed patients.

9.2 Platelet transfusion in marrow failure

Platelet transfusion is usually administered when the platelet count is $\leq 10 \times 10^9$/l in cases of thrombocytopenia due to marrow failure after chemotherapy or radiotherapy. The platelet transfusion threshold may be reduced as a result of clinical criteria such as bleeding, fever, splenomegaly or planned operative procedures.

- Platelet transfusion should not be used in conditions with peripheral platelet destruction (eg idiopathic (immune) thrombocytopenic purpura (**ITP**)), where efforts should be directed to reducing platelet destruction with immunosuppression (except in cases of haemorrhagic emergency).
- Platelet transfusion is contraindicated in TTP and HUS as it will contribute to the microvascular occlusion in the brain and kidneys which is associated with these conditions.
- Platelet preparations are obtained by the thromobocytopheresis of donors who have a high platelet count on the cell separator. One adult unit of platelets contains more than 2×10^{11} platelets.
- Less commonly, the unit of platelets is prepared by pooling the platelets extracted from four to six units of fresh blood.

Platelet refractoriness is defined as an increment of platelet count less than 20 × 10^9/l one hour after transfusion of an adult dose (see above). This may be due to the following:

- non-immune consumption (eg bleeding, DIC, hypersplenism)
- immune due to HLA antibodies directed against class I HLA antigens present on platelets (90%): give HLA-matched cell separator platelets, consider platelet pheresing relatives
- immune platelet-specific antibodies (10%): use double doses of random platelets.

9.3 Indications for the transfusion of fresh frozen plasma

Indications for transfusion of FFP

- Correction of multiple coagulation factor deficits as in DIC or after massive transfusion
- Correction of single coagulation factor deficiency where a heat-detergent virus inactivated concentrate is not available
- Emergency correction of warfarin over anticoagulation associated with bleeding, when II, VII, IX, X concentrate is not available and intravenous vitamin K would be too slow (a few hours)
- Treatment of TTP or HUS with or without large-volume plasma exchange

The 'formula replacement' of coagulation factors by fresh frozen plasma after large-volume blood transfusion is no longer recommended – it is better to perform a coagulation screen and blood count and replace as required.

Chapter 10
Immunology

CONTENTS

9.4 Extractable nuclear antigens
9.5 Anti-neutrophil cytoplasmic antibodies (ANCA)
9.6 Autoantibodies in gastrointestinal and liver disease
9.7 Autoantibodies in thyroid disease
9.8 Antiphospholipid antibodies
9.9 Others

10. Immunodeficiency
10.1 Complement deficiency
10.2 Neutrophil disorders
10.3 B-cell disorders
10.4 T-cell disorders
10.5 Combined B- and T-cell disorders
10.6 Acquired immunodeficiency

11. Immunisation
11.1 Preformed antibody
11.2 Killed organism vaccines
11.3 Live attenuated vaccines
11.4 Subunit vaccines

Immunology

1. COMPLEMENT AND ITS ACTIVATION

This is a plasma protein sequence cascade triggered by one of three distinct pathways: classical, alternative or lectin binding. Each pathway produces protein complexes capable of cleaving the C3 component into its active metabolites, C3a and C3b. These activate the terminal complement components to produce a membrane attack complex (MAC) capable of cell lysis.

The complement cascade slowly 'ticks over' and is never completely inactive. This produces small quantities of active complement components that would cause tissue damage and further complement activation by positive feedback loops but for important regulatory components.

The biologically active complement products have three main effects:

- opsonisation – mediated by C3b
- chemotaxis and inflammation – mediated by C3a, C5a
- cell lysis (MAC) – C5, C6, C7, C8, C9.

1.1 Complement activation

The complement pathways will **all** be activated during infection (bacterial, viral, fungal) and it is unlikely that any particular pathway is predominant. The classical pathway is thought to be the most recently evolved, and is the only pathway to require antibodies for activation. Theoretically, the alternative and lectin pathways therefore can activate complement in the absence of antibody.

Complement activation pathways (see also accompanying figure)

Classical pathway

- Initiated by antigen–antibody complexes containing IgM, IgG1, IgG2 or IgG3
- Components involved: C1q, C1r, C1s, C4, C2, C3
- The C4bC2b complex cleaves and activates C3

Alternative pathway

- Initiated by polysaccharides found in the cell walls of Gram-negative bacteria, pneumococci and yeasts. IgA is also a weak activator of this pathway
- Components involved: properdin, factor D, factor B, C3
- The C3bBb complex cleaves and activates C3

Lectin binding pathway

- Initiated by bacterial cell wall carbohydrate which binds to mannose binding lectin
- Binding activates mannan-binding lectin-associated proteases (MASP1 and MASP2) which cleave C2 and C4
- C4b2a complex cleaves and activates C3

Figure 1 Complement activation pathways

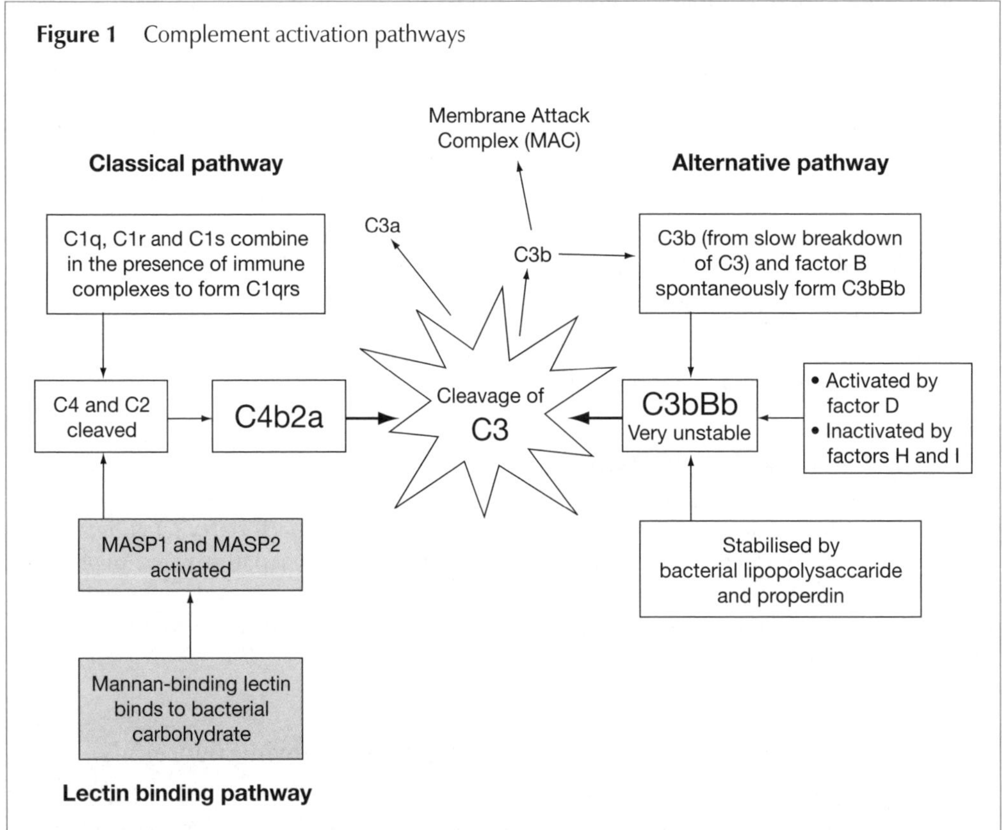

1.2 Terminal membrane attack sequence

Components of C5, C6, C7, C8 and C9 join to form the rosette-like membrane attack complex. This structure forms on cell surfaces and will cause cell lysis unless specific inhibitors are present.

1.3 Regulating proteins

Classical pathway

- C1 inhibitor blocks C1s and C1r irreversibly
- C4 binding protein inhibits cleavage of C3.

Alternative pathway

- Factor H, decay accelerating factor (DAF) and complement receptor 1 inhibit cleavage of C3.

Others

- Factor I and membrane cofactor protein degrade C3b
- Anaphylotoxin inactivator degrades C3a and C5a
- The terminal sequence is regulated by homologous restriction factor (HRF), membrane inhibitor of reactive lysis (MIRL) and S-protein.

2. COMPLEMENT DEFICIENCY

Inherited deficiencies of complement components or regulatory proteins can produce disease states. Complement deficiency is common. Most cases, however, have only partial deficiency and are asymptomatic.

2.1 Deficiency of complement components

- Deficiencies of classical pathway components produce SLE-like disorders in some patients. This may reflect impaired clearance of immune complexes
- C3 deficiency allows life-threatening infections by encapsulated organisms (eg pneumococci)
- Patients with deficiencies of the terminal complement proteins, C5, C6, C7, C8 or C9 are usually healthy but are unable to prevent Neisserial infections becoming disseminated.

2.2 Deficiency of regulatory proteins

- C1 inhibitor deficiency causes **hereditary angio-oedema**, in which there are recurrent acute episodes of non-inflammatory oedema mediated by vasoactive C2 fragments. Uncontrolled complement activation and consumption cause low levels of C2 and C4. Danazol, a synthetic anabolic steroid, can raise levels of the inhibitor sufficiently to prevent attacks. Fifteen per cent of affected patients have normal levels of C1 inhibitor – but functional assays show it to be inactive in these cases.
- **Paroxysmal nocturnal haemoglobinuria** occurs in patients who are unable to bind the regulatory proteins, DAF, HRF or MIRL on their red cell surfaces. Spontaneous complement-mediated lysis of erythrocytes occurs.

2.3 Acquired deficiency

Complement consumption in inflammatory disorders such as lupus nephritis can lead to low levels of C3 and C4. This produces an increased susceptibility to severe infections with encapsulated organisms.

3. IMMUNOGLOBULINS

The functions of immunoglobulins include complement activation, stimulation of phagocytic cells and precipitation of antigen. Immunoglobulins are produced by B lymphocytes and secreted by plasma cells. They are made up of two identical light chains and two identical heavy chains joined covalently by disulphide bonds. Papain splits the Ig molecule into two **a**ntigen **b**inding **f**ragments (Fab) and one Fc fragment containing the complement fixation site. Isotypes (eg IgG, IgM) are due to differences in the heavy chains.

Figure 2 IgCG molecule showing heavy (H) and light (L) chains, constant (C) and variable (V) regions and the antigen-binding site. The fragments produced by the action of papain and pepsin are shown

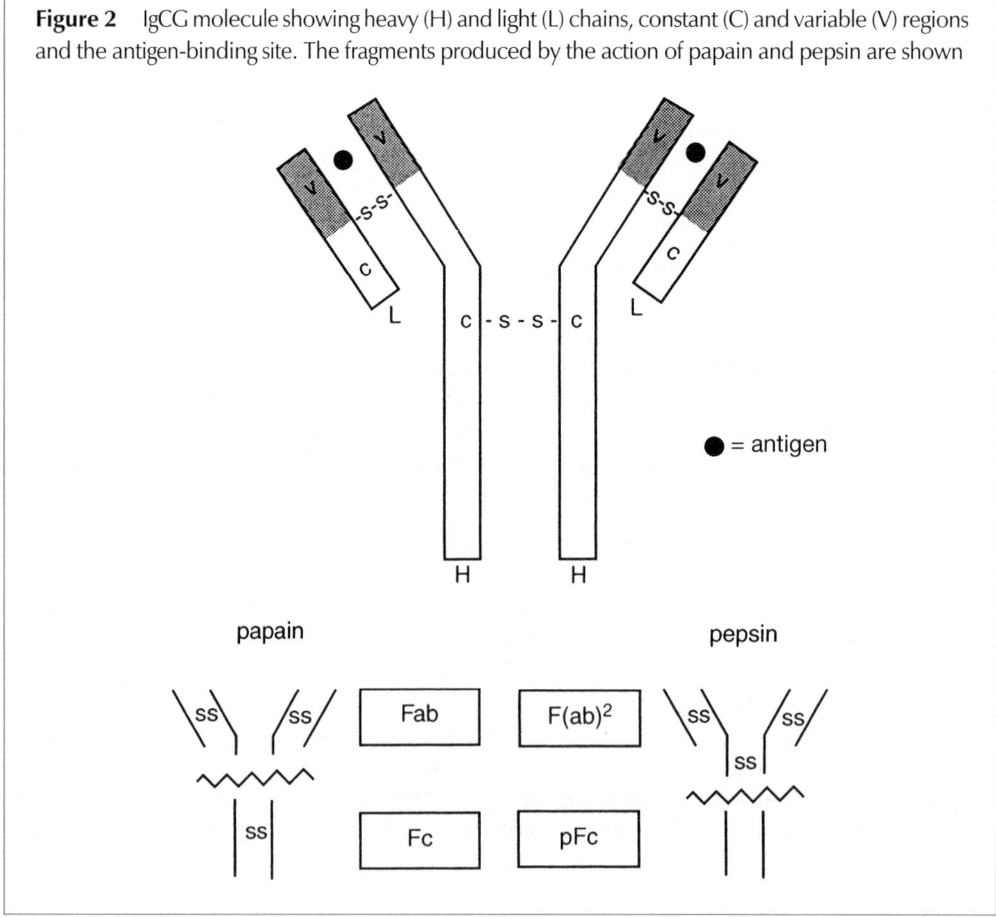

IgG

This is the most abundant immunoglobulin in internal body fluids and it is important in the secondary immune response. It is also the only isotype to cross the placenta and the neonatal intestinal wall; levels fall at age 3 months as maternal IgG is catabolised.

- Fc portion activates complement by the classical pathway
- Four subclasses – differing in Fc portions of the heavy chains
- Molecular weight 150, 000 daltons.

IgA

This is the major immunoglobulin of seromucous secretions, and it is produced predominantly in mucosal-associated lymphoid tissue. It is present in monomeric form in plasma but as a dimer in secretions. Levels are undetectable at birth but reach adult levels by puberty. Deficiency produces autoimmune disorders, chronic diarrhoea and respiratory infections.

- Activates the **A**lternative complement pathway
- Two subclasses – IgA_1 and IgA_2
- Molecular weight 160, 000 daltons.

IgM

This is a pentameric molecule, which is the main immunoglobulin of the primary immune response. It is very effective against bacteria which it agglutinates and then lyses by complement activation. It is undetectable at birth; adult levels are reached at one year of age.

- Secretion does not require help from T_H2 lymphocytes
- Includes blood group antibodies
- Molecular weight 750, 000 daltons.

IgD

- Monomer present on B-cell surface and involved in B-cell activation
- Molecular weight 175, 000 daltons.

IgE

- Immediate (type I) hypersensitivity reactions
- Present on mast cells and basophils, but produced by plasma cells
- Molecular weight 190, 000 daltons.

3.1 Cryoglobulins

These are immunoglobulins (IgM, IgG or IgA) that precipitate when cooled to 4°C, and dissolve when reheated to body temperature. They may be monoclonal or polyclonal. Precipitation in small cool blood vessels in the peripheries and skin produces complement activation and inflammation. In high concentrations they may cause Raynaud's phenomenon or vasculitis. Treatment is of the underlying disorder. Steroids and immunosuppressives may be needed.

Causes

- Thirty-three per cent of cases are essential (ie unexplained)
- Lymphomas
- Hepatitis C
- Paraproteinaemia
- Connective tissue disorders, particularly systemic lupus erythematosus (SLE)

Classification of cryoglobulinaemias

	Type 1	Type 2	Type 3
Frequency*	25%	25%	50%
Nature	Monoclonal (usually IgM, or IgG)	Mixed monoclonal or polyclonal (with rheumatoid factor)	Mixed polyclonal (may have rheumatoid factor activity)
		Monoclone (often IgM) directed against Fc portion of IgG (e.g. rheumatoid factor activity)	IgM 'rheumatoid-like' factors react with IgG
Associations	Waldenstrom's macro-globulinaemia Myeloma Lymphoma	infections (hepatitis C, HIV) Lymphoma CLL	Idiopathic Autoimmune diseases (SLE, RA, Sjögren's)
Clinical features	Vasculitis	'Immune complex disease' (eg vasculitis, arthritis, mesangiocapillary glomerulonephritis)	Purpura
	Cutaneous ulceration Raynaud's		Arthritis Glomerulonephritis

* Of all cryoglobulinaemias

3.2 Cold agglutinins

These are IgM capable of agglutinating red blood cells between 0°C and 4°C. They may be monoclonal or polyclonal. Symptoms are of Raynaud's phenomenon, acrocyanosis and mild haemolytic anaemia.

Causes

- Idiopathic (mainly in the elderly)
- Coxsackie virus
- Mycoplasma
- Lymphoma

4. CELLS AND THE IMMUNE SYSTEM

4.1 Polymorphonuclear cells

Include neutrophils, eosinophils and basophils. Their principal actions are phagocytosis and release of inflammatory mediators.

Neutrophils

- Stored in the bone marrow and rapidly released into the bloodstream in response to infection
- Surface receptors for IgG, IgA and complement components
- Their principal action is phagocytosis and destruction of bacteria.

Basophils and mast cells

- Basophils circulate and mast cells are tissue bound
- Surface receptors for C3, C5 and IgE
- Produce histamine, prostaglandins, leukotrienes and proteases
- Involved in the immune response to parasites
- Interaction of antigen with bound IgE produces immediate hypersensitivity.

Eosinophils

- Commonly increased in patients with allergic disease
- Surface receptors for IgG, C3 and C5
- Also bind IgE but less avidly than mast cells or basophils
- Phagocytose antigen–antibody complexes.

4.2 Lymphocytes

T-lymphocytes

Characteristics of T-lymphocytes

- Form 70–80% of the total lymphocyte population
- Important in intracellular infections, tumour surveillance and graft rejection
- Arise from precursors in the bone marrow and undergo maturation in the thymus
- CD3 (part of the T-cell receptor) is present on all T-cells
- CD4 is a glycoprotein that recognises major histocompatibility complex (MHC) class II antigens on antigen-presenting cells. It is present on the cell surface of T-helper cells and monocytes
- CD8 is a glycoprotein on cytotoxic T-cells which recognises class I antigens on target cells

CD4 (helper) T-cells only recognise antigen presented with class II MHC antigens. They make up 60% of the circulating T-cell population. Important in providing help for B-cell differentiation and type IV hypersensitivity. The following are subsets of CD4 cells:

- **T_H1 (helper) cells** recognise antigen presented by macrophages or other specialised phagocytic cells. When activated they secrete interleukin-2 (IL-2) and interferon and produce type IV cell-mediated immunity. They are suppressed by IL-10.
- **T_H2 (helper) cells** recognise antigen presented by B-lymphocytes. When activated they secrete IL-4, IL-5, IL-6 and IL-10, causing B-lymphocyte proliferation and secretion of IgG, IgA or IgE, contributing to type II and type III immunity. They are suppressed by interferon.

CD8 (cytotoxic) T-cells recognise antigen presented with class I MHC antigens. They make up 35% of the circulating T-cell population. This mechanism is important in eliminating cells infected by viruses.

A schema of antigen recognition by CD4 and CD8 T-cells is shown in figure 3.

Figure 3 Antigen recognition by CD4 and CD8 T-cells

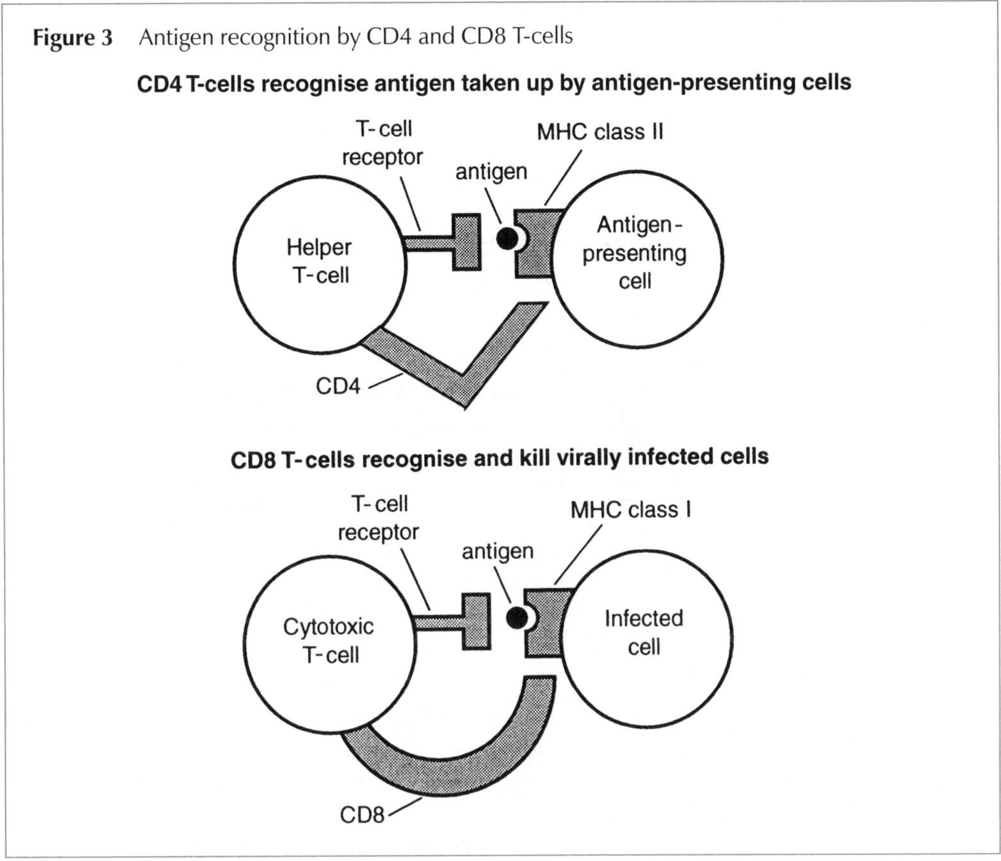

B-lymphocytes

- Develop in the bone marrow with final maturation in the spleen and lymph nodes
- Immunoglobulin is expressed on the cell surface, but immature cells cannot secrete antibody
- Activation requires both antigen and T-helper cells but some antigens, eg bacterial lipopolysaccharide, can produce activation without the need for T-helper cells, but without T-helper collaboration, low affinity antibodies are produced and memory is poor.

Natural killer cells

- Large granular lymphocytes
- Recognise and lyse cells bearing viral or tumour surface markers.

5. TRANSPLANT IMMUNOLOGY

5.1 The major histocompatibility complex

Figure 4 Major histocompatibility complex on chromosome 6

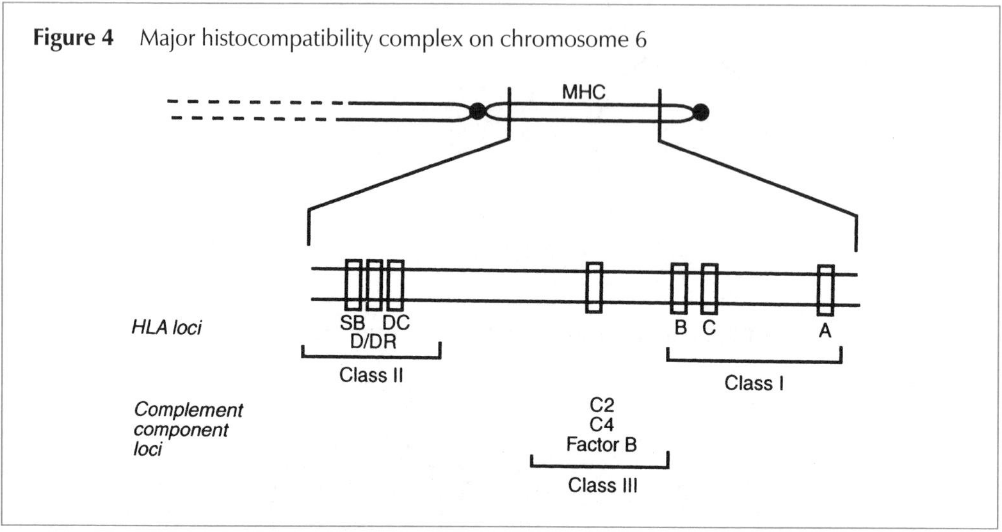

The major histocompatibility complex (MHC) is an area on chromosome 6 containing the genes for HLA antigens and some complement components. The HLA antigens are important in the recognition of self, control of immune reactivity and graft rejection. There are three MHC classes:

- **Class I** (HLA-A, B, C) are expressed as transmembrane peptides associated with β2-microglobulin. They are present on virtually all cells and, with antigen, signal to CD8 cytotoxic T-cells that their carrier cell is a suitable target for destruction.
- **Class II** molecules (HLA-DR, DP, etc) are heterodimers of two α and two β chains. They are present on B cells, macrophages and some endothelial cells. They signal to CD4 helper T-cells, and protect their carrier cells from destruction by cytotoxic T-cells.
- **Class III** includes the complement proteins C4 and factor B.

5.2 The immunology of transplantation

Graft rejection depends on MHC antigens and can be mediated by several mechanisms.

Rejection type	Timing	Mechanism
Hyperacute	Within minutes	Preformed antibody
Acute	Up to 10 days	CD8 lymphocytes
Acute late	After 10 days	Igs and complement
Late	Weeks, months, years	Immune complex deposition?

Privileged sites exist where rejection is rarely a problem even when there is no MHC matching:

- **cornea**: avascular and does not sensitise the patient
- **bone and artery**: even if the grafts die, they provide a structure for host cells to colonise.

In the kidney, HLA-DR and HLA-B matching are the most important. After these, matching for HLA-A, and to a lesser extent HLA-C, produces only small improvements in graft survival (see Chapter 15, Nephrology). Heart and liver grafts survive well with immunosuppression with only limited matching (eg at one HLA site).

6. HYPERSENSITIVITY

Hypersensitivity reactions are immune responses with excessive or undesirable consequences, such as tissue or organ damage. There are five types.

- **Type I: Anaphylactic or immediate**
  Antigen + IgE on mast cells and basophils leads to release of vasoactive substances, histamine, leukotrienes, interleukins and chemotactic factors. Reactions usually occur within 30 minutes of exposure to antigen.
  Clinical significance: asthma, atopy, some acute drug reactions.

- **Type II: Antibody-dependent cytotoxicity**
  Cell-bound antigen + circulating IgG or IgM antibody produces complement activation, phagocytosis, killer cell activation and cell lysis.
  Clinical significance: transfusion reactions, rhesus incompatibility, Goodpasture's syndrome, immune thrombocytopenia.

- **Type III: Immune-complex-mediated or arthus reaction**
  Free antigen + free antibody produces complement activation, platelet aggregation, etc.
  Clinical significance: in *antibody excess* antigen–antibody complexes precipitate close to the site of entry into the body, activate complement and cause localised disease, as in farmer's lung, pigeon fancier's lung and pulmonary aspergillosis.
  In *antigen excess* the complexes remain soluble. They are cleared by binding to red blood cells via CR1 complement receptors. If the classical complement pathway is deficient or becomes overwhelmed, immune complexes continue to circulate and are deposited in the small blood vessels of the kidneys, skin and joints. Complement is activated producing both local tissue damage, eg glomerulonephritis, and systemic illness. The systemic features produced are those seen in serum sickness: pyrexia, lymphadenopathy, urticarial rash, swollen joints and hypocomplementaemia about a week after injection of foreign serum.

- **Type IV: Cell-mediated or delayed type hypersensitivity**
  Antigen (with class II MHC) + sensitised (memory) T-cells – lymphokine release, T-cell activation. Reactions take 24 hours to develop.
  Clinical significance: tuberculin reaction, Kveim test, contact dermatitis, graft versus host disease, graft rejection.

- **Type V: Stimulatory**
  Antibody + cell surface receptor, eg Graves' disease, thyrotoxicosis.

7. CYTOKINES

Cytokines are low-molecular-weight peptides (10–45 kDa) with non-enzymatic biological activity that are produced by lymphocytes (mainly T-cells), macrophages and fibroblasts. They include interleukins, interferons and colony-stimulating factors. The interleukin family is broadly divided into those with local (paracrine or autocrine) effects and those with systemic activity (IL-1, IL-6, tumour necrosis factor (TNF)) which produce fever, increased C-reactive protein (CRP) production, thrombocythaemia and activate osteoclasts, etc. Other actions include enhancement of cytotoxic T-cells and natural killer (NK) cells.

7.1 Some patterns of cytokine production

Immune response	Important cytokines	Derived from
Acute phase response	IL-1, IL-6, TNFα	Macrophage
Cell-mediated immunity	IL-2, IFNγ	T_H1 helper cells
Antibody-mediated	IL-4, IL-5, IL-6, IL-10	T_H2 helper cells

Figure 5 Cytokine production by T-helper cells

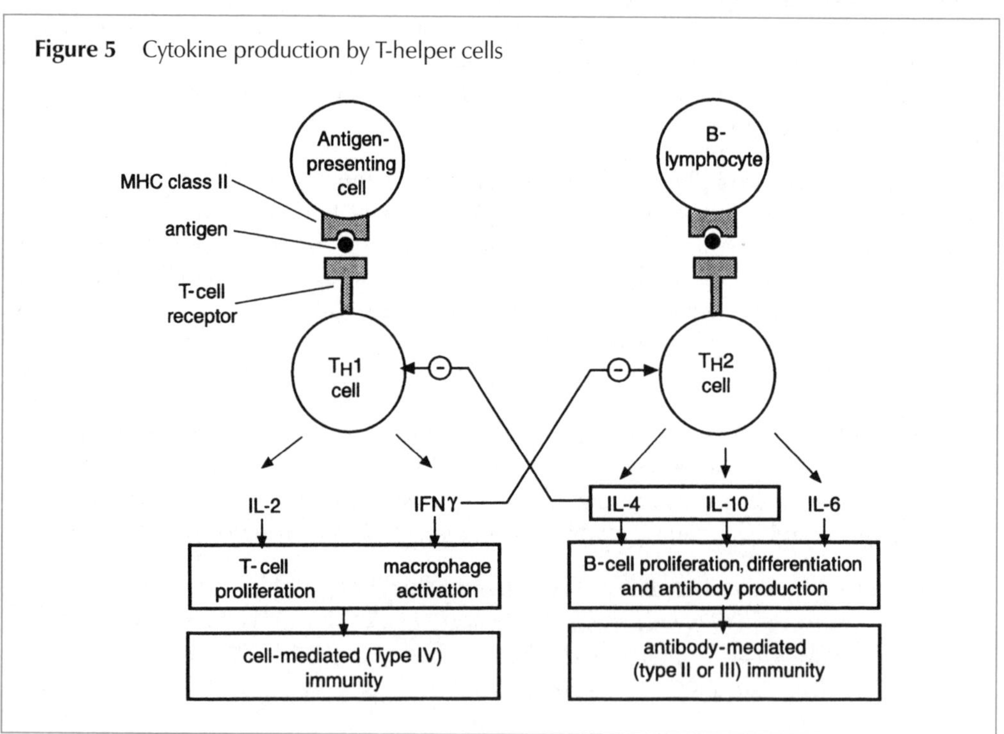

7.2 Therapeutic uses of cytokines

- **Interferon α**
  Hepatitis B
  Hepatitis C
  Kaposi's sarcoma in AIDS
  Hairy cell leukaemia
  Cutaneous T-cell lymphoma
  Recurrent or metastatic renal cell carcinoma
  Condylomata acuminata
- **Interferon β**
  Relapsing/remitting multiple sclerosis or secondary progressive multiple sclerosis
- **Interferon γ**
  Serious infections in chronic granulomatous disease
- **Granulocyte macrophage colony-stimulating factor (GM-CSF)**
  Correction of cytopenias, eg during chemotherapy
- **Interleukin-2**
  Metastatic renal cell carcinoma.

The characteristics of individual cytokines are shown in the following box.

Classification of cytokines and their actions

Cytokine	Produced by	Actions
IL-1	Macrophages	B- and T-cell stimulation Induction of IL-6, GM-CSF Acute phase response Osteoclastic bone resorption
IL-2	T_H1 lymphocytes	Growth of activated B- and T-cells Activation of NK cells
IL-3	T-lymphocytes Mast cells	Proliferation of activated B-, T- and mast cells Isotype switch to IgE and IgG production
IL-4	T_H2 lymphocytes Mast cells Macrophages	Acute phase response Immunoglobulin production
IL-5	T-lymphocytes Mast cells	Proliferation of activated B-cells
IL-6	T_H2 lymphocytes Mast cells Macrophages	Acute phase response Immunoglobulin production

Continues ...

... Continued

Cytokine	Produced by	Actions
IL-7	Bone marrow cells	Proliferation of CD4 and CD8 T-cells
IL-8	Monocytes	Neutrophil chemotaxis Angiogenesis
IL-9	T-lymphocytes	Proliferation of T-cells
IL-10	T_H2 lymphocytes Macrophages	Inhibit production of IFN
IL-11	Bone marrow cells	Acute phase response
IL-12	Macrophages	Activate T_H1 lymphocytes
Interferon α/β	Leukocytes Fibroblasts Others	Anti-viral effects Expression of MHC class I
Interferon γ	T_H1 lymphocytes	Activates macrophages Inhibits T_H2 lymphocytes
TNFα	Macrophages	Stimulates B- and T-lymphocytes Induces IL-6 Acute phase response Angiogenesis
GM-CSF	Mononuclear cells	Stimulates IL-1 production Induction of inflammation Production of granulocytes and macrophages

8. EICOSANOIDS

Eicosanoids are biologically active lipids synthesised in cells by the oxygenation of arachidonic acid. This is released from cellular lipid stores by the action of the enzyme phospholipase-A_2. Omega-3 fatty acids, from fish oils, may act as an alternative substrate. There are two main enzymatic pathways:

- 5-lipoxygenase – producing leukotrienes
- cyclo-oxygenase – producing prostaglandins and thromboxane.

These are shown in the following figure.

Figure 6 The pathway of arachidonic acid metabolism

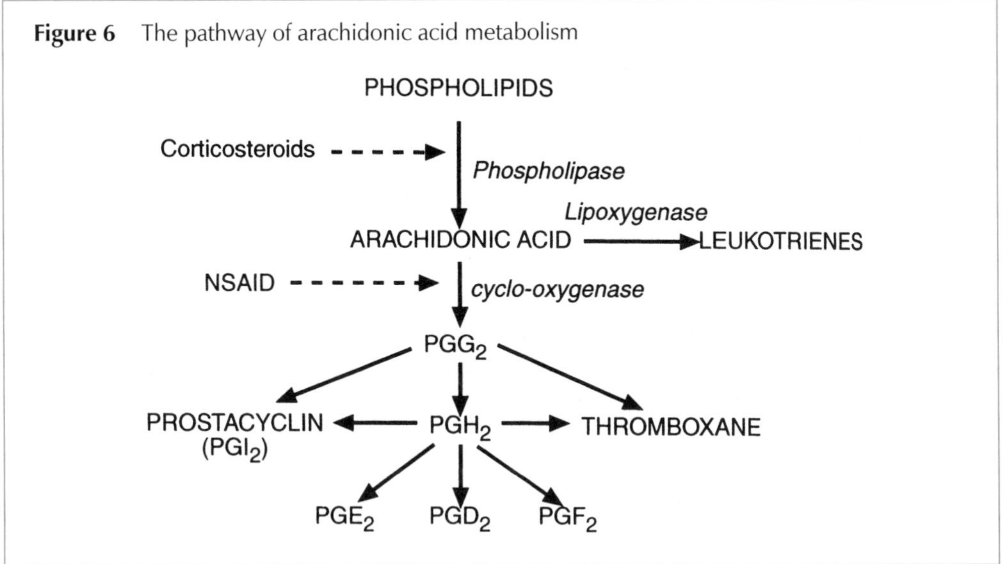

8.1 Prostaglandins

- **PGD_2** is the major cyclo-oxygenase product of mast cells and produces some of the features of anaphylaxis: vasodilatation, bronchoconstriction and inhibition of platelet aggregation.
- **PGI_2** (prostacyclin) is a potent vasodilator and inhibitor of platelet aggregation synthesised in vascular epithelium. Used therapeutically in primary pulmonary hypertension, haemolytic uraemic syndrome and severe Raynaud's disease.
- **PGE_2** has predominantly immunomodulatory effects, inhibiting lymphocyte proliferation, cytokine production and neutrophil function.

Non-steroidal anti-inflammatory drugs (NSAIDs) and aspirin inhibit cyclo-oxygenase (COX) and therefore reduce prostaglandin production. There are two isoenzymes of cyclo-oxygenase: COX-1 and COX-2. COX-1 is a constitutive enzyme present in many tissues, whereas COX-2 is induced at sites of inflammation. NSAIDs which are more specific for COX-2 would be expected to have anti-inflammatory effects with less adverse gastrointestinal effects.

8.2 Leukotrienes

- **LTB_4** causes neutrophil chemotaxis, increased mucus secretion and modulates cell growth.
- **LTC_4, LTD_4, LTE_4** increase vascular permeability, contract intestinal and bronchial wall smooth muscle, increase mucus production and modulate cell growth. These were previously known as slow reacting substances of anaphylaxis.

Leukotriene receptor antagonists are useful for the treatment of asthma (eg montelukast).

9. AUTOANTIBODIES IN DIAGNOSIS

Autoantibodies usually suggest the presence of a disease, or reflect disease activity. Some may be pathogenic through antibody–antigen interaction, such as anti-GBM in Goodpasture's syndrome. Others, such as rheumatoid factors, with cryoglobulin activity have physical properties leading to disease. (This section should be read in conjunction with the relevant sections in Chapter 20, Rheumatology.)

9.1 Rheumatoid factor

- Antibody against human IgG (usually the Fc portion)
- May be of any Ig class but latex and SCAT detect only IgM rheumatoid factors
- Positive in 70% of rheumatoid arthritis (RA) patients, and associated with extra-articular features and more severe articular disease
- Very high titres suggest cryoglobulinaemia.

This topic is covered in detail in Chapter 20, Rheumatology.

9.2 Antinuclear antibodies

Antinuclear antibodies (ANAs) are directed against a variety of nuclear antigens and may be induced by certain drugs (hydralazine). Like rheumatoid factors, ANAs can be of any Ig class (remember that IgG can cross the placenta).

Indirect immunofluorescence is the routine method for detecting ANA. It is highly sensitive and the fluorescence pattern can give some indication of the type of ANA/disease present.

A number of staining patterns are seen. Though these tend to be found in particular disorders, none are specific enough to be diagnostic:

- **homogeneous staining** suggests lupus
- **speckled staining** suggests mixed connective tissue disease
- **nucleolar staining** suggests scleroderma
- **centromere staining** suggests CREST syndrome.

ANAs are found in

- Drug-induced lupus (100%)
- SLE (99%)
- Scleroderma (97%)
- Sjögren's syndrome (96%)
- Mixed connective tissue disease (93%)
- Polymyositis (78%)

ANA in rheumatoid arthritis suggests Felty's syndrome or Sjögren's syndrome. Anti-dsDNA in high titre is virtually diagnostic of SLE.

9.3 Anti-ds-DNA

High titres are specific for SLE; anti-ds-DNA is present in approximately 80% of patients with SLE.

Methods:

- radioimmunoassay (Farr assay)
- *Crithidia lucillae* immunofluorescence
- enzyme-linked immunosorbent assay (ELISA).

9.4 Extractable nuclear antigens

These are specific nuclear antigens and therefore are usually associated with positive ANA tests.

- Anti-Ro – Sjögren's syndrome, congenital heart block, ANA-negative SLE
- Anti-La – primary Sjögren's syndrome
- Anti-Sm – SLE (20%, very specific: conferring a high risk of renal lupus)
- Anti-RNP – mixed connective tissue disease (100%), SLE
- Anti-Jo 1 – polymyositis
- Anti-Scl70 – progressive systemic sclerosis (20%)
- Anti-centromere – CREST syndrome

Method of detection: counter immunoelectrophoresis or ELISA.

9.5 Anti-neutrophil cytoplasmic antibodies (ANCA)

These antibodies are directed against constituents of the neutrophil cytoplasm, proteinase 3 (PR3) and myeloperoxidase (MPO). When neutrophils are activated PR3 and MPO move to the cell surface. Antibodies to either granule will cause activation of the respiratory burst and degranulation, particularly in the presence of TNFα, causing endothelial cell damage. ANCA may therefore play a role in the pathogenesis of its associated disorders. Titres often reflect disease activity. (*See also* Chapter 15, Nephrology.)

- cANCA (cytoplasmic anti-PR3) is found in Wegener's granulomatosis (90% of patients) and microscopic polyangiitis (40%).
- pANCA (perinuclear anti-MPO) is found in microscopic polyangiitis (60%), connective tissue disorders, other vasculitides.

Other inflammatory disorders can be associated with positive ANCA in the absence of vasculitis (eg connective tissue disorders, autoimmune hepatitis and inflammatory bowel disease); in these conditions the immunofluorescent staining may be atypical or appear similar to pANCA patterns.

9.6 Autoantibodies in gastrointestinal and liver disease

- Anti-mitochondrial antibody – primary biliary cirrhosis (96%)
- Anti-smooth muscle antibody – auto-immune hepatitis, cryptogenic cirrhosis
- Gastric parietal cell antibodies – pernicious anaemia (90%), gastric atrophy (40%)
- Intrinsic factor antibodies – pernicious anaemia (70%)
- Anti-tissue transglutaminase, anti-gliadin, anti-endomyseal antibodies – coeliac disease.

9.7 Autoantibodies in thyroid disease

- **Anti-thyroglobulin antibody (anti-Tg)**: high titre in autoimmune thyroiditis (90%)
- **Anti-thyroid peroxidase antibody (anti-TPO)**: previously known as anti-microsomal antibody. It is present in most autoimmune thyroiditis (90%) but also in low titres in Grave's disease (50%) and adenocarcinoma of the thyroid (10%)
- **Anti-thyroid stimulating receptor antibody (Anti-TSHR)**: this is found in 90% of Graves' disease patients and in 20% of autoimmune thyroiditis.

9.8 Antiphospholipid antibodies

Antiphospholipid antibodies have activity against a variety of cell membrane phospholipids, and the most commonly measured are those against cardiolipin. Protein complexes such as β2 glycoprotein-1, which have anticoagulant properties, are found on cell membranes, and it is the interaction between antiphospholipid antibodies and these proteins that is likely to explain the development of thrombosis. Other characteristics of antiphospholipid antibodies include:

- Association with arterial or venous thrombosis, transient neurological deficits, fetal loss, livido reticularis and thrombocytopenia (Hughes' syndrome).
- Anticardiolipin antibodies (ACLA) are measured by ELISA.
- Different isotypes exist; IgG and to a lesser extent IgM isotypes of ACLA are associated with the clinical features.
- Antibodies to β2 glycoprotein-1 itself are found in about 10% of patients with anti-cardiolipin-associated thrombosis.
- Lupus anticoagulant (LA) – prolonged activated partial thromboplastin time (which is not corrected by the addition of normal plasma) – detects some antibodies not picked up by ELISA.
- 80% concordance of ACLA and LA.
- Produce false-negative Wasserman reaction (WR) and venereal disease reference laboratory (VDRL) tests.

- ACLA or LA found in up to 40% of patients with SLE, also in malignancy and HIV infection.
- Poor predictors of first thrombosis (ie most people with ACLA or LA do not develop thrombosis).
- Strongly predict recurrence of thrombosis.

9.9 Others

- Anti-glomerular basement membrane – Goodpasture's syndrome
- Acetylcholine receptor antibody – myasthenia gravis (87%).

10. IMMUNODEFICIENCY

Primary immunodeficiency can be divided into:

- complement deficiency
- neutrophil disorders
- B-cell disorders
- T-cell disorders
- combined B- and T-cell disorders.

10.1 Complement deficiency

May produce angiooedema, SLE-like disease, or disseminated *Neisseria* infection.

- Hereditary angiooedema due to C1 inhibitor deficiency.
- SLE-like syndromes due to deficiencies of classical pathway components.
- Paroxysmal nocturnal haemoglobinuria due to regulator protein defects.

10.2 Neutrophil disorders

Allow recurrent infections with pyogenic bacteria, especially *Staphylococcus aureus*, but also some Gram-negative bacilli and fungi, such as *Aspergillus* and *Candida*. Treatment is with antibiotics.

The following are examples:

- **Chronic granulomatous disease** where there is normal phagocytosis but an inability to kill the micro-organism intracellularly due to an X-linked defect of NADPH oxidase.
- **Chediak–Higashi disease** where there is also normal phagocytosis but inability to kill the intracellular micro-organism because lysosomes lack elastase and cathepsin G.
- **Job's syndrome** – recurrent boils.
- **Myeloperoxidase deficiency**, associated with a susceptibility to systemic candidiasis.
- **Lazy leukocyte syndrome** due to defective responses to chemotactic stimuli.
- **Leukocyte adhesion deficiency** where the β-subunit of β2-integrin is absent.

10.3 B-cell disorders

These lead to failure of antibody synthesis (hypogammaglobulinaemia or agammaglobulinaemia) and recurrent infections with pyogenic bacteria and fungi such as *Candida*. Where necessary, regular immunoglobulin infusions are used to maintain levels of circulating immunoglobulin.

The following are examples:

- **Common variable immunodeficiency** is likely to represent more than one disorder. The marrow contains normal numbers of immature B-cells but there is a failure in maturation. Immunoglobulin levels vary from patient to patient. It is not familial.
- **IgA deficiency** is the commonest isolated Ig deficiency in the UK (1 in 700), and is often asymptomatic. There is an increased susceptibility to giardiasis.
- **Bruton's X-linked agammaglobulinaemia**. No circulating B-cells are found. Usually presents between three months and two years of age.

10.4 T-cell disorders

These produce impaired cell-mediated immunity. There is an increased susceptibility to viruses, mycobacteria and fungi. Though common bacterial infections can be dealt with, infections with measles, vaccinia or even BCG immunisation can prove fatal. Malignancy is increased. Treatment may require bone marrow transplants or thymus grafts.

The following are examples:

- **Di George syndrome** is a primary, non-familial, T-cell deficiency due to a defect in the development of the thymus and third and fourth branchial arches. The parathyroids are absent, causing severe hypocalcaemia, and the usual presentation is with neonatal convulsions. Cardiovascular anomalies may also be present.
- **Nezelof syndrome** is due to an absent thymus though there is often some B-cell involvement.
- **Purine nucleoside phosphorylase deficiency** prevents the development of T-cells.

10.5 Combined B- and T-cell disorders

- **Severe combined immunodeficiency** (SCID) is due in some cases to lack of the enzyme adenosine deaminase. There are several forms, including X-linked recessive.
- **Reticular dysgenesis** leads to lymphopenia, neutropenia and absence of monocytes.
- **Ataxia telangiectasia** is an autosomal recessive disorder presenting in childhood with cerebellar ataxia and telangiectasia. Malignancy is increased due to defective DNA repair mechanisms. There is defective cell-mediated immunity with low levels of IgE and IgA.
- **Wiskott–Aldrich syndrome**, due to lack of sialophorin, produces low IgM levels and impaired cell-mediated immunity. Malignancy is increased and there is thrombocytopenia, lymphopenia and eczema. The disorder is X-linked.

10.6 Acquired immunodeficiency

Causes of acquired immunodeficiency are:

Immunoglobulin deficiency	Cell-mediated immune dysfunction
• **Drugs** Gold (aurothiomalate) Phenytoin Penicillamine Unusual, idiosyncratic reactions	• **Drugs** Ciclosporin Cyclophosphamide Steroids Common and dose-related
• **Haematological malignancy** Chronic lymphocytic leukaemia (CLL)	• **Haematological malignancy** Lymphoma
• **Protein loss** Nephrotic syndrome Protein-losing enteropathy	• **AIDS**

HIV infects T-helper cells leading to a progressive fall in the number of CD4 T-cells. The crucial immunological feature is impaired cell-mediated immunity with increased vulnerability to normally non-pathogenic organisms such as *Pneumocystis* but also viruses (CMV, Herpes simplex and EBV), fungi (*Candida*, *Aspergillus* and *Cryptococcus*) and protozoa (*Toxoplasma*). There is often an associated polyclonal activation of B-cells and hypergammaglobulinaemia.

11. IMMUNISATION

The **benefits of immunisation** depend on several factors.

- **Likelihood of contracting disease**: prevalence of disease, level of immunity in other individuals (herd immunity), presence of immunodeficiency.
- **Severity of disease**: both the disease itself and from the point of view of the host having immune deficiency.
- **Adverse effects**: more common with preformed antibodies and live attenuated vaccines.

There are several ways of enhancing the immune system to produce added protection against infection. Most are used prophylactically to prevent or reduce the severity of infection, but some can prevent the development of disease even after contact with the organism (eg rabies vaccine).

11.1 Preformed antibody

Preformed antibody vaccines

- Tetanus
- Hepatitis B
- Botulism
- Rabies
- Varicella
- Diphtheria

This is obtained from a previously infected individual. Used particularly in immunocompromised patients early after contact with infection and to inhibit the actions of bacterial toxins in tetanus, diphtheria and botulism. Occurs physiologically in the transfer of maternal IgG to the fetus. The antibody is catabolised, however, so protection against infection is temporary. When the source of antibody is a different species there is a risk of serum sickness with repeated doses.

11.2 Killed organism vaccines

Killed organism vaccines

- Cholera
- Pertussis
- Typhoid
- Polio (Salk)
- Influenza
- Rabies

Killed organism vaccines are widely used against both bacteria and viruses. Influenza vaccine is usually offered to those who would fare badly with infection, ie patients with chronic illness such as chronic obstructive pulmonary disease (COPD), heart disease, chronic renal disease, rheumatoid arthritis and the elderly.

11.3 Live attenuated vaccines

Live attenuated vaccines

- BCG
- Vaccinia
- Measles
- Mumps
- Rubella
- Polio (Sabin)

Superior to killed vaccines. They deliver a larger sustained dose of antigen and produce a better immune response. Cytotoxic T-cell memory is acquired which needs viral replication. The immunisation also occurs at the sites of natural infection. The drawback is that attenuation may fail and actual infection occur, especially in the immunocompromised.

11.4 Subunit vaccines

Subunit vaccines

- *H. influenzae*
- *N. meningitidis*
- *S. pneumoniae*
- Hepatitis B

Purified components of the infective organism. Only antigens that produce a protective response are used. The vaccinated host is not challenged with other antigens that may have deleterious effects such as hypersensitivity. Immunisation against Hepatitis B is reserved for high-risk groups such as health workers. Pneumococcal vaccination is important in asplenic patients and those with hypocomplementaemia.

Chapter 11
Infectious Diseases and Tropical Medicine

CONTENTS

6. Specific tropical infections

6.1 Malaria
6.2 Enteric fevers
6.3 Amoebiasis
6.4 Schistosomiasis
6.5 Leprosy

Infectious Diseases and Tropical Medicine

1. BASIC EPIDEMIOLOGICAL CONCEPTS

1.1 Herd immunity

This concept is derived from the recognition that complete protection of a given population against an infectious disease by immunisation does not require 100% coverage. Partial coverage of a population, by reducing the number of susceptible people within it, will reduce the efficiency of transmission to below the levels needed to sustain a particular infectious disease.

1.2 Modes of transmission of infection

Respiratory transmission

Exhaled droplets containing organisms from infected persons will travel for up to 2 metres before falling to the ground. Inhalation of such droplets in sufficient quantity will result in infection.

Respiratory transmission: major pathogens

- *Mycobacterium tuberculosis*
- *Haemophilus influenzae*
- *Streptococcus pyogenes*
- *Neisseria meningitidis*
- *Streptococcus pneumoniae*
- Childhood respiratory viruses (eg measles, chickenpox)

Some pathogens are acquired via the respiratory route but hardly ever from an infected human source, for example:

- ***Legionella pneumophila*** (aerosols from shower heads, cooling towers, air conditioning systems, etc).
- ***Coxiella burnetii*** (aerosols and dust from sheep/goat faeces, also products of conception from same animals).

Faecal–oral transmission

This occurs when gastrointestinal pathogens from the faeces of a human (or animal) case or carrier gain access to food, water or dairy products. The practice of anilingus can transmit many gut pathogens.

A period of amplification prior to consumption is usually required to build up sufficient inoculum to cause disease. However, the level of inoculum required to cause disease is smaller in people with reduced **gastric acid** secretion, such as those on anti-ulcer medications, alcoholics and patients with partial gastrectomy.

- Some organisms are capable of causing disease with very small amounts of infective inoculum. ***Shigella dysenteriae*** can produce severe disease with as few as 12 ingested organisms and so direct transmission from contaminated surfaces, to hands and then to mouth is possible, particularly in children.
- ***Giardia lamblia*** also needs a relatively small inoculum of cysts (approx. 100) to cause disease.
- **Enteroviruses** (eg poliovirus and hepatitis A) are also transmitted by this route.
- **Faeces** (of many bird, mammal and reptile species) may contain human pathogens (eg *Salmonella* spp., *Campylobacter* spp., *Cryptosporidium parvum*, rotavirus).

Sexual transmission

Close apposition of the genito-urinary (GU) mucosa is usually required for transmission of GU tract pathogens because of their fragility. Sometimes oro-genital contact may result in sexually transmitted disease (STD), and it can occasionally occur through oral–oral contact (eg syphilis). A bite from an infected person may also give rise to a primary syphilitic chancre in normal skin.

- Congenital transmission of many STDs can occur either during pregnancy (eg syphilis) or during delivery (eg gonorrhoea, *Chlamydia* infection, Herpes simplex).

(For more information on genito-urinary and HIV infections *see* Chapter 8, *Genito-urinary Medicine and AIDS*.)

Congenital transmission

This may be either transplacental or perinatal. Fetal death or deformity is a variable result of transplacental infection.

Important syndromes associated with particular organisms are given below.

- **Rubella**: heart, eye, CNS. The fetus is nearly always affected if infection occurs in the first 7 weeks of pregnancy; after the 17th week of pregnancy specific deformities are unusual.
- **Toxoplasmosis**: affects the fetus only during maternal primary infection, except in immunocompromised mothers. There is a lower risk of transmission (but more severe disease) in the first trimester. Hydrocephalus, cerebral calcification and choroidoretinitis comprise a classic triad.
- **Chickenpox**: maternal infection in the first trimester can cause limb deformities; later infections cause infant/childhood zoster. Maternal zoster can, very rarely, cause similar problems.

- **Cytomegalovirus (CMV)**: infection may be either transplacental or by perinatal routes, as a result of primary maternal infection or reactivation. At least 75% of infected babies are undamaged. The main syndromes are neurological, including intracranial calcification, microcephaly and cerebral palsy; also cardiac syndromes (septal defects, Fallot's) and GI tract syndromes (hepatosplenomegaly, cleft palate, biliary and oesophageal atresia) can occur.
- **Herpes simplex**: infection is nearly always perinatal and gives rise to severe neonatal disease; 80% are due to type 2 virus.
- **Parvovirus B19**: either fetal death (with abortion or stillbirth) or complete recovery is the rule. Hydrops fetalis is the main intrauterine syndrome.
- **Listeriosis**: both transplacental and perinatal infection can occur. The result is abortion (early) or neonatal septicaemia (late) depending on the stage of pregnancy affected.

Blood-borne transmission

Viruses of the most common infectious agents can be transmitted by this route, but other organisms do feature in certain situations (see below). Examples of blood-borne viral transmission include:

- **Hepatitis B (and delta agent)**: very small amounts of blood are required for transmission of hepatitis B because of the high concentrations of virus present in most carriers or cases. Thus there is a high risk of infection from needle stick injury. In contrast, needle stick transmission is much less likely with HIV because of low virus concentrations.
- **CMV**: transmission in blood is of clinical importance in the immunosuppressed due to the risk of CMV-related disease in such patients (eg in transplant recipients).
- **HTLV-1 and HIV**: transmitted by blood (also by sexual intercourse and breast milk).
- **Other blood-borne viruses**: hepatitis C + G, Epstein–Barr virus.

Blood-borne transmission of bacterial and protozoal infection

This is not a major clinical problem, but some examples are given below.

- **Syphilis**: classically from blood transfusion.
- **Enterobacters**: from contaminated whole blood or platelets stored at room temperature.
- **Q fever**: a few case reports.
- **Protozoa**: transmitted by blood transfusion.
- **Malaria**: all species are transmitted by blood and blood products such as platelets and fresh frozen plasma; infectivity may remain for up to 10 days in stored blood.
- **African and American trypanosomiasis**: both of these may be transmitted by blood transfusion. Chagas' disease is a major (late) complication of blood transfusion in South America.
- **Visceral leishmaniasis**: can be transmitted via transfused blood, particularly in the endemic parts of the Indian subcontinent where the human population acts as the main reservoir of infection and where transmission is usually insect-borne. Various animal species fulfil this role elsewhere in the world.

1.3 Pathogenesis of infection

The basic pathogenesis of infection usually involves a breach of either a mucosal surface or the epithelium:

- Invasion of, or attachment to, the **mucosal surfaces** (ie respiratory, gastrointestinal, genito-urinary) is the usual first step in the establishment of an infection.
- Direct penetration of the **epithelium** may occur by trauma or by insect bite; some organisms (eg leptospires, cercariae (of schistosomes), larvae of hookworm and *Strongyloides*) can penetrate intact skin.

Only a minority (occasionally tiny) of infected individuals develop disease as a consequence of any given infection. The remainder remain asymptomatic and the infection clears spontaneously with an appropriate immune response. This is an almost universal principle across a large spectrum of infections (eg meningococcal infection, poliomyelitis, leprosy).

Predispositions to disease

Host vulnerability or (conversely) resistance to disease is multifactorial. The outcome of any infection depends upon the balance struck between the **inoculum size**, the **virulence** of the pathogen and **host factors**, listed below.

Host factors affecting vulnerability to disease

- **Immunological**
  - *Genetic deficiency*
    - Immunoglobulin/complement/ T-cell deficiencies
  - *Prior immunity*
    - Naturally or artificially acquired
  - *Acquired deficiency*
    - HIV infection; malignant disease; transplant recipients; patients receiving chemotherapy
  - *Miscellaneous influences on immune status*
    - (eg diabetes, pregnancy, splenectomy)
- **Other factors**
  - *Psychological status*
    - (now recognised as an influential factor in the common cold)
  - *Nutritional status*
    - (eg measles in under-nutrition)
  - *Prior antibiotic therapy*
    - (eg *Clostridium difficile*, multi-resistant *Staphylococcus aureus* infections)
  - *Foreign bodies*
    - (eg catheters; artificial heart valves)
  - *Behavioural factors*
    - (eg smokers, alcoholics)

Microbial virulence factors

These include the ability to invade and evade **host immune** defences, often by the production of **enzymes** and **toxins**.

As described above, penetration into host tissues usually occurs via an epithelial surface and certain microbial factors aid this process. **Invasion** through a mucosal surface first requires **attachment**. This can be relatively non-specific, mediated only by the production of a polysaccharide capsule or slime. Alternatively, specific structures on the organism's surface known as **adhesins** attach to specific glycoprotein or glycolipid **receptors** on the host cell.

Examples of receptors and attaching organisms

- **D-Mannose**
  Enterobacteriaceae
- **CD4 T-cell receptors**
  HIV
- **N-Acetyl-D-glycosamine**
  Chlamydiae, group B streptococci, *Plasmodium falciparum and Entamoeba histolytica*
- **Duffy blood group antigen**
  *Plasmodium vivax**

*Duffy blood groups are very rare in Africans, hence there is little vivax in Africa

Following invasion, the pathogenic organism has many survival strategies.

- **Production of spreading enzymes**: (eg hyaluronidase, elastase, collagenase, nucleases).
- **Evasion of immune defences**: by avoidance of phagocytic killing, achieved by a variety of means such as:

  encapsulation (*Staphylococcus aureus, Streptococcus pyogenes/pneumoniae, Neisseria* spp.)
  inhibition of phagolysosome fusion (*Mycobacterium tuberculosis, Chlamydia* spp., *Legionella* spp.)
  antigenic mimicry (*Schistosoma mansoni*)
  antigenic shift (influenza virus, pili of *Neisseria gonorrhoeae*)
  resistance to lysosomal enzymes (*M. leprae, Leishmania* spp.)
  phagocyte destruction (streptolysin from *S. pyogenes*, alpha toxin from *Clostridium perfringens*).

Toxins

These are products of pathogenic bacteria which can be classified into endotoxins and exotoxins.

- **Endotoxin**: an **integral lipopolysaccharide** component of Gram-negative cell walls. Its active component, **lipid A**, induces fever, provokes the coagulation and complement cascades, activates B-lymphocytes and stimulates production of tumour necrosis factor, interleukin-1 and prostaglandins. Heavy exposure as in Gram-negative sepsis causes fever, shock and occasionally death.

- **Exotoxins**: produced by a diversity of organisms, with equally diverse effects:

  Vibrio cholerae – secretory diarrhoea (small bowel)
  Corynebacterium diphtheriae – cardiomyopathy, neuropathy
  Clostridium tetani – tetanus
  Clostridium perfringens – gangrene, secretory diarrhoea
  Clostridium botulinum – paralysis.

2. HOST DEFENCE MECHANISMS

2.1 Non-specific mechanisms ('first line of defence')

Polymorphonuclear neutrophils (PMNs)

Circulate freely in the absence of an infectious process and do not attach to capillary endothelium. Cytokines and complement fragments that are produced at the site of an infection make local capillary endothelium and passing PMNs 'stickier'.

- **Glycoprotein receptors** on PMNs enable them to stick to receptors on the endothelium (**margination**) prior to the process of **diapedesis** (migration through the intercellular gaps in the capillary endothelium).
- PMNs kill by first attaching to the pathogen (with or without the aid of opsonins) and then ingesting the pathogen, to form a **phagosome**.
- **Lysosomes** in the PMN then discharge strong hydrolytic enzymes into the phagosome – known as a **phagolysosome**. The enzymes comprise lysozyme, elastase, a protease and myeloperoxidase. The latter reacts with H_2O_2 and chloride ion to form hypochlorous acid, and oxygen free radicals are produced. These products are highly toxic for micro-organisms.

Natural antibodies

Belong mainly to the IgM class and act against pathogens which the host has not previously encountered. They are probably formed as a result of exposure to antigenically similar but harmless organisms (eg exposure to the commensal *Neisseria lactamica* produces protective antibody against the meningococcus).

Acute phase response

The acute phase response is initiated by cytokines released by cells of the macrophage/monocyte lineage at the site of an infection. They circulate to the liver where they trigger the release of certain proteins. These include **C-reactive protein**, **lipopolysaccharide binding protein** and **serum amyloid A protein**.

- Their concentration may increase 1000-fold or more, whereas that of others, such as complement factor B and alpha-1 antitrypsin, increases by a more modest two- or three-fold.

- These substances have a particular role to play in the control of the immune response to infection; **transferrin** is also a major component of this response. Its major role is to mop up iron and other metals (eg zinc) thus denying them to invading bacteria.

Complement system

The complement system provides protection in many ways but its main functions are:

- direct lysis
- opsonisation
- leukocyte chemotaxis
- promotion of the inflammatory response.

2.2 Humoral immunity

Specific antibodies appear within 7–10 days of primary exposure to an antigen; a significant proportion of these are of the IgM class, making measurement of this antibody useful in serological diagnosis.

Secondary exposure results in an accelerated response, primarily of the IgG class.

Summary of antibody functions

- Opsonisation/lysis (with complement)
- Neutralisation of toxins
- Eosinophil-mediated killing
- Protective coating of host cells
- Facilitation of natural killer (NK) cell activity

'Secretory' IgA antibodies are produced by B-cells in the lamina propria of the gut; they comprise two IgA molecules linked together and as such are resistant to digestion by small bowel enzymes.

2.3 Cellular immunity

Antibodies cannot penetrate infected cells to kill an organism that may be contained within. Sensitised T-cells perform the role of destroying infected cells. They are usually of the CD8 subtype and do so by cytolytic action following direct contact with the target cell; neither complement nor antibody is involved. Such contact can only occur when the target cell and effector cell share the same class 1 histocompatibility antigens.

Sensitised T-cells can also produce lymphokines which specifically stimulate macrophages to destroy organisms against which they are indifferent in the unstimulated state. These macrophages will then be non-specifically more active against a variety of organisms.

3. SPECIFIC ANTIMICROBIALS

3.1 Antibacterial agents

(*See also* Chapter 2, Clinical Pharmacology, Toxicology and Poisoning.)

Penicillins

- **Mechanism of action**: damage to bacterial cell wall by attachment to penicillin binding proteins (PBPs) in the cell wall, inhibiting cross-linking. Resistance can be due to two different mechanisms: beta-lactamase activity which breaks the penicillin beta-lactam ring or the presence of non-penicillin-binding proteins (eg methicillin-resistant *S. aureus* (MRSA); also some pneumococci).
- **Serious side-effects**: anaphylaxis (rare); interstitial nephritis (rare); encephalopathy (very rare, but beware high dosage in acute meningitis).
- **Contraindications**: previous sensitivity; intrathecal injection; nearly always safe in pregnancy.
- **Excretion**: the main excretory route of most penicillins is via the kidneys; dosage adjustment is therefore required in anuria. Nafcillin is metabolised in the liver.

Cephalosporins

- **Mechanism of action**: very similar to penicillins. Most are variably resistant to different beta-lactamases from different bacterial classes. They bind to PBPs and therefore PBP mutations are resistant (as with penicillins).
- **Serious side-effects**: bronchospasm; anaphylaxis; nephrotoxicity (rare).
- **Contraindications**: previous sensitivity, nearly always safe in pregnancy.
- **Excretion**: main excretory route renal. Reduce dose in severe renal failure.

Quinolones

- **Mechanism of action**: inhibition of bacterial DNA synthesis.
- **Spectrum of activity**: broad, but better against Gram-negatives; poor anti-anaerobe activity. Can be used as second-line antituberculous agents (eg ciprofloxacin).
- **Relevant pharmacokinetics**: well-absorbed from the gut; absorption delayed by food and also reduced by magnesium or calcium hydroxide antacids and H_2 blockers. **The quinolones also inhibit cytochrome p450 enzymes, hence they can be responsible for many drug interactions (eg warfarin and ciclosporin A)**.
- **Serious side-effects**: hallucinations, psychotic reactions, convulsions, photosensitivity.
- **Contraindications**: pregnancy and in children (because of effects on growing cartilage in young animals).
- **Excretion**: both renal and hepatic (*see* Chapter 2, Clinical Pharmacology, Toxicology and Poisoning).

Sulphonamides

- **Mechanism of action**: competitive inhibition of enzyme which converts *para*-aminobenzoic acid (PABA) into folic acid.
- **Relevant pharmacokinetics**: well absorbed from the gut.
- **Spectrum of activity**: wide, including chlamydiae, toxoplasma and plasmodia, but resistance common.
- **Serious side-effects**: agranulocytosis, thrombocytopenia, leukopenia, displacement of warfarin from plasma proteins.

Tetracyclines

- **Mechanism of action**: inhibition of bacterial protein synthesis by blocking binding of tRNA to the 30s subunit.
- **Spectrum of activity**: broad, inclusive of rickettsiae, chlamydiae, mycoplasmas.
- **Relevant pharmacokinetics**: well absorbed but food, milk, magnesium, calcium, aluminium and iron compounds tend to reduce this.
- **Serious side-effects**: photosensitivity, exacerbation of renal failure, effects on teeth and bones: discoloration and hypoplasia of enamel (children <8 years), depression of skeletal growth – fetus and premature infant.
- **Excretion**: via kidneys.

Macrolides

- **Mechanism of action**: inhibition of bacterial protein synthesis by binding to the 50s ribosome.
- **Spectrum of activity**: broad, inclusive of mycoplasmas, chlamydiae and rickettsiae. Useful activity against pneumococci, also legionella. **Clindamycin** is particularly effective against anaerobes. **Clarithromycin** is also useful as second-line antituberculous drug.
- **Relevant pharmacokinetics**: moderately absorbed from gut.
- **Serious side-effects**: thrombophlebitis (iv preparation), transient hearing loss, cholestatic hepatitis (erythromycin estolate), pseudomembranous colitis (particularly clindamycin).
- **Excretion**: mainly hepatic; some renal excretion. Reduced dose in severe renal failure.

Aminoglycosides

- **Mechanism of action**: inhibition of bacterial protein synthesis.
- **Spectrum of activity**: predominantly active against Gram-negative aerobic bacilli. Not active against anaerobes. Amikacin has broadest spectrum of activity.
- **Serious side-effects**: ototoxicity, renal tubular damage.
- **Excretion**: via the kidneys. Careful monitoring of plasma levels required to avoid toxicity.

3.2 Antituberculous drugs

Rifampicin

- **Mechanism of action**: inhibition of DNA-dependent RNA polymerase.
- **Spectrum of activity**: broad, inclusive of antituberculous activity. Useful prophylactic against meningococcus, also against legionella infection. Rifabutin is better against *Mycobacterium avium-intracellulare*.
- **Relevant pharmacokinetics**: well absorbed from gut; potent inducer of hepatic enzymes causing accelerated metabolism of many drugs (eg warfarin and contraceptive pill).
- **Serious side-effects**: hepatic toxicity (especially in alcoholics).
- **Excretion**: hepatic and renal. Indeed, orange discoloration of the urine is used to check compliance with treatment.

Isoniazid

- **Mechanism of action**: inhibition of cell wall synthesis.
- **Spectrum of activity**: exclusively antituberculous.
- **Relevant pharmacokinetics**: well-absorbed; must be given with pyridoxine, particularly in slow acetylators, to prevent peripheral neuropathy. Variable activity against other mycobacteria.
- **Serious side-effects**: peripheral neuropathy, psychosis, convulsions, hepatitis-like syndrome, lupus-like syndrome.
- **Excretion**: hepatic.

Pyrazinamide

- **Mechanism of action**: poorly understood, but works best in more acid environment, ie inside phagosomes.
- **Spectrum of activity**: exclusively antituberculous, not effective against *Mycobacterium bovis*.
- **Relevant pharmacokinetics**: well absorbed.
- **Serious side-effects**: hepatotoxicity (dose-related) and **gout**.
- **Excretion**: hepatic.

Ethambutol

- **Mechanism of action**: inhibits bacterial RNA synthesis.
- **Spectrum of activity**: good range of activity against other mycobacteria.
- **Relevant pharmacokinetics**: well absorbed.
- **Serious side-effects**: retrobulbar neuritis, impairment of colour vision or visual acuity. (Careful monitoring of visual acuity necessary during **treatment**.)
- **Excretion**: renal.

Streptomycin

- **Mechanism of action**: inhibits bacterial protein synthesis by binding to the 50s ribosome. Now rarely used (mainly for drug resistance or in cases of toxicity with other agents); parenteral use only, and can be given intrathecally.
- **Serious side-effects**: ototoxicity, renal tubular damage.
- **Excretion**: via the kidneys.

3.3 Antiviral drugs

Aciclovir

- **Mechanism of action**: selective activity against **herpes viruses** that encode a **thymidine kinase**. The latter phosphorylates the drug (to monophosphate), the process being continued by host cell enzymes to triphosphate. Aciclovir triphosphate competes with guanosine triphosphate causing termination of the growing viral DNA chain. Thus only virus infected cells convert aciclovir to an active form; it remains virtually inert in uninfected healthy cells.
- **Spectrum of activity**: very useful for Herpes simplex and Herpes varicella-zoster infections, the important principle being early commencement of therapy.
- **Serious side-effects**: renal failure (usually reversible); neurotoxicity (rare) with hallucinations, psychosis, convulsions and/or coma. May occur with drug accumulation in severe renal failure.
- **Contraindications**: very safe in most situations, including pregnancy.
- **Excretion**: excreted unchanged by the kidneys.

Ganciclovir

Similar mechanism of action, metabolism and side-effects as for aciclovir. However, ganciclovir has a greater effect against CMV; it is used to treat AIDS patients with retinitis, and also for the CMV infections which are common in transplanted patients.

Ribavirin

- **Mechanism of action**: analogue of the nucleoside guanosine; inhibits nucleoside biosynthesis, mRNA capping and other processes essential to viral replication.
- **Spectrum of activity**: useful as an aerosol in severe respiratory syncytial virus (RSV) infection. It is also used for Lassa fever (early treatment is important) and it is one of the main drugs used to treat hepatitis C infection.
- **Serious side-effects**: bone marrow depression.

3.4 Anthelmintic agents

Benzimidazoles

- (eg albendazole, thiabendazole, mebendazole).
- **Mechanism of action**: the net effect of various biochemical activities is a reduction or paralysis of parasite motility.
- **Spectrum of activity**: broad against intestinal nematodes (eg *Trichuris*, *Necator*, *Ascaris*, *Ancylostoma*, *Enterobius*; also cestodes such as *Hymenolepis*, *Taenia* and *Echinococcus*).

Piperazines

- **Mechanism of action**: induction of paralysis in target worms.
- **Spectrum of activity**: piperazine is useful against *Ascaris* and *Enterobius*. Diethylcarbamazine (DEC) is also active against the microfilariae of *Onchocerca volvulus* (cause of river blindness), *Wuchereria bancrofti* and *Brugia malayi* (both causes of lymphatic filariasis).

Praziquantel

- **Mechanism of action**: acts as calcium agonist; causes elevated intracellular calcium, tetanic muscular contraction and destruction of the tegument. This allows hitherto unexposed antigens to be attacked by host antibody.
- **Spectrum of activity**: has particularly useful activity against *Schistosoma* and *Taenia*.

3.5 Other agents used to counteract infection

Immunoglobulins

Normal human immunoglobulin has many applications, particularly in passively immunising patients with humoral immunodeficiency. Kawasaki disease (possibly due to an infectious agent) is one clear-cut application. There are also a number of specific immunoglobulins for specific situations (eg tetanus, rabies, diphtheria, hepatitis B and zoster immune globulin).

Vaccines

- **Inactivated/killed vaccines**: the predominant vaccine type for bacterial disease, eg toxoids (diphtheria, tetanus); killed cell (pertussis, typhoid); capsular polysaccharide (*Haemophilus influenzae* b, meningococcal, pneumococcal).
- **Attenuated/live vaccines**: the predominant vaccine type for viral disease (with exceptions), eg attenuated (measles, mumps, rubella, yellow fever, polio); subunit (hepatitis B); inactivated (rabies, Japanese encephalitis, influenza, hepatitis A).
- **Attenuated bacterial vaccines**: BCG, oral typhoid vaccine.

(*See also* Chapter 10, Immunology.)

4. INFECTIONS IN SPECIFIC SITUATIONS

4.1 Pregnancy

Because **the fetus is antigenically different from the mother**, modulation of selected aspects of the maternal immune response is necessary for the fetus to be tolerated. The placenta is responsible for this modulation.

Infections exacerbated by pregnancy

- Urinary tract infection (*see* Chapter 12, Maternal Medicine)
- Listeria
- Varicella (pneumonitis life-threatening, especially in third trimester)
- Candidiasis
- Pulmonary tuberculosis
- *Salmonella* spp.
- Hepatitis E (25% mortality)
- HIV disease
- Falciparum malaria (especially primigravidae in second trimester)

For more information on congenital infection, *see* Modes of transmission in Section 1.2.

4.2 Alcoholism

Alcoholics are more vulnerable to a number of infections because of the **immunosuppressive effects of excessive alcohol intake**, and they are at an increased risk of **septic shock**. The neutropenia of alcoholism is probably due to toxic effects on the bone marrow; studies show the neutrophils themselves are less effective and less able to phagocytose foreign particles.

Important infections to which alcoholics are particularly vulnerable

- Pulmonary tuberculosis
- Legionella
- Inhalational pneumonias
- Amoebic abscess
- Salmonella
- Pneumococcal pneumonia
- *Klebsiella* pneumonia
- Typhoid fever
- Listeria

4.3 Splenectomy

The spleen accounts for approximately 25% of the body's lymphatic tissue; absence of its function causes particular vulnerability to capsulate organisms such as:

- Pneumococcus
- *Haemophilus influenzae*
- Meningococcus
- DF-2 'Dysgonic fermenter 2' (now known as *Capnocytophaga canimorsus*) characteristically acquired from dog bites.

Splenectomised patients are also vulnerable to malaria and to **babesiosis**, a protozoal infection transmitted by ixodid ticks from an animal reservoir comprising small rodents such as field mice. The merozoite stage of the parasite invades blood cells directly after being injected under the skin by the tick. It causes a mild malaria-like disease in the immunocompetent, but is potentially life-threatening in splenectomised individuals. Diagnosis is by blood film.

4.4 Sickle cell disease

Sicklers (ie SS homozygotes) often have functional hyposplenism and also a reduction in complement-mediated serum opsonising activity. This gives rise to vulnerability to:

- pneumococcal infection (in particular)
- other forms of bacterial sepsis
- osteomyelitis (due to *Salmonella* spp.)
- falciparum malaria (in contrast to AS heterozygotes who are resistant to malaria).

5. MAJOR CLINICAL SYNDROMES

In the following section short notes and lists of infective organisms are included for the more important clinical syndromes associated with infectious diseases.

5.1 Respiratory infections

Upper respiratory tract

Clinical symptoms of upper respiratory tract infections

- The common cold (coryza)
- Mastoiditis
- Pharyngitis (± tonsillitis)
- Otitis media
- Sinusitis
- Laryngitis

Both viruses and bacteria may cause infection in these sites but viral infection usually 'prepares the ground' for a bacterial infection to follow.

Viruses responsible for upper respiratory tract infections

- Rhinoviruses
- Coronaviruses
- Adenoviruses (conjunctivitis is an occasional extra feature)
- Parainfluenza viruses
- Coxsackie groups A+B
- Respiratory syncytial virus (RSV)

Bacteria responsible for upper respiratory tract infections

- β haemolytic group A streptococcus
- *H. influenzae*
- *Neisseria meningitidis* (usually asymptomatic)
- *Neisseria gonorrhoeae* (as above)
- *Branhamella catarrhalis*
- *Mycoplasma pneumoniae*

Lower respiratory tract

Clinical syndromes include: tracheitis, bronchiolitis, pneumonia, bronchitis and alveolitis.

Organisms responsible for lower respiratory tract infections

- **Common**
  Streptococcus pneumoniae
  Haemophilus influenzae
  Streptococcus pyogenes
  Legionella pneumophila
  Staphylococcus aureus
  Mycoplasma pneumoniae
  Klebsiella pneumoniae
- **Uncommon**
  Chlamydia spp.
  Coxiella burnetii
  Leptospira icterohaemorrhagiae
  Fusobacterium necrophorum
  Salmonella typhi
  Francisella tularensis
  Yersinia pestis
- **Immunocompromised**
  Pseudomonas spp.
  Pneumocystis
  Aspergillus
  CMV
- **Viral**
  RSV
  Influenza
  Parainfluenza

For a description of specific pneumonias *see* Chapter 19, Respiratory Medicine.

5.2 Neurological infections

The brain and spinal cord, despite being well protected from the external environment, are prone to a large range of infections from viruses to helminths. The two main clinical syndromes are meningitis and encephalitis. Routes of access are:

- Haematogenous
- Via skull fractures/direct penetration
- Via the cribriform plate
- Via infected sinuses, mastoids or middle ear
- Via peripheral nerves

The **peripheral nerves** tend to be less susceptible to direct bacterial infection (with the exception of leprosy). Most bacterial infections that affect peripheral nerves do so by the action of specific toxins (eg botulinum, diphtheria). Guillain–Barré syndrome may follow several different viral and bacterial infections. A number of viruses (particularly enteroviruses (eg poliovirus)) may seriously damage peripheral nerves.

Causes of Meningitis

- **Acute bacterial**
  Common in adults:
    Meningococcus
    Pneumococcus
    Haemophilus influenzae
  Common in neonates:
    Group B streptococcus
    Escherichia coli
  Rarities (characteristically with **lymphocytic CSF**):
    Listeria monocytogenes
    Leptospirosis
    Syphilis
    Lyme disease (due to *Borrelia burgdorferi*)
  Rarities (characteristically with **polymorphs in CSF**):
    Mycobacterium tuberculosis (acute onset with CSF polymorphs)
    Staphylococcus aureus

- **Chronic bacterial**
  Mycobacterium tuberculosis

- **Chronic fungal**
  Cryptococcosis (particularly in the immunosuppressed)

- **Acute viral**
  Mumps, enteroviruses (eg polio), Herpes simplex (mainly type 2)

- **Miscellaneous**
  Cysticercal meningitis (chronic, eosinophilic CSF)
  Amoebic meningitis (can be acute or chronic); acquired from contaminated water gaining access through cribriform plate

Causes of Encephalitis

- **Viral**
  Herpes simplex (high mortality/morbidity, mainly type 1)
  Enteroviruses, flaviviruses (eg Japanese encephalitis)
  Varicella
  HIV
  Rabies
- **Other**
  Toxoplasmosis
  Cysticercosis
  African trypanosomiasis

(*See also* Chapter 16, Neurology.)

5.3 Gastrointestinal infections

Bowel

The majority of gut infections cause diarrhoea; as a general rule, small bowel infection usually manifests toxin-mediated watery diarrhoea with no blood whilst large bowel infections (with exceptions) are invasive of colonic mucosa and cause bloody diarrhoea with mucus and sometimes pus – 'dysentery'. (*See also* Chapter 6, Gastroenterology.)

Small bowel, toxin-mediated, 'secretory' infective agents

- ***Salmonella* spp.**
  Can occasionally be invasive
  Acquired mainly from eggs and chickens
- **Enterotoxigenic *E. coli* (ETEC)**
  Major cause of traveller's diarrhoea
- ***Vibrio cholerae***
- **Some campylobacters**
  With salmonellas account for most acute gastroenteritis in UK
- ***Yersinia enterocolitica***
- ***Aeromonas* spp.**

Large bowel, invasive infective agents

- ***Shigella* spp.**
- ***Yersinia enterocolitica***
- **Enteroinvasive *E. coli* (EIEC)**
- ***Entamoeba histolytica***
  NB. Amoebic dysentery is occasionally mistaken for ulcerative colitis; steroids are lethal in this situation

Large bowel, toxin-mediated infective agents

- *Clostridium difficile*
- **Enterohaemorrhagic *E. coli* (EHEC)** (Typical serotype is O157) – verotoxin secreting; may lead to epidemic form of haemolytic–uraemic syndrome

Liver

Viral hepatitis is described in Chapter 6, Gastroenterology.

5.4 Specific soft tissue infections

Staphylococcus aureus and *Streptococcus pyogenes* (beta-haemolytic streptococci) are mainly responsible for community-acquired soft tissue infection in otherwise healthy patients.

- **Necrotising fasciitis**: this is a rare complication of *Streptococcus pyogenes* infection. It requires aggressive surgical debridement as well as antibiotics (iv cefotaxime, metronidazole and benzylpenicillin). Necrotising fasciitis can also be due to mixed **facultative anaerobes and anaerobic streptococci**. In addition to the above therapeutic measures, this type of infection will require hyperbaric oxygen therapy.
- Anaerobic soft tissue infection often arises as a complication of severe trauma with destruction of tissue, including that due to human and animal bites. Dog and cat bites may result in *Pasteurella multocida*, also DF-2 infection (see Section 4.3). Anaerobes are also the predominant organism in sepsis arising from the gastrointestinal tract, from dental and gum sepsis to peri-anal abscesses.

6. SPECIFIC TROPICAL INFECTIONS

6.1 Malaria

Four species affect mankind: *Plasmodium falciparum, vivax, ovale* and *malariae. P. falciparum* is potentially lethal, the others are usually more benign.

Complications of falciparum malaria

- **Cerebral malaria**: depression of consciousness is the main feature; other neurological syndromes include seizures, focal neurological disorders and acute psychosis.
- **Blackwater fever**: may cause renal failure due to massive intravascular haemolysis; the haemolysing red cells have not been parasitised but appear to become fragile through some other (unknown) mechanism. Parasites are typically scanty or even absent on blood films.

- **Pulmonary oedema**: has many features in common with the adult respiratory distress syndrome of Gram-negative sepsis; neither left ventricular failure nor fluid overload contributes primarily to the pathogenesis of the oedema. Mortality is severe (80%).
- **Severe anaemia**: partly due to haemolysis, also marrow suppression, the mechanism of the latter being poorly understood.
- **Hyper-reactive malarious splenomegaly**: previously known as 'tropical splenomegaly' syndrome.
- **Other complications**: these include splenic rupture, glomerulonephritis and a malarial hepatitis syndrome (easily mistaken clinically for 'viral hepatitis').

Treatment or prophylaxis of falciparum malaria

Treatment of falciparum malaria comprises quinine and Fansidar®, the other species still being sensitive to chloroquine (except for a few vivax strains found in Papua New Guinea and Indonesia). Newer drugs include artemesinin and atovaquone.

Drugs used for **prophylaxis** of malaria when travelling to endemic areas include: doxycycline, mefloquine, malarone, chloroquine and proguanil.

Complications of infection with other malaria species: these include nephrotic syndrome, particularly in children with *Plasmodium malariae* infection (Quartan nephropathy). The latter is the commonest worldwide cause of nephrotic syndrome. Splenic rupture may also occur in other forms of malarial infection.

6.2 Enteric fevers

Both typhoid and paratyphoid are included in this category. Blood cultures are usually positive in the first two weeks of illness; stool cultures in the second two weeks. The Widal test is unreliable.

Quinolones are now the treatment of choice, with most *S. typhi*, particularly from the Indian subcontinent, being chloramphenicol-resistant. High-dose steroids have been shown to be beneficial in fulminant disease, unlike other forms of Gram-negative sepsis.

6.3 Amoebiasis

The majority of infections with *Entamoeba histolytica* are benign, as evidenced by the very high asymptomatic cyst excretion rate found in many parts of the world. Factors which convert this benign state into disease are not known. The latter can vary from mild diarrhoea to fulminant colitis.

- Diagnosis is by microscopy of fresh warm stool or by serology for invasive disease (colitis or liver abscesses). The latter are usually single and unloculated, unlike pyogenic abscesses which tend to be multiple and loculated.
- **Amoebic liver abscesses hardly ever require a drainage procedure whilst pyogenic ones usually do.**

- Both types of abscess can present 'chronically', resembling malignant disease of the liver with the potential for misdiagnosis.
- Treatment comprises metronidazole or tinidazole with diloxanide furoate to eradicate intestinal cyst carriage.

6.4 Schistosomiasis

These infections are due to **trematodes** and they cause much morbidity worldwide. According to species, the adult worms live in the venous plexuses of the portal tract or in those of the bladder. The adult worms tend not to inflict much damage. They release huge numbers of eggs which make their way through the wall of the blood vessel into the surrounding tissue; the principal pathological feature is a **granuloma around the egg**. The three principal species affecting humans are:

- *Schistosoma mansoni* (bowel and liver)
- *S. haematobium* (urinary tract)
- *S. japonicum* (bowel and liver).

The granulomatous reaction results in fibrosis on a macroscopic scale giving rise to **obstructive uropathy** or **liver fibrosis** with portal hypertension. **Bladder cancer** is also a well-recognised complication of urinary schistosomiasis.

- Sometimes the eggs gain access to the pulmonary and systemic circulations with extra consequences such as **pulmonary hypertension** (eg *S. haematobium*), **paraparesis** (eg *S. mansoni*), or **seizures** (eg *S. japonicum*).
- **Diagnosis** is by identification of ova in the urine or faeces or in tissue biopsy. Serological diagnosis is a useful alternative.
- The **treatment** of choice is praziquantel (*see* Section 3.4).

6.5 Leprosy

This is a very indolent inflammatory disease of skin and nerves with a natural history measurable in years. Most infection is subclinical without progression to disease; this can be demonstrated by positive serology in asymptomatic contacts.

Only 5% of healthy spouses of lepromatous leprosy patients (the most infective kind) eventually get the disease. Clinical expression in a given patient depends on the degree of T-cell-mediated immune response to *Mycobacterium leprae*.

- The immunological spectrum in the patient population varies from lepromatous (LL), with no measurable T-cell responses, to tuberculoid (TT), with brisk T-cell responses. There are intermediate stages termed borderline (BB), borderline lepromatous (BL) and borderline tuberculoid (BT). These immunological variants can be closely correlated with the clinical expression of the disease.

- **Diagnosis** requires appropriate diagnostic suspicion of any longstanding rash or neuropathy in a patient from an indigenous area (most tropical countries, including SE Asia, India, Africa, West Indies, South America).
- **Treatment** comprises remedial and protective advice (relating to anaesthetic feet and hands, etc), as well as drugs.
- Rifampicin, dapsone and clofazimine currently comprise the WHO-recommended multi-drug regime. **Reactions** to drug therapy are due to a shift in the individual's immune status either up or down the spectrum.

Type 1 (reversal reactions) occur in patients who have a TT immunological response. They give rise to acute inflammatory, often painful episodes involving affected nerves and skin. These sometimes resemble acute cellulitis but need to be recognised and treated quickly (with steroids) because of the rapidity of the nerve damage which ensues.

Type 2 reactions occur in patients with an LL-type immunological response. They comprise fever, erythema nodosum leprosum and occasionally life-threatening glomerulonephritis and renal failure.

Chapter 12
Maternal Medicine

CONTENTS

Maternal Medicine

1. PHYSIOLOGY OF NORMAL PREGNANCY

Pregnancy impacts upon every system in the body, and each system adapts in order to accommodate the demands of the feto-placental unit. Consequently, pregnancy can adversely affect many pre-existing medical conditions and, likewise, many pregnancy complications arise because physiological adaptation does not occur.

1.1 Cardiovascular system

- There is an increase in plasma volume from 2600 ml to approximately 3800 ml, reaching a plateau by 32 weeks' gestation.
- Cardiac output rises by about 40%, from about 4.5 l/min to 6 l/min, reaching a plateau by 24–30 weeks' gestation. This occurs because of an increase in heart rate (from approximately 80 beats per minute to 90 beats per minute) and an increase in stroke volume.
- There is a decrease in total peripheral resistance which outstrips the increase in cardiac output, and this results in a fall in blood pressure. This generalised vasodilatation accommodates the increased blood flow to the uterus and other organs.

1.2 Respiratory system

Vital capacity does not change during pregnancy but the tidal volume expands into the expiratory and inspiratory reserve volume. Consequently, ventilation increases by 40% in pregnancy. This increase in ventilation exceeds the increase in oxygen consumption and there is a proportional fall in pCO_2. The bicarbonate level falls to maintain a normal pH and there is a concomitant fall in sodium.

1.3 Haematological system

- There is an increase in red cell mass, from a non-pregnant level of 1400 ml to 1650–1800 ml.
- Plasma volume increases proportionately more than red cell mass, resulting in a fall in the haematocrit and haemoglobin concentration in normal pregnancy, such that a haemoglobin level of 10.5 g/dl may be within normal limits.
- There is an increased demand for iron, mainly to meet the demands of the increased red cell mass and to a lesser extent the requirements of the developing fetus and placenta.
- There are increases in the levels of factors VII, VIII and X, and in the level of plasma fibrinogen, such that in late pregnancy the fibrinogen concentration is at least double that in the non-pregnant state.

1.4 Renal system

- Kidneys increase in length by about 1 cm in pregnancy.
- Ureters become dilated, secondary to increased progesterone and to the obstructive effect of the gravid uterus.
- Renal blood flow increases from about 1.2 l/min in the non-pregnant state to at least 1.5 l/min in pregnancy. This results in an increase in glomerular filtration rate (GFR).
- Increased GFR leads to a fall in blood urea (from 4.3 to 3.1 mmol/l) and creatinine (from 73 to 47 μmol/l).
- Increased GFR also increases the filtered load of glucose and benign glycosuria is common in pregnancy.

2. PHARMACOKINETICS IN PREGNANCY

The physiological changes of normal pregnancy profoundly affect pharmacokinetics.

Physiological changes in pregnancy which affect drug pharmacokinetics

- Renal blood flow increases and leads to increased renal clearance
- Increased plasma volume and fluid retention lead to an increased volume of distribution and decreased plasma concentration
- Induction of liver enzyme pathways increases the hepatic metabolism of certain drugs and results in a decreased plasma concentration

The concept of placental transfer is unique to pregnancy. Essentially, every drug (with the exception of heparin) crosses the placenta and has the potential to cause unwanted side-effects, including teratogenic effects in the unborn fetus. Under most circumstances, drugs cross the placenta and will equilibrate between the fetal and maternal compartments. In view of this, drug therapy is best avoided unless absolutely necessary, during the period of organogenesis in the first trimester (ie between conception and 12 weeks). If unavoidable, older drugs with established safety data should be the agents of first choice. Specific drugs are discussed in more detail later in this chapter.

3. PRE-EXISTING MEDICAL DISORDERS AND PREGNANCY

3.1 Diabetes and pregnancy

Before the advent of insulin, women with type I diabetes who survived to the age of reproduction and were then able to become pregnant had a less than 50% chance of having a successful pregnancy. Today maternal mortality is rare, but both fetal and neonatal morbidity and mortality remain higher compared to the general pregnant population. In 1989 the St Vincent Task Force, together with the WHO, endeavoured to 'achieve pregnancy outcomes in women with diabetes that approximate to those in women without diabetes'. This necessitates achieving normogylcaemia.

Terminology and definitions

Pregnancy induces profound metabolic alterations. To maintain stable concentrations of plasma glucose, insulin secretion must double from the end of the first to the third trimester. In pregnancy glucose concentrations:

- increase post prandially
- decrease with fasting
- decrease with gestation.

Pregnancy is associated with insulin resistance. This is a post-receptor defect, mediated by an increase in pregnancy-associated hormones and cortisol. Changes in insulin also cause an accelerated starvation, with an increase in triglyceride breakdown resulting in raised free fatty acids and ketone bodies.

The diagnosis of diabetes in pregnancy is based on a 75-g oral glucose tolerance test (GTT):

Interpreting the oral glucose tolerance test in pregnancy

Diagnosis	Fasting blood glucose (mmol/l)	Two-hour blood glucose (mmol/l)
Diabetes	> 7.8	> 11.1
Impaired glucose tolerance	> 7.8	> 8 but < 11

Women with gestational diabetes are those who are found, during pregnancy, to have a GTT that meets the threshold for diagnosing diabetes (see Table). A small proportion of these women will inevitably have true, previously undiagnosed, diabetes.

Effects of diabetes on the fetus

Congenital malformations

- Overall there is a 4- to 10-fold increase in the incidence of congenital abnormalities in infants of diabetic mothers compared to the normal pregnant population.
- Cardiac and neural tube defects are among the commonest abnormalities.
- Caudal regression. (This is an embryological defect that occurs during the third week of intrauterine development and is strongly associated with maternal diabetes. Although the syndrome is highly variable in severity, it can result in fusion of the lower limbs and urogenital and anorectal abnormalities.)
- The exact mechanism underlying the increase in congenital abnormalities is unknown but may reflect an abnormal metabolic environment around the time of organogenesis.

Spontaneous miscarriage

- Poorly controlled diabetes is associated with an increased risk of miscarriage, but women with moderately well controlled diabetes have only a minimally increased risk.

Perinatal mortality

- In a multidisciplinary setting, excluding deaths from congenital malformations, perinatal mortality rates are similar between infants of diabetic mothers and those of normal pregnant women.

Unexplained fetal death in utero

Despite improvements in care, death in utero of a normally formed fetus still occurs. The aetiology of these deaths is complex but includes alterations in:

- placental oxygen transfer (reduced red cell oxygen release mediated through 2,3-DPG)
- fetal acid–base balance (tendency toward metabolic acidosis, worsened by increasing maternal glucose concentrations)
- organomegaly (results in increased metabolic demand)
- fetal thrombosis (more likely because of fetal polycythaemia).

Effects of diabetes on the neonate

Birth weight

- There is an increased incidence of both small and large for gestational age fetuses born to diabetic mothers.
- Approximately 25–40% of infants of mothers with diabetes have birth weights above the 90th centile and as many as 35% have birth weights greater than the 95th centile. This leads to an increase in intrapartum complications, including an increase in both the Caesarean section rate and the incidence of shoulder dystocia.
- Increased growth rates may be seen as early as 20–24 weeks' gestation.
- Subcutaneous fat deposits correlate with maternal plasma glucose concentrations and glycosylated haemoglobin levels, amniotic fluid C-peptide levels and fetal serum insulin/glucose ratios.

Respiratory dysfunction

- Reduced phosphatidylglycerol production results in surfactant deficiency; this in turn predisposes the infant to hyaline membrane disease.

Hypoglycaemia

This arises because of:

- endogenous hyperinsulinaemia developed in utero
- reduced hepatic phosphorylase activity
- reduced glucagons and catecholamines resulting in reduced glucose release from the liver.

Polycythaemia and jaundice

Polycythaemia occurs in 29% of infants of diabetic mothers, compared to 6% of infants of normal pregnant women; there is a direct correlation with diabetic control. Polycythaemia results in an increased viscosity, which may cause the following:

- increased cardiac work
- microvascular abnormality, leading to respiratory distress, renal vein thrombosis and necrotising enterocolitis
- jaundice occurs in about 19% of infants due to increase in red cell destruction as well as liver immaturity and poor handling of bilirubin.

Hypocalcaemia and hypomagnesaemia

Calcium and magnesium levels are lower in infants born to diabetic mothers, predisposing to neonatal seizures; the exact mechanism is unknown.

Hypertrophic cardiomyopathy

As many as 30% of infants may have an enlarged heart, and 10% of these may have associated cardiac dysfunction. This correlates with maternal diabetic control. The heart shows features similar to that of hypertrophic obstructive cardiomyopathy, but the dysfunction tends to resolve in the neonatal period.

Management of pregnancy in the diabetic patient

All patients should be counselled regarding the risks of pregnancy and the need for vigilant clinical management. The following are necessary:

Pre-pregnancy

- Switch to insulin if patient on oral hypoglycaemics.
- Encourage tight glucose control (eg pre-prandial levels 4–6 mmol/l).
- HbA_{1c} <6% should be maintained.
- Treat any retinopathy.
- Screen for nephropathy.

Antenatal care

It is very important to involve the multidisciplinary team in the care of the patient. Patients should be booked in the antenatal clinic at a very early stage with organisation of a dating scan to confirm the gestation. Patients should be given dietary advice and baseline renal function should be assessed. Other important aspects of management include:

- Maintain tight glucose control; the patient should be warned about the possibility of hypoglycaemic episodes.
- Serum screening should be interpreted with care as α-feto-protein (AFP) levels are lower in diabetic pregnancies.
- A detailed anomaly scan, including fetal echocardiography, should be performed.
- Regular review with BP measurement and urinalysis.
- Serial fetal growth and liquor volume assessment.
- Cardiotocograph (CTG) may be useful after 36 weeks to assess fetal well-being, in the light of possible risk of fetal death in utero.

- In view of the increased risk of pre-term delivery (induced or spontaneous) patients may require high-dose intramuscular steroids. A sliding scale of insulin would be necessary during this treatment. Tocolytics are used to stop uterine activity (ie in the treatment of pre-term labour). Ritodrine and salbutamol have been used in the recent past for this indication and can interfere with glycaemic control. These agents have largely been superseded by nifedipine and atosiban (an oxytocin receptor antagonist).

The timing and mode of delivery will be individualised according to the patient and health of the fetus.

Labour

Good diabetic control should be maintained for patients often requiring a sliding scale for insulin administration. The following are also important:

- continuous CTG
- watch for obstructed labour
- beware possible shoulder dystocia
- high Caesarian section rate (as high as 60–65%).

Post-partum

- Reduce insulin back to pre-pregnancy levels following delivery of placenta.
- Encourage breast feeding.
- Discuss contraception (see below).

Gestational diabetes/impaired glucose tolerance in pregancy

Initially, glycaemic control may be achieved through diet (total calories between 1800 and 2000/day). Fibre intake should be increased and > 50% of energy should be derived from carbohydrates.

- If pre-prandial blood glucose levels are > 6 mmol/l then insulin is introduced, usually twice daily.
- The fetus is at risk of macrosomia and hence birth trauma.
- Insulin requirements cease following delivery of placenta.
- It is vital that a glucose tolerance test (GTT) is performed at 6 weeks after delivery

The patient should be counselled with regard to their weight, diet and exercise output. Without attention to this, more than 50% of women with gestational diabetes will develop true diabetes over the next 20 years.

Contraception for patients with diabetes

The following are important considerations:

- Combined pill (COP): associated with an increased risk of thrombosis, both venous and arterial. Nevertheless this would be suitable for the young, well controlled diabetic with no evidence of vascular disease.

- Progesterone-only pill: lower efficacy compared to the COP; greater likelihood of menstrual irregularities.
- IUCD: an effective method of contraception in diabetics. No evidence of reduced efficacy.
- Sterilisation: this is suitable for diabetic women who have completed their family, or wish to avoid pregnancy because of associated microvascular complications (severe retinopathy or nephropathy).

3.2 Cardiac disease and pregnancy

The overall incidence of heart disease in pregnancy is approximately 1% and is increasing, reflecting recent advances in cardiac management that have allowed greater numbers of women with congenital heart disease to reach childbearing age. The haemodynamic changes that occur in pregnancy can be dangerous for women with cardiac disease. However, although the prognosis for pregnancy is generally good, in women with cardiac disease the exact level of risk posed by the pregnancy depends upon the underlying pathology:

- In general, regurgitant valvular lesions and mild/moderate left-to-right shunts are well tolerated due to the decrease in total peripheral vascular resistance which occurs in pregnancy.
- Conversely, stenotic valvular lesions, pulmonary hypertension and right-to-left shunts are poorly tolerated.

It is therefore helpful to categorise heart disease in terms of mortality risk, as this will optimise accurate counselling, evaluation and management.

Risk	Condition
High (mortality 25–50%)	Eisenmenger's complex Cyanotic heart disease (tetralogy of Fallot, Ebstein's anomaly, transposition of the great vessels) Pulmonary hypertension Acute myocardial infarction Hypertrophic obstructive cardiomyopathy Heart failure (including peripartum cardiomyopathy)
Moderate to high (mortality 5–15%)	Valvular stenosis Coarctation of the aorta History of myocardial infarction Marfan's syndrome Mechanical prosthetic valve
Low (mortality < 1%)	Acyanotic heart disease Mild to moderate valvular regurgitation Mitral valve prolapse Small VSD Small ASD

Symptoms and signs in normal pregnancy

Symptoms of pregnancy may mimic cardiac disease and dyspnoea, peripheral oedema and palpitations are all common complaints in normal pregnancy. A benign ejection systolic murmur occurs in 96% of pregnant women.

ECG and echocardiographic changes in normal pregnancy include

ECG changes

- Sinus tachycardia
- Leftward or rightward shift of the QRS axis
- Premature atrial or ventricular beats

Echocardiographic changes associated with normal pregnancy include

- An increase in heart size and left ventricular mass
- A small pericardial effusion
- Mild valvular regurgitation

Management of the pregnant woman with cardiac disease

Pre-conception

Management should take place in a multidisciplinary setting, preferably in a tertiary centre, and this should involve the obstetrician, cardiologist, anaesthetist and if necessary the cardiothoracic surgeon.

Pre-conception evaluation will allow for appropriate counselling regarding maternal and fetal risks, optimisation of drug therapy or pre-pregnancy surgery if indicated.

- Most cardiac drugs are safe, but angiotensin-converting enzyme inhibitors should be avoided as they are associated with fetal and neonatal renal failure and death.
- **Anticoagulation**: due to the hypercoagulable state of pregnancy, there is an increased risk of valve thrombosis and embolism in women with prosthetic valves. Warfarin is teratogenic, particularly in the first trimester, and is also associated with fetal haemorrhage throughout pregnancy. Heparin does not cross the placenta, but is associated with maternal bone demineralisation and thrombocytopenia. In addition, heparin has also been associated with a higher risk of thromboembolic complications. Anticoagulation in these patients should be determined on an individual risk basis.

Antenatal management

Consideration should be given to the genetic implications of maternal cardiac disease. Congenital heart disease has a multifactorial inheritance. There is a small increase in the risk of congenital heart disease occuring in the fetus but this risk increases sharply if more than one member of the family is affected. Consequently, high-resolution ultrasound with fetal echocardiography is advised in the second trimester.

- Once pregnant, the majority of women will have no haemodynamic problems. Cardiac decompensation, however, is an indication for termination of pregnancy.
- Fetal growth should be assessed regularly, particularly in women with severe heart disease and cyanotic congenital heart conditions.
- Indications for cardiac surgery are the same as for the non-pregnant woman.
- If surgery is required, it should be performed with the patient in the left decubitus position with provision for Caesarean section if the gestation is greater than 24 weeks.
- Standard cardiopulmonary bypass may compromise the placenta and fetus due to hypothermia, reduced arterial perfusion and alterations in coagulation and acid–base balance. To avoid these complications, cardiopulmonary support should be high-flow, normothermic and initiated without hyperkalaemic arrest.

Intrapartum management

In general, spontaneous vaginal delivery is preferred but selected patients with severe heart disease may benefit from elective Caesarean section. In labour, care must be taken to avoid supine hypotension due to aorto-caval compression by the gravid uterus.

- In the majority of patients with adequate cardiac reserve, epidural anaesthesia is effective and well tolerated. It should, however, be used with extreme caution in women with restricted cardiac outputs such as in primary pulmonary hypertension or right-to-left shunts. Under these circumstances, general anaesthesia and abdominal delivery may be preferred.
- Fluid balance requires special attention and high-risk cases may warrant pulmonary wedge pressure monitoring with a pulmonary catheter.
- Under certain circumstances, ergometrine should be avoided during the third stage of labour. The tonic contraction of the uterus caused by this drug will force approximately 500 ml of blood into the circulation causing a rise in left atrial pressure. This would be particularly detrimental in patients with significant mitral stenosis.
- Delivery is associated with a transient asymptomatic bacteraemia. Therefore, women with structural heart disease may benefit from antibiotic prophylaxis. This is mandatory in women with prosthetic valves.

3.3 Renal disease and hypertension in pregnancy

Pregnancy outcome in women with renal disease has improved markedly in recent years. The main risks of pregnancy in a patient with renal disease are of **adverse pregnancy outcome** and **deterioration of renal function** accompanying the pregnancy. The risks depend upon the:

- degree of renal impairment at conception
- presence of hypertension at conception or in early pregnancy
- degree of proteinuria.

Risk is best determined by accurate assessment of renal function.

Mildly impaired renal function

In the presence of mildly impaired renal function (serum creatinine <125 μmol/l or GFR 50–70 ml/min), the live birth rate approaches 95%. There is a slightly increased risk of pre-term delivery, pre-eclampsia and intra-uterine growth retardation (IUGR), but pregnancy does not seem to adversely influence renal function. Therefore, women in this category should not be discouraged from becoming pregnant.

Moderately impaired renal function

In the presence of moderately impaired renal function (serum creatinine 125–265 μmol/l or GFR 25–50 ml/min), there is a significantly increased risk of pre-term delivery, pre-eclampsia and IUGR. The success of the pregnancy depends upon adequate control of blood pressure.

- Uncontrolled hypertension is associated with significantly increased rates of fetal and neonatal loss.
- There is a 25–50% chance of decline in renal function, which may be permanent.
- Nevertheless, in a multidisciplinary setting and with rigorous control of blood pressure, the live birth rate approaches 84%.

Severely impaired renal function

In the presence of severly impaired renal function (serum creatinine > 265 μmol/l or GFR < 25 ml/min), fertility is reduced. Spontaneous conception may occasionally occur. Again, the key to successful outcome is largely dependent upon adequate control of maternal blood pressure. However, the risks to both the fetus and mother are such that termination of pregnancy may be offered.

- In women who continue with the pregnancy, there is a 90% chance of antenatal complications.
- Uncontrolled hypertension is associated with a 10-fold increase in perinatal mortality.
- The live birth rate is 50–80% (depending on underlying diagnosis and management).

End-stage renal disease

Patients who are receiving dialysis have very low fertility, and even if conception is successful, there is a high rate of miscarriage. There have only been a handful of reported cases of successful pregnancies in women receiving dialysis.

- In patients with functioning renal transplants, the outcomes are again determined by the level of graft (ie renal) function, as described above. Most of the commonly used immuno-suppressant agents (eg ciclosporin A, tacrolimus, micophenolate (MMF), prednisolone and azathioprine) are considered to be safe for administration during pregnancy. Again, optimal blood pressure control is the key to a successful pregnancy.

Specific renal diseases and pregnancy

Renal disease	Effects and outcome	Risk of pre-eclampsia
Chronic glomerulonephritis	Usually no adverse effect in absence of hypertension UTI more frequent The renal lesion may be affected by the coagulation changes of pregnancy	Mild
IgA nephropathy	Risk of hypertension and worsening of renal function	Moderate-severe
Pyelonephritis	Bacteriuria in pregnancy may lead to exacerbation Multiple organ dysfunction can occur	Mild
Reflux nephropathy	Risks of hypertension/worsening or renal function	Mild-moderate
Urolithiasis	UTI more frequent Avoid lithotripsy Natural history not affected	Mild
Diabetic nephropathy	Increased UTI, oedema Natural history not affected	Moderate-severe
Polyarteritis nodosa	Poor fetal prognosis Risk of maternal death	Severe
Polycystic disease	Minimal risk of functional impairment and hypertension	Mild at most
Systemic lupus erythematosus	More favourable prognosis if in remission > 6 months prior to conception Controversies regarding steroid dosing	Severe
Scleroderma	If onset during pregnancy; rapid deterioration may occur Reactivation of quiescent scleroderma may occur postpartum	Severe
Previous urinary tract surgery	Possible associations with other urinary tract malformations Renal function may worsen	Mild

Specific renal diseases and pregnancy *continued*

Renal disease	Effects and outcome	Risk of pre-eclampsia
After nephrectomy, solitary kidney and pelvic kidney	Possible associations with other malformations of urogenital tract Pregnancy well tolorated	Mild
Wegener's granulomatosis	Proteinuria (+_hypertension) is common from early pregnancy Avoid cytotoxics but immunosupressives safe	Moderate/severe
Renal artery stenosis	May present as chronic hypertension or recurrent isolated preeclampsia Transluminal angioplasty in pregnancy if appropiate	Mild-moderate

The table above has been reproduced from *Hypertension in Pregnancy*, Belfont M et al 2003, by kind permission of Marcel Dekker.

Management of pregnancy in patients with pre-existing renal disease

The patients with pre-existing renal disease should be managed in a multidisciplinary setting. Where possible, the patients should be referred for pre-conception evaluation and counselling prior to embarking upon a pregnancy. At this stage, there needs to be a consideration of possible genetic causes of renal impairment (eg polycystic kidney disease or Alport's syndrome) which may affect the fetus. Once pregnant, the patient with renal disease should undergo the following management:

- Early referral for antenatal clinic booking with dating ultrasound scan.
- Baseline biochemistry and urinalysis (including urea, creatinine, electrolytes, urate, lactate dehydrogenase and 24-hour urine protein excretion). These investigations should be repeated at least every 4 weeks.
- Preferred anti-hypertensive drugs include labetalol, methyldopa and long-acting nifedipine.
- ACE inhibitors should be discontinued pre-conceptually or at the earliest opportunity (see earlier).
- The patient should be assessed frequently (fortnightly until 28 weeks, then weekly until delivery).
- Regular fetal surveillance with growth scans, commencing at 24 weeks (particularly if on anti-hypertensive medication).
- Indications for pre-term delivery are deteriorating renal function, the development of superimposed pre-eclampsia and/or severe IUGR. Hence, appropriate specialised paediatric services will be required.

3.4 Antiphospholipid syndrome and pregnancy

The antiphospholipid syndrome is defined as a clinical disorder with recurrent arterial and venous thrombotic events, pregnancy wastage and/or thrombocytopenia in the presence of the lupus anticoagulant and/or a moderate to high positive anticardiolipin test.

- **The lupus anticoagulant** is an inhibitor of the coagulation pathway. Its presence is a good predictor of poor fetal outcome.
- **Anticardiolipin antibodies** are antibodies active against certain phospholipid components of cell walls. They may be IgG or IgM.
- Both a **primary form** (patients without clinical or serological evidence of autoimmune disorders), and a secondary form (usually in patients with SLE) of the antiphospholipid syndrome are recognised.

The mechanism of pregnancy loss/adverse pregnancy outcome is not clearly elucidated. Current theories include damage to placental vascular endothelium, platelet deposition, imbalance in the thromboxane: prostacyclin (PGI_2) ratio and inhibition of protein C and tissue plasminogen.

Treatment

The treatment options include oral therapy with low-dose aspirin and/or low-molecular-weight heparin (LMWH). Even with treatment the pregnancies can be complicated by hypertension and fetal growth restriction, and hence they require careful monitoring.

- Clinical trials indicate a take home baby rate of 70% with combined therapy versus 40% with aspirin alone. With no treatment success is in the region of only 10%.

See also Chapter 9, Haematology.

3.5 Thyroid disease and pregnancy

Thyroid disease is relatively common in women of child bearing age. Physiological changes during normal pregnancy include:

- increased thyroxine-binding globulin (TBG)
- increase in triiodothyronine (T_3) and thyroxine (T_4)
- relative iodine deficiency, increased renal excretion
- free T_4/T_3 falls in the third trimester
- thyroid-stimulating hormone (TSH) falls in first/second trimester, increases in third trimester.

Serum screening is less accurate in hypothyroidism. Raised fetal TSH concentrations may falsely elevate both fetal and maternal serum α-feto-protein (AFP). This results in false-positive screening for neural tube defects and false-negative for Trisomy 21 screening.

Hyperthyroidism

Untreated hyperthyroidism is associated with subfertility and reduced libido. It occurs with an incidence of approximatedly 2/1000 pregnancies and is most frequently due to autoimmune thyrotoxicosis (Graves' disease).

Effect of pregnancy on hyperthyroidism

- Flares are seen in both the first trimester and the puerperium
- Typically remits in the second and third trimester, which results in a reduction in medication for many, and cessation of therapy in about 30%
- The change in disease activity reflects the maternal immune state and titres of thyrotropin receptor-stimulating antibodies

Effect of hyperthyroidism on pregnancy

- If hyperthyroidism is well controlled before and throughout pregnancy, outcomes are good for mother and baby
- Poor control is associated with congestive cardiac failure, pre-eclampsia, pre-term labour, IUGR and stillbirth

Treatment

The treatment of choice is propylthiouracil or carbimazole. The dose is titrated against biochemical results (free T_4 at the upper limit of normal) and the maternal condition:

- about 30% of women require dose reduction or discontinuation in the second/third trimester, with possible increase/recommencement in the puerperium
- a blocking/replacement regime should be avoided in pregnancy.

Fetal and neonatal risks in thyrotoxicosis

In pregnancy the aim of therapy is to reduce the dose of any drugs to the minimum required to control maternal disease. However, both propylthiouracil and carbimazole cross the placenta. High dosage may be associated with fetal goitres which usually resolve post-natally.

- 10-20% of babies have transient biochemical hypothyroidism which is rarely symptomatic and resolves on day 4–5.
- The fetal and neonatal risk of Graves' disease is proportional to the titre of maternal TSH receptor stimulating antibodies. These should be measured in the first and third trimester in women with active disease, or in those with a history of disease treated with surgery and/or radioactive iodine.

Fetal hyperthyroidism develops between 20 and 24 weeks' gestation.

Complications of fetal hyperthyroidism

- Fetal tachycardia (>160 beats/min)
- Increased fetal movements
- IUGR
- Fetal goitre
- Craniosynostosis
- Hydrops
- Polyhyramnios
- Pre-term labour

Treatment is dependent upon gestation and is either delivery or anti-thyroid agents, titrated against fetal heart rate, movements and growth rate.

Neonatal hyperthyroidism occurs in 1% of cases of maternal thyrotoxicosis. The clinical presentation may be delayed. However, treatment with anti-thyroid drugs or beta blockers is rarely needed for more than a few months.

Clinical features of neonatal hyperthyroidism

- Jitteriness
- Failure to gain weight
- Poor feeding
- Poor sleeping
- Bossing of frontal bones
- Liver dysfunction
- Jaundice

Hypothyroidism

Hypothyroidism is the commonest pre-existing endocrine disorder in pregnancy. The incidence is 9 in 1000 pregnancies. The commonest cause is Hashimoto's thyroiditis.

Treatment

Thyroxine is the mainstay treatment, as it is safe in pregnancy and in breast-feeding.

- Thyroid function tests should be measured at 8–12 weeks if stable, and every 4–6 weeks if the dosage is being adjusted.
- Thyroxine should be altered according to the free T_4 levels; TSH may remain raised after the correct dosage has been achieved (especially in third trimester).
- If the patient is stable pre-pregnancy, they are likely to remain stable without requiring any dose adjustment during the pregnancy.
- Sub-optimal maternal treatment (ie a low free T_4 in first trimester) may be associated with adverse neurodevelopment in the child.
- Neonatal hypothyroidism is rare and transient and is caused by TSH-receptor-blocking antibodies.

Post-partum thyroiditis

This has an autoimmune aetiology and hence it is associated with other autoimmune diseases. Thyroid antiperoxidase antibodies are seen in 90% of sufferers. The histology of the thyroid gland is typical of autoimmune thyroiditis with focal/diffuse thyroiditis, lymphocytic infiltration, follicular destruction and hyperplasia.

There are three phases of post-partum thyroiditis:

- **Thyrotoxicosis**: 1–3 months post-partum. This is associated with low uptake of radioactive iodine (unlike Graves' disease). Treatment is rarely required, but if needed involves only beta-blockers.
- **Hypothyroidism**: 3–8 months post-partum. This may be associated with symptoms which include lethargy, poor memory and cold intolerance, and treatment with thyroxine may be indicated.
- **Normal thyroid function**: by l year post-partum.

The mother may experience one, two or all of these phases. The recurrence risk in another pregnancy is about 70%. Patients will need long-term surveillance as the risk of permanent hypothyroidism is about 3–5% per year.

3.6 Epilepsy and pregnancy

Epilepsy occurs in 1 in 200 women of childbearing age, and is the commonest neurological disorder in pregnancy. In general, the longer a woman has been free of fits prior to pregnancy the less likely it is that her epilepsy will deteriorate during pregnancy.

Factors influencing fit frequency in pregnancy

- Disease pattern pre-pregnancy
- Sleep deprivation, especially in the third trimester
- Vomiting in pregnancy
- Altered protein binding, and increased volume of distribution of anticonvulsants
- Altered drug compliance
- Altered metabolism and excretion of anti-convulsant drugs

Effect of maternal epilepsy upon the fetus

The fetus is very tolerant of isolated, short-lived fits. Repeated fits can result in fetal hypoxia and lactic acidosis, which may be associated with fetal bradycardia. In rare instances, fetal intraventricular haemorrhages and death have been attributed to maternal convulsions. The effect may be remote and only detected in developmental delay years later. Status epilepticus doubles the risk of maternal death and is associated with a 50% miscarriage rate.

- **Birth defects**: epilepsy is associated with an increased incidence of certain congenital malformations (3.5–4.4%); the risk is multifactorial and increases with the number of anticonvulsants used.
- **Risk of epilepsy in the newborn**: about 4% if one parent is affected, rising to 10% if both are affected.
- **Neonatal coagulopathy**: associated with maternal use of phenytoin, phenobarbital and primidone; maternal coagulation studies are usually normal.

Management of the epileptic in pregnancy

Pre-pregnancy counselling should be given to the patient regarding the risks of pregnancy. Where possible, anticonvulsant monotherapy should be used.

- A detailed fetal anomaly scan should be performed.
- If fits occur during pregnancy, the anticonvulsant levels should be monitored.
- If the patient is receiving phenytoin, then vitamin K should be administered to the mother from 36 weeks' gestation in order to counteract possible neonatal coagulopathy.

4. MEDICAL COMPLICATIONS OF PREGNANCY

4.1 Hypertensive disorders of pregnancy

Definitions

Hypertension in pregnancy is defined as:

- diastolic BP ≥ 110 mmHg on any one occasion **or**
- diastolic BP ≥ 90 mmHg on two or more consecutive occasions ≥ 4 hours apart.

Blood pressure should be measured in the sitting position with a sphygmomanometer cuff size appropriate for the size of the patient's arm.

Phases I and V of the Korotkoff sounds identify the systolic and diastolic limits, respectively, correlating more accurately with outcome than phase IV.

Proteinuria in pregnancy is defined as:

- total protein excretion ≥ 300 mg per 24 hours **or**
- two 'clean-catch – midstream' or catheter specimens of urine collected ≥ 4 hours apart with ≥ 2+ on reagent strip.

Hypertension is associated with between 6% and 8% of pregnancies and can have serious repercussions for both fetal and maternal well-being. Hypertension can predate the pregnancy (**essential** or **chronic hypertension**) or arise in pregnancy (**pregnancy-induced hypertension** or PIH).

- The majority of women with PIH have non-proteinuric PIH, a condition associated with minimal maternal or perinatal mortality/morbidity.
- Approximately 2% of pregnancies, are complicated by proteinuric PIH (**pre-eclampsia**).

Pre-eclampsia is a serious pregnancy complication that causes significant maternal and perinatal morbidity and it remains one of the leading causes of maternal and fetal/neonatal deaths. It is therefore imperative that every effort is made to accurately classify the nature of hypertension occurring in pregnancy as the aetiology and management of the three conditions, chronic hypertension, non-proteinuric PIH or pre-eclampsia, are very different.

The ISSHP classification (modified and abbreviated)

1. **Gestational hypertension and/or proteinuria developing during pregnancy, labour or the puerperium in a previously normotensive non-proteinuric woman:**
   Gestational hypertension (without proteinuria)
   Gestational proteinuria (without hypertension)
   Gestational proteinuric hypertension (pre-eclampsia)
2. **Chronic hypertension (before the 20th week of pregnancy) and chronic renal disease (proteinuria before the 20th week of pregnancy):**
   Chronic hypertension (without proteinuria)
   Chronic renal disease (proteinuria with or without hypertension)
   Chronic hypertension with superimposed pre-eclampsia (new-onset proteinuria)
3. **Unclassified hypertension and/or proteinuria**
4. **Eclampsia**

Pre-eclampsia

Although the primary events leading to pre-eclampsia are still unclear, it is now thought that the pathophysiology involves a cascade of events which leads to the clinical syndrome.

Pathophysiology of pre-eclampsia

- Genetic predisposition
- Faulty interplay between invading trophoblast and decidua
- Decreased blood supply to feto-placental unit
- Release of circulating factor(s)
- Endothelial cell alteration

Pre-eclampsia is associated with hypertension, proteinuria and IUGR.

Maternal mortality rate is about 2% in the UK and world-wide 100,000 women die of pre-eclampsia each year. Perinatal mortality is also increased, and this is associated with IUGR and iatrogenic pre-term delivery.

Screening for pre-eclampsia

It is important to take a full history, as several factors can be associated with an increased risk of pre-eclampsia.

Risk factors associated with pre-eclampsia

Increased risk

- Family history 4–8 times higher in first-degree relatives
- Primigravidas 15 times higher than multiparus
- Longer pregnancy interval
- Change in partner
- Teenage pregnancy
- Donor insemination
- Medical disorders such as chronic hypertension, renal disease

Decreased risk

- Previous termination of pregnancy
- Previous miscarriage
- Non-barrier contraception
- Increased duration of sexual cohabitation

- **Biophysical tests**: all currently available tests are of limited clinical value. The uterine artery may appear 'notched'. Doppler waveforms may be of significance but they are only of sufficient sensitivity and specificity when used in a pre-selected high-risk population.

Prophylaxis of pre-eclampsia

Several agents have been investigated:

- **Aspirin** (and other anti-platelet agents): a cyclooxygenase inhibitor. A Cochrane review of 42 randomised trials demonstrated a 15% relative risk reduction in the risk of pre-eclampsia associated with the use of aspirin or other anti-platelet agents.
- **Calcium**: 10 randomised trials have investigated the role of calcium in prophylaxis of pre-eclampsia. A moderate reduction in incidence could be demonstrated with calcium supplementation but only in women with an inadequate calcium intake prior to the study.
- **Fish oils**: fish oils containing omega-3 fatty acids are thought to inhibit platelet thromboxane A_2. However, trials to date have not shown any reduction in pre-eclampsia.
- **Vitamins C and E**: in patients at high risk of developing pre-eclampsia, a 50% reduction could be demonstrated with the use of these agents. Multicentre trials in high- and low-risk populations are now ongoing to determine whether the potential benefit extends to all pregnant women, particularly primigravida.

Maternal and fetal assessment in pre-eclampsia

Maternal assessment

Several different organ systems can be affected in the pregnant woman:

- **Platelets**: are consumed due to the endothelial activation. Although a platelet count of $> 50 \times 10^9/l$ will support normal haemostasis, a falling platelet count, particularly to $< 100 \times 10^9/l$ may indicate a need to deliver.
- **Hypovolaemia**: results in an increased haematocrit, with an apparent rise in the haemoglobin.
- **Clotting disorders**: pre-eclampsia can cause disseminated intravascular coagulation, and clotting disorders must be assessed, particularly in the face of falling platelet numbers.
- **Renal tubular function**: uric acid is a measure of 'fine' renal tubular function. It is used to assess the disease severity, although severe disease can still occur with a normal uric acid level. Spuriously high levels of uric acid are associated with acute fatty liver of pregnancy (see below).
- **Renal impairment**: raised urea and creatinine are associated with late renal involvement hence are not useful as an early indicator of disease severity. However, serial measurements will identify renal disease progression. Proteinuria is a hallmark of pre-eclampsia; protein excretion may increase progressively as the pre-eclamptic process evolves.
- **Liver involvement**: pre-eclampsia can cause sub-capsular haematoma, liver rupture and hepatic infarction. Aspartate aminotransferase (AST) and other transaminases indicate hepatocellular damage. Elevated levels may again indicate a need to deliver. It should be remembered that the normal range for transaminases is approximately 20% lower than the non-pregnant range.

The circulating albumin may fall especially if urinary protein excretion is high (eg > 3 g/24 hours); hypoalbuminaemia increase the risk of pulmonary oedema. Note that a raised AST can be associated with either **haemolysis** or liver involvement; lactate dehydrogenase levels (LDH) are also elevated in the presence of haemolysis (see HELLP syndrome, overleaf).

Fetal assessment

Fetal well-being must be carefully assessed in all cases of pre-eclampsia. This involves:

- **Clinical assessment**: the symphyseal-fundal height should be carefully measured and an enquiry as to fetal movements undertaken.
- **Investigations**: Regular ultrasound assessment of fetal growth and amniotic fluid volume should be performed. Umbilical artery Doppler waveforms may be of use (see above).

Suspected fetal compromise is a frequent indication for delivery in pre-eclampsia.

Management of pre-eclampsia

Pre-eclamptic hypertension can cause direct arterial injury which can, in turn, predispose to possibly fatal cerebral haemorrhage. In order to prevent this injury severe hypertension should be avoided. Blood pressures greater than 170/110 mmHg (mean arterial pressure (MAP) of ≥140 mmHg) require urgent therapy. The rationale for treating moderate hypertension (BP > 140/90 mmHg but < 170/110 mmHg) is less clear. Treatment at this level may, by reducing placental blood flow, compromise fetal growth, without affording any maternal benefit.

- Choice of anti-hypertensive agents: methyldopa, labetalol and nifedipine are the mainstay in therapy. In practice, the choice of agent probably matters less than the clinician's familiarity with it.
- **Timing of delivery**: in women with established pre-eclampsia, delivery should be considered once fetal lung maturity has been achieved. However in asymptomatic women with pre-eclampsia, presenting between 26 and 32 weeks, management can often be conservative in an attempt to achieve improved perinatal survival, without substantial risk to the mother. This does, however, require close inpatient supervision, in a unit with adequate numbers of appropriately skilled staff. Trials have confirmed the advantages of this cautiously expectant approach. As stated previously, fetal compromise will indicate the need for delivery.

Indications for delivery in pre-eclampsia

- Inability to control hypertension
- Deteriorating liver or renal function
- Progressive fall in platelets
- Neurological complication
- Abnormal CTG
- Deteriorating fetal condition

HELLP syndrome

HELLP (haemolysis, elevated liver enzymes and low platelets) syndrome is a severe form of pre-eclampsia, associated with:

- haemolysis
- elevated liver enzymes (ALT/LDH)
- low platelets.

It complicates about 10–15% of cases of pre-eclampsia. Mortality rates vary from 0 to 25%, and mortality is associated with cerebral haemorrhage, DIC and correlates with the extent of thrombocytopenia. HELLP syndrome and acute fatty liver of pregnancy are two conditions which are very similar and there is a recognised degree of overlap in both aetiology and pathophysiology, such that a definitive diagnosis can be difficult to make.

Acute fatty liver of pregnancy

Acute fatty liver of pregnancy typically occurs in obese women or in the third trimester of pregnancy. It is associated with pre-eclampsia (30–100% of cases), twin pregnancy and in women with male fetuses.

Symptoms develop acutely and include abdominal pain, nausea/vomiting, headache and jaundice. Other clinical features which may occur include pruritus, fever, enterocolitis, ascites or pancreatitis.

Investigations in acute fatter liver of pregnancy

Laboratory findings

- Neutrophil leukocytosis
- Increased fibrin degradation products
- Low platelets
- Microangiopathic haemolytic anaemia
- Increased bilirubin
- Raised AST (3–10 times above normal)
- Hypoglycaemia
- Increased uric acid

Liver pathology

- The liver is small and yellow
- Histology reveals microvesicular steatosis with intrahepatic cholestasis and canalicular plugs of bile. Distribution is panlobar with sparing of periportal areas
- Extramedullary haematopoiesis

Imaging

- Increased reflectivity of liver on ultrasound scanning and lower attenuation on MR imaging are both indicative of 'fat' within the liver
- Infarction appears as multiple non-enhancing lesions of low attenuation, with mottled appearance

Management of acute fatty liver of pregnancy

Early diagnosis is important, followed by transfer of the patient to tertiary care. The patients may need to be transferred to intensive care for correction of hypertension, hypoglycaemia and bleeding diathesis. The baby needs to be delivered as a matter of urgency.

The neonate is at risk of fatty infiltration of the liver and this is associated with impaired liver function, hypoglycaemia, thrombocytopenia and neutropenia.

Eclampsia

Eclampsia is defined as convulsions occurring in a woman with pre-eclampsia in the absence of any other neurological cause. The maternal mortality rate associated with eclampsia in the UK is approximately 1 in 50. It complicates 1 in 2000 pregnancies in the UK. In about 40% of cases it is totally or partially unheralded by prodromal signs or symptoms. In 10% of cases the only warning sign is proteinuria, and in another 20% there is hypertension only. Most cases occur during labour or after delivery. Such cases are usually at term and in hospital. Pre-term eclampsia is more likely to be antepartum.

Management of eclampsia

The aim of management is to protect the maternal airway, control the convulsions and extreme hypertension, as well as to expedite delivery.

- **Choice of anticonvulsant**: most fits stop quickly and spontaneously. In the Collaborative Eclampsia Trial (1995) magnesium sulphate was shown to be the anti-convulsant of first choice. A bolus of 4 mg is given intravenously over 10 minutes. About 10% of all fits will not be controlled by magnesium sulphate. A brain scan should be performed if presentation is atypical, if any focal signs develop, or in the case of repeated or prolonged seizures.

Magnesium sulphate treatment in eclampsia

- **Toxic side-effects**: muscular weakness; respiratory paralysis; heart failure and death
- **Monitor**: check deep tendon reflexes
- **Therapeutic levels**: 2–3.5 mmol/l
- **Antidote**: calcium gluconate 1 g over 10 minutes, intravenously

Chronic hypertension

Chronic hypertension (CHT) is detected either by an antecedent medical history or by a raised blood pressure in the first half of pregnancy. The physiological decline in the blood pressure in early pregnancy is exaggerated in women with CHT so that they may be normotensive. Conversely, in later pregnancy the normal rise in blood pressure is exaggerated in patients with CHT. Hence a woman with CHT may be normotensive initially, with hypertension only appearing in the third trimester.

- CHT in pregnancy is a major predisposing factor for pre-eclampsia. This risk is about 5 times greater than in normotensive women.
- Women with CHT who do not develop pre-eclampsia can usually expect a normal, uncomplicated perinatal outcome, although there is some evidence for a modest increase in the incidence of IUGR in these women. Perinatal morbidity and mortality is related to treatment and so cautious discontinuation of pharmacological agents may be appropriate (see later).
- **Antihypertensive treatment**: ACE inhibitors should be avoided, as this class of drug is associated with fetal and neonatal renal failure and death. Women with mild to moderate hypertension should discontinue treatment prior to conception because of the risk of IUGR. There is no evidence that treating CHT reduces the risk of superimposed pre-eclampsia, and nor is there any evidence to support a particular fetal benefit. Long-term use of antihypertensives has been associated with IUGR; it is uncertain whether this is a specific drug effect (eg beta-blockers) or a consequence of a reduction in placental perfusion following a lowering of arterial pressure.

4.2 Thrombotic complications in pregnancy

Thromboembolic disease

Pulmonary embolism is the commonest cause of maternal mortality in the UK. Pregnancy increases the risk of thromboembolism by about 6-fold. The absolute incidence varies widely between 0.1% and 1.2% of all pregnancies. Deep vein thrombosis (DVT) is about twice as common as pulmonary embolism.

Aetiology

Pregnancy is a hypercoagulable state due to an increase in Factors VII, VIII and X as well as fibrinogen and prothrombin. This is exacerbated by venous stasis as the gravid uterus obstructs the inferior vena cava, causing a decrease in venous tone in the lower limbs, which is greater on the left than the right. Immobility during labour and in the postpartum period, particularly after operative delivery, further exacerbates the situation.

Other factors increasing the risk of thromboembolism in pregnancy

- Increased with age (>35 years)
- Increased with rising parity
- Increased BMI (3 times increased risk if >29)
- Smoking, as it causes inhibition of fibrinolysis
- Sickle cell disease
- Anaemia
- Dehydration
- Blood group other than O
- Thrombophilic conditions (see below)

Thrombophilia

Thrombophilic tendencies are of particular significance in women of reproductive age as pregnancy may uncover a hitherto unrecognised condition. The main conditions to consider are:

- antithrombin deficiency
- antiphospholipid deficiency/lupus anticoagulant syndrome
- protein C deficiency
- protein S deficiency
- factor V Leiden
- homocystinuria.

All thrombophilic states are associated with an adverse pregnancy outcome including an increased risk of miscarriage, stillbirth, pre-eclampsia and IUGR.

Antithrombin deficiency

Two types of antithrombin deficiency exist:

- type I – is a deficiency of a normal molecule
- type II – is associated with an abnormal molecule.

The risk of thromboembolism is as high as 40–70% and necessitates life-long warfarin. The risk is greater in type I than type II antithrombin deficiency.

In pregnancy, patients with types I and II antithrombin deficiency (plus additional risk factors see other factors increasing the risk of thromboembolism on previous page) should receive therapeutic levels of low-molecular-weight heparin (LMWH). Antithrombin concentrate may be required to cover labour and if thrombosis occurs earlier in pregnancy. Cord blood should be taken to assess neonatal status at birth; it should be repeated at 6 months.

Antiphospholipid sydrome

Antiphospholipid deficiency/lupus anticoagulant have been considered earlier (see Section 3.4).

Protein C deficiency

Protein C deficiency may be inherited in autosomal dominant and recessive forms. Thrombosis is more likely to occur in the post-natal than in the antenatal period. Treatment (administration of therapeutic levels of protein C) is usually reserved for the puerperium if no additional factors exist. Warfarin is avoided because it is associated with skin necrosis (purpura fulminans in the homozygous form). Prenatal diagnosis is achieved by cordocentesis in the second trimester.

Protein S deficiency

Protein S is a co-factor for protein C and levels normally fall in pregnancy, making diagnosis difficult. Deficiency of protein S is associated with a 0–6% risk of thrombosis antenatally and 7–22% postnatally. The usual approach is to treat (with prophylactic doses of LMWH) in the post-partum period only, unless additional risk factors exist.

Factor V Leiden

Factor V Leiden is caused by a single point mutation. It is resistant to activated protein C, causing thrombosis. Two forms of Factor V Leiden exist:

- **heterozygous**: more common; risk of thrombosis 0.25%
- **homozygous**: rare; risk of thrombosis 50–80 times greater than non-carriers.

Homocystinuria

Homocystinuria is an inborn error of metabolism that is associated with increased risk of both arterial and venous thrombosis.

Diagnosis of thromboembolic disorders in pregnancy

Disorder	Diagnostic tool	Description
Deep vein thrombosis	Clinical and laboratory	The clinical diagnosis of DVT in pregnant women is as difficult as it is in non-pregnant women (50% of pregnant women with a tender, swollen painful leg do not have a DVT) D-dimers are raised in normal pregnancy and therefore of minimal use in aiding the diagnosis of thromboembolism
	Plethysmography	Used in left lateral position to detect blood flow in the limb. Normal blood flow is reduced in pregnancy; a negative test excludes DVT; but a positive test requires further evaluation
	Doppler ultrasound	Most widely used technique; effective in diagnosis of symptomatic, proximal DVT. If clot is present the vein is incompressible and does not dilate during Valsalva manoeuvre; sensitivity/specificity about 97%. Insensitive for thrombosis within the calf, or above the inguinal ligament
	Venography	Can be performed with adequate shielding of uterus with minimal risk to the fetus. Useful for confirming femoral and more distal vein thrombosis
Pulmonary embolism	Chest X-ray	Confers minimal risk to fetus. Often normal but may demonstrate an effusion, decreased vascularity
	ECG	Note that changes can occur within normal pregnancy. In PE the ECG may be normal, or it may demonstrate a sinus tachycardia, right heart strain or the classical features of deep S wave in I, Q wave and inverted T wave in III
	Blood gas analysis	May be normal but in the presence of a PE will typically demonstrate hypoxia with reduced PaO_2, and normal or reduced $PaCO_2$
	V/Q scan	The isotopes used have short half-lives and so exposure of the fetus is minimal. The *V/Q* scan can be safely performed in breast-feeding mothers. False-negatives are rare and hence a normal scan excludes PE. The typical features are perfusion defect, with normal ventilation

Treatment of thromboembolic disorders

Warfarin is generally avoided in pregnancy. In the first trimester it is associated with an increased risk of miscarriage and teratogenic side-effects which include chondrodysplasia punctata, splenism and diaphragmatic hernia. In the second and third trimester it is associated with retroplacental and intracerebral fetal haemorrhage, as well as fetal microcephaly, optic atrophy and developmental delay.

LMWH is the mainstay of treatment (but also note use of aspirin in antiphospholipid syndrome). LMWH is preferred to unfractionated heparin as it is associated with less bleeding, thrombocytopenia and osteopenia.

Chapter 13
Metabolic Diseases

CONTENTS

Metabolic Diseases

1. DISORDERS OF AMINO ACID METABOLISM

Most of the inherited metabolic diseases are mendelian, single-gene defects, transmitted in an autosomal recessive manner. Disease expression requires the affected individual to be homozygous – inheriting a mutant gene from each of their parents, who are both heterozygous for the defect. Although heterozygotes may synthesise equal amounts of normal and defective enzymes they are usually asymptomatic.

- Even the major inborn errors of amino acid metabolism are rare – phenylketonuria, one of the most common, has an incidence of 1/20, 000.
- Complete penetrance is common and the onset is frequently early in life.
- The consequences of these enzyme deficiencies are varied and frequently multisystem but expression tends to be uniform.

The more common of these conditions are listed in the box below and the major inborn errors of amino acid metabolism are then discussed.

Inborn errors of amino acid metabolism

- Albinism
- Cystinosis
- Homocystinuria
- Maple syrup urine disease
- Phenylketonuria
- Alkaptonuria
- Cystinuria
- Histidinaemia
- Oxalosis

1.1 Alkaptonuria (ochronosis)

This is a rare autosomal recessive disease with an incidence of 1/100, 000. Homogentisic acid accumulates as a result of a deficiency in the enzyme homogentisic acid oxidase.

- The homogentisic acid polymerises to produce the black–brown product alkapton, which becomes deposited in cartilage and other tissues (ochronosis).
- Classical features include pigmentation of the ears, arthritis, inter-vertebral disc calcification and dark sweat-stained clothing.
- Rarer manifestations include renal stone disease as well as aortic valve and ocular involvement.

- The urine darkens on standing because homogentisic acid conversion to alkapton is accelerated in alkaline conditions.
- There is a high prevalence of alkaptonuria in Slovakia (1:19, 000) due to novel mutations which have resulted in geographical clustering.
- The molecular basis of the disorder is known but there is no specific treatment. Arthritis may require symptomatic therapy.

1.2 Cystinosis

In cystinosis, cystine accumulates in the reticuloendothelial system, kidneys and other tissues. There is a defect of cystine transport across the lysosomal membrane resulting in widespread intra-lysosomal accumulation of cystine. The causative gene (CTNS), which encodes for an integral membrane protein called cystinosin, has been identified on chromosome 17p13. Unlike cystinuria, stones do not occur in this condition.

Clinical features of cystinosis

- Severe growth retardation
- Lymphadenopathy
- Bone marrow failure
- Corneal opacities and photophobia
- Hypothyroidism
- Central nervous system involvement
- Fanconi syndrome (often with severe hypophosphataemia and consequent vitamin-D-resistant rickets)
- Insulin deficiency
- Abnormalities of cardiac conduction

Onset is usually in the first year of life and the renal disease is progressive often resulting in end-stage renal disease by the age of 10 years. Corneal or conjunctival crystals usually suggest the diagnosis, which can be confirmed by measuring the cystine content of neutrophils. Specific therapy with cysteamine bitartrate is effective at reducing cystine accumulation and delaying renal failure. However, this treatment is unpleasant and rarely tolerated. Supportive care, including dialysis and transplantation, is usually needed. Cystinosis does not recur in the transplant but extra-renal disease is progressive.

- **Ocular non-nephropathic cystinosis**: this is a variant of the classical disease and is due to different mutations of the cystinosis gene CTNS. It is an autosomal recessive lysosomal storage disorder characterised by photophobia due to corneal cystine crystals.

1.3 Cystinuria

Cystinuria is an autosomal recessive disorder with a prevalence of about 1/7000. The transport of cystine and the other dibasic amino acids lysine, ornithine and arginine is abnormal in the proximal renal tubule and the jejunum.

- No malnutrition occurs as sufficient dietary amino acids are absorbed as oligopeptides.
- Presentation is usually in the second or third decade of life with renal stones.

- Cystine accumulates in the urine. It is highly insoluble at acid pH and this results in the formation of radio-opaque calculi.

A urinary cystine concentration >1 mmol/l (at pH 7.0) is supersaturated and leads to calculi formation.

Diagnosis requires measurement of urinary cystine and/or chromatographic analysis of the stone.

Management

Large fluid intake, alkalinisation of urine and D-penicillamine (which chelates cystine and increases its solubility). Captopril also binds to thiol groups of cystine and increases its solubility.

1.4 Homocystinuria

This autosomal recessive abnormality results from reduced activity of cystathionine β-synthase. The resulting homocysteine and methionine accumulation interferes with collagen cross-linking.

Clinical features of homocystinuria

- Downward lens dislocation
- Spontaneous retinal detachment
- Osteoporosis
- Venous and arterial thromboses
- Developmental and mental retardation
- Seizures and psychiatric syndromes

Diagnosis is established by the cyanide-nitroprusside test that detects elevated urinary homocysteine.

Management

Early detection (of younger siblings). Methionine restriction and cystine-supplemented diets. Pyridoxine supplements (effective in 50%). Some variants are responsive to folate or vitamin B_{12} supplements.

1.5 Oxalosis

There are two inborn errors of metabolism that cause overproduction of oxalate. Both are autosomal recessive and can lead to hyperoxaluria with stones and tissue deposition of oxalate.

- Type I is due to a deficiency of hepatic peroxisomal alanine:glycoxylate aminotransferase.
- Type II is due to a deficiency of D-glyceric acid dehydrogenase.

Clinical features of oxalosis

- Oxalate renal stones
- Bone disease
- Cardiac disease
- Nephrocalcinosis
- Severe arterial disease (due to deposition of oxalate crystals in the vessel wall)

Diagnosis

Oxalosis should be suspected if there is increased urinary oxalate excretion, but the latter can also occur with pyridoxine deficiency (as this is a necessary co-enzyme in oxalate metabolism), ileal disease, ethyl glycol poisoning and excess oxalate ingestion.
Confirmation of diagnosis requires:

- liver biopsy to demonstrate enzyme deficiency in type I
- demonstration of enzyme deficiency in peripheral blood leukocytes in type II
- genetic testing by mutation and linkage analysis is useful for identifying other affected family members, as well as in prenatal diagnosis and carrier testing.

Treatment of oxalosis

This initially involves high fluid intake and the use of pyridoxine. In primary hyperoxaluria type I early diagnosis and pre-emptive isolated liver transplantation can be curative. In patients who already have advanced renal failure, dialysis therapy is appropriate. Concomitant liver and renal transplantation is often performed, but in this situation the renal transplants are often lost due to rapid oxalate crystal deposition (prior liver transplantation is preferable as it would allow clearance of the oxalate load before consideration of renal transplantation).

1.6 Phenylketonuria (PKU)

There are several variants of PKU due to different allelic mutations. For example, mutations of the gene that encodes phenylalanine hydroxylase (and associated enzymes) are found on chromosome 12. Only severe deficiency of the enzyme results in classic PKU with neurological damage. PKU affects between 1:10, 000 and 1:14, 000 live births.

The biochemical abnormality is an inability to convert phenylalanine into tyrosine due to lack of phenylalanine hydroxylase. This results in hyperphenylalaninaemia and increased excretion of its metabolite, phenylpyruvic acid ('phenylketone'), in the urine.

Clinical features of PKU

- Affects children usually manifesting by 6 months of life
- Eczema
- Mental retardation
- Irritability
- Decreased pigmentation* (pale skin, fair-haired and blue-eyed phenotype)

* This is due to reduced melanin formation

Diagnosis

The Guthrie screening test is a bacterial inhibition assay named after its inventor. Blood applied from a heel-prick is applied to filter paper that is subsequently incubated with *Bacillus subtilis* in the presence of β-2-thienylalanine (an analogue that inhibits utilisation of phenylalanine). The amount of bacterial growth is proportional to the phenylalanine concentration in the neonatal blood.

Phenylalanine levels can also be measured by spectrofluorometric methods or using a form of mass spectrometry which has the ability to analyse many amino acids, fatty acids and short-chain organic acid metabolites simultaneously.

Management

Diet low in phenylalanine, with tyrosine supplementation, in infancy and childhood. PKU females should be advised to reinstitute strict dietary control prior to conception and throughout pregnancy and breast-feeding. Fish oil supplementation can also improve symptoms.

2. DISORDERS OF PURINE METABOLISM

Uric acid is the end product of purine metabolism. Purines can be synthesised de novo or salvaged from the breakdown of nucleic acids of endogenous or exogenous origin. Increased de novo synthesis of purines is thought to be responsible, at least partly, for primary gout. Deficiency of hypoxanthine guanine phosphoribosyl transferase (HGPRT), which is involved in the salvage pathway, results in the Lesch–Nyhan syndrome.

Disorders of purine metabolism

- Primary gout
- Secondary hyperuricaemia
- Lesch–Nyhan syndrome

(See *also* Chapter 20, Rheumatology.)

2.1 Gout

More than 10% of the population of the Western world has hyperuricaemia, which can be due to a variety of genetic and environmental factors. Gout develops in fewer than 0.5% of the population. (*See also* Chapter 20, Rheumatology.)

- Primary hyperuricaemia is more common in males and post-menopausal females than in pre-menopausal females.
- It is rare in childhood.
- It is probably polygenic, involving both increased purine synthesis and reduced renal tubular secretion of urate.
- Gout can be precipitated by thiazide diuretics, alcohol and high purine intake.
- Hyperuricaemia is associated with increased cardiovascular risk and can also be a marker of pre-eclamptic toxaemia of pregnancy.

2.2 Lesch–Nyhan syndrome

Lesch–Nyhan syndrome is an uncommon X-linked recessive disease (therefore seen only in males) due to complete lack of hypoxanthine guanine phosphoribosyl transferase (HGPRT). This results in accumulation of both hypoxanthine and guanine both of which are metabolised to xanthine and subsequently uric acid.

Clinical features of Lesch–Nyhan syndrome

- Mental retardation
- Athetosis
- Gout
- Spasticity
- Self-mutilation
- Renal calculi
- Renal failure due to crystal nephropathy

- Neurological manifestations are usually present in early infancy; death from renal failure in adolescence is common.
- Kelley–Seegmiller syndrome is a variant, with mild neurological symptoms, due to a partial deficiency of HGPRT.
- Carrier and pre-natal diagnosis is possible by mutation detection and linkage analysis for probands and their families. Biochemical measurement of HGPRT is also possible for at-risk pregnancies.

3. DISORDERS OF METALS AND METALLOPROTEINS

Iron and copper play central roles in the function of a number of metalloproteins, including cytochrome oxidase, which is essential in cellular aerobic respiration; haem, based on iron, is the key molecule in oxygen transport. Excessive accumulation can, however, promote free radical injury (eg Wilson's disease and haemochromatosis) and disorders of haem synthesis result in porphyria.

Disorders of metals and metalloproteins

- Wilson's disease
- Haemochromatosis
- Secondary iron overload
- The porphyrias

3.1 Wilson's disease

This autosomal recessive disorder has a gene frequency of 1/400 and a disease prevalence of approximately 1/200, 000. The responsible defective gene (*ATP 7B*) is on chromosome 13, and this codes for a copper-transporting P-type adenosine triphosphate.

In normal subjects 50% of ingested copper is absorbed and transported to the liver loosely bound to albumin. Here copper is incorporated into an alpha-2-globulin to form caeruloplasmin, which is the principal transport protein for copper, and necessary for biliary excretion. In Wilson's disease copper absorption is normal but intrahepatic formation of caeruloplasmin is defective. Total body and tissue copper levels rise due to failure of biliary excretion and urinary excretion of copper is increased.

Clinical features of Wilson's disease

- **Onset in childhood or adolescence**
- **Hepatic dysfunction**
  Acute hepatitis
  Cirrhosis
  Chronic hepatitis
  Massive hepatic necrosis
- **Hypoparathyroidism**
- **Haemolysis**
- **CNS involvement**
  Behavioural problems/psychosis
  Mental retardation
  Tremor/chorea
  Seizures
- **Kayser–Fleischer corneal rings**
  Due to copper deposition in Descemet's membrane
- **Fanconi syndrome**
- **Arthropathy**

Diagnosis

This is based on a decrease in serum caeruloplasmin and increases in hepatic copper content and urinary excretion of copper. However, biochemical diagnosis is increasingly recognised to have low sensitivity. Molecular diagnosis is now available to identify pre-symptomatic individuals. Serum copper levels are of no diagnostic value.

Management

Early detection permits long-term use of copper chelators (eg penicillamine) to prevent the accumulation of copper. Fulminant hepatic failure and end-stage liver disease necessitate liver transplantation which is curative (but CNS sequelae may persist). (*See also* Chapter 6, Gastroenterology.)

3.2 Haemochromatosis

In the normal adult the iron content of the body is closely regulated. Haemochromatosis is the excessive accumulation of iron. Primary (or idiopathic) haemochromatosis is a common autosomal recessive disorder in which iron accumulates in parenchymal cells, leading to damage and fibrosis. Haemosiderin is an insoluble iron protein complex found in macrophages (it is relatively harmless to them) in the bone marrow, liver and spleen. Secondary iron overload, which has many causes, is often referred to as haemosiderosis.

- The gene for haemochromatosis (HFE) is located on chromosome 6 close to the HLA locus. HFE codes for a transmembrane glycoprotein that modulates iron uptake.
- The gene frequency is 6% and disease frequency 1/220 people, but the severity of the disease seems to vary.
- Males are affected earlier and more severely than females (as menstrual loss/pregnancy protects females).
- Heterozygotes are at greater risk of secondary haemosiderosis than non-carriers if they have a predisposing condition.
- Thirty per cent of patients with cirrhosis develop hepatocellular carcinoma. (*See also* Chapter 6, Gastroenterology.)

Clinical features of haemochromatosis

- Presentation above the age of 40 years
- Hepatomegaly preceding micronodular cirrhosis
- Chondrocalcinosis and pseudogout
- Bronze skin pigmentation
- Diabetes mellitus and (rarely) exocrine pancreas failure
- Hypopituitarism, hypogonadism and testicular atrophy
- Cardiomyopathy and arrhythmias

Diagnosis

Serum iron is elevated with greater than 60% transferrin saturation. Serum ferritin >500 μg/l. Liver iron concentration >180 μmol/g is also indicative of haemochromatosis. Molecular genetic diagnosis is now available.

Management

- Venesection
- Chelation therapy with desferrioxamine
- Screening of first-degree relatives (serum ferritin)
- Liver transplantation (for end-stage liver disease).

3.3 Secondary iron overload

Secondary haemochromatosis is due to iron overload which can occur in a variety of conditions. The pattern of tissue injury is similar to that in primary haemochromatosis. In the inherited haemolytic anaemias iron overload can present in adolescence; the features are often modified by the underlying disease. Treatment is with desferrioxamine.

Secondary causes of iron overload

- **Anaemia due to ineffective erythropoiesis**
  Beta-thalassaemia
  Sideroblastic anaemia
  Aplastic anaemia
  Pyruvate kinase deficiency
- **Parenteral iron overload**
  Transfusions
  Iron–dextran
- **Liver disease**
  Alcoholic cirrhosis
  Chronic viral hepatitis
  Porphyria cutanea tarda
- **Increased oral iron intake**
  (Bantu siderosis)
- **Congenital transferrinaemia**

3.4 The porphyrias

The porphyrias are a rare heterogeneous group of abnormalities of enzymes involved in the biosynthesis of haem, resulting in overproduction of the intermediate compounds called porphyrins. Excess production of porphyrins can occur in the liver or bone marrow and is classified as acute or non-acute. The haem metabolic pathway and the type of porphyria resulting from different enzyme deficiencies are shown in the following figure. The two most important porphyrias are porphyria cutanea tarda and acute intermittent porphyria – these are described in more detail.

Porphyria cutanea tarda

This is the most common hepatic porphyria. There is a genetic predisposition but the pattern of inheritance is not established. Many sporadic cases are due to chronic liver disease, usually alcohol related.

- There is reduced uroporphyrinogen decarboxylase activity.
- Uroporphyrinogen accumulates in blood and urine.
- Manifests as photosensitivity rash with bullae.

Diagnosis

Based on elevated urinary uroporphyrinogen (urine is normal in colour).

Figure 1 Haem synthesis and the porphyrias

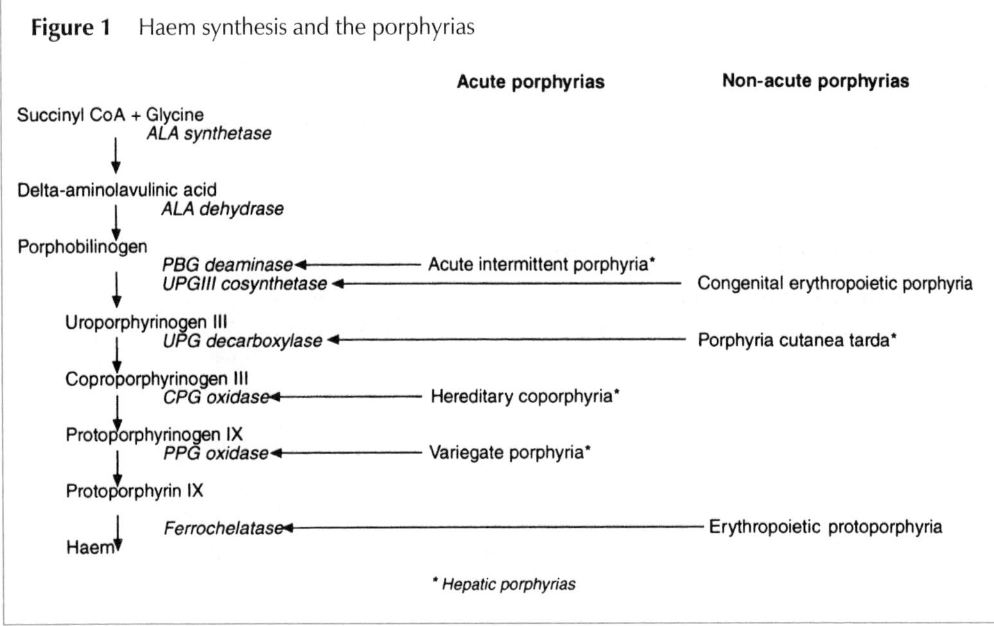

Treatment

- The underlying liver disease
- Chloroquine
- Venesection.

Acute intermittent porphyria

This causes attacks of classical acute porphyria often presenting with abdominal pain and/or neuropsychiatric disorders. It is an autosomal dominant disorder.

- There is reduced hepatic porphobilinogen deaminase activity.
- The gene (and disease) frequency is between 1/10, 000 and 1/50, 000.

- Episodes of porphyria are more common in females (?due to the effects of oestrogens).
- There is no photosensitivity or skin rash.
- There is increased urinary porphobilinogen and aminolaevulinic acid especially during attacks.
- Urine turns deep red on standing.

Clinical features of acute intermittent porphyria

- Onset in adolescence
- Females more affected
- Polyneuropathy (motor)
- Hypertension and tachycardia
- Episodic attacks
- Abdominal pain, vomiting, constipation
- Neuropsychiatric disorders
- Tubulointerstitial nephritis

Precipitating drugs:

- alcohol
- benzodiazepines
- rifampicin
- oral contraceptives
- phenytoin
- sulphonamides.

Management

- Supportive: maintain high carbohydrate intake; avoid precipitating factors
- Gonadotrophin-releasing hormone analogues to prevent cyclical attacks
- Sertraline and other psychotropic drugs have been used without precipitating acute porphyria, but care is advisable with use of all drugs.

4. DISORDERS OF LIPID METABOLISM

Hyperlipidaemia, especially hypercholesterolaemia, is associated with cardiovascular disease.

Total cholesterol (mmol/l)	Relative risk of myocardial infarct
5.2	1
6.5	2
7.8	4

Although lipid metabolism is complex, and many inherited or acquired disorders can disrupt it, the end result is usually elevated cholesterol and/or triglyceride concentrations. These can be managed by dietary and pharmacological means.

4.1 Lipid metabolism

Cholesterol and triglycerides are insoluble in plasma and circulate bound to lipoproteins. The lipoproteins consist of lipids, phospholipids and proteins. The protein components of lipoproteins are called apolipoproteins (or apoproteins) and they act as cofactors for enzymes and ligands for receptors. A schemata of lipoprotein structure is shown below.

Figure 2 Schemata of lipoprotein structure

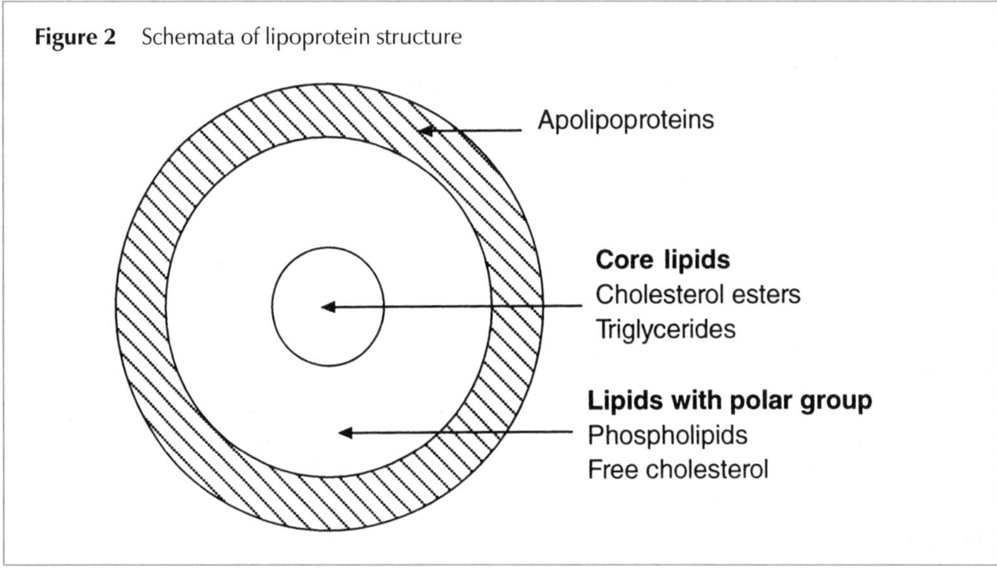

There are four major lipoproteins:

- **Chylomicrons**: large particles that carry dietary lipid (mainly triglycerides) from the gastrointestinal tract to the liver. In the portal circulation lipoprotein lipase acts on chylomicrons to release free fatty acids for energy metabolism.
- **Very low density lipoprotein (VLDL)**: carries endogenous triglyceride (60%), and to a lesser extent cholesterol (20%), from the liver to the tissues. The triglyceride core of the VLDL is also hydrolysed by lipoprotein lipase to release free fatty acids. The VLDL remnants are called intermediate density lipoprotein.
- **Low density lipoprotein (LDL)**: is formed from the intermediate density lipoproteins by hepatic lipase. LDL contains a cholesterol core (50%) and lesser amounts of triglyceride (10%). LDL metabolism is regulated by cellular cholesterol requirements via negative feedback control of the LDL receptor.
- **High density lipoprotein (HDL)**: carries cholesterol from the tissues back to the liver. HDL is formed in the liver and gut and acquires free cholesterol from the intracellular pools. Within the HDL, cholesterol is esterified by lecithin cholesterol acyl-transferase (LCAT). HDL is inversely associated with ischaemic heart disease.

Figure 3 Lipid metabolism

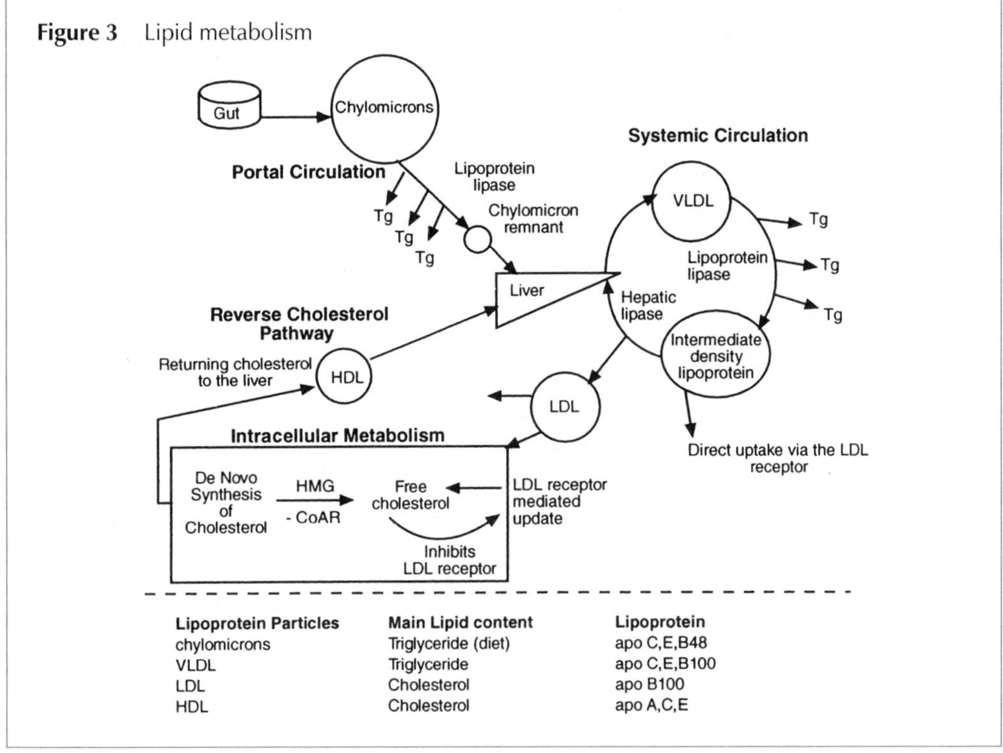

Lipoprotein Particles	Main Lipid content	Lipoprotein
chylomicrons	Triglyceride (diet)	apo C,E,B48
VLDL	Triglyceride	apo C,E,B100
LDL	Cholesterol	apo B100
HDL	Cholesterol	apo A,C,E

The LDL receptor

Circulating LDL is taken up by the LDL receptor. Cells replete in cholesterol reduce LDL receptor expression. In contrast, inhibition of 3-hydroxy-3-methylglutaryl coenzyme A (HMG CoA) reductase, the enzyme that controls the rate of de novo cholesterol synthesis, leads to a fall in cellular cholesterol and an increase in LDL receptor expression.

Lipoprotein (a)

Lp(a) is a specialised form of LDL. Lp(a) inhibits fibrinolysis and promotes atherosclerotic plaque formation. It is an independent risk factor for ischaemic heart disease.

4.2 The hyperlipidaemias

Population studies have consistently demonstrated a strong relationship between both total and LDL cholesterol and coronary heart disease. HDL is protective. A total cholesterol:HDL ratio of >4.5 is associated with an increased risk. Intervention trials have now established that reduction in LDL cholesterol is associated with improvement in outcome.

Triglycerides are also associated with cardiovascular risk; very high triglycerides are also associated with pancreatitis, lipaemic serum and eruptive xanthomata. Triglycerides must be measured fasting.

A genetic classification of lipid disorders has now replaced the Fredrickson (WHO) classification, which was based on lipoprotein patterns. The primary hyperlipidaemias can be grouped according to the simple lipid profile. Secondary causes of hyperlipidaemia need to be excluded and are discussed opposite.

Primary hypercholesterolaemia (without hypertriglyceridaemia)

Familial hypercholesterolaemia (FH) is a monogenic disorder resulting from LDL receptor dysfunction.

- There are many different mutations in different families all resulting in LDL receptor deficiency/dysfunction and producing isolated hypercholesterolaemia.
- Heterozygote prevalence is 1/500; these individuals have cholesterol levels of 9–15 mmol/l and sustain myocardial infarctions at about age 40 years (M = F).
- Homozygous FH is rare. Cholesterol levels are in excess of 15 mmol/l and patients suffer myocardial infarction in the second or third decades.
- Other typical clinical features are Achilles tendon xanthomata (can also occur in other extensor tendons) and xanthelasma.

In **polygenic hypercholesterolaemia** the precise nature of the metabolic defect(s) is unknown.

These individuals represent the right-hand tail of the normal cholesterol distribution. They are at risk of premature atherosclerosis. Depressed HDL levels are a risk factor for vascular disease.

Factors modifying HDL levels

- **Decreasing**
  Familial deficiency of HDL
  Hyperandrogenic state
  Post-pubertal males
  Obesity
  Hypertriglyceridaemia
  Diabetes mellitus
  Sedentary states
  Cigarette smoking
- **Increasing**
  Familial hyper-α-lipoproteinaemia
  Low triglyceride levels
  Thin habitus
  Exercise
  Oestrogens
  Alcohol

Primary hypertriglyceridaemia (without hypercholesterolaemia)

- **Polygenic hypertriglyceridaemia** is analogous to polygenic hypercholesterolaemia. Some cases are familial but the precise defect is not known. There is elevated VLDL.
- **Lipoprotein lipase deficiency** and **apoprotein CII deficiency** are both rare. They result in elevated triglycerides due to a failure to metabolise chylomicrons.
- These patients present in childhood with eruptive xanthomata, lipaemia retinalis, retinal vein thrombosis, pancreatitis and hepatosplenomegaly.
- Chylomicrons can be detected in fasting plasma.

Primary mixed (or combined) hyperlipidaemia

- **Familial polygenic combined hyperlipidaemia** results in elevated cholesterol and triglycerides
- The prevalence is 1/200
- There is premature atherosclerosis
- **Remnant hyperlipidaemia** is a rare cause of mixed hyperlipidaemia (palmar xanthomas and tuberous xanthomas over the knees and elbows are characteristic). It is associated with apoprotein E_2. There is a high cardiovascular risk.

Secondary hyperlipidaemias are usually mixed but either elevated cholesterol or triglycerides may predominate.

Causes of secondary hyperlipidaemias

- **Predominantly increased triglycerides**
  Alcoholism
  Obesity
  Chronic renal failure
  Diabetes mellitus
  Liver disease
  High-dose oestrogens
- **Predominantly increased cholesterol**
  Hypothyroidism
  Renal transplant
  Cigarette smoking*
  Nephrotic syndrome
  Cholestasis

* Cigarette smoking reduces HDL

4.3 Lipid-lowering drugs

Cholesterol and triglyceride levels should be considered in combination with other risk factors. Potential secondary causes of hyperlipidaemia should be corrected.

Dietary intervention can be expected to reduce serum cholesterol by a maximum of 30%. Dietary measures should be continued with pharmacological therapy. The following table shows the impact that can be expected with the various agents.

Impact of lipid-lowering drugs

Drug class	↓LDL (%)	↑HDL (%)	↓TGs (%)
HMG CoA reductase inhibitors	20–40	5–10	10–20
Fibric acid derivatives	10–15	15–25	35–50
Bile acid sequestrants	15–30	No change	No change
Nicotinic acid	10–25	15–35	25–30
Probucol	10–15	↓20–25	No change
Neomycin	20–25	No change	No change
Fish oil	↑5–10	No change	30–50

The side-effect profile of the older agents (see following box) made them unpopular and reduced compliance. In the majority of cases, hypercholesterolaemia will respond to dietary intervention and statin therapy; and mixed or isolated hypertriglyceridaemia, to diet and a fibrate.

Side-effects and drug interactions of lipid-lowering drugs

Drug class	**Side-effects/interactions**
HMG CoA reductase inhibitors	Headache, nausea, insomnia, abnormal LFTs. Myositis and rhabdomyolysis (when in combination with gemfibrozil or ciclosporin A) Simvastatin (but not pravastatin) potentiates warfarin and digoxin
Fibric acid derivates	
Gemfibrozil Bezafibrate	Potentiates warfarin. Gemfibrozil absorption is impaired by bile acid sequestrants
Bile acid sequestrants	
Cholestyramine Cholestipol	GIT side-effects: nausea, cramping, abnormal LFTs Impaired absorption of digoxin, warfarin, thyroxine and fat-soluble vitamins
Nicotinic acid	Flushing, headaches, upper GIT symptoms, acanthosis nigricans and myositis
Probucol	Diarrhoea, eosinophilia, long QT syndrome, angioneurotic oedema
Neomycin	Ototoxicity, nephrotoxicity
Fish oil	Halitosis, bloating, nausea Impaired glycaemic control in NIDDM

4.4 Rare lipid disorders

A multitude of rare inborn errors of lipid metabolism can lead to multisystem diseases. The most common (all very rare) are shown in the following table.

Disorder	Serum lipid abnormality	Clinical features	Pathogenesis	Treatment
Abetalipoproteinaemia	Low cholesterol Low triglycerides	Onset in childhood Fat malabsorption Acanthocytosis (of RBCs) Retinitis pigmentosa Ataxia and peripheral neuropathy	Defective Apo B synthesis	Vitamin E
Tangier disease	Low cholesterol	Onset in childhood Large orange tonsils Polyneuropathy No increased IHD risk	Increased Apo A catabolism	None
LCAT deficiency	↑ Triglycerides Variable cholesterol	Affects young adults Renal failure	Reduced LCAT activity	Low-fat diet
Cerebro-tendinous xanthomatosis	None	Affects young adults Cerebellar ataxia Dementia Tendon xanthomas Cataracts	Not known	None
β-Sitosterolaemia absorption	None	Affects adults Tendon xanthomas	Increased β-sitosterol absorption	Low plant fat diet
Fabry's disease	None	Affects young male adults (mild disease in females) Angiokeratomas Periodic crises Thrombotic events Chronic renal failure	Deficiency of α-galactosidase A	Human recombinant α-galactosidase A therapy Renal replacement therapy if end-stage renal failure develops

5. DISORDERS OF BONE, MINERAL METABOLISM AND INORGANIC IONS

Bone is a unique type of connective tissue that mineralises. Biochemically it is composed of matrix (35%) and inorganic calcium hydroxyapatite (65%). Bone and mineral homeostasis are tightly regulated by numerous factors, so as to maintain skeletal integrity and control plasma levels.

5.1 Calcium homeostasis

Calcium homeostasis is linked to phosphate homeostasis to maintain a balanced calcium phosphate product.

- Hypocalcaemia activates parathyroid hormone (PTH) release to restore serum ionised calcium; other stimuli to PTH release include hyperphosphataemia and decreased vitamin D levels.
- Hypercalcaemia switches off PTH release.
- Vitamin D promotes calcium and phosphate absorption from the GI tract.
- Bone stores of calcium buffer the serum changes.

The metabolism and effects of vitamin D, and the actions of PTH are shown schematically in the figures opposite.

5.2 Hypercalcaemia

In over 90% of cases hypercalcaemia is due to either hyperparathyroidism or malignancy. Hypercalcaemia normally suppresses PTH and so PTH is therefore the best first test to identity the cause of hypercalcaemia – if it is detectable (in or above the normal range) the patient must have hyperparathyroidism.

- Primary hyperparathyroidism is common, especially in women aged 40–60 years. It is usually due to an adenoma of one of the four parathyroid glands.
- PTH-related protein (PTH-rP) is responsible for up to 80% of hypercalcaemia in malignancy.
- PTH-rP acts on the same receptors as PTH and shares the first (N-terminal) 13 amino acids with PTH; however, they are coded from two separate genes.
- Common malignancies secreting PTH-rP are squamous cell tumours, breast and kidney.

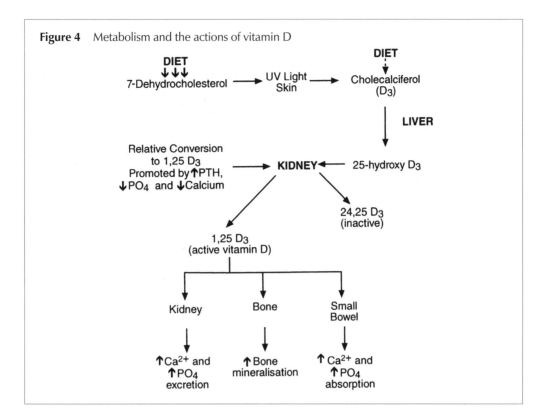

Figure 4 Metabolism and the actions of vitamin D

DIET ↓↓↓
7-Dehydrocholesterol → UV Light Skin → Cholecalciferol (D_3)
DIET ↓
LIVER ↓
25-hydroxy D_3 → KIDNEY
Relative Conversion to 1,25 D_3 Promoted by ↑PTH, ↓PO_4 and ↓Calcium → KIDNEY
KIDNEY → 24,25 D_3 (inactive)
KIDNEY → 1,25 D_3 (active vitamin D)
Kidney → ↑Ca^{2+} and ↑PO_4 excretion
Bone → ↑Bone mineralisation
Small Bowel → ↑Ca^{2+} and ↑PO_4 absorption

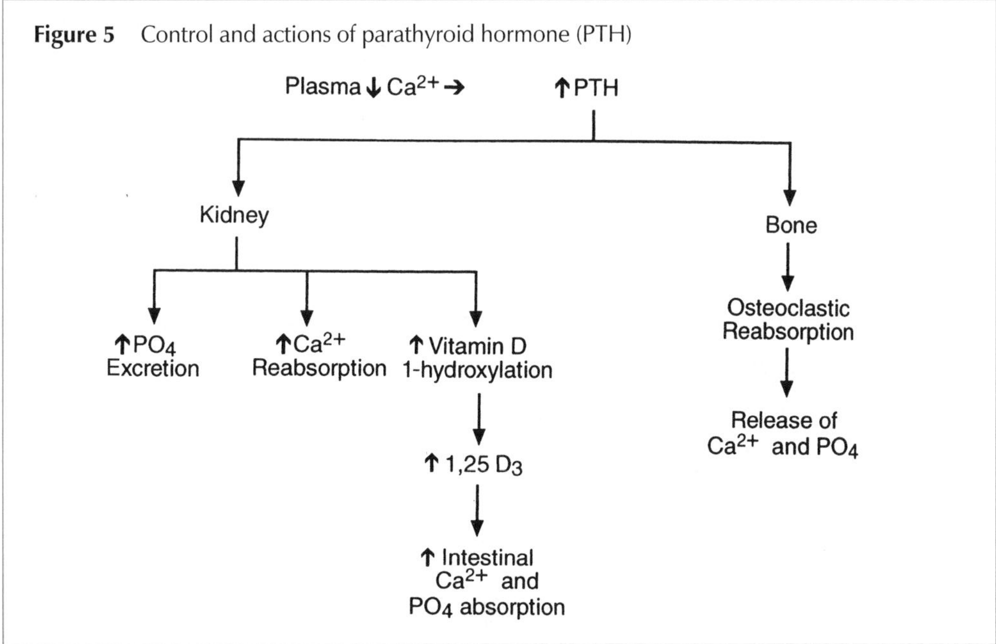

Figure 5 Control and actions of parathyroid hormone (PTH)

Causes of hypercalcaemia

- **Increased calcium absorption**
  Increased calcium intake
  Increased vitamin D
- **Increased bone reabsorption**
  Primary and tertiary hyperparathyroidism
  Malignancy
  Hyperthyroidism
- **Miscellaneous unusual causes**
  Lithium
  Thiazide diuretics
  Addison's disease
  Sarcoidosis*
  Phaeochromocytoma
  Familial hypocalciuric hypercalcaemia
  Theophylline toxicity
  Milk–alkali syndrome**
  Vitamin A toxicity

* Sarcoidosis causes hypercalcaemia due to excess production of 1,25-D_3 by macrophages in the sarcoid lesions

** Hypercalcaemia can be seen in patients who consume excess quantities of 'Rennies' bought over the counter

The symptoms of hypercalcaemia are often mild but a range of manifestations can occur as shown below.

Clinical manifestations of hypercalcaemia

- Malaise/depression
- Lethargy
- Muscle weakness
- Confusion
- Peptic ulceration**
- Pancreatitis
- Constipation
- Nephrolithiasis
- Nephrogenic diabetes insipidus
- Distal renal tubular acidosis (RTA)
- Renal failure*
- Short QT syndrome
- Band keratopathy
- Diabetes insipidus

* Renal failure is due to chronic tubulo-interstitial calcification and fibrosis

** Peptic ulceration is due to excess gastrin secretion

The **management** of acute hypercalcaemia (serum calcium >3 mmol/l) involves:

- adequate rehydration – 3–4 litres saline/day
- intravenous diphosphonates (eg pamidronate disodium)
- identification of the cause, and its subsequent specific treatment (eg corticosteroids for sarcoid) if indicated.

5.3 Hyperparathyroid bone disease

Hyperparathyroidism has a prevalence of about 1/1000. It results in bone reabsorption due to excess PTH action.

Primary hyperparathyroidism is caused by a single (80% +) or multiple (5%) parathyroid adenomas or by hyperplasia (10%). Parathyroid carcinoma is rare (<2%). It results from abnormal regulation of PTH by calcium because of an increase in the calcium set point. Familial cases (as seen in MEN type I) have a higher incidence of hyperplasia and, like parathyroid carcinoma, can be associated with abnormalities of chromosome 11 (usually deletions in the little q13 region).

Biochemically there is increased PTH, serum and urinary calcium, reduced serum phosphate and increased alkaline phosphatase. Histologically there is an increase of both osteoblasts and osteoclasts resulting in 'woven' osteoid, increased resorption cavities ('osteastitis fibrosa cystica') and marrow fibrosis. The definitive treatment of primary hyperparathyroidism is by surgical parathyroidectomy.

Secondary hyperparathyroidism is physiological compensatory hypertrophy of all four glands due to hypocalcaemia (eg renal failure, malabsorption). PTH levels are raised, calcium is low or normal. The secondary hyperparathyroidism in renal failure is controlled by phosphate restriction, phosphate binders and with use of 1-α-hydroxylated vitamin D preparations (*see also* Chapter 15, Nephrology).

Tertiary hyperparathyroidism is the development of autonomous parathyroid hyperplasia in the setting of long-standing secondary hyperparathyroidism – usually in renal failure. Calcium levels are raised and parathyroidectomy is the only appropriate treatment.

5.4 Hypocalcaemia

Hypocalcaemia is usually secondary to renal failure (increased serum phosphate), hypoparathyroidism or vitamin D deficiency.

Causes of hypocalcaemia

- **Decreased calcium absorption**
  Hypoparathyroidism
  Hypovitaminosis D
  Malabsorption
  Sepsis
  Fluoride poisoning
  Hypomagnesaemia*
- **Acute respiratory alkalosis**
- **Hyperphosphataemia (by reduction in ionised calcium)**
  Renal failure
  Phosphate administration
  Rhabdomyolysis
  Tumour lysis syndrome
- **Deposition of calcium**
  Pancreatitis
  Hungry bone syndrome
  EDTA infusion
  Rapidly growing osteoblastic metastases

*Cause of functional hypoparathyroidism

Hypoparathyroidism can be spontaneous (autoimmune), post-surgical or due to a receptor defect (pseudo-hypoparathyroidism). Autoimmune hypoparathyroidism may be part of **autoimmune polyglandular failure type I** (mucocutaneous candidiasis, with adrenal, gonadal and thyroid failure).

Recombinant human 1-34PTH is available but is not used in routine clinical practice because of cost, need for parenteral administration and short half-life.

In **pseudo-hypoparathyroidism** there is a characteristic phenotype with short stature, short metacarpals and intellectual impairment. The disorder is due to a G-protein abnormality (*see* Chapter 14, Molecular Medicine).

Vitamin D deficiency can occur in several settings, including:

- dietary deficiency/lack of sunlight
- malabsorption
- renal failure (failure of 1-α-hydroxylation)
- I-OHase deficiency (vitamin-D-dependent rickets type I)
- vitamin D receptor defect (vitamin-D-dependent rickets type II).

Rickets without vitamin D deficiency and with normal calcium may be due to hypophosphataemia, as in X-linked dominant hypophosphataemic vitamin-D-resistant rickets.

The symptoms of hypocalcaemia are mainly those of neuromuscular irritability and neuropsychiatric manifestations. Signs include Chvostek's (tapping the facial nerve causes twitching) and Trousseau's (precipitation of tetanic spasm in the hand by sphygmomanometer-induced ischaemia).

Clinical manifestations of hypocalcaemia

- **Neuromuscular**
  Tetany
  Seizures
  Confusion
  Extrapyramidal signs
  Papilloedema
  Psychiatric
  Myopathy
  Prolonged QT syndrome
- **Ectodermal**
  Alopecia
  Brittle nails
  Dry skin
- **Cataracts**
- **Dental hypoplasia**

The **management** of hypocalcaemia involves:

- intravenous calcium gluconate if severe (tetany/seizures)
- oral calcium supplements
- vitamin D (for hypoparathyroidism, vitamin D deficiency and renal failure)
- thiazide diuretic and low-sodium diet.

5.5 Osteomalacia

Osteomalacia results from inadequate mineralisation of osteoid. The biochemical features are elevated alkaline phosphatase (95%), hypocalcaemia (50%) and hypophosphataemia (25%). The childhood equivalent is rickets. It is usually caused by a defect of vitamin D availability or metabolism.

Causes of osteomalacia

- **Vitamin D deficiency**
  Dietary
  Sun exposure*
  Malabsorption
  Gastrectomy
  Small bowel disease
  Pancreatic insufficiency
- **Defective 25-hydroxylation**
  Liver disease
  Anticonvulsant treatment**
- **Loss of vitamin D binding protein**
  Nephrotic syndrome
- **Defective 1-α-hydroxylation**
  Hypoparathyroidism
  Chronic renal failure
- **Defective target organ response**
  Vitamin-D-dependent rickets (type II)
- **Mineralisation defects**
  Abnormal matrix
  Osteogenesis imperfecta
  Chronic renal failure
  Enzyme deficiencies
  Hypophosphatasia
- **Inhibitors of mineralisation**
  Fluoride
  Aluminium
  Bisphosphonates
- **Phosphate deficiency**
  Decreased GI intake
  Antacids (reduce absorption)
  Impaired renal reabsorption
  Fanconi syndrome
  X-linked hypophosphataemic rickets (vitamin-D-resistant rickets)

*Asian immigrants in Western countries are at increased risk because melanin in skin decreases D_3 formation; as vegans they may not benefit from dietary vitamin D and certain foods (eg chapattis) bind calcium unmasking vitamin D deficiency

** Especially phenytoin

The **management** of osteomalacia involves:

- diagnosis and treatment of the underlying disorder
- vitamin D therapy to correct hypocalcaemia and hypophosphataemia
- beware iatrogenic hypercalcaemia when alkaline phosphatase begins to fall at the time of bone healing.

5.6 Paget's disease

Paget's disease is a focal (or multifocal) bone disorder characterised by accelerated and disorganised bone turnover resulting from increased numbers and activity of both osteoblasts and osteoclasts. A viral aetiology has not been confirmed.

- Rare in patients aged under 40 years.
- Prevalence of 4% over the age of 40 years.
- Familial clustering and HLA linkages.
- Biochemically characterised by raised alkaline phosphatase, osteocalcin and urinary hydroxyproline excretion.

Paget's disease is usually diagnosed because of asymptomatic sclerotic changes (which can mimic sclerotic bone metastases) but a number of complications can arise.

Clinical manifestations of Paget's disease

- Bone pain
- Secondary arthritis
- Bone sarcoma (rare)
- High output congestive cardiac failure
- Skeletal deformity
- Fractures (and pseudofractures)
- Neurological compression syndromes*
- Hypercalcaemia (only with immobilisation)

*Including deafness, other cranial nerve palsies and spinal stenosis

Treatment is indicated for bone pain, nerve compression, disease impinging on joints and immobilisation hypercalcaemia. Options include:

- bisphosphonates
- calcitonin
- mithramycin
- surgery.

Causes of a raised bone alkaline phosphatase

- **With high calcium**
  Hyperparathyroidism
- **With high or normal calcium**
  Malignancy
  Paget's disease
- **With normal calcium**
  Puberty
  Fracture
  Osteogenic sarcoma
- **With low calcium**
  Osteomalacia

5.7 Osteoporosis

A very common disorder characterised by reduced bone density and increased risk of fracture. The most common form is post-menopausal osteoporosis, which affects 50% of women aged 70. Common sites of fracture are the vertebrae, neck of femur (trabecular bone) and the distal radius and humerus (cortical bone); these fractures may occur with minimal trauma.

Diagnosis is by bone mineral densitometry, measured by DEXA, SPA or QCT. The measured bone density is compared to the mean population peak bone density (ie that of young adults of the same sex) and expressed as the number of standard deviations from that mean, the T score. The bone mineralisation and serum biochemistry are normal.

- T scores down to –1 are regarded as normal.
- T scores between –1 and –2.5 represent osteopenia.
- T scores below –2.5 are osteoporotic.

Fracture risk

The risk of future fractures is dependent on both bone quality (strength and resilience) and the risk of falling. Fractures increase twofold with each standard deviation of the T score and independently with age by 1.5-fold per decade.

Aetiology

From the age of 30, bone loss occurs at about 1% per year. This is accelerated to about 5% per year in the five years after the menopause. Persistent elevations of parathyroid hormone will accelerate bone loss further. This occurs both in primary hyperparathyroidism but also in secondary hyperparathyroidism arising in vitamin D deficiency, or in negative calcium balance (eg hypocalcaemia, hypercalciuria).

Aetiology of osteoporosis

- **Primary**
  Type 1: post-menopausal
  Type 2: age-related or involutional
  Osteoporosis of pregnancy

- **Secondary**
  Endocrine: premature menopause, Cushing's syndrome, hypopituitarism, hyperparathyroidism, prolactinomas, hypogonadism, hyperthyroidism
  Drugs: steroids, heparin, ciclosporin A, anticonvulsants
  Malignancy: multiple myeloma, leukaemia
  Inflammatory: rheumatoid arthritis, ulcerative colitis
  GI: gastrectomy, malabsorption, primary biliary cirrhosis

continued overleaf

Aetiology of osteoporosis *(continued)*

Renal failure
Immobilisation: eg space flight
Other: osteogenesis imperfecta, homocystinuria, Turner's syndrome (oestrogen deficiency, rheumatoid arthritis*, scurvy)

- **Additional risk factors**
  Race: white/Asian
  Short stature and low body mass index
  Positive family history
  Multiparity
  Amenorrhoea >6 months (other than pregnancy)
  Poor calcium and vitamin D intake
  Excess alcohol and smoking

* In rheumatoid arthritis osteoporosis is multifactorial but corticosteroids and immobility are major contributors

In the absence of a recent fracture, or secondary cause of osteoporosis, bone biochemistry should be normal.

Treatment of osteoporosis

- **General measures**
  Correct any secondary cause
  Weight bearing exercise
  Adequate dietary calcium and vitamin D intake
- **Other**
  Fluoride (increases bone density, but can increase peripheral fractures)
  Calcitonin
- **Specific drug treatments**
  (These may reduce fractures by approximately 50%)
  Oestrogens (HRT)
  Vitamin D
  Testosterone (in males)
  Bisphosphonates*

*Prophylaxis with bisphosphonates is now recommended for patients receiving high-dose (eg relapsing nephrotic syndrome) or long-term (eg asthma) steroids

5.8 Disorders of magnesium

Magnesium is principally found in bone (50–60%) and as an intracellular cation plasma levels are maintained within the range 0.7–1.1 mmol/l. Disorders of magnesium balance usually occur in association with other fluid and electrolyte disturbances.

Hypomagnesaemia

Hypomagnesaemia is frequently accompanied by hypocalcaemia and hypokalaemia. Patients are often asymptomatic but may complain of weakness or anorexia, and features of neuromuscular irritability have been described. Hypomagnesaemia is an important risk factor for ventricular arrhythmias.

Causes of hypomagnesaemia

- **Gastrointestinal losses**
  Diarrhoea
  Malabsorption
  Small bowel disease
  Acute pancreatitis**
- **Loop of Henle dysfunction**
  Acute tubular necrosis†
  Renal transplantation
  Post-obstructive diuresis
  Bartter's syndrome
  Gitelman syndrome
- **Primary renal magnesium wasting††**
- **Renal losses**
  Loop and thiazide diuretics
  Volume expansion
  Alcohol*
  Diabetic ketoacidosis
  Hypercalcaemia***
- **Nephrotoxins**
  Aminoglycosides
  Amphotericin B
  Cisplatin
  Pentamidine
  Ciclosporin A

* Alcohol acutely increases urinary magnesium excretion, in chronic alcoholism this is compounded by ketoacidosis and phosphate depletion

** Due to the formation of magnesium soaps in the areas of fat necrosis

*** Hypercalciuria increases magnesium excretion; if saline and diuretics are given to treat hypercalcaemia then the three stimuli together predispose to hypomagnesaemia

† Diuretic phase

†† Primary magnesium wasting is a rare familial disorder

Hypermagnesaemia

Hypermagnesaemia is rare. It is usually due to magnesium ingestion or infusion in the setting of renal failure (ie when the kidney cannot excrete a magnesium load).

- At concentrations above 4 mmol/l symptoms develop including lethargy, drowsiness, areflexia, paralysis, hypotension, heart block and finally cardiac arrest.
- Toxic effects can be temporarily reversed by intravenous calcium.

Causes of hypermagnesaemia

- Renal failure
- Magnesium infusion
- Oral ingestion
- Magnesium enemas
- Familial hypocalciuric hypercalcaemia
- Adrenal insufficiency
- Milk–alkali syndrome
- Lithium
- Theophylline intoxication

5.9 Disorders of phosphate

Serum phosphate is maintained between 0.8 and 1.4 mmol/l largely by renal regulation of excretion. Bone accommodates 85% of body stores, the rest is found extracellularly as inorganic phosphate and intracellularly as phosphate esters, eg phospholipids, nucleic acids and high energy compounds such as adenosine triphosphate (ATP).

Hypophosphataemia

Hypophosphataemia can occur in a variety of settings, due to redistribution, renal losses or decreased intake.

- Symptoms rarely develop unless phosphate is below 0.6 mmol/l; below 0.3 mmol/l rhabdomyolysis is likely.
- Hypophosphataemia leads to reduced oxygen delivery (via reduced 2,3-DPG levels) and also impairs intracellular metabolism (by depleting ATP).
- Symptoms include weakness (especially respiratory muscles – a particular problem when weaning certain ICU patients from respiratory support), confusion, coma, heart failure and rhabdomyolysis.

Causes of hypophosphataemia

- **Internal redistribution**
  Hyperinsulinaemia
  Acute respiratory alkalosis
- **Decreased intestinal absorption**
  Inadequate intake (especially alcoholism)
  Antacids containing aluminium or magnesium
  Steatorrhoea and chronic diarrhoea
- **Increased urinary excretion**
  Primary and non-renal secondary hyperparathyroidism
  Vitamin D deficiency/resistance
  Fanconi syndrome
  X-linked hypophosphataemic rickets
  Miscellaneous – osmotic diuretics, thiazide diuretics
  Acute volume expansion

Hyperphosphataemia

Hyperphosphataemia is common in renal failure. It can also occur in massive tissue breakdown (eg rhabdomyolysis) and if there is increased tubular reabsorption of phosphate.

- It is usually asymptomatic. If symptoms do occur, they are secondary to a reduction in ionised calcium.
- In acute hyperphosphataemia, saline infusion and acetazolamide (a carbonic anhydrase inhibitor) can be used to increase phosphate excretion.
- In chronic renal failure a low-phosphate diet, phosphate binders and dialysis are required. The high serum phosphate (and consequently elevated $[Ca^{2+}] \times [PO_4]$ product) in chronic kidney disease is a major vascular risk factor in this population.

Causes of hyperphosphataemia

- **Massive acute phosphate load**
  Tumour lysis syndrome*
  Rhabdomyolysis
  Lactic and ketoacidosis
  Exogenous phosphate
- **Renal failure**
- **Increased tubular reabsorption of phosphate**
  Hypoparathyroidism
  Acromegaly
  Thyrotoxicosis
  Bisphosphonates

*The tumour lysis syndrome results in release of phosphate, potassium, purines (metabolised to uric acid) and proteins (metabolised to urea). It can result in acute renal failure due to uric acid crystal deposition.

6. NUTRITIONAL AND VITAMIN DISORDERS

In the developed countries the most common nutritional problem is obesity (*see also* Chapter 4, Endocrinology). In contrast, in the developing countries, protein-energy malnutrition is common.

- Body mass index (BMI) = weight (kg) / (height in metres)^2.
- Obesity is defined as a BMI of >30 in males and >28.6 in females.
- Obesity is associated with increased risks of cardiovascular disease, diabetes mellitus, osteoarthritis and gall stones.
- In developed countries the long-term sequelae of fetal and childhood undernutrition are increased cardiovascular disease in adult life.

6.1 Protein-energy malnutrition (PEM)

Starvation is common in the developing world. In the developed countries PEM frequently complicates severe sepsis, cachexia, renal failure and malabsorption. In these circumstances undernutrition is a risk factor for death.

Protein-energy malnutrition in both adults and children can be divided into undernutrition, kwashiorkor and marasmus.

Wellcome Trust classification of protein-energy malnutrition

Weight (% of standard for age)	Oedema present	Oedema absent
60–80	Kwashiorkor*	Undernutrition
<60	Marasmic kwashiorkor	Marasmus

*Kwashiorkor literally means 'disease of the displaced child'

- Marasmus results from severe deficiency of both protein and calories.
- Kwashiorkor results primarily from protein deficiency (ie diet entirely of carbohydrate).
- Oedema is the cardinal sign separating marasmus from kwashiorkor; fatty liver also develops in kwashiorkor.
- Growth failure is more severe in marasmus.

6.2 Vitamin deficiencies

Multiple vitamin deficiencies frequently accompany protein-energy malnutrition (PEM). Isolated or grouped vitamin deficiencies (for example, of fat-soluble vitamins) can also occur in specific circumstances.

Deficiencies of fat-soluble vitamins

Vitamin	Causes of deficiency	Roles of vitamin	Deficiency syndromes
Vitamin A	Severe PEM*	Component of visual pigment Maintenance of specialised epithelia	Night blindness Xerophthalmia** Follicular hyperkeratosis Keratomalacia***
Vitamin D	Vegans† Elderly with poor diet Renal failure	Absorption of calcium and phosphate Bone mineralisation	Rickets Osteomalacia
Vitamin E	Severe (near total) fat malabsorption†† Abetalipoproteinaemia	Antioxidant Scavenger of free radicals	Spino-cerebellar degeneration
Vitamin K	Oral antibiotics‡ Biliary obstruction	Cofactor in carboxylation of coagulation cascade factors	Bleeding tendency

* Although vitamin A is fat-soluble and deficiency can occur in any chronic malabsorptive state, this is rare unless there is severe protein-energy malnutrition

** Xerophthalmia – dryness of the cornea

*** Keratomalacia – corneal ulceration and dissolution

† Vitamin D_3 is produced in the skin by photoactivation of 7-dehydrocholesterol. If sun exposure is sufficient, dietary vitamin D is not essential

†† Vitamin E deficiency is rare. It can complicate biliary atresia. In abetalipoproteinaemia (see earlier section) chylomicrons cannot be formed

‡ Antibacterial drugs interfere with the bacterial synthesis of vitamin K

Deficiencies of water-soluble vitamins

Vitamin	Causes of deficiency	Roles of vitamin	Deficiency syndromes
Vitamin B_1* (thiamine)	Alcoholism Dietary	Nerve conduction Coenzyme in decarboxylation	Dry beri-beri – symmetrical Polyneuropathy Wernicke-Korsakoff syndrome Wet beri-beri** – peripheral vasodilatation, heart failure
Vitamin B_2 (riboflavin)	Severe PEM***	Enzyme cofactor	Angular stomatitis Glossitis Corneal vascularisation
Niacin (nicotinic acid)	Carcinoid syndrome† Alcoholism Low-protein diets Isoniazid††	Incorporated into NAD and NADP	**Pellagra** – dermatitis and diarrhoea (the three Ds)
Vitamin B_6‡ (pyridoxine)	Isoniazid Hydralazine	Enzyme cofactor	Peripheral neuropathy Dermatitis Glossitis
Vitamin B_{12} (cyano-cobalamin)	Pernicious anaemia Post-gastrectomy Vegan diet Terminal ileal disease Blind loops	Coenzyme for DNA synthesis; coenzyme in myelin metabolism	Pernicious anaemia Subacute combined degeneration of the spinal cord
Vitamin C‡‡	Dietary	Redox reactions	Scurvy – bleeding, joint swelling, hyperkeratotic hair follicles, gingivitis

* Thiamine deficiency is confirmed by reduced red cell transketolase activity

** In alcoholics, wet beri-beri must be distinguished from alcoholic cardiomyopathy

*** Riboflavin deficiency usually occurs with multiple deficiencies

† In the carcinoid syndrome (and to a lesser extent in phaeochromocytoma) tryptophan metabolism is diverted from nicotinamide to form amines

†† Isoniazid can lead to deficiency of pyridoxine which is needed for the synthesis of nicotinamide from tryptophan

‡ Dietary deficiency of pyridoxine is extremely rare

‡‡ Deficiency of vitamin C is confirmed by low white cell (buffy coat) ascorbic acid levels

7. METABOLIC ACID–BASE DISTURBANCES (NON-RENAL) AND HYPOTHERMIA

The kidneys and the lungs are intimately involved in the regulation of hydrogen ion concentration. Metabolic acid–base disturbances arise from abnormalities in the regulation of bicarbonate and other buffers in the blood. Acidosis results from an increase in hydrogen ion concentration and alkalosis from a fall in H^+. pH is the negative logarithm of H^+ – a small change in pH represents a large change in H^+ concentration – this is often poorly appreciated in clinical practice.

7.1 Metabolic acidosis

The metabolic acidoses are conveniently divided on the basis of the anion gap.

$$\text{Anion gap} = Na^+ + K^+ - (Cl^- + HCO_3^-).$$

The normal anion gap is 10–18 mmol/l and represents the excess of negative charge (unmeasured anions) present on albumin, phosphate, sulphate and other organic acids.

Relationship of metabolic acid to anion gaps

- **Normal anion gap**
  Diarrhoea (or other GI loss)
  Renal tubular acidosis
  Hypoaldosteronism
  Treatment of ketoacidosis
- **Increased anion gap**
  Lactic acidosis
  Ketoacidosis
  Renal failure
  Hepatic failure
  Toluene ingestion
  Ingestion of methanol, aspirin (eg ethylene glycol)

Specific metabolic acidoses

Metabolic acidosis with diarrhoea

The gastrointestinal secretions (below the stomach) are relatively alkaline and have a high potassium concentration. There is usually hypokalaemia, low urinary potassium loss (<25 mmol/l) and low urine pH (<5.5). Causes include:

- villous adenoma
- enteric fistula
- obstruction
- laxative abuse.

Metabolic acidosis with ureteric diversion

This results in hyperchloraemic acidosis in 80% of ureterosigmoid diversions. The mechanism is due to urinary chloride exchange for plasma bicarbonate which is then lost in the urine. Urinary ammonia is also absorbed across the sigmoid epithelium.

Metabolic acidosis accompanying poisoning

Metabolic acidosis often accompanies poisoning (eg toluene, ethylene glycol, salicylates, paracetamol). These are covered in detail in Chapter 2, Clinical Pharmacology, Toxicology and Poisoning.

7.2 Metabolic alkalosis

Metabolic alkalosis is less common than metabolic acidosis because metabolic processes produce acids as by-products, and also because renal excretion of excess bicarbonate is very efficient.

Metabolic alkaloses

- **Gastrointestinal hydrogen ion loss**
  Vomiting/pyloric stenosis
  Nasogastric suction
  Antacids (in renal failure)
- **Intracellular shift of hydrogen ion**
  Hypokalaemia
- **Alkali administration**
- **Renal hydrogen ion loss**
  Mineralocorticoid excess
  Loop or thiazide diuretics
  Post-hypercapnic alkalosis
  Hypercalcaemia and the milk–alkali syndrome
- **Contractional alkalosis**
  Volume depletion

Specific metabolic alkaloses

Gastric loss of hydrogen ions

In protracted vomiting (eg pyloric stenosis) or nasogastric suction there can be complete loss of up to three litres of gastric secretions per day. The gastric secretions contain:

- hydrogen ion: 100 mmol/l
- potassium: 15 mmol/l
- chloride: 140 mmol/l.

Alkalosis will result but, paradoxically, acid urine is produced due to renal tubular sodium bicarbonate reabsorption to maintain plasma volume. Patients respond to volume expansion with normal saline and correction of hypokalaemia.

Milk–alkali syndrome

This is defined as the triad of hypercalcaemia, metabolic alkalosis and ingestion of large amounts of calcium with absorbable alkali (traditionally for peptic ulcer pain). The hypercalcaemia increases renal bicarbonate reabsorption exacerbating the alkalosis. Clinical presentation is with symptoms of hypercalcaemia or metastatic calcification.

Post-hypercapnic alkalosis

Chronic respiratory acidosis leads to a compensatory increase in urinary hydrogen ion secretion resulting in a rise in plasma bicarbonate concentration. Rapid lowering of a raised pCO_2 (usually by mechanical ventilation) is not immediately accompanied by a fall in plasma bicarbonate. There is often an accompanying chloride loss that must be replaced before bicarbonate can fall to normal.

7.3 Hypothermia

Hypothermia is defined as a fall in core temperature to below 35°C. It is frequently fatal if the core temperature falls below 32°C.

Causes of hypothermia

- Elderly with inadequate heating
- Hypothyroidism
- Immersion in cold water
- Alcoholism
- Hypoglycaemia
- Exposure to low external temperatures (eg unconscious patients, mountaineers, etc)

Mild hypothermia (32–35°C) causes shivering and intense feeling of cold.
Severe hypothermia (<32°C) causes impairment in judgement and reduced awareness of the cold.

- **Clinical features of hypothermia**: include bradycardia, hypoventilation, muscle stiffness, hypotension and loss of reflexes. The pupils can be fixed and dilated in recoverable hypothermia.
- **Metabolic acidosis**: due to lactate accumulation is common, pancreatitis can complicate hypothermia.
- **Electrocardiograph changes**: include J waves, prolonged PR interval, prolonged QT and QRS complexes. Death results from ventricular arrhythmias or asystole.

Chapter 14
Molecular Medicine

CONTENTS

10. The molecular basis of some important diseases
- 10.1 Amyloidosis
- 10.2 Alpha-1 antitrypsin deficiency
- 10.3 Alzheimer's disease
- 10.4 Trinucleotide repeat disorders
- 10.5 Mitochondrial disorders
- 10.6 Myasthenia gravis
- 10.7 Duchenne muscular dystrophy
- 10.8 Sickle cell disease

11. Glossary of terms in molecular medicine

Molecular Medicine

1. MOLECULAR DIAGNOSTICS

The diagnostic process in medicine is entering a new and important historical phase. Increasingly, diagnostic entities are being reclassified according to the molecules that are central to the disease process and also according to changes in the expression of genes which code for these molecules. With the advent of the complete human gene sequence we now have the tools for a complete understanding of how cells develop and how they function in health and disease.

1.1 Genomes, transcriptomes and proteomes

The genome of an organism is its complete complement of coding genes. Comparing the organisms in the table overleaf reveals that the level of complexity of an organism is not explained by the number of genes predicted to code for protein. Fruitflies (*Drosophila melanogaster*, a favourite organism for geneticists) have more complex behaviours than nematode worms (*Caenorhabditis elegans*) but fewer genes. One reason for this is that flies process genes in a more complex way. Humans and mice have the same number of predicted genes and 98% of these are **orthologues** (have a common ancestral gene and code for equivalent proteins). Biological complexity is explained by:

- The **transcriptome**: this is the name given to the total complement of expressed mRNA sequences in an organism. In lower organisms this will be the same as the number of genes. In mammals genes are transcribed in a more complex way with transcription being initiated from different exons in different tissues and alternative splicing (post-transcriptional processing). The temporal (*when* in development) and spatial (in *which* cells) expression of genes allows significant diversity which is not evident just from looking at gene number. It is likely therefore that the transcriptomes of mouse and humans contain significant differences.
- Processed mRNA is translated into protein. Similarly, differences in mRNA transport, localisation and stability mean that the **proteome** cannot be inferred directly from the transcriptome.
- **Post-translational processing**: proteins can be modified by glycosylation, sialydation, etc. Protein stability and turnover may be very different in different cell types and between similar cells in different organisms.
- Finally, the progressive diversity of the proteome with evolution leads to an exponential amplification of combinatorial possibilities between proteins. Therefore, while the human genome may have 30, 000 information units (genes) the final number of information units needed to explain human biological complex is theoretically several orders of magnitude greater.

Organism	Number of proteins	Approx genome size	Introns	Splicing
Human	30, 000	3×10^9 (3 Gb)	Yes	Highly complex
Mouse	30, 000	3 Gb	Yes	Complex
Fruitfly	13, 500	40×10^6 (40 Mb)	Yes	Yes
Nematode	19, 000	96 Mb	Very few	Very little
Fission yeast	6000	12 Mb	Rare	Absent
Bacterium	2000–6000	2–6 Mb	Absent	Absent

Transcriptomics

The gene expression profile (**transcriptome**) of a particular tissue is the key to understanding the cell phenotype in health and disease. An average cell expresses about 16, 000 genes throughout its lifetime but clearly the range of genes expressed in the lifetime of an individual cell will vary during development, maintenance and ultimately cell death. Inevitably the genes expressed by a neurone in the cerebellum will be very different from those expressed by a lymphocyte, though **housekeeping genes** are common to many cells and encode constitutive cellular processes.

The **transcriptome** of a cell can be captured using a technique known as **microarray analysis**. This depends on the same hybridisation reaction as other nucleic acid techniques but represents dramatic scaling up of the procedure such that many thousands of hybridisation reactions occur on a single medium and changes in transcription in many genes can be assessed simultaneously. RNA is prepared from the tissue of interest (for example, a tumour biopsy specimen) and from a control sample (eg normal tissue from the same organ from which the biopsy was obtained). The RNA is hybridised to a 'DNA chip'. This consists of a silicon slide 1–2 cm in size onto which have been spotted oligonucleotides, 20–30 base pairs long. Each oligonucleotide represents a particular gene. The RNAs from the abnormal and control tissues are labelled with different colour fluorescent dyes (eg red and green) and the level of expression of many thousands of genes can then be analysed by computer software which compares the differences in intensity generated by the hybridisation reaction.

- The power of this technology is such that it is not necessary to know anything about the function of the particular gene spotted onto the chip.
- As the sequence of every gene is now known, DNA chips with a representative coverage of the whole human genome can be produced commercially.
- It is also possible to produce tissue-specific chips (eg human CNS) or chips with a limited number of genes of interest for use in diagnostics, when a specific question is being asked.
- DNA microarrays can in principle identify a whole array of downstream genetic consequences of a particular gene mutation and provide a **molecular profile** of a disease state that can act as a marker of therapeutic effect.

Practical applications

- Rapid sequencing for many genetic mutations can be performed simultaneously in a high throughput approach. For example, specific oligonucleotides that recognise all of the mutations responsible for a particular disease can be spotted onto a chip and DNA from an affected individual analysed.
- Tumours or other abnormal tissue can undergo molecular profiling in order to identify patterns of gene expression. For example, it is now possible in clinical practice to use microarrays to analyse the expression of panels of key genes that determine the clinical response to chemotherapeutic agents in lymphoma. Also, tissue or fluid from infections can be analysed for the expression of genes conferring antibiotic resistance before organisms have even been cultured.
- Though still a research tool it is likely that microarrays will be routinely used in the near future in **genotyping** large numbers of genes simultaneously to look at specific disease risk (eg cardiovascular) associated with single nucleotide polymorphisms (SNPs) or other genetic variants.
- Individual responses to common drug treatments (eg anti-hypertensive agents) are likely to have a basis in genetic variation. The application of knowledge acquired through genetic profiling such as with microarrays is known as **pharmacogenomics**.

Proteomics

As discussed above the total protein content of a cell or tissue may be a more meaningful target for analysis in certain situations than either the genome or transcriptome. Protein from whole tissue or from subcellular fractions (eg membrane, nuclear, mitochondrial, etc) can be separated by physical methods, such as on a **2-D gel**, in which proteins are resolved by charge and mass to produce individual spots on a polyacrylamide gel which can then be silver stained. Individual spots of interest can be removed and eluted from the gel. The protein within can then be identified using **tandem mass spectrometry** which can sequence short peptides. A known protein can then be identified by reference to protein sequence databases.

Where the oligopeptide does not produce a match, a search can be made of the **human genome sequence databases** – computer programmes have been used to predict genes and therefore protein sequences from the primary data (an example of what is known as **bio-informatics**). Currently, proteomics is largely a research tool, but with time and improved technology it will inevitably be used in clinical practice.

Potential applications include:

- The identification of all of the proteins expressed in a particular cell, groups of cells or whole tissues throughout the whole development of an organism from conception to death. Ultimately a complete description of the ontogeny of the cell will be possible allowing virtual modelling and computer-based drug design.
- Comparisons can be made between healthy and diseased tissue in the same way as for mRNA with microarrays. However, the advantage with proteomics is that it may be possible to detect differences at the protein level which are not reflected at the transcriptional level

due to changes in turnover or post-translational processing. As with RNA techniques, protein from different sources can be differentially labelled with fluorescent dyes to aid the detection of differences.

- **Protein chips** contain antibodies spotted onto silicon-based media similar to microarrays. Several hundred targeted proteins can be analysed in this way.

1.2 The polymerase chain reaction (PCR)

PCR is an amplification reaction in which a small amount of target DNA (the **template**) is amplified to produce enough to perform analysis. This might be the detection of a particular DNA sequence, such as that belonging to a pathogenic microorganism or an oncogene, or the detection of differences in genes, such as mutations causing inherited disease. Therefore, the template DNA might consist of total human genomic DNA derived from peripheral blood lymphocytes, amniocentesis or chorionic villous sampling; alternatively, it might consist of a tumour biopsy or a biological fluid from a patient with an infection.

- Two unique oligonucleotide sequences, known as **primers**, are mixed with a DNA template and a thermostable DNA polymerase (***Taq* polymerase**, derived from an organism that inhabits thermal springs). Sometimes more than two primers can be used if more than one gene is to be amplified (multiplex PCR) or the region of DNA to be amplified needs special definition ('nested' PCR); for example, if it is similar to other sequences in the genome which may give spurious reaction products.
- In the initial stage of the reaction the DNA template is heated (typically for about 30 seconds) to make it single stranded and then as the reaction cools the primers will anneal to the template if the appropriate sequence is present.
- Then the reaction is heated to 72°C (for about a minute) and the DNA polymerase synthesises new DNA between the two primer sequences. During 30 or so cycles (each typically lasting a few minutes) the target sequence will have been amplified exponentially.

The crucial feature of PCR is that to detect a given sequence of DNA it only needs to be present in one copy (ie one molecule of DNA): this makes it extremely powerful.

Clinical applications of PCR

- Mutation detection
- Detection of viral and bacterial sequences in tissue (Herpes simplex virus in CSF, hepatitis C, HIV in peripheral blood, meningococcal strains)
- Single-cell PCR of in vitro fertilised embryo to diagnose genetic disease before implantation

In the example below, some CSF from a patient suspected of having Herpes simplex encephalitis is used in a PCR reaction in an effort to detect the presence of the virus directly.

Figure 1 The polymerase chain reaction (PCR)

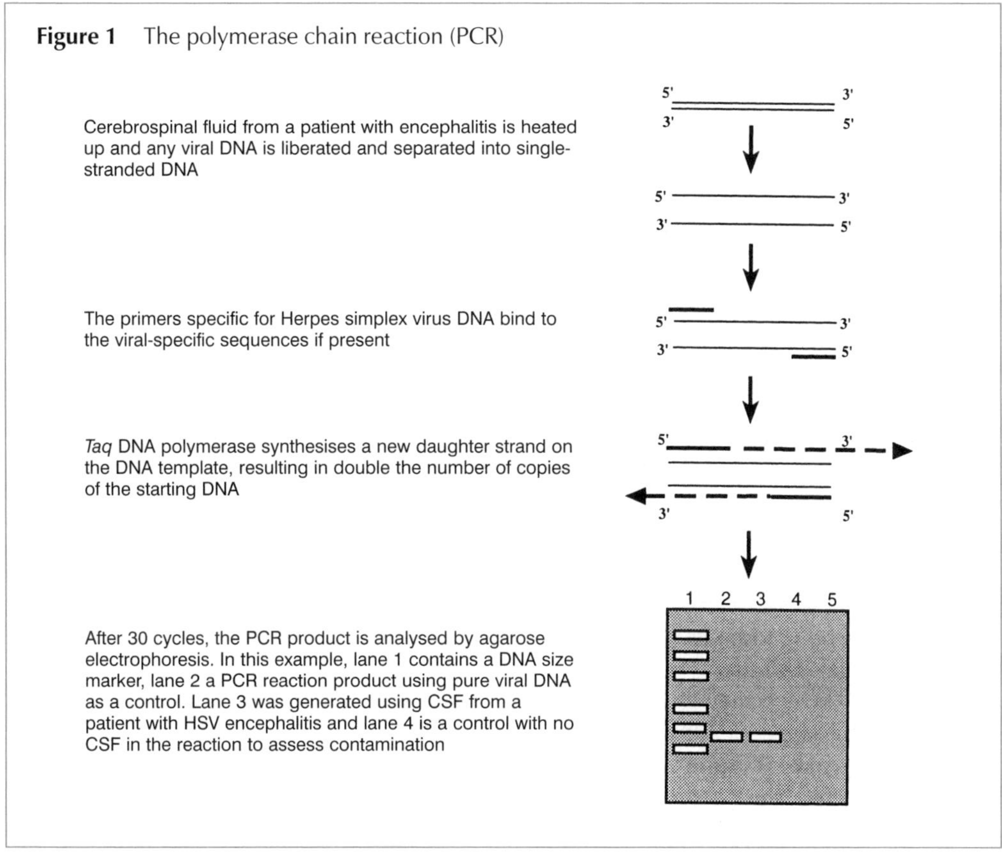

Cerebrospinal fluid from a patient with encephalitis is heated up and any viral DNA is liberated and separated into single-stranded DNA
The primers specific for Herpes simplex virus DNA bind to the viral-specific sequences if present
Taq DNA polymerase synthesises a new daughter strand on the DNA template, resulting in double the number of copies of the starting DNA
After 30 cycles, the PCR product is analysed by agarose electrophoresis. In this example, lane 1 contains a DNA size marker, lane 2 a PCR reaction product using pure viral DNA as a control. Lane 3 was generated using CSF from a patient with HSV encephalitis and lane 4 is a control with no CSF in the reaction to assess contamination
5'
3'
1 2 3 4 5

Small amounts of target DNA are amplified with a thermostable DNA polymerase.

1.3 Reverse transcription PCR (rt PCR)

Conventional PCR looks at genomic DNA. Every cell in our body contains our total genome in two copies. However, the phenotype of a cell (what makes a hepatocyte different from a Purkinje cell) depends on which genes are being expressed at any one time. To look at the expression of genes we must therefore analyse only those genes that are being transcribed into mRNA.

- RNA is too unstable to be used in PCR so it must first be converted to complementary DNA (cDNA) using **reverse transcriptase**, a retroviral enzyme that makes a precise copy of the mRNA.
- PCR is then performed in the normal way but, because the template reflects the mRNA of the starting material, this technique can look at **gene expression** in individual tissues.

Clinical applications of rt PCR

- Detection of the expression of particular genes in tumour tissue carries important prognostic information
- Basic scientific research into normal function of disease genes by understanding their spatial and temporal expression

1.4 Monoclonal antibodies

The detection of specific proteins in molecular diagnosis relies on the fact that the antibody used has a high specificity for the target protein. An immune response to an antigen consists of a polyclonal proliferation of cells giving rise to antibodies with a spectrum of specificity for the target. Therefore, useful diagnostic and therapeutic antibodies must be selected from this complex immune response before they can be used.

Myeloma is a malignantly transformed B-cell lineage that secretes a specific antibody. This fact is used to produce unlimited amounts of specific antibodies directed toward an antigen of choice.

- A laboratory animal is injected with the antigen of choice, it mounts an immune response and its spleen, which contains B-cell precursors with a range of specificity for the antigen, is harvested.
- The spleen cells are fused en masse to a specialised myeloma cell line that no longer produces its own antibody.
- The resulting fused cells, or **hybridomas**, grow in individual colonies, are immortal and produce antibodies specified by the lymphocytes of the immunised animal. These cells can be screened to select for the antibody of interest which can then be produced in limitless amounts.

Clinical applications of monoclonal antibodies

- Diagnosis of cancer and infections
- Imaging of tumours, radiotherapy
- As a 'magic bullet' to direct drugs to target
- Transplantation and other immune modulations (eg OKT3).

Figure 2 Monoclonal antibody production from mouse B-cell precursors fused with myeloma cells in culture

Polyclonal immune response
BALB cells selected for immunoglobulin deficiency
+
Spleen cells from the mouse are harvested and fused with a mouse myeloma cell line to form a HYBRIDOMA
The hybridoma can be grown in culture indefinitely and produces antibody of a defined specificity

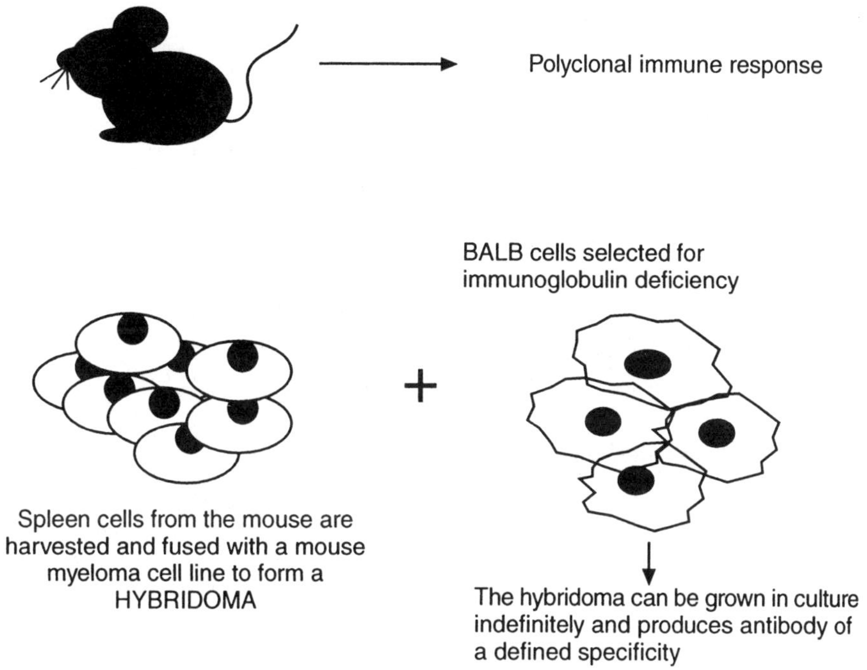

2. CELL SIGNALLING

Central to all cellular processes is the conversion of external signals (first messengers) via intermediates (second messengers) into changes that alter the state of that cell. This often involves adjustment in the expression of genes in the cell nucleus and new protein synthesis. In the following example (see figure overleaf) a photon of light is the external stimulus that produces, via second messengers, a change in the resting state of the rod cell leading it to transmit a signal to the visual cortex.

2.1 Types of receptor

The chief function of the cell membrane is to provide a barrier to ion flux and therefore to maintain the internal milieu of the cell. There are, as described below, certain lipophilic modules which travel freely into the cell. However, most external signals can only effect changes inside the cell by interaction with membrane-bound receptor modules. This biologically ubiquitous system of signal transduction by receptors underlies the action of many hormones, growth factors and drugs.

Figure 3 A typical signalling pathway (the rod photoreceptor). This involves a G-protein-coupled membrane receptor which activates a second messenger pathway

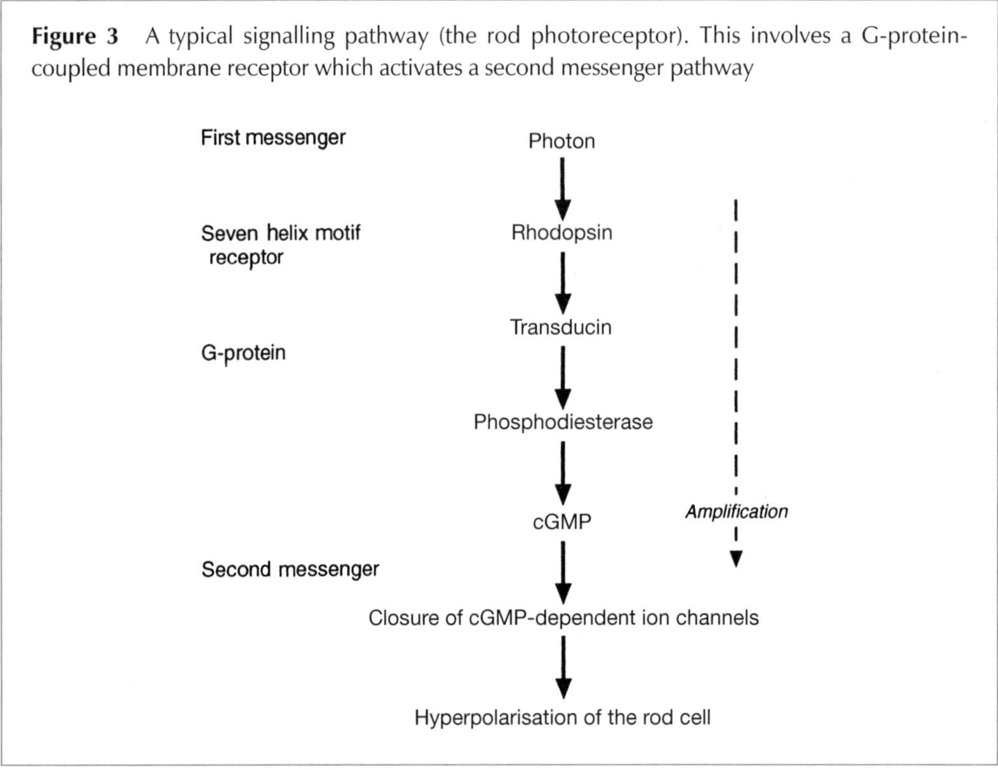

Ligand-gated ion channel

For example, **acetylcholine receptor** (nicotinic).

- Five non-covalently assembled subunits ($\alpha_2\beta\gamma\delta$) are located at the post-synaptic neuromuscular junction.
- Each subunit is coded for by a different gene which enables mixing and matching of subunits between different tissues and in embryological development to generate a repertoire of responses.
- On binding of acetylcholine to the α subunits the whole complex undergoes a conformational change leading to the passage of sodium ions into the cell and cellular depolarisation.

Other examples include some **glutamate** receptors (excitatory), γ-aminobutyric acid (GABA) and **glycine** (inhibitory: the passage of chloride ions into the cell renders it more resistant to depolarisation).

Receptors that contain cytoplasmic domains with protein-tyrosine-kinase activity

- **Insulin** binds to its receptor which then undergoes dimerisation and autophosphorylation at a tyrosine residue.
- The tyrosine kinase activity intrinsic to the receptor is then activated and the result is the phosphorylation of cytoplasmic proteins and initiation of an intracellular cascade.
- This ultimately leads to the action of insulin on glucose uptake, etc.

Other examples include platelet-derived growth factor, insulin-like growth factor 1 (IGF-1), macrophage-colony stimulating factor, nerve growth factor.

G-protein-coupled receptors

Guanine nucleotide binding proteins are a ubiquitous cellular mechanism for coupling an extracellular signal to a second messenger, such as cyclic AMP.

Figure 4 G-proteins are activated by ligand binding to a transmembrane receptor

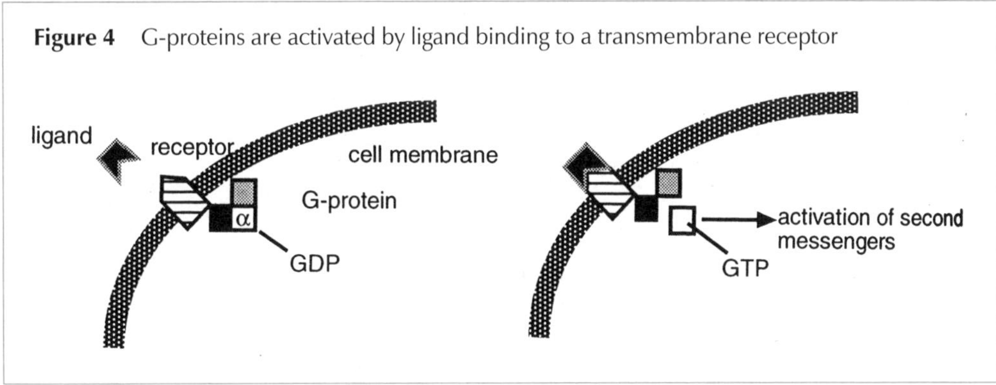

- G-proteins have three non-covalently associated subunits: α, β, γ. In the inactive state GDP is bound to the α subunit of the G-protein.
- When the receptor is activated by ligand binding, the G-protein is activated by the hydrolysis of GTP to GDP.
- In this active state the α subunit dissociates from the β and γ subunits. Either of these two complexes (the GTP-α or the β-γ) can then interact with second messengers.
- The α subunit is rapidly inactivated by hydrolysis of GDP to GTP (this is an intrinsic property of the α subunit, which is therefore known as a GTPase) and then re-associates with the β and γ subunits resetting the whole system to the inactive state.

G-proteins can be inhibitory (Gi) or stimulatory (Gs) and the overall activity of a second messenger such as adenylate cyclase is likely to be regulated by the differential activation of these different forms. The **muscarinic acetylcholine receptor**, the α and β **adrenergic receptor** and the retinal photoreceptor **rhodopsin** are all G-protein-coupled receptors. These can be linked to a variety of second messenger systems or sometimes directly to ion channels.

Diseases associated with G-protein abnormalities

- **Cholera**: *Vibrio cholerae* secretes an exotoxin which catalyses ADP-ribosylation of an arginine residue on Gsα. This makes the subunit resistant to hydrolysis and the second messenger (in this case cAMP) remains activated and this ultimately leads to the fluid and electrolyte loss characteristic of the disease.
- **Pituitary adenomas**.
- **McCune-Albright syndrome**.
- **Albright's hereditary osteodystrophy** (or pseudohypoparathyroidism).

} *See* Chapter 4, Endocrinology.

2.2 Protein kinases and phosphatases

Protein kinases catalyse the transfer of a phosphate group from ATP to a serine, threonine or tyrosine residue on a target protein (the substrate). Phosphorylation of this amino acid residue results in an alteration in the conformation of the target protein and thus leads to its activation or inactivation. Many **growth factor receptors** are protein tyrosine kinases (see above). Many of the 'downstream' intracellular pathways which are initiated by the activation of a second messenger system involve protein kinases (usually serine kinases in the cytoplasm). In this way an external signal can, through the activation of one receptor, influence a vast array of cellular processes due to a cascade of protein interactions.

2.3 Nuclear hormones

Not all extracellular signals use second messenger systems to effect changes to the cell. Important exceptions are **steroid hormones** that bind to an intracellular receptor allowing the receptor to be freed from its cytosolic membrane-bound anchor. The receptor hormone complex then travels to the nucleus where it binds to specific regions of DNA called **hormone responsive elements**, thereby effecting alterations in the transcription of DNA.

Examples of nuclear hormones

- Corticosteroids
- Vitamin D
- Retinoic acid
- Sex steroids.

Figure 5 The nuclear hormone superfamily of receptors act by controlling gene transcription in the nucleus

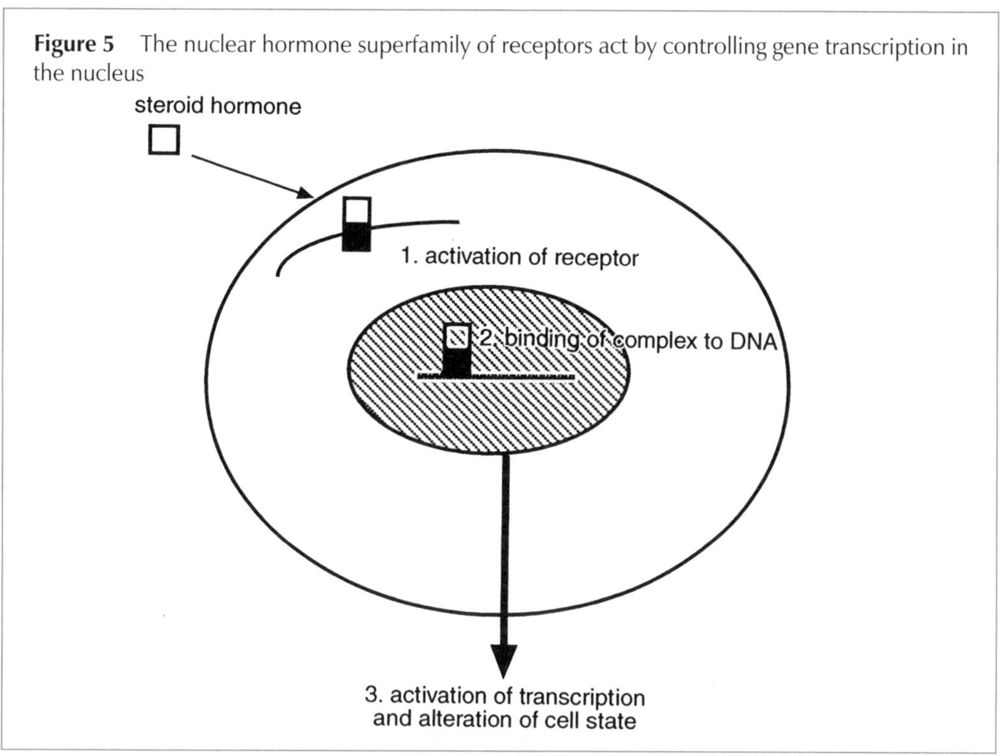

2.4 Transcription factors and the regulation of gene expression

The human genome is present in two copies in every cell in the body, and is estimated to consist of around 30, 000 genes. The spatial and temporal expression of a proportion of these genes (typically 10, 000–15, 000 genes are expressed in any one cell at any time) determines the differentiation, morphology and functional characteristics of each cell type (the **cellular phenotype**). Clearly, for cells to maintain a specific identity, this process must be very tightly regulated.

Eukaryotic genes consist of **exons**, which are transcribed into the mRNA template which is translated into protein. Exons are separated by **introns**, which do not code for protein but have a role in mRNA stability and are spliced out of the pre-mRNA prior to translation. Sometimes exons are also spliced out to produce variant forms of the protein with tissue-specific functional elements (splice variants).

Clearly some genes have a fundamental biological role and will be expressed in all cells at all times ('housekeeping genes'). However, the transcription of most genes only proceeds when a macromolecular complex (the initiation complex) binds to a region of the 5′ end of genes called the **promoter**. The assembly of this complex is directed by the presence of transcription factors and facilitates the binding of RNA polymerase, which leads to transcription. Muscle, for example, will contain specific transcription factors that lead to the expression of muscle-specific genes which determine the muscle phenotype.

Figure 6 Structure of a typical gene

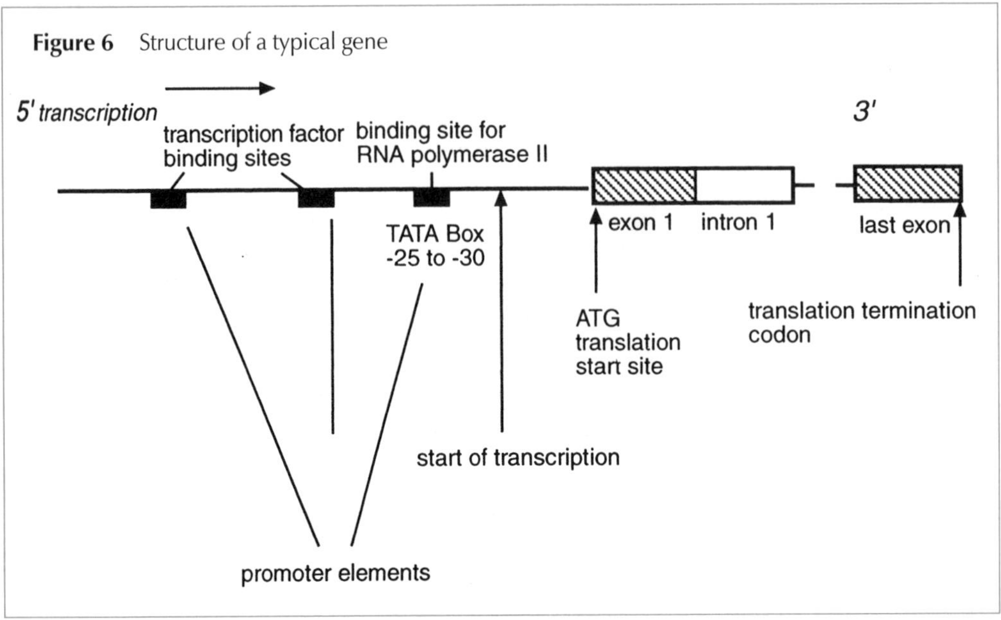

The promoter

- A modular arrangement of different elements that act as a binding site for RNA polymerase II and the initiation of transcription.
- The initiation of transcription involves a large complex of multimeric proteins (RNA polymerase II plus the general transcription factors (GTFs): TFII A–H).
- The GTFs can activate transcription of any gene that has a TATA box (see below).

Enhancers

- Elements that can be at the 5′ or the 3′ end of genes and can vary in distance from the coding sequence itself.
- Enhancers are not obligatory for the initiation of transcription but alter its efficiency in such a way as to lead to an increase in gene expression.

Transcription factors

Transcription factors are proteins that bind to sequence-specific regions of DNA at the 5′ end of genes called **response elements** to regulate gene expression. These elements can form part of promoters or enhancers. They can be divided into:

- basal transcription factors – involved in the constitutive activation of so-called housekeeping genes
- inducible transcription factors – involved in the temporal and spatial expression of genes that underlie tissue phenotype and developmental regulation.

They fall into a number of groups based on their structure:

- helix-loop-helix
- helix-turn-helix
- zinc finger
- leucine zipper.

The **TATA box** is a promoter element that is always located 25–30 base pairs from the start of transcription and serves to anchor RNA polymerase II.

Clinical applications of transcription factors

- An increasing number of diseases are being described where an inherited mutation in transcription factors leads to a developmental disorder. These are usually complex congenital malformations
- Transcription factors can be oncogenes, eg c-myc, p53 (*see* Section 3.2)
- Many future drugs will be developed to alter gene transcription by acting directly or indirectly on gene transcription in the manner described above for steroids

3. THE MOLECULAR PATHOGENESIS OF CANCER

3.1 Somatic evolution of cancer

Cancer cells are a clonal population. The accumulation of mutations in multiple genes results in escape from the strictly regulated mechanisms that control the growth and differentiation of somatic cells. It will be evident that some of these genetic 'errors' will be inherited and form the basis of a familial tendency to cancer. For cancer to develop, in most cases, an environmentally driven genetic mutation is necessary. Genotoxic damage from ionising radiation and some of the constituents of tobacco smoke fall into this category. In addition, all somatic cell division requires the copying of DNA and this can result in the spontaneous mutations of genes. It is a combination of these three types of genetic mutation (inherited, spontaneous and environmentally determined) which leads to cancer. Therefore, cancer evolution is a complex, multifactorial process.

Most tumours show visible abnormalities of chromosome banding on light microscopy, suggesting that as tumours develop they become more bizarre and more prone to genetic error. Although there are some cancer genes that lead to Mendelian (ie monogenic) inheritance of specific tumours, most cancers result from a complex mixture of polygenetic and environmental influences.

3.2 Oncogenes

Originally identified as genes carried by cancer-causing viruses that are integrated into the host genome and, when expressed, lead to loss of growth control (viral oncogenes are denoted v-onc). They have cellular homologues, **proto-oncogenes** (denoted c-onc), found in the normal human genome and expressed in normal tissue, that are usually highly conserved in evolution and have central roles in the signal-transduction pathways that control cell growth and differentiation. They can be thought of as exerting a dominant effect in that they cause cancer in the presence of the normal gene product because, in mutating, they have gained a new function.

- **Ras** is a small, monomeric, G-protein and is likely to be involved in the transduction of growth-promoting signals. The relative abundance of the active and inactive forms of **ras** is controlled by positive and negative regulators of GTP–GDP exchange (GAP and GNRF). Mutations affecting the GTP binding site prevent GTP hydrolysis and prolong **ras** activation. At least a third of sporadic tumours contain acquired somatic mutations in **ras**.
- Further downstream, after a number of protein kinase steps have been activated, the transduction of growth signals culminates in the activation of the transcription factors **fos** and **jun** which in turn induce the transcription of the proto-oncogene **myc** which commits the cell to a round of DNA replication and cell division. Mutant forms of these proteins can induce tumour growth.
- The 9:22 balanced translocation (Philadelphia chromosome) found in chronic myeloid leukaemia (**CML**) generates a composite gene comprising exons from the **bcr** locus on chromosome 22 and the **c-abl** locus on chromosome 9, generating a **fusion protein** with distinct biochemical properties which presumably promote tumour growth.

Figure 7 Activation of the oncoprotein ras is under reciprocal control by GNRF and GAP

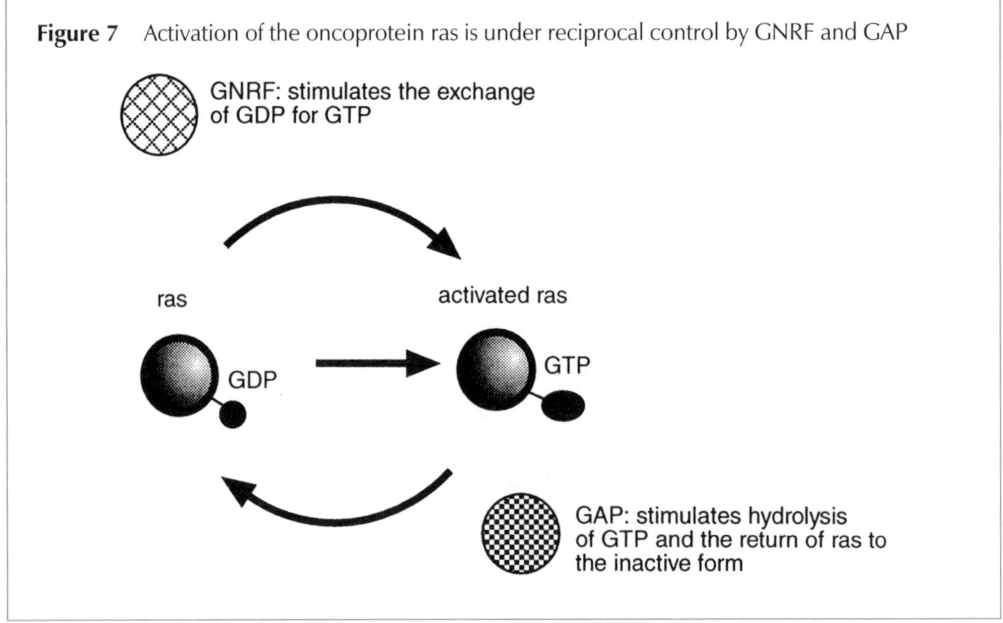

- In **Burkitt's lymphoma** the **c-myc** gene is transposed from its normal position into the immunoglobulin heavy chain locus on chromosome 14, resulting in a gross increase in its expression and a potent molecular signal for cells to undergo mitosis (see figure below).

Figure 8 In CML the Philadelphia chromosome leads to the production of an oncoprotein

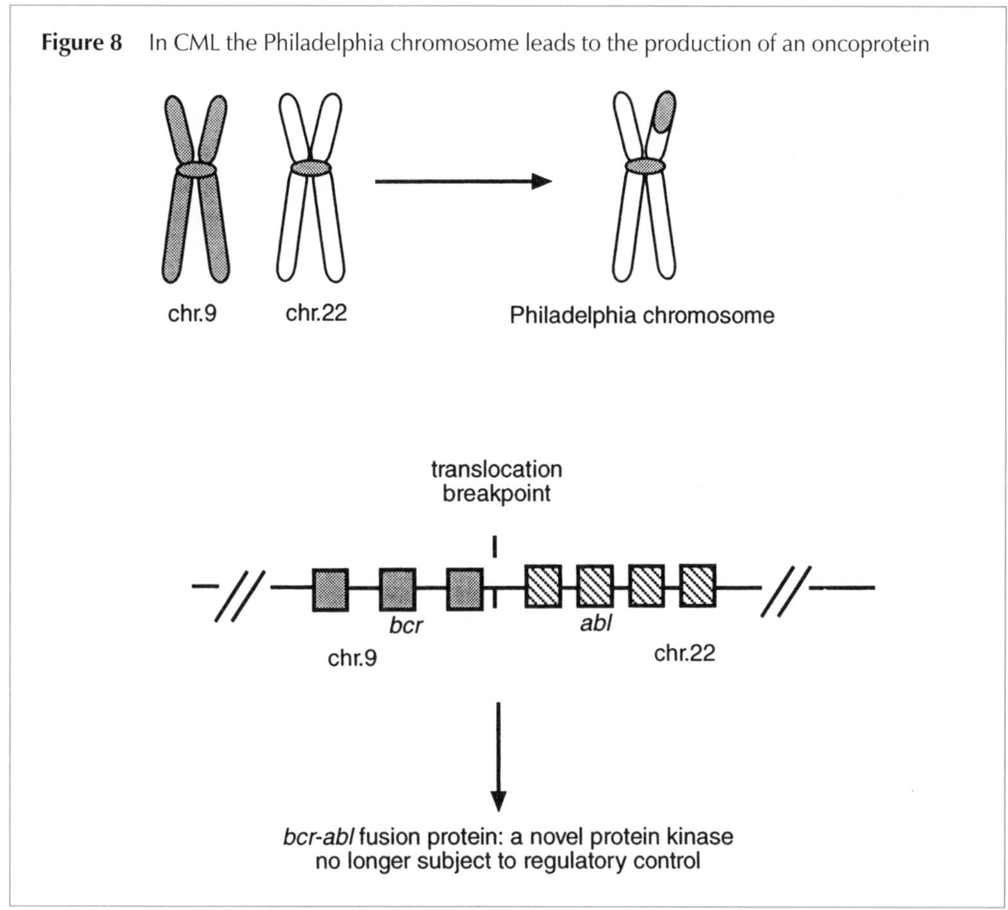

3.3 Tumour suppressor genes

- In contrast to oncogenes these exert a recessive effect, in that both copies must be mutated before tumorigenesis occurs.
- Mutation results in loss of function.
- These genes normally function to inhibit the cell cycle and therefore, when inactivated, lead to loss of growth control.

p53 is a protein that occupies a pivotal role in the cell cycle and is the most commonly mutated gene in tumours (breast, colon, etc). It encodes a transcription factor, the normal function of which is to downregulate the cell cycle. Inactivation of **p53** is the primary defect in the Li–Fraumeni syndrome (a dominantly inherited monogenic cancer syndrome characterised by breast carcinoma, sarcomas, brain and other tumours), and is a central regulator of **apoptosis** (see below).

4. APOPTOSIS AND DISEASE

It has only recently been fully appreciated that widespread cell death occurs in human development and in the normal regulation of cell number in the adult organism. In embryonic development cells are lost, for example, as finger webbing disappears or as neurones are 'selected' for survival by making the appropriate synaptic contact. In post-natal life, the expansion of lymphocyte numbers in response to antigen stimulation must be regulated by the subsequent death of these cells or clonal proliferation would continue unabated. It turns out that this process of naturally occurring cell death is regulated by the activation of a specific set of genes in response to external signals in a process referred to as **programmed cell death**. The morphological change that accompanies this process is called **apoptosis**.

- Cells undergo shrinkage, compaction of chromatin, nuclear and cytoplasmic budding to form membrane-bound apoptotic bodies and finally phagocytosis by surrounding macrophages.
- The activation of intracellular nucleases can be detected by the 'laddering' of DNA on electrophoresis gels, which serves as a marker for apoptosis.

In contrast to necrosis, apoptosis does not induce the release of destructive proteolytic enzymes and free radicals and is thus a non-inflammatory process. Therefore, collateral damage to neighbouring cells is not seen. Most cells seem to rely on a constant supply of survival signals without which they will undergo apoptosis. These are provided by neighbouring cells and the extracellular matrix. The absence or withdrawal of these molecular signals is a trigger to apoptosis.

The 'cell death programme' is genetically regulated and there are specific proteins that promote or inhibit apoptosis.

- A family of proteases called **caspases** (ICE, or interleukin-1β converting enzyme, is the best-studied example) is central to apoptosis in mammals and is responsible for driving all the structural changes in the nucleus that accompany apoptosis. Caspases have been shown to be present in all cells and thus to prevent apoptosis there must be specific inhibitors of these proteases.
- The **bcl-2** family of molecules inhibit apoptosis by a variety of mechanisms and are thus cytoprotective survival signals. Over-expression of bcl-2 specifically prevents cells from entering apoptosis and its high expression has been correlated with poor survival from cancer.
- **fas**, or CD95, is a transmembrane receptor that belongs to the tumour necrosis factor (TNF) receptor family. The binding of TNF-like ligands to fas is coupled to the activation of intracellular caspases. Some tumours express the fas ligand on their surface, thus activating fas on cytotoxic T-lymphocytes leading to their death (a way of evading immune surveillance).

- **p53** is required for the apoptosis of cells in which DNA has been damaged. The failure of tumour cells to die in the face of genotoxic damage may be due to the accumulation of p53 mutations.

Programmed cell death can be stimulated by a variety of triggers and leads to the activation of proteases such as ICE that initiate a cascade of morphological changes (collectively known as apoptosis) which result in inevitable phagocytosis.

Figure 9 Apoptosis (programmed cell death)

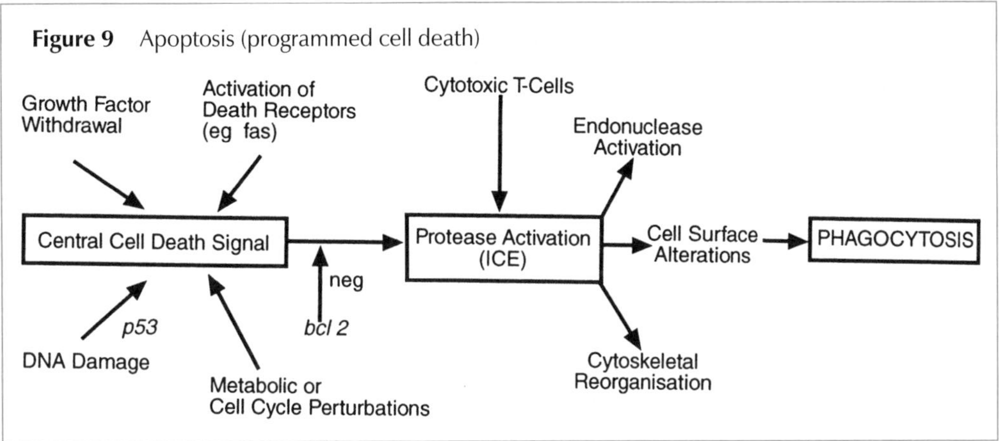

- Certain disorders (cancer, autoimmunity and some viral illnesses) are associated with increased cell survival (and therefore a failure of programmed cell death). Metastatic tumour cells have circumvented the normal environmental cues for survival and can survive in foreign environments.
- Physiological cell death is necessary for the removal of potentially autoreactive T-cells during development and for the removal of excess cells after the completion of the immune response. Animal models of SLE (CD95/fas knockout mice) have implicated apoptosis genes in the pathogenesis of autoimmunity.
- Death by apoptosis can be seen as an evolutionary adaptation to prevent the survival of virally infected cells. Therefore, viruses have developed strategies for circumventing this. Pox viruses appear to inhibit apoptosis by producing an inhibitor of ICE.
- Excessive cell death due to an excess of signals promoting apoptosis has been hypothesised to occur in many degenerative disorders where cells have been observed to die by apoptosis. Direct evidence that this actually occurs has yet to be found.

5. MOLECULAR REGULATION OF VASCULAR TONE

Both the regulation of systemic arterial blood pressure and the local control of the microcirculation in organs such as the kidney and the brain are vital for the maintenance of homeostasis. Recently there has been an explosion of knowledge concerning the molecular mediators of blood flow and this is already having an impact in the therapy of some common disorders.

Two important principles should be kept in mind:

- the regulation of vascular tone is predominantly a **paracrine** process, where molecules are released to act in adjacent cells
- vascular control is often a balance between competing vasodilators and vasoconstrictors.

5.1 Nitric oxide (NO)

Previously called endothelium-derived relaxant factor (EDRF), NO is an important transcellular messenger molecule that is involved in a diverse range of processes.

NO is synthesised from the oxidation of nitrogen atoms in the amino acid L-arginine by the action of NO synthase (NOS).

Figure 10 Formation of nitric oxide

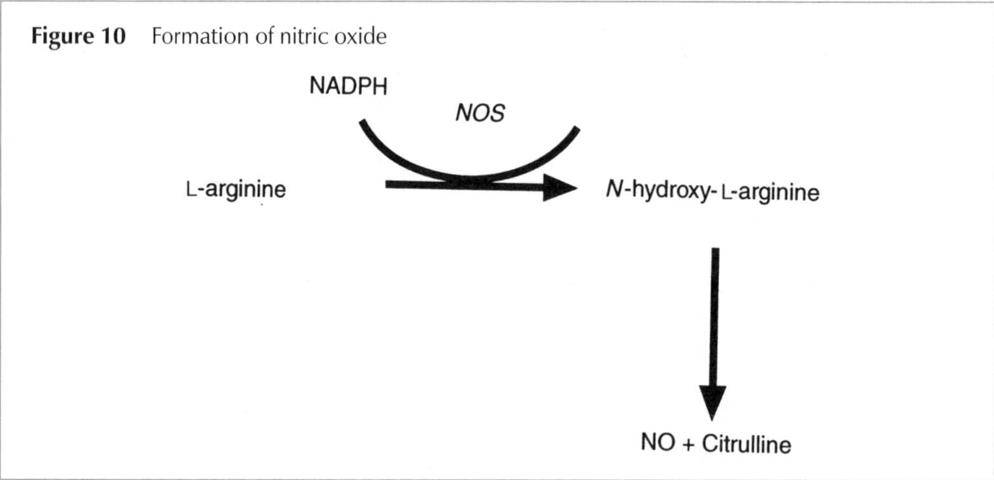

Cell types which synthesise nitric oxide

- Vascular endothelium
- Macrophages
- Neutrophils
- Central and peripheral nerve cells
- Platelets
- Vascular smooth muscle
- Hepatocytes

NO acts on target cells close to its site of synthesis where it activates guanylate cyclase leading to a rise in intracellular cGMP, which acts as a second messenger to modulate a variety of cellular processes. It has a very short half-life.

There are at least three distinct **isoforms** of NO synthase:

- neuronal (constitutive)
- endothelial (constitutive)
- macrophage (inducible).

Constitutive NO production is involved in regulation of vascular tone and neurotransmission and is calcium/calmodulin dependent. **Inducible NO production** is mainly involved in cell-mediated immunity and is activated by cytokines.

Synthetic nitrates, such as GTN and sodium nitroprusside, act after their conversion into NO.

Functions of nitric oxide

- Vasodilator tone modulation in the regulation of systemic blood pressure
- CNS neurotransmission, including the formation of new memories
- Inhibition of platelet aggregation
- Cytotoxic action utilised in the generation of the host immune response in activated macrophages
- Organ-specific microregulatory control (eg kidney)
- Peripheral nervous system 'non-adrenergic, non-cholinergic neurotransmission' (NANC), mediating neurogenic vasodilatation

Diseases related to abnormalities in the generation or regulation of NO

- **Septic shock**: NO is released in massive amounts and correlates with low blood pressure.
- **Atherosclerosis**: NO synthesis may be impaired more than endothelin synthesis leading to tonic vasoconstriction and vasospasm.
- **Primary and secondary pulmonary hypertension**: inhaled NO reverses pulmonary hypertension.
- **Hepatorenal syndrome** and the **hypertension of chronic renal failure**: failure of breakdown and secretion of endogenous antagonists of NO leads to a microcirculatory imbalance between NO and endothelin (see below).
- **Excitotoxic cell death in the CNS**: glutamate is the principal excitatory neurotransmitter in the CNS. NO is the transduction mechanism when glutamate binds to NMDA (*N*-methyl-D-aspartate) receptors on neurones. The final event in the presence of excess glutamate is a rise in intracellular calcium and the cell becomes vulnerable to dying. This process, in which NO is now implicated, is thought to be important in neuronal loss in many neurodegenerative conditions such as Alzheimer's disease and also in acute brain injury such as stroke.
- **Tissue damage** in acute and **chronic inflammation** (probably by interacting with oxygen-derived free radicals).
- **Adult respiratory distress syndrome** (ARDS).

5.2 Endothelin-1

This is the most potent vasoconstrictor substance yet described. It is manufactured following vascular endothelial 'stress' (shear, hypoxia, growth factors, expansion of plasma volume). It is produced from pre-pro ET by the action of endothelin converting enzyme (ETCE). Very little endothelin reaches the circulation and serum levels do not generally carry any diagnostic significance.

There are endothelin receptors:

- on the vascular endothelium and on some smooth muscle cells (gut and heart), including coronary arteries where they cause constriction
- on capillary endothelium where they cause vasodilatation.

When ET-1 is infused intravenously it causes a transient vasodilatation followed by a long period of intense vasoconstriction lasting up to two hours. The normal function of endothelin is in the regulation of vascular tone. ETCE inhibitors and receptor blockers are under development as agents for systemic arterial hypertension. More diverse functions of endothelin are indicated by the recent finding of mutations in the endothelin-B receptor in some patients with Hirschsprung's disease.

Disorders whose pathogenesis may be related to endothelin

- Essential hypertension
- Primary pulmonary hypertension
- Renovascular hypertension
- Hepatorenal syndrome
- Acute renal failure
- Chronic heart failure
- Raynaud's phenomenon
- Vasospasm after subarachnoid haemorrhage

6. MOLECULAR MEDIATORS OF INFLAMMATION, DAMAGE AND REPAIR

The process of tissue injury, inflammation and subsequent repair is highly conserved in evolution and represents part of the 'primitive' repertoire of protective mechanisms against invasion by foreign organisms and other insults. This is in contrast to the more sophisticated mechanisms of defence mediated by the immune system. Some of the same molecules are involved in both processes but they are considered here to emphasise the enormous importance of inflammation as a pathological process central to many diseases. These molecular interactions are to a certain extent therefore independent of the immune system.

The principal molecules involved are termed **cytokines**, because they function in the immune system as products secreted by one cell to act on another cell to direct its movement ('kinesis'). In the context of inflammation it is the **proinflammatory cytokines** that are relevant. (*See also* Chapter 10, Immunology.)

6.1 Interleukin-1 (IL-1)

This molecule has a broad spectrum of both beneficial and harmful biological actions and, as a central regulator of the inflammatory response, has been implicated in many diseases.

There are three structurally related polypeptides in the interleukin-1 family:

- IL-1α
- IL-1β
- IL-1 receptor antagonist.

IL-1α and IL-1β are synthesised by mononuclear phagocytes that have been activated by microbial products or inflammation:

- IL-1α stays in the cell to act in an autocrine or paracrine fashion.
- IL-1β is secreted into the circulation and cleaved by interleukin-1β-converting enzyme (ICE).

IL-1β levels in the circulation are undetectable except:

- after strenuous exercise
- with sepsis
- with acute exacerbation of rheumatoid arthritis
- in ovulating women
- with acute organ rejection.

IL-1 in disease

- **Rheumatoid arthritis**: IL-1 is present in the synovial lining and fluid of patients with rheumatoid arthritis and it is thought to activate gene expression for collagenases, phospholipases and cyclo-oxygenases. It is thus acting as a molecular facilitator of inflammatory damage in the joint but is not an initiator.
- **Atherosclerosis**: the uptake of oxidised LDL by vascular endothelial cells results in IL-1 expression, which stimulates the production of platelet-derived growth factor. IL-1 is thus likely to play a role in the formation of the atherosclerotic plaque.
- **Infection**: IL-1 has some host defence properties, inducing T- and B-lymphocytes, and reduces mortality from bacterial and fungal infection in animal models.
- **Septic shock**: IL-1 acts by increasing the concentration of small mediator molecules such as platelet activating factor (PAF), prostaglandins and nitric oxide, which are potent vasodilators.

6.2 Tumour necrosis factor (TNF)

This is a pro-inflammatory cytokine that has a wide spectrum of actions. Either through neutralising antibodies (anti-TNFα) or inhibitor drugs it is the target of therapy in disorders such as rheumatoid arthritis and multiple sclerosis.

Two non-allelic forms of TNF, α and β, are expressed in different cells:

- TNFα is produced by macrophages, eosinophils and NK cells
- TNFβ is made by activated T-lymphocytes.

Its name is derived from the early observation that it can have a cytotoxic effect on tumour cells in vitro. Trials with TNFα as a therapeutic agent were soon stopped due to the severe toxicity of the substance. In fact in certain situations it can promote tumour growth.

Its action in diseases such as **rheumatoid arthritis** depends on a synergistic effect with IL-1. Both are found in the synovial membrane of patients with the disease. TNFα strongly induces monocytes to produce IL-1 at a level comparable to that stimulated by bacterial lipopolysaccharide (LPS).

Activations of TNF

- TNFα is a potent stimulator of prostaglandin production
- TNF is a key cytokine in the pathogenesis of multi-organ failure
- It induces granulocyte-macrophage colony stimulating factor (GM-CSF) and thus is an activator of monocytes and macrophages in diseased tissue

6.3 Transforming growth factor β (TGFβ)

A key cytokine that initiates and terminates tissue repair and whose sustained production underlies the development of tissue fibrosis.

TGFβ is released by platelets at the site of tissue injury and is strongly chemotactic for monocytes, neutrophils, T-cells and fibroblasts. It induces monocytes to begin secreting fibroblast growth factor (FGF), TNF and IL-1, but inhibits the functioning of T- and B-cells and their production of TNF and IL-1. It also induces its own secretion. This **autoinduction** may be important in the pathogenesis of fibrosis.

TGFβ in disease

- TGFβ-deficient (knockout) mice die of an autoimmune disease in which levels of TNF and IL-1 are very high.

- It has a potent effect on cells to induce the production of extracellular matrix (a dynamic superstructure of self-aggregating macromolecules including fibronectin, collagen and proteoglycans to which cells attach by means of surface receptors called **integrins**). Extracellular matrix is continually being degraded by proteases which are inhibited by TGFβ.
- In **mesangioproliferative glomerulonephritis**, glomerular immunostaining for TGFβ correlates well with the amount of mesangial deposition.
- In **diabetic nephropathy**, increased TGFβ is found in the glomeruli, and TGFβ may be central to the pathogenesis of progression of many chronic renal diseases.
- Elevated plasma levels of TGFβ are highly predictive of **hepatic fibrosis** in bone marrow transplant recipients. mRNA for TGFβ is found in areas of active disease in liver biopsy samples of patients with chronic liver disease.
- In patients with **idiopathic pulmonary fibrosis**, TGFβ is increased in the alveolar walls. It is also implicated in **bleomycin lung**.

6.4 Heat shock proteins (HSPs)

The **heat shock response** is a highly conserved and phylogenetically ancient response to tissue stress that is mediated by activation of specific genes leading to the production of specific heat shock proteins that alter the phenotype of the cell, and enhance its resistance to stresses.

Some HSPs are extremely similar to constitutively activated proteins that have essential roles in unstressed cells. Their diverse functions include:

- export of proteins in and out of specific cell organelles (acting as **molecular chaperones**)
- catalysis of protein folding and unfolding
- degradation of proteins (often by the pathway of ubiquitination).

As well as heat, HSP expression can be triggered by cytotoxic chemicals, free radicals and other stimuli. The unifying feature that leads to the activation of HSPs in these situations is thought to be the accumulation of damaged intracellular protein.

Clinical relevance

- Tumours have an abnormal thermotolerance which is the basis for the observation of the enhanced cytotoxic effect of chemotherapeutic agents in hyperthermic subjects.
- Stress proteins are prominent amongst the bacterial antigens recognised by the immune response of humans to bacterial and parasitic infections and are thought to be involved in some autoimmune diseases.
- Mutations in small heat shock proteins (sHSPs) have been associated with diseases as diverse as cataract (alpha-crystallin) and forms of motor neurone degeneration (sHSPs 22 and 27).

6.5 Free radicals and human disease

Free radicals have been implicated in a large number of human diseases and are currently the subject of much interest. Therapeutic trials have been undertaken with putative free radical scavengers such as vitamin E. A free radical is literally any atom or molecule that contains one or more unpaired electrons, making it more reactive than the native species.

Free radical species produced in the human body

- $-O\mathring{O}H$ (peroxide radical)
- $-\mathring{O}_2$ (superoxide radical)
- $-\mathring{O}H$ (hydroxyl radical)
- $-N\mathring{O}$ (nitric oxide)

The hydroxyl radical is by far the most reactive species but the others can generate more reactive species as breakdown products.

When a free radical reacts with a non-radical a chain reaction ensues which results in the formation of further free radicals and direct tissue damage by lipid peroxidation of membranes. This is particularly implicated in **atherosclerosis**, and **ischaemia-reperfusion injury** (eg acute tubular necrosis within the kidney) within tissues. Hydroxyl radicals can cause mutations by attacking purines and pyrimidines. Also:

- Activated phagocytes generate large amounts of superoxide within lysosomes as part of the mechanism whereby foreign organisms are killed. During chronic inflammation this protective mechanism may become harmful.
- **Superoxide dismutases** (SOD) convert superoxide to hydrogen peroxide and are thus part of an inherent protective antioxidant strategy. **Catalases** remove hydrogen peroxide. **Glutathione peroxidases** are major enzymes that remove hydrogen peroxide generated by SOD in cytosol and mitochondria.
- **Free radical scavengers** bind reactive oxygen species. Alpha-tocopherol, urate, ascorbate and glutathione remove free radicals by reacting directly and non-catalytically. Severe deficiency of alpha-tocopherol (vitamin E deficiency) causes neurodegeneration.

Clinical relevance

There is growing evidence that cardiovascular disease and cancer can be prevented by a diet rich in substances that diminish oxidative damage.

Principal dietary antioxidants

- Vitamin E
- Beta carotene
- Vitamin C
- Flavonoids

Epidemiological studies have demonstrated an association between increased intake of vitamins C and E and morbidity and mortality from coronary artery disease. This supports models where atherogenesis is initiated by lipid peroxidation of LDL.

Patients with dominant familial forms of amyotrophic lateral sclerosis (motor neurone disease) have mutations in the gene for Cu-Zn SOD-1, suggesting a link between failure of oxidative damage and neurodegeneration.

7. TRANSMISSIBLE SPONGIFORM ENCEPHALOPATHIES (TSEs)

The transmissible spongiform encephalopathies (TSEs) are a group of diseases that are characterised by progressive spongiform degeneration in the brain and neuronal loss. While these conditions are rare, they are the subject of intense interest because of an epidemic of human infection which is linked to the cattle disease bovine spongiform encephalopathy (BSE). The biologically unique features of these diseases are, firstly, that they can be simultaneously inherited and also infectious, and, secondly, that the agent of transmission is thought to be a protein only rather than an 'organism' containing DNA or RNA. This protein has been called a **prion**; it is encoded by the host genome and cannot replicate.

Diseases caused by TSEs

- **Sporadic Creutzfeldt–Jakob disease (CJD)**: rare ($1/10^6$), causes rapid dementia with myoclonus and characteristic EEG.
- **Variant CJD (vCJD)**: approximately 150 cases had occurred in the UK by mid-2004. This affects young people and has a slower course than sporadic CJD; it has characteristic pathological features.
- **Autosomal dominant CJD**: familial form of classical CJD.
- **Gerstmann-Straussler-Scheinker Syndrome (GSS)**: familial spongiform encephalopathy with prominent ataxia.
- **Fatal familial insomnia**.
- **Kuru**: previously endemic in New Guinea Highlanders who performed ritual cannibalism. This condition is now disappearing.

Molecular features of TSEs

The accidental or deliberate inoculation of affected brain tissue from a case of inherited or sporadic TSE results in the passage of the disease to the recipient. Procedures that destroy nucleic acid do not prevent this passage, which has led to the proposition that the prion protein itself causes the disease by interacting with the host encoded protein, leading to its conversion to the mutant form of the protein. Other important considerations for the TSEs are:

- **Prion protein**: this is encoded by a gene on chromosome 20, exact function unknown. Curiously, mice lacking this gene only have subtle neurological defects. Prion proteins are not destroyed by boiling, UV irradiation or formaldehyde, nor do they elicit an immune response of any recognisable kind.

- **Species barrier**: this means that the diseases are, to some extent, species specific. For example, scrapie in sheep has never been passed on to humans as far as is known. Similarly, the transmission of a spongiform encephalopathy from one species to another is very difficult. If CJD brain tissue is injected into the brain of a monkey then there is very little cell death, but if brain tissue from that same monkey is injected into another monkey (second passage) then there is severe neuronal loss. This suggests that the pathological process leading to spongiform change depends on the host protein.
- **Susceptibility polymorphism**: at codon 129 of the prion protein the amino acid can either be a valine or a glycine residue. Given that there is one copy of the gene on each chromosome we can either be heterozygous (valine/glycine) or homozygous (valine/valine or glycine/glycine). It turns out that homozygosity at this residue is vastly over-represented in affected individuals in sporadic CJD and in variant CJD. It would appear that the one amino acid can confer susceptibility to the disease.
- **Strain type**: when the protein from affected brains is electrophoretically separated and blotted onto a membrane (Western blotting) and then incubated with anti-prion protein antibody, different patterns can be seen. This is what is referred to as the 'strain' of the infective agent but is really a surrogate marker. It is the fact that the observed pattern with variant CJD is identical to that observed with BSE, and different to sporadic CJD, that provides the strongest evidence of a link between the two.

8. ADHESION MOLECULES

The way in which cells communicate with each other is fundamental to the maintenance of homeostasis in the developing and adult organism. In particular, the molecular basis of neural connectivity, the immune response and the prevention of cancer are all dependent on **adhesion molecules**. Adhesion involves the interaction of one molecule, for example a cell surface molecule, with a specific ligand which may be on another cell or a part of the extra-cellular matrix. These can be divided into four groups on the basis of structure and function:

- the immunoglobulin superfamily
- the cadherin superfamily
- integrins
- selectins.

The **immunoglobulin superfamily** is so-called because at the genetic level it has a sequence similarity that suggests that it arose from the same set of ancestral genes by duplication. These molecules are involved as cofactors in antigen presentation and are present as cell surface receptors on leukocytes (eg CD2, CD3, T-cell receptor) and some function as **integrin ligands** (eg ICAM, NCA: intercellular and neural cell adhesion molecule, respectively).

Cadherins are involved in the interaction between muscle and nerve in the developing embryo.

Integrins are heterodimeric (two subunits, different from each other) transmembrane glyco-proteins which are widely distributed in different tissues and serve to interact with molecules of the extracellular matrix (laminin, fibronectin, collagen).

Selectins are expressed on leukocytes and are thought to be involved in leukocyte adherence to endothelium during acute inflammation and coagulation.

Expression of adhesion molecules is dynamic and can be upregulated by proinflammatory cytokines (IL-1, TNF), viral infection, T-cell activation and many other stimuli.

Clinical relevance of adhesion molecules

Adhesion molecule expression is upregulated in many forms of solid organ inflammation (eg autoimmune and viral hepatitis, and also in organ rejection after transplantation). The adhesion molecule intercellular adhesion molecule-1 (ICAM-1) is a receptor for the integrin lymphocyte function associated molecule-1 (LFA-1) and may be involved in the recruitment and maintenance of activated lymphocytes in tissue inflammation.

- It is theoretically possible to block these molecules to treat inflammation (eg in acute renal failure and in transplant rejection).
- The integrin $\alpha_{IIb}\beta$ is the platelet receptor for fibrinogen.
- Mutations in its gene lead to the congenital bleeding disorder **Glanzmann's thrombasthenia.**
- In another genetic disease, **leukocyte adhesion deficiency** (LAD), lack of $\beta 2$ integrins leads to failure of leukocyte migration to sites of infection and hence to recurrent bacterial sepsis.
- Conversely, antibodies against $\alpha_{IIb}\beta$ are routinely used in clinical practice (ie abciximab) as anti-thrombotic agents in coronary artery disease.

9. STEM CELLS

A number of tissues in the body contain progenitor cells which are capable of producing progeny, or daughter cells, to replenish cell populations. The most obvious example is the bone marrow where red and white cells are constantly being replaced to match turnover in the peripheral blood. It is now known that a number of other tissues contain stem cells:

- **Embryonic stem cells** are totipotential and hence can give rise to any tissue type. There are ethical difficulties in the acquisition and use of these cells which may limit their therapeutic use. Embryonic stem cells from mice are a powerful investigative tool in basic science.
- **Bone marrow stem cells** can be easily accessed and purified by antigen sorting with CD34 antibodies. If these cells undergo **transdifferentiation** they can then function as a replacement for degenerating cells of non-haematological origin (eg neurones).

10. THE MOLECULAR BASIS OF SOME IMPORTANT DISEASES

The following conditions have been highlighted either because their molecular basis is well understood (eg **myasthenia gravis, alpha-1 antitrypsin deficiency**) or because they are caused by novel mechanisms (eg **trinucleotide repeat disorders**). Others are included because the identification of their molecular basis is historically important as for dystrophin in

Duchenne muscular dystrophy, which was the first disease to be worked out by identifying the gene through positional cloning. Overall, the following diseases serve to illustrate the importance of the molecular mechanisms of disease outlined in the above sections.

10.1 Amyloidosis

A pathological process characterised by the accumulation of extracellular fibrils of insoluble protein. The aggregated protein is specific to the different amyloid diseases listed below, but in all cases the fibrillar component is associated with a non-fibrillar constituent called **amyloid-P component** which is derived from the acute phase protein **serum amyloid P** (SAP). (*See also* Section 12.1, Chapter 15, Nephrology.)

Pathogenesis

Whilst the inherited forms of amyloid are rare, the accumulation of amyloid fibrils is a central part of the pathological process of a number of common diseases such as Alzheimer's and type II diabetes, where amyloid is found in the islets of Langerhans. Many individuals on

Figure 11 Classification of amyloidosis. The individual protein that associates with serum amyloid P is shown in italics

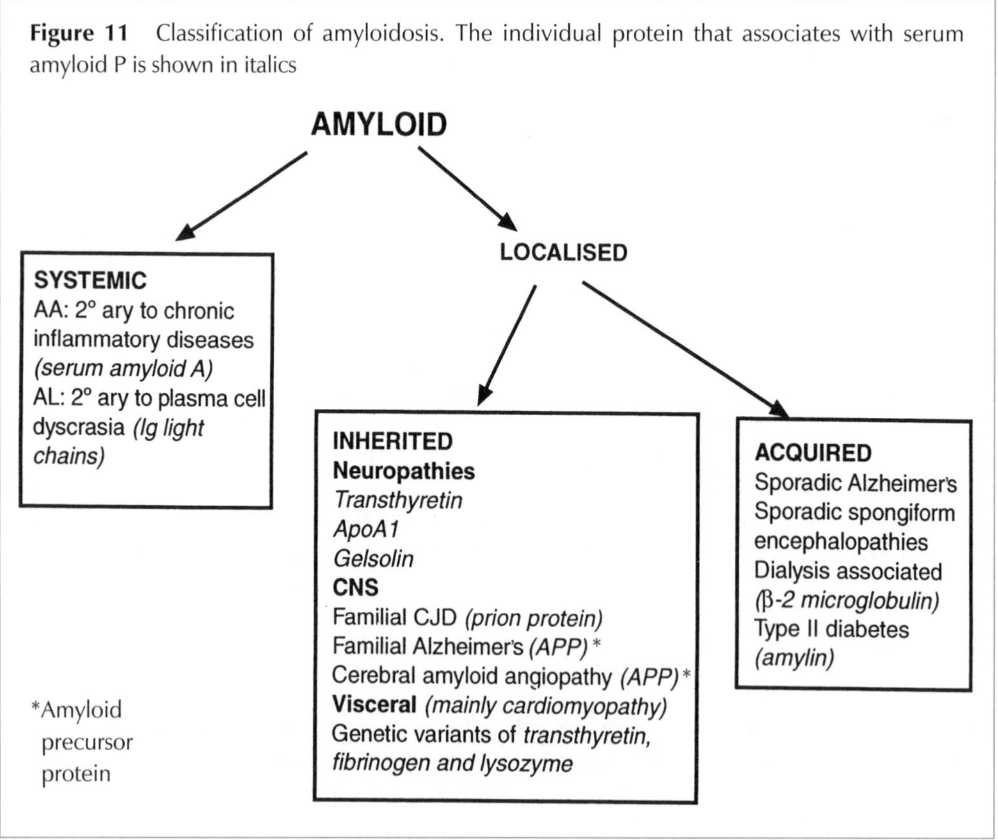

long-term haemodialysis eventually develop amyloid arthropathy. The key event in amyloid fibril formation is a change in conformation of the respective precursor protein which leads to its aggregation into an insoluble fibrillar form. The exact mechanism of this conformational change is unclear but it is thought to involve partial proteolytic cleavage of the precursor, and/or its overproduction. Using ^{131}I-labelled SAP amyloid deposits can be localised using scintigraphy. Amyloid may cause organ dysfunction by progressive replacement of functional parenchyma or it may possibly be inherently cytotoxic.

10.2 Alpha-1 antitrypsin deficiency

Deficiency of alpha-1 antitrypsin is one of the most common hereditary diseases affecting Caucasians. The prime function of the enzyme is to inhibit neutrophil elastase and it is one of the serpin superfamily of protease inhibitors. Patients with deficiency present with emphysema (*see* Chapter 19, Respiratory Medicine) because low protein levels fail to protect the lung from proteolytic attack. A proportion of individuals also develop liver cirrhosis, but this does not appear to be directly due to enzyme deficiency.

- The most common mutation that changes a glutamate residue to a lysine at position 342 of the protein (the Z mutation) results in the accumulation of protein in the endoplasmic reticulum of the liver.
- The formation of these hepatic inclusions results from a protein–protein interaction between the reactive centre loop of one molecule and the beta-pleated sheet of a second.
- This leads to polymerisation and aggregation. Similar mechanisms have been found to be responsible for deficiency of C-1 esterase inhibitor (hereditary angioneurotic angio-oedema) and anti-thrombin III.
- Since not all patients who are homozygously deficient develop liver damage, other factors, such as the way the mutant protein is broken down in the liver, must be relevant to the manifestation of the liver component.

10.3 Alzheimer's disease

A neurodegenerative disease of inexorable cognitive decline characterised histologically by intra-neuronal **neurofibrillary tangles** and extracellular **amyloid plaques**. Most cases are sporadic.

- About five per cent of cases are inherited as an autosomal dominant with at least three genes responsible.
- Mutations in the amyloid precursor protein (APP) gene on chromosome 21 are a rare cause of familial Alzheimer's disease (AD). The βA4 protein is a proteolytic product of APP and the principal constituent of senile plaques.
- Mutations in two closely related genes, the presenilins PS-1 and PS-2, are responsible for other cases of AD.
- Inheritance of the ε-4 allele of apolipoprotein E is an important determinant of age of onset in familial AD and a risk factor for sporadic AD. (*See also* Chapter 16, Neurology.)

Molecular markers

Neurofibrillary tangles consist of highly ordered intraneuronal structures called paired helical filaments (PHF) which are assembled from the microtubule associated protein **tau**.

This suggests that neurones die because tau is handled in some abnormal way which leads to dysfunction of the microtubular network. Tau protein from PHFs is abnormally phosphorylated but it is not yet known whether this is part of the primary pathological process leading to AD. APP is cleaved into a β and a γ fragment. It is thought that plaque formation occurs when the Aβ fragment becomes insoluble and aggregates. Aggregated Aβ has been shown to induce free-radical-mediated damage to neurones.

10.4 Trinucleotide repeat disorders

A new class of genetic disease has been recognised in recent years, in which the responsible genetic mutation is a repetitive sequence of three nucleotides which can undergo expansion (and occasionally contraction). It has therefore become known as a dynamic mutation.

Examples of trinucleotide repeat disorders

- Huntington's disease
- Fragile X syndrome*
- X-linked bulbospinal neuronopathy (Kennedy's syndrome)
- Myotonic dystrophy
- Friedreich's ataxia
- Spinocerebellar ataxias (there are a number of variants)

*See Chapter 7, Genetics

As a consequence of dynamic mutation, mutant alleles arise from a population of pre-mutant alleles that have a repeat number at the upper limit of the normal range (usually < 35) which then become unstable and undergo sudden expansion into the mutant range (> 50). Two key genetic characteristics are illustrated by trinucleotide repeat disorders.

Anticipation

The phenomenon whereby the severity of a disease becomes worse, and the age of onset earlier, in successive generations.

Somatic instability

The length of the expansion continues to increase as cells divide throughout life. This may partly explain why a disease such as myotonic dystrophy gets worse as the patient gets older.

For a particular disease the length of the expansion corresponds with the age of onset of the disease.

There are two main types of trinucleotide repeats.

Figure 12 Trinucleotide repeats

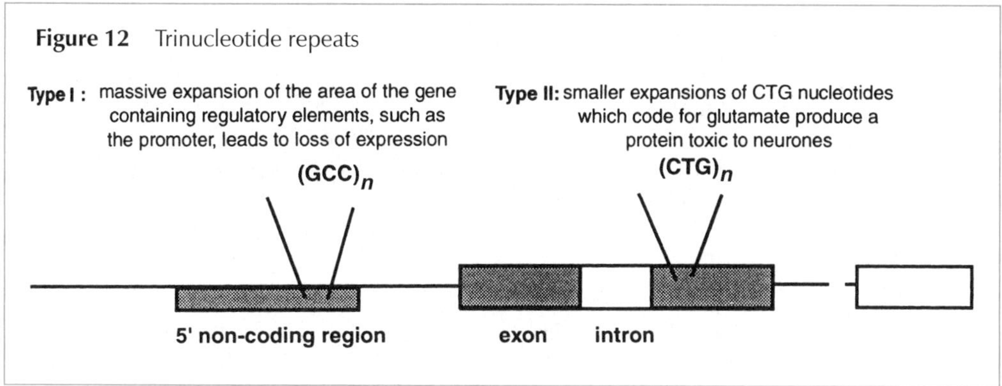
Type I : massive expansion of the area of the gene containing regulatory elements, such as the promoter, leads to loss of expression
Type II: smaller expansions of CTG nucleotides which code for glutamate produce a protein toxic to neurones
(GCC)n
(CTG)n
5' non-coding region
exon
intron

Trinucleotide repeats can occur in the non-coding region or within exons, giving different effects.

It will be evident from the above diagram that the consequence of a type I expansion is loss of gene expression because the gene cannot be transcribed due to stereochemical interference from the expanded region. Type II disorders are thought to be so-called '**gain of function**' dominant mutations. That is, the trinucleotide expansion leads to the accumulation of an abnormal protein which is toxic to cells. In several of these disorders it has now been demonstrated that toxic protein accumulates in intraneuronal inclusions which stain positive for ubiquitin. (*See also* Chapter 7, Genetics.)

10.5 Mitochondrial disorders

The mitochondrial genome is circular and approximately 16.5 kb in length. It encodes genes for the mitochondrial respiratory chain and for some species of transfer RNA. Nucleic acids cannot move in and out of mitochondria, thus all of the mRNA synthesised from the mitochondrial genome must be translated in the organelle itself. However, many nuclear encoded proteins are transported into mitochondria and are absolutely necessary for mitochondrial function. (*See also* Chapter 7, Genetics.)

- Mitochondrial DNA (mtDNA) mutates 10 times more frequently than nuclear DNA; as there are no introns, a mutation will invariably strike a coding sequence.
- **Maternal inheritance**: no mitochondria are transferred from spermatozoa at fertilisation and so each individual only inherits mtDNA from the mother.
- Because there are 10^3–10^4 copies of mitochondrial DNA in each cell (each mitochondrion has 2–10 copies of mtDNA) normal and mutant mtDNA may coexist within one cell (known as heteroplasmy). This may be one explanation why mitochondrial diseases show a **poor genotype-phenotype correlation**.
- There is evidence that mtDNA mutations are accumulated throughout life, as mitochondrial DNA has no protective DNA repair enzymes, and that this may contribute to the changes of ageing.

Phenotypes due to mitochondrial DNA mutations

- Sensorineural deafness
- Optic atrophy
- Stroke in young people
- Myopathy
- Cardiomyopathy and cardiac conduction defects
- Diabetes mellitus
- Chronic progressive external ophthalmoplegia
- Lactic acidosis
- Pigmentary retinopathy

Virtually all tissues in the body depend on oxidative metabolism to a greater or lesser extent and thus these phenotypes can often occur together (for example, diabetes and deafness). As mentioned above the relationship between the mutations and the clinical features is poorly understood.

10.6 Myasthenia gravis

This relatively rare disease (incidence 1 case per 8000–20, 000) has a molecular pathogenesis that is well understood, and it serves as a model for other autoimmune diseases. Specific antibodies are directed against the nicotinic acetylcholine (ACh) receptor which is present on the post-synaptic membrane of the neuromuscular junction. This results in:

- Complement-mediated destruction of acetylcholine receptors and a loss of the normal convolution of the muscle membrane (an important morphological hallmark of the disease); this leads to the loss of surface area for ACh to interact with its receptors.
- Accelerated endocytosis and degradation of receptors.
- Functional blockade of receptors.

These abnormalities lead to fatigable weakness (*see also* Chapter 16, Neurology). Ptosis and diplopia are the commonest symptoms. In 10–15% of sufferers, symptoms are confined to the eyes (ocular myasthenia). Fatigability occurs because of a combination of the normal rundown of ACh release which occurs physiologically, and a decreased number of ACh receptors.

Over 80–90% of patients have detectable antibodies to the ACh receptor and the others are presumed to have antibodies not detectable by current assays. Antibody negativity is more common in the ocular form.

- Passive transfer of antibodies from patients to mice reproduces the disease features.
- Reduction of antibody levels by plasmapheresis or treatment with immune globulin ameliorates the disease.
- The antibody titre in patients does not always correlate with disease severity, suggesting that anti-ACh receptor antibodies have different functional consequences depending on the exact epitope to which they are directed.

The origin of the autoimmune process is controversial but 75% of patients have thymic abnormalities (hyperplasia in 85% and thymoma in 15%).

Figure 13 The neuromuscular junction in myasthenia gravis. There is loss of acetylcholine receptors and a decrease in post-synaptic folds.

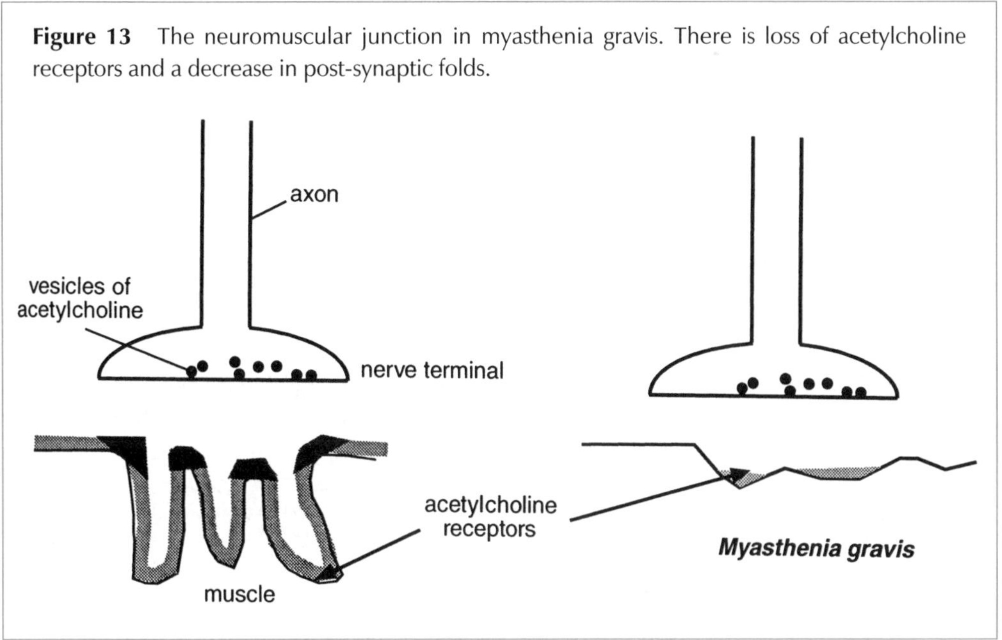

10.7 Duchenne muscular dystrophy

This is a genetic disease which is X-linked; it has the highest new mutation rate of any X-linked gene. It is caused by mutations in a protein called **dystrophin** which is part of a large complex of membrane-associated proteins, defects in most of which can cause forms of muscular dystrophy.

Dystrophin is a very large protein indeed (>400 kDa) which is attached at its C-terminus to laminin on the inner aspect of the muscle membrane and at its N-terminus to actin, thus providing a connection between the extracellular matrix and the muscle cytoskeleton. Therefore, its role is probably structural.

The most common mutations are large deletions which can be either of the following:

- **In frame** in which the C-terminus and N-terminus of the molecule are preserved and a truncated form of dystrophin missing some of the rod domain is produced leading to Becker dystrophy, a milder form of the disease compatible with a normal lifespan and prolonged ambulation.
- **Out of frame** which results in total abolition of dystrophin production because one or both of the binding sites for actin or laminin is disrupted. This is the abnormality which leads to typical Duchenne muscular dystrophy.

Figure 14 Dystrophin is an extremely large protein which links the cytoskeleton (actin) to the extracellular matrix of muscle

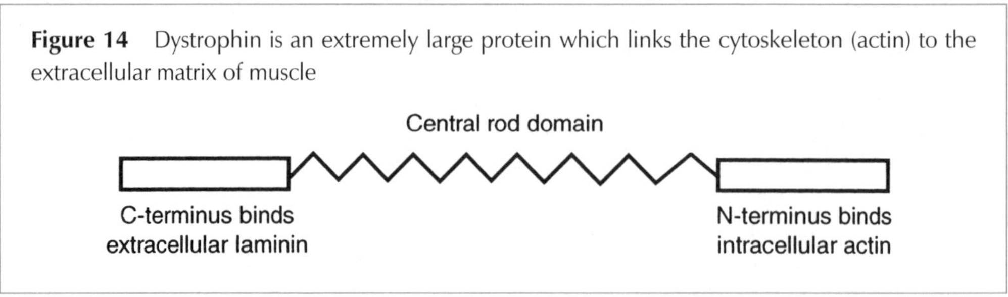

The very occasional finding of affected females can be due to the following:

- **Lyonisation**: X-chromosome inactivation occurring non-randomly and leading to preferential inactivation of the normal chromosome.
- Very rarely, **X-autosome translocation**. The presence of a fragment of an autosome in the region where dystrophin is normally found leads to the preferential activation of this chromosome and inactivation of the normal chromosome.

The clinical features of Duchenne muscular dystrophy are described in Chapter 16, Neurology.

10.8 Sickle cell disease

It has been known for five decades that haemoglobin from patients with this disease undergoes abnormal electrophoretic mobility. The basis for this is the presence, in all patients with the disease, of a single amino acid substitution of valine for glutamic acid in the haemoglobin (HbS) β-globin subunit. Haemoglobin has to be highly soluble to pack into red cells at high concentrations and the sickle mutation leads to polymerisation of HbS and consequent loss of solubility. The reason that polymerisation takes place is that, in its deoxygenated form, the HbS β-globin subunit can bind to a partner β-subunit on another strand leading to the formation of large polymers (see diagram), which deform the

Figure 15 Sickle cell disease. In sickle cell disease HbS undergoes abnormal depolymerisation when deoxygenated

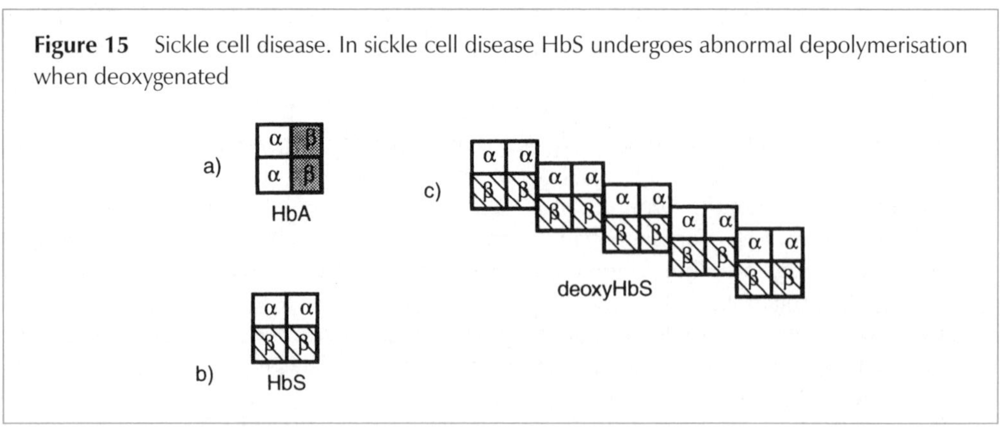

red cell by damaging the membrane and interfering with ion flux. The polymerisation process is a dynamic event under the influence of the oxygenation state of the cell and the intracellular concentration of Hb which accounts in part for the variable clinical manifestations of the disease.

- The unpredictable nature of the vaso-occlusive events observed in patients has been explained because the SS red cells have a greater propensity for attachment to vascular endothelium. The degree of stickiness to endothelium is determined primarily by the rapidity of polymer formation which in turn is dependent on the rapidity of deoxygenation.
- The binding of sickle red cells to endothelium appears to be mediated by the interaction between integrins on the cell membrane and adhesion molecules expressed on the vascular endothelial surface.
- The presence of proinflammatory cytokines such as TNF stimulates this process, which explains why infection of any kind can provoke a sickle crisis.
- One factor that has been shown to modify the rate of polymer formation is the presence of fetal haemoglobin (HbF), which slows the rate of polymer formation.
- Certain ethnic subpopulations have higher amounts of fetal Hb persisting in the circulation and milder SS disease.
- This suggests that pharmacological upregulation of HbF could ameliorate the disease. Hydroxyurea has been shown to increase the amount of HbF and is now widely used in the prevention of sickle crises. The risk of tumours from this cytotoxic drug appears to be small and any myelosuppression is reversible.

The clinical features of sickle cell disease are discussed in Chapter 9, Haematology.

11. GLOSSARY OF TERMS IN MOLECULAR MEDICINE

Allele: one of several different forms of a gene occupying a given genetic locus.

Annealing: the pairing of complementary strands of DNA to form a double helix.

Apoptosis: the morphological changes accompanying the process of programmed cell death.

Autocrine: secretion of substances by cells which then act on the cells themselves rather than on a distant target.

cDNA: a single-stranded DNA complementary to an RNA, synthesised from it by the enzyme reverse transcriptase in vitro.

Cell cycle: the period from one cell division to the next.

Cytokines: act locally and their effect can be positive or negative depending on the environment, other cytokines, the physiological state of the cell and the extracellular matrix. This variable response of cytokines underlies the ability of the organism to maintain a wide repertoire of responses to tissue injury.

DNA polymerase: an enzyme that synthesises a daughter strand of DNA on a DNA template.

Exon: any segment of an interrupted gene which is represented in the mature RNA product.

Gene family: consists of a set of genes the exons of which are related; the members were derived from a common ancestral gene by duplication and subsequent variation.

Gene targeting: the creation of animals (usually mice) which are null mutants for a particular gene. That is, the gene has been 'knocked out' and the 'knockout' mouse contains no copy of the gene at all.

G-protein: heterotrimeric membrane protein that is activated by the exchange of GDP for GTP and dissociates on activation into an α and $\beta\gamma$ subunits. It has intrinsic GTPase activity which mediates its inactivation.

Growth factor: a hormone that induces cell division and differentiation.

Heterozygote: an individual with different alleles on each chromosome at a given locus.

Housekeeping genes: constitutively expressed genes in all cells because they provide basic functions needed for survival of all cell types.

Hybridoma: a cell line produced by fusing a myeloma with a lymphocyte; it can indefinitely express the immunoglobulin of both cells, unless the myeloma has been selected to be deficient in Ig expression.

Introns: sequences of DNA that are transcribed but removed from nascent mRNA by splicing.

Isoform: one of a number of different forms of a protein that may be derived from one gene by splicing or from separate closely related members of a gene family.

Oligonucleotide: a short sequence of (synthetic) DNA, typically 18–22 base pairs in length, which acts as a primer for PCR reactions or a molecular probe when detecting gene sequences.

Oncogene: a gene whose protein product (the oncoprotein) has the ability to transform eukaryotic cells so that they grow in a manner analogous to tumour cells.

Paracrine: secretion by one cell of substances that act on adjacent cells.

Programmed cell death: the process whereby unwanted cells die under the control of a genetic programme.

Promoter: a region of DNA involved in the binding of RNA polymerase to initiate transcription.

Protein kinase: an enzyme that phosphorylates (adds a phosphate group) to a substrate (an amino acid in another protein).

Protein phosphatase: an enzyme that removes phosphate groups from substrates.

Proto-oncogene: the normal counterpart in eukaryotic genomes of retroviral genes which can transform cells.

Response elements: specific nucleotide recognition sequences in the 5′ regulatory regions of genes which recognise transcription factors that have been activated by upstream signals such as steroid hormones.

Somatic cells: all the cells of an organism except the germ cells.

Transcription factor: a protein that binds to the promoter region of a gene to influence its transcription.

Tumour suppressor gene: a gene that, when activated, will produce a protein that inhibits cell division. Mutations of these genes therefore lead to loss of control of cell division and contribute to tumorigenesis.

Chapter 15
Nephrology

CONTENTS

Nephrology

1. RENAL PHYSIOLOGY

The chief functions of the kidneys are:

- Excretion of water-soluble waste
- Maintenance of electrolyte balance
- Maintenance of water balance
- Acid–base homeostasis
- Endocrine: Renin–angiotensin–aldosterone system, erythropoietin, vitamin D activation.

1.1 Glomerular filtration rate (GFR)

Glomerular filtration is a passive process which depends upon the net hydrostatic pressure acting across the glomerular capillaries, countered by the oncotic pressure, and also influenced by the intrinsic permeability of the glomerulus (K_f); the latter may vary due to mesangial cell contraction, such as in response to angiotensin II. The mean values for GFR in normal young adults are 130 $ml \cdot min^{-1} \cdot 1.73\ m^{-2}$ (men) and 120 $ml \cdot min^{-1} \cdot 1.73\ m^{-2}$ (women), the 1.73 m^2 being mean body surface area of young adults. However, variation between individuals is large and accepted ranges of GFR at this age are 70–140 $ml \cdot min^{-1} \cdot 1.73\ m^{-2}$. In health, GFR remains stable until around 40 years of age but thereafter declines at a rate of approximately 1 $ml \cdot min^{-1} \cdot year^{-1}$; by the age of 80 years the mean GFR is approximately 50% of that of a young adult.

- GFR increases by 50% in the first trimester of pregnancy (*see* Chapter 12, Maternal Medicine).
- GFR has a diurnal rhythm, values being 10% greater in the afternoon than at midnight. This may be partly related to protein intake (which increases GFR).
- GFR falls transiently during exercise.

There are several means of calculating GFR:

- **Plasma creatinine**: creatinine is produced from muscle cells at a constant rate, and so its plasma concentration at steady state depends upon its excretion, which reflects GFR. Plasma creatinine is therefore useful to crudely assess GFR. However, when renal function is well preserved, small changes in creatinine are associated with large changes in GFR, and so plasma creatinine is an insensitive marker of early renal disease.

When considering plasma creatinine values, the patient's age, sex and weight should be taken into account (see below) – the elderly and malnourished patients may have low GFR but plasma creatinine close to the normal range.

- **Creatinine clearance**: usually calculated from a 24-hour urine collection with a consecutive blood sample.

$$\text{Creatinine clearance} = \frac{\text{Ucr} \times \text{Uv} \times 1000}{\text{Pcr} \times 24 \times 60} \text{ ml/min,}$$

where U = urine, P = plasma, v = volume and cr = creatinine concentration (μmol/l). This tends to overestimate GFR as creatinine is not just filtered, but also secreted into the tubule from the post-glomerular circulation; the error increases with declining renal function. Note that certain drugs (eg trimethoprim and cimetidine) compete for this secretion mechanism, and so will increase plasma creatinine.

- **Cockcroft and Gault formula**: a useful means of estimating GFR; it only requires knowledge of the patient's age, weight and plasma creatinine.

$$\text{GFR (ml/min)} = \frac{(140 - \text{age in years}) \times \text{weight (kg)}}{\text{plasma creatinine } (\mu\text{mol/l})} \times 1.23 \text{ (men) or } 1.04 \text{ (women).}$$

This formula overestimates creatinine clearance in obese patients and in those patients adhering to a strict low-protein diet (in both of these groups the endogenous creatinine production will be less than that predicted by overall body weight). A correction should be undertaken for body surface area.

The most accurate laboratory techniques for assessing GFR are:

- **inulin clearance**: inulin is a small molecule, freely filtered by the glomerulus, and with no tubular secretion
- **chromium-labelled EDTA**: the most frequently used isotopic technique.

1.2 Tubular physiology

The renal tubule has many reabsorptive and secretory functions (see figure below); these are energy-consuming and hence tubular cells are those most vulnerable to ischaemic damage (the acute tubular necrosis (ATN) of ischaemic acute renal failure).

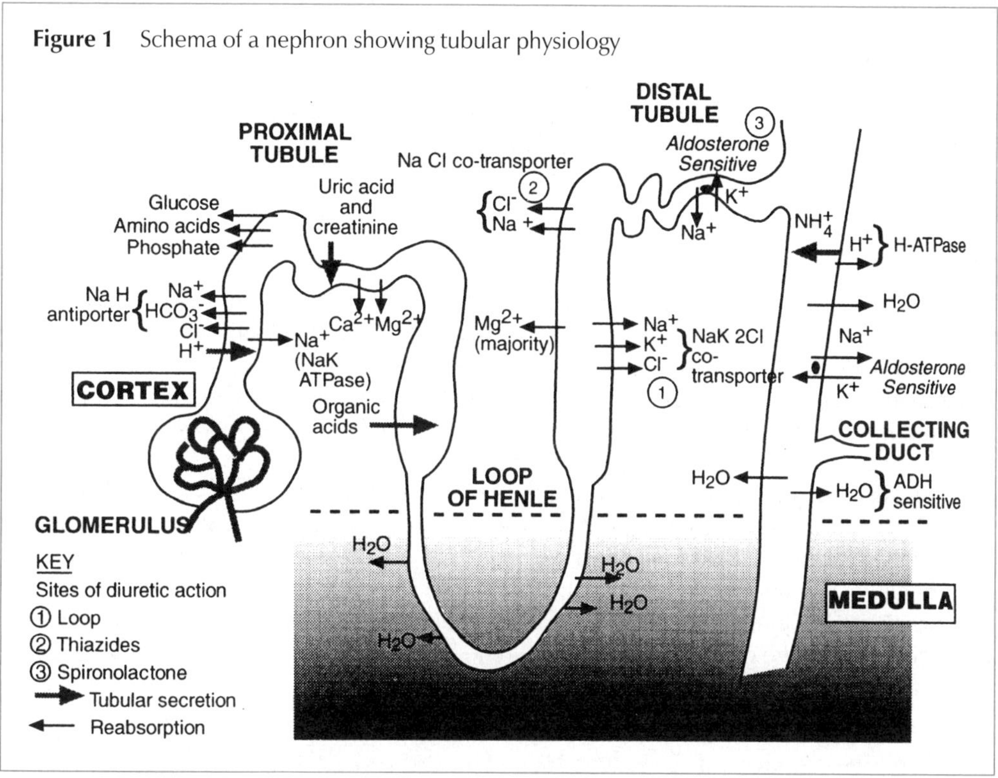

Figure 1 Schema of a nephron showing tubular physiology

Proximal tubule

Fifty per cent of filtered sodium is reabsorbed within the proximal tubule (via Na K ATPase); the Na H antiporter secretes H^+ into the lumen and is responsible for 90% of bicarbonate and some chloride reabsorption. All of the filtered glucose and amino acids are reabsorbed here. Other important characteristics are as follows:

- Phosphate reabsorption occurs under the influence of parathyroid hormone (PTH).
- Some important drugs are secreted into the tubular filtrate here: trimethoprim, cimetidine, most β-lactams and most diuretics (note that diuretics such as thiazides, amiloride and loop diuretics are highly protein-bound and are not filtered at the glomerulus).
- Creatinine and urate are secreted into the lumen.

Loop of Henle

The medullary concentration gradient is generated here; the medullary thick ascending limb (mTAL) is impermeable to water. Forty per cent of sodium is reabsorbed (via the Na K 2Cl co-transporter). Loop diuretics compete for chloride-binding sites on this transporter.

Distal tubule

In this segment of the nephron 5% of sodium is reabsorbed (Na Cl co-transporter); thiazide diuretics compete for these chloride-binding sites. As loop diuretics increase sodium delivery to the distal tubule, their combination with a thiazide (eg metolazone) can provoke a massive diuresis in resistant oedema. There are aldosterone receptors in both the distal and collecting tubules (see below).

Collecting duct

Aldosterone-sensitive sodium channels are responsible for 2% of all sodium re-absorption; spironolactone binds to the cytoplasmic aldosterone receptor. Atrial natriuretic peptide (ANP) is also anti-aldosterone in action (and hence is increased in renal failure and in patients with congestive cardiac failure (CCF), where it is thought to be counteractive against secondary hyperaldosteronism). Other important collecting duct functions are as follows:

- H^+ is secreted into lumen by H-ATPase, so forming ammonia/NH_4^+ (urinary acidification).
- Antidiuretic hormone (ADH, or vasopressin) increases water reabsorption by opening 'water channels'. G-protein-coupled receptors on the basolateral membrane (non-luminal) of the collecting duct cell are stimulated by ADH, leading to insertion of **aquaporins** into the luminal membrane. The aquaporins then allow water uptake by the cell.
- Lithium enters the collecting duct cells via the sodium channels and inhibits the response to ADH (hence, nephrogenic diabetes insipidus (NDI) results).

1.3 Renin–angiotensin–aldosterone (RAA) system

This is covered in Chapter 4, Endocrinology. The RAA system has a central role in the pathogenesis of many cases of secondary renal hypertension (see below). Remember that intra-renal perfusion will become critically dependent upon the RAA when hypovolaemia and hypotension supervene; this explains why patients can be vulnerable to acute renal failure induced by angiotensin converting enzyme (ACE) inhibitors (and now, angiotensin II receptor blockers, AIIRB) even in the absence of renovascular disease.

- As well as the effects of the RAA in provoking renal-related hypertension, the system (and particularly, angiotensin II) is also of key importance in the pathogenesis of progressive renal disease, irrespective of the primary disease aetiology.
- Angiotensin is not only a vasoconstrictor; it also stimulates scarring, and indirectly (due to hyperfiltration), further nephron loss within damaged renal tissue.
- This is the reason why ACE inhibitors and/or AIIRBs are now considered to be essential therapy in patients with a variety of chronic nephropathies.

2. RENAL INVESTIGATION

2.1 Urinalysis

Urinary dipstick

Standard dipsticks assess the presence of protein, blood and glucose. 'Multi-stix' will also assess pH (range 4.5–8 but normally 5–6; pH>8 suggests renal tubular acidosis, for example) and leukocytes (most commonly raised because of vaginal contamination of urine or urinary tract infection).

- The sticks register positive for 'blood' in the presence of erythrocytes, as well as free myoglobin (eg in rhabdomyolysis) and haemoglobin. Many cases of 'dipstick +ve, microscopy –ve (absence of red cells on MSU) haematuria' are seen, and these are presumably due to haemoglobinuria (eg exercise, low-grade haemolysis).
- Standard dipsticks do not detect Bence–Jones proteins, and so if free urinary light chains are to be identified immunoelectrophoresis of urine is necessary.
- Microalbuminuria (see below) may not be detected either.

Proteinuria

Normal urinary protein excretion is <150 mg/day, and this consists of <30 mg albumin, tubular secreted proteins (40–60 mg), such as the Tamm–Horsfall or tubular glycoprotein and immunoglobulin, and various filtered low-molecular-weight proteins.

- **Microalbuminuria**, which is the hallmark of early diabetic nephropathy but which is also prognostically important when present in hypertensive patients, is defined as albumin excretion of 30–300 mg/day.
- The urinary **albumin (mg): creatinine (mmol) excretion ratio (ACR)** is often used to quantify proteinuria in clinical practice – normal ACR <2.5, microalbuminuric range 2.5–33, nephrotic range >400.

Significant non-nephrotic proteinuria (eg dipstick + to +++, 0.2–3.5 g/24 h) is usually indicative of renal parenchymal disease (unless due to urinary tract infection). **Nephrotic** range proteinuria (>3.5 g/24 h, dipstick ++++) is always due to glomerular disease.

Non-renal causes of proteinuria:

- fever
- severe exercise
- skin disease (eg severe exfoliation, psoriasis)
- lower urinary tract infection (eg cystitis).

Orthostatic proteinuria

This describes proteinuria detectable after the patient has spent several hours in the upright posture; it disappears after recumbency, and so the first morning urine should test negative. Proteinuria is usually <1 g/24 h, there is no haematuria and renal function and blood pressure are normal. Renal biopsy samples are usually normal and nephrological consensus suggests this is a benign condition.

Urine microscopy

Microscopic examination of a fresh specimen of urine may yield many helpful pointers to intrinsic renal pathology.

- **Red cells**: >2–3/high power field is pathological (microscopic haematuria); cells are usually dysmorphic in glomerular bleeding, but appear normal when derived from the lower urinary tract.
- **Leukocytes**: infection, and some cases of glomerular and interstitial nephritis.
- **Crystals**: eg oxalate, struvite (*see* Section 10.1 on renal calculi), cystine and, with polarised light, uric acid.
- **Casts**: there are several types of cast:
  Tubular cells – acute tubular necrosis (ATN) or interstitial nephritis
  Hyaline – Tamm–Horsfall glycoprotein (ie in normals)
  Granular – non-specific
  Red cell – glomerulonephritis or tubular bleeding
  Leukocytes – pyelonephritis or ATN.

Causes of urinary discoloration

- Haematuria
- Myoglobinuria (brown)
- Beetroot consumption
- Alkaptonuria (urine brown on exposure to the air)
- Obstructive jaundice (yellow)
- Haemoglobinuria
- Drugs (eg rifampicin, para-aminosalicylic acid)
- Porphyria (urine dark brown or red on standing)

2.2 Renal radiology

The essential first-line radiological investigation for acute (ARF) or chronic (CRF) renal failure, and most other nephrological conditions, is **renal ultrasound**. This will demonstrate:

- **Bipolar renal length**: in most cases of **CRF**, the kidneys are small (<8 cm) – the exceptions are polycystic kidney disease (very large with multiple cysts), and sometimes in diabetic renal disease and amyloid (normal size). In **ARF** the kidneys are usually normal size (8.5–13.5 cm), but slight enlargement is common due to swelling. Asymmetry

(>1.5 cm disparity) is seen in unilateral renal artery stenosis (RAS), but also in chronic pyelonephritis and other causes of renal atrophy.

- **Obstruction**.
- **Cortical scarring**: for example in reflux nephropathy or following segmental ischaemic damage.
- **Calculi**: within the substance of the kidney and collecting systems.
- **Mass lesions and cysts**: (eg renal tumour, polycystic disease or simple renal cysts).

Doppler ultrasound is useful to assess renal blood flow and to measure the resistive index within the kidney; specific patterns are observed in eg RAS, acute tubular necrosis and acute transplant rejection.

Intravenous urography (IVU) is reserved for investigation of urinary tract bleeding (eg to detect urothelial tumours of the renal pelvis, ureters and bladder), UTI and for some cases of obstructive uropathy. IVU can exacerbate ARF (*see* Section 4.3 Radio-contrast nephropathy), and has very limited value in advanced CRF (eg creatinine >250 μmol/l) because of poor concentration of the dye.

Isotope renography

Two major types of renograms are commonly utilised:

- **Static scans (eg DMSA)**: the isotope is concentrated and retained within the renal parenchyma, and elimination is slow. DMSA will therefore demonstrate aspects of structure (eg scars in reflux nephropathy) and split function of the two kidneys.
- **Dynamic scans (eg MAG_3, DTPA, Hippuran)**: these isotopes are rapidly taken up and eliminated by the kidneys; such scans are used to assess renal blood flow, split function and also to investigate obstruction (eg to show whether urinary tract dilatation is due to obstruction).

Captopril renography: this involves a dynamic scan (eg MAG_3) which is then repeated 1 hour after an oral dose of captopril (utilised because it is the shortest acting ACE inhibitor). Changes in the renographic curves (eg delay in time-to-peak, cortical retention of isotope) can be indicative of significant RAS.

Renal angiography

The most frequently used techniques are:

- **MRA**: non-invasive and now an excellent screening investigation for RAS. Gadolinium (non-nephrotoxic when given iv) is used as the 'contrast' agent.
- **CT angiography (CTA)**: non-invasive and readily available, but risk of contrast nephropathy in renal impairment, diabetics, etc.
- **i.a. angiography**: provides excellent detail of intra-renal vasculature; invasive and risk of contrast nephropathy. Now less frequently used because of the availability of MRA and CTA.

Renal tract CT and MR

These imaging modalities are commonly used in nephro-urology in the investigation of many conditions including:

- delineation of cause of obstruction
- assessment of renal tract tumours, including staging
- assessment of renal cyst structure.

3. ACID–BASE, WATER AND ELECTROLYTE DISORDERS

3.1 Acidosis and alkalosis

Respiratory acidosis (eg carbon dioxide retention due to chronic or acute-on-chronic lung disease) and **alkalosis** (eg due to hyperventilation) are common, and well understood by all.

Metabolic alkalosis and **metabolic acidosis** are covered in detail in Chapter 13, Metabolic Diseases. The width of the anion gap can help differentiate the likely causes of a metabolic acidosis; the HCO_3 will be low, and the anion gap can be either wide (normal chloride and exogenous acid) or normal (increased chloride and, hence, hyperchloraemic acidosis). Renal failure is associated with a wide gap acidosis (due to excess ammonia and organic acids), whereas **renal tubular acidosis** is worth consideration as a cause of a normal gap acidosis.

3.2 Renal tubular acidosis (RTA)

Distal or **type 1** RTA is fairly common, and can complicate many renal parenchymal disorders, particularly those which predominantly affect the medullary regions. Note that the latter may also be associated with nephrogenic diabetes insipidus, and sometimes with salt-wasting states. **Proximal** or **type 2** RTA is uncommon. GFR is usually normal in both conditions.

- **Nephrocalcinosis and renal calculi formation**: urinary calcium excretion is increased in severe acidosis, and calcium salts are more insoluble in alkaline urine, and hence calculi develop frequently in distal but not in proximal RTA (which is usually associated with a lower urinary pH and less severe acidosis).

The two types of RTA can be differentiated by several parameters, but the hallmark associations are severe acidosis, hypokalaemia and renal calculi/nephrocalcinosis in **distal RTA**, and proximal tubular dysfunction, osteomalacia/rickets and less severe acidosis in **proximal RTA**.

	Type 1 (Distal)	Type 2 (Proximal)
Defect	Impaired urinary (H^+) acidification	Failure of HCO_3 reabsorption
Urine pH	>5.3 (ie urine never 'acidifies')	Variable
Plasma HCO_3	<10 mmol/l	14–20 mmol/l
Plasma K	Usually ↓	Normal or ↓
Complications	Nephrocalcinosis Calculi	Osteomalacia (phosphate wasting) Rickets
Other features	Growth failure Urine infection	Fanconi syndrome (ie phosphaturia, glycosuria, aminoaciduria)

Treatment of RTA: this is usually straightforward (compared to an understanding of the condition!), and consists of oral potassium and bicarbonate replacement therapy. Close monitoring is needed to prevent major imbalances in electrolyte concentrations, especially during inter-current illness.

Causes of distal RTA

- **Primary**
  Genetic (dominant) or idiopathic
- **Secondary to autoimmune diseases**
  Systemic lupus erythematosus (SLE), Sjögren's syndrome, chronic active hepatitis
- **Tubulointerstitial disease**
  Chronic pyelonephritis, transplant rejection, obstructive uropathy, chronic interstitial nephritis
- **Nephrocalcinosis**
  Medullary sponge kidney, hypercalcaemia
- **Drugs and toxins**
  Lithium, amphotericin, toluene

Causes of proximal RTA

- **Occurring alone**
  Idiopathic
- **With Fanconi syndrome**
  Wilson's disease, cystinosis, fructose intolerance, Sjögren's syndrome
- **Tubulointerstitial disease**
  Interstitial nephritis, myeloma, amyloidosis
- **Drugs and toxins**
  Outdated tetracyclines, streptozotocin, lead and mercury (and other heavy metals), acetazolamide, sulphonamides

Type 4 RTA

This describes a metabolic acidosis that is associated with hyperkalaemia and mild renal impairment (GFR usually >30 ml/min). It is commonly due to **mineralocorticoid deficiency**:

- Low renin, low aldosterone (hyporeninaemic hypoaldosteronism): diabetes mellitus, and drugs (NSAIDS and ciclosporin).
- High renin, low aldosterone: adrenal destruction, congenital enzyme defects and drugs (ACE inhibitors and AIIRBs).

Abnormal collecting duct function (eg due to absent/defective mineralocorticoid receptor, chronic tubulointerstitial disease or drugs such as spironolactone or amiloride) is responsible for other cases.

3.3 Polyuria

Polyuria (urine output >3 l/day) may result from:

- diuretic usage
- large fluid intake (eg alcohol): inhibits ADH release
- cranial diabetes insipidus: osmolality high
- nephrogenic diabetes insipidus: osmolality high; note that the polyuria (often manifest as nocturia) is often the first symptom of CRF
- psychogenic polydipsia: osmolality usually low
- atrial natriuretic peptide release: post-arrhythmia, cardiac failure.

The causes of **cranial** and **nephrogenic diabetes insipidus** are listed in Chapter 4, Endocrinology; hyponatraemia as well as other disorders of water balance, including syndrome of inappropriate ADH (**SIADH**), are also discussed in that chapter.

3.4 Hypokalaemia

Acute hypokalaemia can lead to muscle weakness and direct renal tubular cell injury (vacuolation). Chronic hypokalaemia is a cause of interstitial nephritis. The causes can be classified according to the **presence** or **absence** of **hypertension** with reference also to the **plasma renin activity** and **urinary potassium excretion**.

Causes of hypokalaemia

- **With hypertension** (potassium excretion usually >30 mmol/day)

High plasma renin activity	*Low plasma renin activity*
Renovascular disease	Primary hyperaldosteronism (including Conn's syndrome)
Accelerated-phase hypertension	Carbenoxolone*
Cushing's syndrome	Liquorice excess*
Renin-secreting tumour	11-β-hydroxy steroid dehydrogenase deficiency* ('apparent mineralocorticoid excess')
	Liddle's syndrome (see text)
	Glucocorticoid suppressible hyperaldosteronism (GSH)**

- **Without hypertension** (usually high plasma renin activity)

  High plasma renin activity
  Diuretic usage (urinary potassium excretion may be high or low)
  Gastro-intestinal tract losses (potassium excretion <30 mmol/day)
  Salt-wasting CRF (high potassium excretion)
  Bartter's syndrome (high potassium excretion – see text)
  Gitelman syndrome (see text)
  Secondary hyperaldosteronism (eg cardiac or hepatic failure – increased potassium excretion)

*11-β-hydroxy steroid dehydrogenase metabolises cortisol and prevents it from binding to the mineralocorticoid receptor. Acquired or congenital conditions in which this enzyme is inhibited have a Conn's phenotype (including patients taking liquorice in excess, and carbenoxolone). Patients may have acidosis rather than alkalosis
**GSH is rare and is due to a gene fusion which makes the hyperaldosteronism completely ACTH sensitive. The clue to diagnosis is a strong family history (autosomal dominant). Treatment is with glucocorticoids which lower the blood pressure

Bartter's syndrome

Severe hypokalaemia is consequent upon a salt-wasting state (increased sodium delivery to the distal tubule) that is due to defective chloride reabsorption (at the Na K 2Cl co-transporter) in the loop of Henle; inheritance is usually autosomal recessive. Patients have normal or low blood pressure and severe hyper-reninaemia (with hypertrophy of the juxtaglomerular apparatus) with consequent hyperaldosteronism; GFR is usually normal. Treatment is with large-dose potassium replacement; NSAIDs may also be beneficial.

Liddle's syndrome

This is an autosomal dominant syndrome of hypertension and variable degrees of hypokalaemic metabolic alkalosis. The patient appears to have primary hyperaldosteronism, but renin and aldosterone are suppressed and there is no response to spironolactone. The pathogenesis is associated with enhanced reabsorption of sodium in the distal nephron (amiloride-sensitive sodium channel). Treatment consists of salt restriction, potassium supplements and use of either amiloride or triamterene.

Gitelman syndrome

This condition can be either autosomal recessive or dominant, and is characterised by hypokalaemic metabolic alkalosis and also with hypocalciuria and hypomagnesaemia. Patients present at a later age than those with classic Bartter's syndrome and, like the latter, the blood pressure is low or normal and patients have hyper-reninaemic hyperaldosteronism. The metabolic abnormalities may lead to muscular weakness and tetany. Treatment is with magnesium and potassium supplements.

4. ACUTE RENAL FAILURE

4.1 Pathogenesis and management of acute renal failure

Acute deterioration of renal function is seen in up to 5% of all hospital admissions. The incidence of severe ARF (eg creatinine >500 μmol/l) increases with age; the overall annual incidence is approximately 150 per million in the UK, but this figure is six times greater in the >80-year-old group. Dialysis-requiring ARF occurs in 70 per million of the population annually. Oliguria is usual, and is defined as a daily urine output of <400–500 ml; this is the minimum volume to enable excretion of the daily waste products of metabolism.

Non-oliguric ARF occurs in 10%; this may be associated with drug toxicity (eg gentamicin or amphotericin), radio-contrast nephropathy and acute interstitial nephritis.

The majority (55%) of cases of ARF result from renal hypoperfusion and ischaemic damage; the resulting renal histopathological lesion is **acute tubular necrosis** (**ATN**). Many other patients may have similar ischaemic insults to the kidneys, with an initial period of oliguria, but renal perfusion can then be restored by vigorous haemodynamic management before severe tubular injury ensues; this is termed **pre-renal uraemia** and most cases can be managed without dialysis. In the latter, physiological mechanisms (ie stimulation of the RAA system) are preserved within the kidney, and so the urinary manifestations of sodium and water reabsorption allow differentiation from established ATN. In practice, the two conditions may sometimes only be differentiated by the clinical response to fluid resuscitation – patients with ATN will remain oliguric, whereas those with pre-renal uraemia will usually start diuresing.

Urinary findings	ATN	Pre-renal uraemia
Urine sodium	>40 mmol/l	<20 mmol/l
Urine: plasma osmolality	<1.1:1	>1.5:1
Fractional sodium excretion (FeNa)*	>1%	<<1%
Urine: plasma urea	<7:1	>10:1
Urine volume	Oligo-anuric or polyuria (recovery phase)	<1.5 litres

*FeNa is the percentage of sodium that is filtered at the glomerulus (normally 1000 mmol/h) which actually appears in the urine (normal <6 mmol/h, ie <0.6%)

Many patients with pre-existing chronic renal impairment or CRF present with acute deterioration of renal function ('**acute-on-chronic renal failure**') and require similarly intensive support and clinical management, although strictly they do not have ARF.

The causes of ARF, with approximate relative frequency, are summarised below.

Classification of ARF

- **Pre-renal factors leading to renal hypoperfusion and ATN (55%)**
  Reduced circulating volume: blood loss; excess GI losses; burns
  Low cardiac output states: toxic or ischaemic myocardial depression
  Systemic sepsis
  Drugs inducing renal perfusion shutdown: (eg ACE inhibitors; NSAIDs)
- **Toxic ATN (5%)**
  Rhabdomyolysis with urinary myoglobin
  Drugs: (eg gentamicin; amphotericin)
  Radio-contrast nephropathy
- **Structural abnormalities of renal vasculature (5%)**
  Large vessel occlusion (renovascular disease)
  Small vessel occlusion: accelerated-phase hypertension; DIC; haemolytic–uraemic syndrome; thrombotic thrombocytopenic purpura; pre-eclampsia; systemic sclerosis
  Acute cortical necrosis
- **Acute glomerulonephritis and vasculitis (15%)**
  Idiopathic crescentic glomerulonephritis
  ANCA-positive vasculitis
  Goodpasture's syndrome
  Other proliferative glomerulonephritis (eg SLE; endocarditis; Henoch–Schönlein nephritis)
- **Interstitial nephritis (5%)**
  Idiopathic, immunologically mediated
  Drug-induced hypersensitivity
  Infection (eg pyelonephritis; leptospirosis; Hanta virus)
- **Myeloma/tubular cast nephropathy (<5%)**
- **Urinary tract obstruction (10%)**

Pathophysiology of ATN

After an ischaemic insult there is intense afferent arteriolar vasoconstriction, mediated by the release of vasoconstrictors (particularly endothelin) and by loss of intrinsic vasodilators (nitric oxide and prostaglandin I_2 (PGI_2)); this contributes to the loss of GFR and the redistribution of blood flow within the kidney. Hypoxic injury to the energy-consuming cells of the proximal tubule and thick ascending limb of Henle occurs; calcium- and oxygen-free-radical-mediated cell necrosis results in cell shedding from the tubular basement membrane, with the formation of casts that block urine flow.

Investigation of ARF

The history may point to the cause of ARF (eg drugs, skin rash); assessment of the haemodynamic status is imperative, and appropriate fluid resuscitation should be given.

- **Urinary examination**: ATN and pre-renal uraemia can be differentiated by urinary biochemistry (see above); microscopic haematuria and red cell casts will point to acute glomerulonephritis as the cause.
- A **renal ultrasound** scan will usually show normal-sized (or swollen) kidneys, and will identify obstruction (the latter should be urgently treated to reduce irreversible renal injury).
- **Autoantibody profile**: ANF, ANCA, anti-GBM, complement and plasma and urinary electrophoresis should all be routinely performed (unless the cause of ARF is obvious, eg post-myocardial infarction or renal obstruction).
- **Percutaneous renal biopsy** is essential if an intrinsic lesion (eg vasculitis, glomerulonephritis, interstitial nephritis) is suspected, or if no ischaemic cause is apparent.

Management of ARF

The mainstay of treatment involves **optimisation of fluid balance** and avoidance of either hypovolaemia or fluid overload. Patients with single-organ ARF are best managed in an HDU setting. Blood pressure should be controlled, haemoglobin maintained around 10 g/dl and sepsis should be promptly and vigorously treated. 'Renal dose' dopamine and loop diuretics are often given in ATN, although there is no evidence that they alter the outcome of ARF in humans. Some cases of ATN can be managed without dialysis, with the adoption of careful fluid balance and dietary control; however, many patients with ATN also have multi-organ failure (MOF) and they can only be managed on an ICU.

The most important advances in ARF management have involved attention to **intensive nutritional support** of the sicker patients, and the use of **continuous renal replacement therapies** (eg CVVH: continuous veno-venous haemofiltration) which are less likely to provoke haemodynamic instability.

Other more specific treatments in ARF depend upon the causative condition and include the following:

Specific **immunosuppressive therapy**, and sometimes plasma exchange, may be appropriate for some conditions (eg Goodpasture's syndrome, ANCA +ve vasculitis).

Obstruction: bladder catheterisation for bladder outflow obstruction; nephrostomy drainage for renal obstruction.

Other: eg steroids in acute interstitial nephritis (AIN), plasma exchange in HUS and TTP, chemotherapy in myeloma.

Indications for urgent dialysis in ARF

- **Severe uraemia**
  (eg vomiting, encephalopathy, urea > 60 mmol/l)
- **Severe acidosis**
  pH <7.1
- **Pulmonary oedema**
- **Hyperkalaemia**
  K >6.5 mmol/l (or less, if ECG changes apparent)
- **Uraemic pericarditis**

Prognosis of ARF

The survival prognosis for patients with ARF remains only moderate; 55–60% of patients who require dialytic therapy survive, but this figure partly reflects the very poor outcome of patients who have ATN as a component of MOF who are managed on the ICU. For example, only 10–20% of those with three- or four-organ failure will survive, yet 90% of patients with ARF in isolation survive.

The prognosis for **recovery of renal function** varies according to the causative condition; > 90% show full renal recovery in AIN, but this is the case in <50% of cases with autoimmune vasculitis. In survivors of ATN, renal function will return to the normal range in 60%, whereas 30% will be left with CRF and 10% will be dialysis-dependent.

4.2 Rhabdomyolysis

Muscle damage with release of myoglobin can cause severe, hypercatabolic ARF. Serum potassium and phosphate (released from muscle) rapidly rise, calcium is typically low and the creatine kinase massively elevated; serum creatinine may be disproportionately higher than urea. Primary management involves intravascular fluid expansion with the encouragement of diuresis; there is some evidence that alkalinisation of the urine (with IV bicarbonate) helps to solubilise the myoglobin pigment within the renal tubules. Sometimes the source of the rhabdomyolytic process requires specific therapy (eg fasciotomy for compartment syndrome, debridement of dead tissue and amputation of non-viable limbs).

Causes of rhabdomyolysis

- **Crush injury**
  Trauma; unconsciousness with compression
- **Metabolic myopathies**
  (eg McArdle's syndrome)
- **Infections**
  Viral necrotising myositis, infectious mononucleosis (eg Coxsackie influenza)
- **Uncontrolled fitting**
- **Drugs**
  (eg statins)
- **Overdose**
  Barbiturates, alcohol, heroin
- **Severe exercise, heat stroke, burns**
- **Inflammatory myopathies**
  Polymyositis
- **Malignant hyperpyrexia**

Prognosis of rhabdomyolysis

Patient survival in rhabdomyolysis depends upon the nature and extent of the underlying causative pathology. However, in survivors the prognosis for full renal functional recovery is usually good.

4.3 Radio-contrast nephropathy

Mild renal dysfunction may complicate up to 10% of angiographic procedures and IVUs. Radio-contrast nephropathy is manifest by non-oliguric ARF, typically occurring 1–5 days after the procedure. Intra-renal vasoconstriction, mediated largely by endothelin, and tubular cell toxicity (with ATN) are important in the pathogenesis. The ARF is fully reversible. Recent attention has been directed to prevention of radio-contrast nephropathy with:

- Pre-hydration of patients at greatest risk (eg with N-saline infusion before and during the procedure).
- *N*-Acetyl cysteine (given orally for 2–3 days, from before to 24 hours post-procedure).

Risk factors for radio-contrast nephropathy

- High contrast load
- Hypovolaemia
- Myeloma
- Age
- Hyperuricaemia
- High iodine content of contrast
- Diabetes mellitus*
- Hypercalcaemia
- Pre-existing CRF

*Especially if the patient is taking metformin – this should be withdrawn before injection of radio-contrast

5. CHRONIC RENAL FAILURE (CHRONIC KIDNEY DISEASE) AND RENAL REPLACEMENT THERAPY

5.1 Chronic renal failure (CRF)

A changing nomenclature now sees the term chronic kidney disease (CKD) used interchangeably with CRF. When describing the epidemiology of CRF, distinction has to be made between:

- end-stage renal failure (ESRF, also termed end-stage renal disease, ESRD) at which stage patients require renal replacement therapy (RRT, ie dialysis or transplantation) and
- less severe, but often progressive, degrees of chronic renal disease (CRF or CKD).

CRF is very common, and the prevalence is thought to be at least 2000 patients per million. The incidence of ESRD patients joining RRT programmes in the UK is 80–125/million each year; the figure is almost 300/million in parts of the USA (because of racial factors and increased population prevalence of diabetes mellitus and hypertension). The prevalence of patients on UK RRT programmes is around 600/million, but as ageing constitutes one of the major risk factors for CRF and ESRD, the prevalence is greatest in people aged >65 years (eg 1000/million, or 0.1%, receiving RRT).

There are several recognised stages of **CRF/CKD**:

- CKD stage 1: Loss of renal reserve – GFR >90 ml/min*.
- CKD stage 2: Mild renal impairment – GFR 60–89 ml/min*. Note that creatinine may be at the **top end of the normal range**. Hypertension control should be optimally treated and use of ACE inhibitors considered (see below).
- CKD stage 3: **moderate CRF** – GFR 30–59 ml/min; this (and stage 4) is also referred to as 'azotaemia' in the USA, as plasma urea and creatinine exceed normal levels. Renal anaemia and secondary hyperparathyroidism begin to complicate this level of renal dysfunction.
- CKD stage 4: **severe CRF** – GFR 15–29 ml/min; patients may have uraemic symptoms. Patients should receive counselling on the need for future RRT at this stage, and elective commencement of dialysis planned (ie rather than allowing development of severe uraemia which would need emergency dialysis). Dialysis access should be planned; transplant work-up should occur at a GFR of around 20 ml/min with the aim of transplant listing (for a pre-emptive transplant) at GFR 15 ml/min.
- CKD stage 5: **ESRD** – GFR <15 ml/min. The patient will require RRT, unless conservative treatment agreed. If RRT is commenced late (eg when GFR <5 ml/min) then there is a risk of developing a life-threatening uraemic syndrome.

*With evidence of renal disease (eg abnormal renal imaging or urinalysis).

Although many cases of CRF progress insidiously, so that very abnormal biochemistry is relatively well-tolerated by the patient, about one-third of dialysis patients initially present as uraemic emergencies (which carries a twofold worse prognosis). The key parameters that **differentiate CRF from ARF** are:

- small kidneys at imaging
- anaemia
- renal bone disease
- clinical tolerance of very severe uraemia.

Causes of CRF (approximate relative frequencies)

- **Most common causes of ESRD in UK***
  Diabetic nephropathy (25%)
  Chronic glomerulonephritis (15%)
  Hypertension (15%) – renovascular disease may co-exist in >1/2 of cases
  Chronic pyelonephritis (12%) – most often due to reflux nephropathy, but also renal calculi (nephrolithiasis) with infection
  Polycystic kidney disease (8%)
  Obstructive uropathy (5%)
  Chronic interstitial nephritis (4%) – eg sarcoidosis, lithium toxicity, myeloma
  Post-acute renal failure (3%)
  Amyloidosis (1%)
- **Rarer causes of CRF**
  Analgesic nephropathy
  Other hereditary disorders – eg Alport's syndrome
  Toxic nephropathy
  Following nephrectomy for renal tumours

*In at least 10% of cases of ESRD, the aetiology remains unknown. These are patients presenting with small kidneys on ultrasound, and in whom renal biopsy will be diagnostically unhelpful. Most likely diagnoses are hypertension, chronic glomerulonephritis or pyelonephritis, or dysplastic kidneys

Pathogenesis and management of progressive renal dysfunction in CRF

Although the majority of cases of CRF are slowly progressive towards ESRD, patients with particular pathologies (eg post-obstructive atrophy, and hypertension – when controlled) may manifest stable CRF for many years. The pathogenesis of the progressive renal dysfunction is multifactorial. It is thought that angiotensin plays a major role; this vasoactive mediator not only exacerbates the intraglomerular hypertension seen in remaining nephrons, but it also stimulates fibrosis within the tubulointerstitium (see Section 1.3 on renin–angiotensin–aldosterone axis). Proteinuria may also directly damage tubular cells. Hence the **management** of patients with CRF requires attention to:

- **Control of blood pressure**: it is imperative to optimise blood pressure control. Target blood pressures for patients with CRF are equivalent to those required for treatment of diabetic nephropathy (eg <125/75 mmHg if significant proteinuria). Hypertension control can slow the progression towards ESRD, and **ACE inhibitors and angiotensin II blockers** are logical agents to choose because of their effects upon angiotensin. The importance of optimal blood pressure control has been shown in observational studies; for example, diabetic patients with optimal control may lose GFR at a rate of only 1–2 ml/min per year whereas those with poor blood pressure and glycaemic control deteriorate rapidly towards ESRD, losing GFR at 8–16 ml/min per year.

- **Reduction of proteinuria**: heavy urinary protein losses (eg > g/day) are associated with an increased rate of progression in many cases of CRF. Amelioration of proteinuria by use of ACE inhibitors and AIIRB may also slow progression.
- **Dietary modification**: it is now widely accepted that patients with advanced CRF should maintain a normal protein and high calorie intake to avoid malnutrition (and a consequent increased likelihood of morbidity) in the phase leading up to RRT. Very severely restricted protein intakes (eg the 18–21 g/day Giovannetti diet) are only used as a conservative means of limiting uraemia in a minority of patients. However, phosphate restriction and dietary modification of salt and potassium intake should be instituted at an early stage of CRF.
- **Endocrine complications**: anaemia and renal osteodystrophy may begin during CKD stages 2 and 3, and hence early attention should be directed to these endocrine complications (see below).
- **Cardiovascular disease prevention**: CRF creates a pro-atherosclerotic environment due to factors such as hypertension, mixed hyperlipidaemia, hyperhomocystinaemia, anaemia, hyperparathyroidism and, when present, diabetes mellitus. Major complications include congestive cardiomyopathy, left ventricular hypertrophy (LVH), vascular calcification, coronary artery disease, stroke and peripheral vascular disease. Patients with CRF therefore have a marked increase in CVS mortality compared to the general population; the importance of early treatment with statins and aspirin is now the subject of a multi-centre trial.

5.2 Anaemia of CRF

The anaemia of CRF usually first appears when GFR is <50 ml/min; if untreated, it is a major contributor to morbidity in patients with advanced CRF. The major cause is the lack of endogenous erythropoietin (EPO) secretion by the damaged kidneys, but other factors which predispose to the anaemia are listed below:

- Reduced dietary iron intake due to anorexia
- Uraemia has toxic effect upon precursor cells in bone marrow
- Blood loss due to capillary fragility and platelet dysfunction (probably of minor importance)
- Impaired intestinal absorption of iron
- Reduced RBC survival (particularly in haemodialysis patients)

Patients with polycystic kidney disease are less likely to be anaemic as they tend to have greater intrinsic EPO levels than other patients with similar degrees of CRF. In general, haemodialysis patients have more severe anaemia, and a poorer response to EPO therapy, than their counterparts receiving continuous ambulatory peritoneal dialysis (CAPD). This may be because haemodialysis represents an 'inflammatory state' with cytokine release being stimulated by interaction of blood cells with the artificial dialysis membranes.

Recombinant erythropoietin

Endogenous EPO is normally synthesised by renal peritubular cells; it stimulates proliferation and maturation of erythroid lines within the marrow. Recombinant EPO preparations are now widely available and are used to correct anaemia in patients with CKD (ie pre-dialysis and patients with failing transplants) as well as those receiving dialysis. It is imperative that these patient groups avoid repeated blood transfusion, so that future renal transplantation will not be precluded by allo-sensitisation. The recombinant EPOs are:

- α-Erythropoietin: now only given iv, and hence to haemodialysis patients only, because of risk of pure red cell aplasia (PRCA, see below).
- β-Erythropoietin.
- Darbepoetin: a novel erythrocyte-stimulating protein; it has a long duration of action and hence the dosing interval can be twice as long. This may be beneficial for patients in their pre-dialysis phase, as once-weekly or once-fortnightly dosing may be possible.

The usual initiation dose of EPO is approximately 100 iu/kg per week (α- and β-erythropoietin) or 0.5 μg/kg per week (darbepoetin) in dialysis patients who have been shown to be iron replete; maintenance doses (once target haemoglobin achieved) are usually lower. The serum ferritin and the transferrin saturation need monitoring as most patients require supplemental iv iron. Key targets of these parameters are:

- Target haemoglobin: 11–13 g/dl; one of the key aims of therapy is to limit or reverse the left ventricular hypertrophy (LVH) which is prevalent in RRT patients. Haemoglobin correction will also have a positive effect upon sexual function and other quality of life measures.
- Ferritin: >200 μg/l in haemodialysis patients, or >100 μg/l in CAPD and pre-dialysis patients.
- Transferrin saturation: >20% (a figure of less than this may indicate functional iron deficiency).

Causes of resistance to EPO therapy

- Iron deficiency
- Sepsis or chronic inflammation
- Occult GI tract blood loss
- Hyperparathyroidism
- Aluminium toxicity (rare)
- PRCA

Main side-effects of EPO therapy: accelerated hypertension with encephalopathy (aim for a monthly Hb increase of <1.5 g/dl), bone aches, flu-like syndrome, fistula thrombosis (rare) and, most recently, PRCA (see below).

Pure red cell aplasia (PRCA)

A few cases of unresponsive and progressive severe anaemia have recently been identified in patients treated with EPO. Such patients have antibodies directed at endogenous and exogenous EPO, and they become transfusion dependent. Other marrow functions remain intact. The number of cases of PRCA has been greatest in α-erythropoietin-treated patients, and it is thought that previous defects in industrial production and storage of the EPO might have been important in pathogenesis. New cases of PRCA are now very rare.

5.3 Hyperparathyroidism and renal bone disease (renal osteodystrophy)

The regulation of vitamin D and parathyroid hormone (PTH) metabolism are discussed in Chapter 13, Metabolic Diseases. Renal bone disease (osteodystrophy) is common in patients with CRF and those receiving dialysis. The pathogenesis is fairly intricate but the most important components are:

- **High serum phosphate**: phosphate clearance is reduced in renal failure.
- **Low plasma ionised calcium**: due to several factors. There is lack of 1,25 di-hydroxy vitamin D (the 1α hydroxylation, which markedly increases activity of vitamin D, normally occurs in the kidney). Malnutrition may contribute, but hyperphosphataemia (imbalancing the ionic product of Ca × P) is also very important.
- **Stimulation of PTH release**: in CRF and ESRD **secondary hyperparathyroidism** is very common and is the direct response of the glands to hypocalcaemia, hyperphosphataemia and low 1,25 di-hydroxy vitamin D levels. The latter three factors feed back independently on the parathyroid glands to stimulate PTH release, and hence correction of all of them (phosphate perhaps the most important) is necessary before the hyperparathyroidism can be optimally controlled. PTH has end-organ effects upon bones (leading to osteoclastic resorption cavities) and also the heart, contributing to LVH, and it is also a major cause of EPO resistance. **Tertiary hyperparathyroidism** is defined by the presence of elevated PTH and non-iatrogenic hypercalcaemia; it is due to autonomous PTH secretion from generally hyperplastic parathyroid glands (90%) or an adenoma (10%). Note that **primary hyperparathyroidism** is only rarely associated with renal failure (due to the nephrotoxic effects of hypercalcaemia or to renal calculus disease).
- **Low vitamin D levels**: this not only results in reduced absorption of calcium by the gut, but also in osteomalacia.
- **Acidosis**: increases the severity of bone disease.

Histological findings at bone biopsy in osteodystrophy

Several different histological lesions often co-exist in the same patient:

- **Osteomalacia**: due to 1,25 di-hydroxy vitamin D deficiency.
- **Hyperparathyroid bone disease**: osteoporosis and cystic resorption; also termed 'osteitis fibrosa cystica' (von Recklinghausen's disease of bone). Sub-periosteal erosions on the radial border of phalanges are characteristic.
- **Osteoporosis**: due to relative malnourishment; steroid use.
- **Osteosclerosis**: a component of the 'rugger jersey' spine appearance at X-ray (bone denser at the vertebral end-plates and thin in the middle of the vertebrae).
- **Adynamic bone disease**: bone with low turnover; PTH levels (and serum alkaline phosphatase) are usually sub-normal. Over-treatment of secondary hyperparathyroidism with excess vitamin D (totally suppressing PTH release) may be contributory. Although the exact clinical significance is uncertain there is perhaps a greater likelihood of fracturing.
- **Aluminium bone disease**: now much less common with the use of specially treated water supplies for dialysis (reverse osmosis) and non-aluminium-containing phosphate binders.

Prevention and treatment of renal osteodystrophy

The basic principles are to improve the diet, reduce hyperphosphataemia and acidosis, and to reduce the PTH level (see below). This is brought about by use of phosphate binders, oral bicarbonate, dialysis where necessary, and by giving the maximum dose of vitamin D that does not provoke hypercalcaemia:

- **Phosphate binders**: aluminium-containing binders are now rarely used and the mainstay of treatment has been calcium-based binders (calcium carbonate or calcium acetate). However, practice is changing, and with the awareness that CRF and dialysis patients are at risk of vascular calcification and aortic valve calcification, non-calcimimetic agents (eg sevelamer (Renagel®), a polymer, and, in the near future, lanthanum carbonate) will be increasingly used.
- **Treatment targets**: serum phosphate <1.7 mmol/l, calcium low–normal range (2.2–2.45 mmol/l) and PTH <3 times above the normal range (ie <200 pg/ml).

Most cases (>97%) of secondary hyperparathyroidism can be controlled with medical treatment. Parathyroidectomy may be necessary in resistant cases (usually those with large parathyroid gland mass (eg >1 cm^3), who have had chronic and poorly treated secondary hyperparathyroidism) and in patients with tertiary disease.

5.4 Maintenance dialysis

In the UK, the dialysis population is approximately 25, 000, or 450/million. In other Western countries (eg Germany and the USA) approximately 85% of patients receive **haemodialysis**, and only a minority of ESRD patients are treated with continuous ambulatory peritoneal dialysis (**CAPD**). In the UK there has been a historical over-reliance upon CAPD, owing to lack of haemodialysis resources, but this is gradually being addressed with a strategy to increase the availability of haemodialysis (currently haemodialysis 65%). Ideally, a patient should be given the opportunity to choose dialysis modality according to lifestyle factors (employment, home environment), their capability and local resources. The dose of dialysis delivered to a patient can now be quantified. Hence, Renal-Association-derived standards for dialysis adequacy are:

- CAPD: Kt/V (an estimate of solute clearance) of >1.7 or weekly creatinine clearance >50 litres.
- Haemodialysis: urea reduction ratio (URR) of >65%, where URR =

$$\frac{(\text{pre-dialysis urea} - \text{post-dialysis urea})}{\text{pre-dialysis urea}} \times 100\%.$$

Factors which would favour haemodialysis in preference to CAPD

- Recent abdominal surgery, or irremediable hernias
- Recurrent or persistent (eg pseudomonas or fungal) peritonitis
- Peritoneal membrane failure: inability to ultra-filtrate the necessary fluid volume to maintain fluid balance in the patient
- Age and general frailty (ie physically or mentally incapable of CAPD)
- Severe malnutrition: protein losses in the dialysis effluent may be 3–10 g/day on CAPD (>15 g/day during peritonitis)
- Intercurrent severe illness with hypercatabolism
- Chronic severe chest disease: respiratory function may be compromised by CAPD
- Loss of residual renal function: it is now recognised that many patients only obtain adequate dialysis with CAPD during the early stages after development of ESRD. As residual function is lost, underdialysis becomes a reality, especially in larger body weight patients

Peritoneal dialysis

A standard CAPD regime would involve four 2-litre exchanges/day. The concentration of dextrose within the dialysate can be altered so that differing ultrafiltration requirements, or patient characteristics, can be addressed. Although a few patients manage CAPD for many years, in most there is a finite length of time (eg 3–6 years) for its efficacy as a form of RRT. This is determined by gradual loss of **residual renal function** (ie a patient will commence CAPD with a GFR of 10–15 ml/min, which is a major contributor to waste product clearance; over time, the GFR falls to zero, with corresponding inadequacy of the CAPD technique) and deterioration of peritoneal membrane function. **Automated peritoneal dialysis (APD)** is performed overnight, and can maintain fluid homeostasis in patients with ultrafiltration failure (see overleaf). APD may also be chosen for its convenience by some patients with normal peritoneal membrane characteristics.

The main **complications of CAPD** treatment are:

- **Bacterial peritonitis**: most cases are treatable. The most common infecting organisms are coagulase-negative staphylococci, Gram-negative bacteria and *Staphylococcus aureus*. With use of disconnect CAPD systems the rate of CAPD-peritonitis should be no greater than 1 episode/30 patient months. Patients who have repeated episodes of peritonitis, and hence several courses of intraperitoneal antibiotics, are prone to develop resistant organisms (eg *Pseudomonas* or fungal peritonitis) and catheter loss, necessitating switch to haemodialysis. If the dialysis fluid culture yields more than one organism (especially Gram-negative and anaerobes) during a peritonitis episode, then intra-abdominal pathology (eg bowel perforation, diverticular abscess) should be suspected and expediently diagnosed and treated.
- **Ultrafiltration failure**: some patients are identified as 'high transporters' of glucose; the osmolar benefit of their CAPD dialysate is rapidly lost and hence these patients have difficulty with fluid removal (ultrafiltration). The latter may also develop after several years of CAPD treatment. APD may help maintain fluid balance in such patients, but polymer-based dialysis solutions can also be beneficial.
- **Sclerosing peritonitis**: a rare complication of long-term CAPD, perhaps triggered by repeated peritonitis. The peritoneal membrane thickens and encases the bowel. Clinical features include CAPD ultrafiltration failure, but in more severe cases, life-threatening bowel obstruction and malnutrition. Surgery can be of benefit in some cases.
- **Malnutrition**: renal failure is an anorexic condition; patients often need nutritional supplements.

Haemodialysis

This therapy has been available for several decades; it is an intrinsically more efficient means of RRT than CAPD and so many patients have lived for >20 years whilst being supported by haemodialysis. As this is an intermittent therapy (typically, 4 hours of dialysis 3 times each week) water restriction and dietary modification are even more important than for patients receiving CAPD (which gives continuous dialysis). Successful haemodialysis relies upon adequate **vascular access**:

- This is ideally provided by arterio-venous fistulae. An appropriate blood-flow rate would be 250–400 ml/min into the dialyser circuit. Fistulae take 4–6 weeks to mature and so vascular access surgery should be planned in timely fashion, when at all possible.
- Patients who present late with severe uraemia and patients with fistula complications inevitably require use of temporary or semi-permanent (tunnelled) vascular access catheters. The most frequent complication is line-related sepsis (in particular, *S. aureus* and coagulase-negative staphylococci), and the incidence of bacterial endocarditis is increased in haemodialysis patients.
- The other main complication of haemodialysis catheters is venous stenosis or occlusion, most commonly seen after subclavian insertion. Consequently, most temporary catheters are now inserted into the femoral or right internal jugular veins, and the jugular veins are the preferred sites for tunnelled catheter insertion.

- Complications relating to insertion can be minimised by using ultrasound scanning to locate the vein for all insertions, and the use of fluoroscopy with left internal jugular vein insertion (as anatomical variants are common).

Long-term complications in dialysis patients

Although dialytic therapies will keep patients alive and, with the additional use of EPO, relatively well, many of the metabolic abnormalities of the uraemic condition persist and these patients are at increased risk of:

- **Vascular disease**: dialysis patients have a much greater incidence of cardiovascular events, and higher relative mortality, than the general population. The relative risk of mortality is almost 100-fold in dialysis patients aged <35 years, and it remains 3-fold that of the general population even in dialysis patients aged >80 years. The risk is increased further in diabetic dialysis patients (eg mean survival of 2 years) and in those with atherosclerotic renovascular disease. Pathogenetic factors have been discussed earlier in this section. The majority of deaths are due to cardiac disease but this is more often due to arrhythmia or congestive cardiomyopathy (which is exacerbated by fluid overload) than to overt myocardial infarction. **Vascular calcification** is a major component of the vascular disease affecting patients with renal failure; it is associated with arterial stiffness (assessed with aortic pulse wave Doppler) and LVH, which in turn correlate with increased mortality. Its prevention may be improved with use of non-calcimimetic phosphate-binding agents, and this is currently under investigation.
- **Cardiac valve calcification**: this affects the aortic valve in particular, and is frequently seen in haemodialysis patients. As with vascular calcification, it is thought to be associated with perturbations in serum phosphate and calcium product.
- **Dialysis-related amyloid**: β_2 microglobulin is a small molecular weight (about 11,000 Da) protein normally metabolised and excreted by the kidney. Plasma levels increase greatly in patients on long-term (eg >10 years) haemodialysis, and the protein is deposited as amyloid within carpal tunnels, joints and bones. Dialysis with more biocompatible membranes (eg polyacrylonitrile or polysulphone) can alleviate the β_2 microglobulin burden.
- **Arthritis**: pyrophosphate arthropathy (pseudogout) and gout (*see* Section 5.5 on transplantation below) are common in patients with renal failure.

5.5 Renal transplantation

About 2000 UK patients benefit from renal transplantation each year, and the vast majority of transplants derive from **cadaveric donors**. With the overall shortage of organs available for transplantation the rate of **live-related transplants** (currently 15% of all grafts) is being increased and non-related live renal donation (often from the spouse) is now occurring; such potential donors require careful counselling before the donor operation. All potential live renal donors have to be screened carefully to ensure that they are clinically fit; absolute contraindications include pre-existing renal disease, a disease of unknown aetiology (eg multiple sclerosis or sarcoidosis), recent malignancy and overt ischaemic heart disease. Hypertensive patients may be considered provided that they have no evidence of end-organ damage, and the blood pressure is well controlled.

Screening and preparation of potential recipients

All dialysis patients and those with advanced CRF are considered for transplantation. However, less than half will be suitably fit for listing.

- Exclusion criteria include current or recent malignancy (eg <2 years) and severe co-morbidity (eg debilitating COPD or stroke, dementia, etc). Although advanced age is not an absolute contraindication, few patients aged >70 years are eventually listed.
- As the transplant is inserted in the iliac fossa, anastomosed to the iliac vessels, vascular calcification of the latter should be sought with pelvic X-ray. This is especially important in patients with a history of peripheral vascular disease.
- Patients with major risk factors (long-standing diabetes, previous IHD, heavy smoking) should undergo **CVS screening** prior to referral. This would include echocardiography (LV ejection fraction must be >30%) and non-invasive imaging for reversible coronary ischaemia (eg dipyridamole radio-nuclide 'myoview' scan or stress echocardiograph). Selected patients then undergo coronary angiography and, if necessary, angioplasty or coronary artery bypass grafting (CABG) prior to transplantation.
- Patients with obstructed and persistently or recurrently infected urinary tracts (eg severe reflux, patients with spina bifida) need bilateral native nephrectomy prior to transplantation.

HLA typing

The majority of cadaveric organs are transplanted to the best available tissue match, although occasionally preference is given to less well-matched patients who are highly sensitised to the majority of HLA allotypes, or to those with dialysis (eg no remaining vascular access) or co-morbid problems.

- HLA antigens are coded from chromosome 6 (*see also* Chapter 10, Immunology).
- Class 1 antigens are A, B and C; class 2 are the D group antigens.
- Relative importance of HLA matching: DR>B>A>C; most centres accept 1 DR or 1 B mismatch.
- Beneficial match: defined as a 0 DR with 0 or 1 B mismatch.

Combined kidney–pancreas transplantation

This is now increasingly performed for patients with type I diabetes mellitus. HLA matching criteria tend to be less strict than for kidney-alone transplantation, as only a limited number of suitable pancreases become available, but recipient fitness is of paramount importance. The pancreas is usually transplanted onto the opposite iliac vessels to the kidney, with its duct draining into the bladder.

- Acute rejection of the pancreas usually follows (rather than precedes) kidney rejection; it is manifest by worsening of glycaemic control and by a rise in urinary amylase, but responds well to pulsed-steroid therapy.
- Long-term results are encouraging – normalisation of glycaemic status is expected, and most diabetic microvascular complications (particularly retinopathy and neuropathy) can be stabilised, but not reversed.

Indications for recipient nephrectomy prior to transplantation

- Pyonephrosis or any suppuration within the urinary tract (see above). If this is due to bladder dysfunction (eg spina bifida) a resting ileal conduit will need to be created prior to transplantation
- Massive polycystic kidneys (very unusual)
- Uncontrollable hypertension (rare with modern drug therapies)
- Renal/urothelial malignancy: patients must remain free of recurrence for >2 years before transplantation

Post-transplantation renal function

It is common to see **acute renal transplantation dysfunction**, especially in the first 2 weeks after engraftment. Nevertheless, overall graft survival is 90% at 1 year, 70% at 5 years and 50% at 10 years. **Chronic graft dysfunction** is common and is responsible for the majority of these renal graft losses beyond 1 year after transplantation. The causes of acute and chronic graft dysfunction are shown in the following table.

Causes of graft dysfunction after transplantation

Acute graft dysfunction (1 day to 4 months after transplantation)

- **Delayed graft function** (ATN of the graft): increased with prolonged cold ischaemia time (seen in 20–50% of all transplants – usually resolves by 2–3 weeks)
- Ureteric leakage (breakdown of anastomosis)
- Vascular thrombosis (arterial or venous thrombosis of the transplant vessels – usually irremediable); this may be associated with **primary non-function** (ie the transplant never functions)
- Urinary tract infection
- Acute ciclosporin or tacrolimus toxicity – resolves rapidly with alteration in dosage
- CMV infection (diagnosed with PCR for the virus)
- **Acute rejection**: occurs in 25–50% of all transplants (see below)

Chronic graft dysfunction (4 months after transplantation onwards)

- **Chronic allograft nephropathy**: by far the most common cause of chronic dysfunction of the transplant (see overleaf)
- Recurrent primary disease within the graft (see overleaf)
- Calcineurin inhibitor (ciclosporin or tacrolimus) nephrotoxicity: changes on transplant biopsy are rarely pathognomonic. Withdrawal of the calcineurin inhibitor in such patients will often stabilise graft function

Acute transplant rejection

This is very common, and should be anticipated in the early weeks after transplantation. The risk of acute rejection episodes may be less with use of tacrolimus rather than ciclosporin A. Most cases respond rapidly to pulsed iv methylprednisolone therapy. Steroid-resistant rejection occurs in about 5% and usually requires therapy with monoclonal antibody therapy (eg ATG or OKT3).

Chronic allograft nephropathy (CAN)

This accounts for >90% of graft losses occurring after the first year after transplantation. It is usually manifest by the development of proteinuria and slowly progressive graft dysfunction. It is thought to be due to both immunological and non-immunological (hypertension, hypercholesterolaemia, vascular disease within the graft) factors. Management involves:

- Optimising hypertension control.
- Limiting proteinuria (use of ACE inhibitors and AIIRBs).
- **Modification of immunosuppressive therapy**: calcineurin inhibitors (CNI) may increase the risk of CAN, partly because of their tendency to provoke vasoconstriction and vasculopathy (and consequent ischaemia) within the graft. There is increasing evidence that reduction in CNI dose, or complete withdrawal, with introduction of mycophenolate mofetil (MMF) or sirolimus (see below) can ameliorate, or even stabilise, progressive graft dysfunction in patients with CAN.

Post-transplantation: non-renal complications

Although the quality of life of most patients is improved after transplantation, patients are still at risk of:

- **Malignancy**: **non-Hodgkin's lymphoma** (usually EB virus-associated) is 20–50 times and **skin cancer** 5–20 times commoner in transplant recipients than in age-matched general populations, and the increased incidence is thought to be due to the effects of immunosuppression (especially azathioprine with skin and ciclosporin with lymphoma). All other malignancies are slightly more prevalent (1.5-fold increased).

- **Cardiovascular**: ischaemic heart disease is 10–20 times more prevalent (due to effects of immunosuppression and hyperlipidaemia, as well as persistence of the CVS risk accompanying the patients' previous 'uraemic state') than in an age/sex-matched equivalent population. Mortality is 2% in the first year after transplantation, half of which is due to CVS disease, and half to infection (see below).

- **Infections**: all infections are commoner but patients are also at risk from opportunistic infections such as *Pneumocystis carinii* pneumonia (PCP), and especially cytomegalovirus (CMV).
  –**CMV** occurs in about 30% and is anticipated in CMV antibody-negative recipients of a CMV-positive graft at 6–12 weeks after transplantation. Patients at risk of CMV are prophylaxed with oral ganciclovir, and oral valganciclovir is used to treat mild infections (leukopenia and mild pyrexia are typical). Severe infections occur in 10%, and can be associated with myocarditis, encephalitis, retinitis and renal dysfunction; these cases require treatment with systemic ganciclovir.

-**PCP** is uncommon, but patients now receive cotrimoxazole prophylaxis for the first 6 months post-transplantation.
-Patients of Asian origin, or those with a previous TB history, are given anti-tuberculous prophylaxis with isoniazid for the first year after transplantation.

- **Osteoporosis**: the risk is increased because of immunosuppressant (particularly steroid) usage. Many patients receive prophylaxis in the form of weekly or daily bisphosphonates.
- **Gout**: all patients with reduced renal clearance are at increased risk of hyperuricaemia and acute gout. However, prophylaxis with allopurinol is not generally given to all patients, largely because this agent has many unwanted effects. Treatment of acute gout in patients with renal impairment presents a major problem – there are no truly non-nephrotoxic NSAIDs available, and patients with transplants (or with CRF) are at risk of serious renal dysfunction with their usage. Colchicine can be used, but it also has frequent GI side-effects; temporary treatment with moderate-dose steroids (eg a single im injection of 125 mg methylprednisolone, or 30 mg prednisolone orally for one month) will provide an excellent anti-inflammatory effect and provides cover for the introduction of allopurinol.
- **Post-transplantation diabetes mellitus (PTDM)**: the incidence is increased in transplanted patients (3–5% may develop it per year); immunosuppressants (particularly tacrolimus) are thought to be responsible.

Recurrent renal disease after transplantation

Patients with Alport's syndrome are at risk of developing anti-glomerular basement membrane antibody syndrome after transplantation, as they have no prior tolerance to the Goodpasture antigen. Vasculitis may recur, but this can be prevented by monitoring autoimmune antibody levels (eg ANCA). All types of primary glomerulonephritis may recur in the graft, but particularly:

- Focal segmental glomerulosclerosis (FSGS) – 15% recurrence rate, with graft loss in 50% of these.
- IgA nephropathy – 30–60% have evidence of histologic recurrence; graft loss in 15% of these.
- Membranous glomerulonephritis – <10% recurrence rate, but 50% graft loss if affected.
- Mesangiocapillary glomerulonephritis: 30–80% risk of recurrence.

Commonly used immunosuppressants for renal transplantation

Immunosuppressive regimes vary from centre to centre. Historically, a combination of ciclosporin with azathioprine and prednisolone was the favoured regime, but this has changed with the advent of newer agents (particularly tacrolimus, MMF and sirolimus). Most now involve induction with monoclonal antibody (eg basiliximab, directed against CD25, given at induction and day 4), followed by a CNI-based regime. Patients who have at least two steroid-responsive acute rejections will usually receive oral corticosteroids for up to 12 months after transplantation. Particular considerations with immunosuppressants are:

- **Ciclosporin A**: this agent inhibits a T-cell phosphatase, calcineurin, which is needed for T-cell activation, and hence its status as a CNI. Its introduction around 1980 completely revolutionised the outcome of transplantation. Common side-effects include hirsutism, liver dysfunction and gum hypertrophy, but recent attention has focused on the hypertension and chronic graft dysfunction that often accompany its long-term use (*see* Chronic allograft nephropathy (CAN) section above). Some centres now try to tailor immunosuppressive regimes in order to maximise the chances of good long-term graft function, but with limitation of recipient vascular risk; this involves reducing or complete withdrawal of CNI dose, and introducing either MMF or sirolimus (*see* 'Optimal immunosuppressive regime' below).

- **Tacrolimus (FK506)**: this is also a CNI which acts to reduce T-cell activation. When compared to ciclosporin, it appears to be associated with a lower incidence of acute rejection episodes in the initial post-transplant period. Also, the number of steroid-resistant rejection episodes is seen to be reduced, and hypertension may be less frequent or severe. However, the risk of CAN with long-term use appears to be similar to that of ciclosporin, and the considerations regarding CNI dose reduction/withdrawal also apply to tacrolimus. Approximately 5% of patients receiving this agent develop diabetes mellitus per year.
- **Azathioprine**: this traditional anti-proliferative agent is commonly associated with mild bone marrow suppression. Unfortunately, many transplant patients have hyperuricaemia, but the use of azathioprine in conjunction with allopurinol is contraindicated because of the risk of life-threatening bone marrow suppression.
- **Mycophenolate mofetil (MMF)**: this is a newer anti-proliferative agent whose chief side-effects are gastro-intestinal, in particular diarrhoea, and bone marrow suppression (but less frequently than azathioprine). It is usually used in combination with a CNI; it has a major role in the management of CAN, being used when the CNI dose is withdrawn or reduced.
- **Sirolimus (rapamycin)**: this is related to erythromycin, but it inhibits T-cell division by blocking interleukin-2-mediated signal transduction. When used in combination with a CNI it markedly reduces the incidence of acute rejection (by 85–90%). It is not associated with nephropathy, but it can provoke hyperlipidaemia.
- **Corticosteroids**: although these agents have played a large role in immunosuppressive regimes for several decades, there is concern about dosing with steroids. This is particularly relevant to cardiovascular complications after transplantation, as well as to post-transplant bone metabolism (osteoporosis). Some centres now have regimes that involve steroid withdrawal at 6–12 months post-transplantation.

Optimal immunosuppressive regime

Although there is no current consensus view, the following would be a logical strategy that gives more clarity for the reader:

- Induction with monoclonal antibody and large CNI dose.
- Maintenance therapy with CNI coupled with either MMF or sirolimus.
- If more than one steroid-sensitive acute rejection episode, prednisolone for 6–12 months.
- At 1 year post-transplant, reduce CNI dose.
- If CAN develops, then reduce/withdraw CNI, and introduce MMF or sirolimus (if not receiving one or other). Both of these agents should be used with a low-dose steroid.

6. GLOMERULONEPHRITIS AND ASSOCIATED SYNDROMES

6.1 Clinical presentation of glomerulonephritis

The broad definition of glomerulonephritis would be inflammatory disease primarily affecting the glomeruli (but note that no inflammation is seen in minimal change disease) – but other glomerular diseases exist which do not involve glomerulonephritis (eg diabetic nephropathy). Most glomerulonephritis develops as a result of **immune dysregulation**, either due to an inappropriate immune response to a 'self-antigen' (autoimmunity, eg anti glomerular basement membrane (anti-GBM) disease, ANCA +ve vasculitis), or to an ineffectual response to a foreign antigen (eg membranous glomerulonephritis secondary to hepatitis B infection).

- This 'immune dysregulation' pathogenesis explains why there is a genetic predisposition to some forms of glomerulonephritis (eg IgA nephropathy).
- Immune complexes are often deposited in the glomeruli (eg SLE nephritis), but in some glomerulonephritides immune complexes form in situ within the glomerulus (eg anti-GBM disease).
- Inflammation often leads to proliferation of cellular structures (mesangial, endothelial or epithelial cells) and/or scarring.
- Glomerulonephritis may be **idiopathic** (**primary**), or **secondary** to systemic disease, drugs, etc.
- The long-term clinical outcome often depends more upon the severity of tubulointerstitial damage rather than the extent of glomerular injury.
- The type of glomerulonephritis is defined by light microscopic, immunofluorescent and electron microscopic (ultrastructural) characteristics (see below).

Screening for glomerulonephritis

- Dipstick for proteinuria; 24-hour quantification of proteinuria
- Dipstick for haematuria; urine microscopy for red cells and casts
- Hypertension.

Attenuation of progression of glomerulonephritis

- Control blood pressure: for all types of glomerulonephritis
- ACE inhibitors and angiotensin II blockers: decrease proteinuria and blood pressure, and may ameliorate progressive scarring (*see* Section 1.3 on RAA system and also Section 5 on CRF)
- The target blood pressure for patients with chronic renal disease and persistent proteinuria is <130/80 mmHg (*see* Section 5 on CRF)
- Progression depends upon degree of co-existent scarring in the tubulointerstitium.

Classification of glomerulonephritis

Diabetes mellitus is the most common cause of glomerular pathology within the Western world. It causes glomerulosclerosis and is therefore not truly a 'glomerulonephritis'. The commoner forms of glomerulonephritis (GN) that are encountered are:

- minimal change disease
- membranous glomerulonephritis
- focal segmental glomerulosclerosis (FSGS)
- mesangioproliferative (IgA nephropathy) glomerulonephritis
- crescentic glomerulonephritis (eg associated with Goodpasture's syndrome or vasculitis)
- focal segmental proliferative glomerulonephritis (eg associated with vasculitis or endocarditis)
- mesangiocapillary glomerulonephritis
- diffuse proliferative glomerulonephritis (eg post-streptococcal).

Renal syndromes and their relationship to glomerulonephritis

There is often confusion regarding the relationship of the various glomerulonephritides to the different renal syndromes. A particular type of glomerulonephritis may manifest several different clinical syndromes (see Table below). For example, membranous glomerulonephritis may be responsible for CRF, persistent proteinuria, nephrotic syndrome and hypertension; any combination of these may be present during the course of the disease. However:

- Certain glomerulonephritides are characteristically associated with typical clinical presentations (eg minimal change disease and nephrotic syndrome, IgA nephropathy and recurrent macroscopic haematuria).
- It should also be borne in mind that a particular syndrome may be due to many conditions other than glomerulonephritis (eg the nephrotic syndrome can be due to accelerated phase hypertension, pre-eclamptic toxaemia or amyloid, as well as various forms of glomerulonephritis, etc).

Clinical presentation of glomerulonephritis

	Proteinuria	Nephrotic	Nephritic	Haematuria	ARF	CRF
Minimal change disease	+	+++	–	–	–	–
Membranous GN	+++	++	–	±	–	++
Focal segmental glomerulosclerosis	++	++	±	–	±	++
Mesangial IgA	+	+	+	+++	±	++
Mesangiocapillary GN	++	++	+	+	+	+
Diffuse proliferative GN	+	±	+++	++	++	+
Diabetic glomerulosclerosis	+++	++	–	–	–	+++
Crescentic nephritis	+	±	+++	++	+++	+
Focal segmental proliferative GN	+	++	++	++	++	+

+++ = Very common presentation; – = Never seen/extremely rare

Definitions of the common renal syndromes

- **Asymptomatic proteinuria**
  <3 g/day
- **Nephritic syndrome**
  Characterised by hypertension, oliguria, haematuria and oedema
- **Hypertension**
- **Nephrotic syndrome**
  > 3 g proteinuria/day with serum albumin <25 g/l; oedema; hypercholesterolaemia
- **Haematuria**
  Microscopic or macroscopic
- **Acute and chronic renal failure**
  (Discussed in previous sections)

Causes of the nephrotic syndrome

- **Common**
  Primary glomerulonephritis
  Diabetes mellitus
  Basement membrane nephropathy (eg Alport's syndrome)
  Infections (eg leprosy, malaria, hepatitis B)
  Pre-eclampsia
  Accelerated hypertension
  Myeloma
  Amyloidosis
  Drugs (eg gold, penicillamine, captopril, NSAIDs, mercury)
  Connective tissue disease (eg SLE)
- **Rare**
  Vesico-ureteric reflux
  Constrictive pericarditis
  Sickle cell disease
  Allergies (eg bee sting, penicillin)
  Hereditary glomerulonephritis (eg 'Finnish type' nephrotic syndrome)

Causes of macroscopic haematuria*

- Urinary infections
- Acute glomerulonephritis
- IgA nephropathy
- Renal calculi
- Urinary tract malignancy
- Renal papillary necrosis
- Loin-pain haematuria syndrome
- Prostatic hypertrophy (dilated prostatic veins)

*It is usually imperative to exclude urinary tract malignancy (urine cytology, cystoscopy, IVU and ultrasound) in patients aged > 40 years presenting with macroscopic haematuria

6.2 Notes on particular glomerulonephritides

Minimal change disease

The clinical presentation is almost always nephrotic. Although most common in children (causing 80% of nephrotic syndrome due to glomerulonephritis in under 15-year-olds), it also accounts for 28% of nephrotic syndrome in adults. Highly selective proteinuria (IgG/transferrin <0.1) is typical, and the majority of cases are steroid-responsive. Other features include:

- normal renal function and renal histology (by light microscopy – but epithelial cell foot-process fusion on EM)
- may be due to NSAIDs or gold; rare associations are with Hodgkin's lymphoma and thymoma
- may frequently relapse (10%), but renal prognosis is excellent.

Monitoring: patients with frequently relapsing disease (especially children) are taught to dipstick their urine on a regular basis; three consecutive days of +++ proteinuria is the trigger to commence steroids, which are continued at high dose until urinalysis has remained negative for three consecutive days.

Treatment: the mainstay is with short courses of high-dose prednisolone. Most relapses are steroid-sensitive; cyclophosphamide (usually orally in children, pulsed iv in adults) is used for frequent relapsers or steroid-resistant disease. A distinct sub-group of frequently relapsing (eg 2–4 relapses/year) teenagers enter adult nephrological care and prove quite difficult to manage. Avoidance of long-term steroid side-effects (particularly osteoporosis) is important and so the relapse rate can be reduced by treatment with ciclosporin (taken for several years), in the knowledge that, in the majority of these patients, the presumed underlying immune perturbation resolves by their late 20's. However, a small group of these patients are eventually found to have FSGS (see below).

Urinary protein selectivity

The index of urinary protein selectivity is used mainly in paediatric nephrological practice; highly selective proteinuria is likely to result from minimal change disease, and so its detection may obviate the need to perform renal biopsy of the child. In adults the range of possible renal diagnoses in patients with significant proteinuria usually makes biopsy essential. The index is calculated from the respective concentrations of different molecular weight proteins within the urine:

$$\frac{\text{IgG (mol. wt. 150 kDa)}}{\text{Transferrin (mol. wt. 40 kDa)}}.$$

Highly selective (ie minimal change) proteinuria is defined as an index of <0.1; unselective proteinuria >0.3.

Membranous glomerulonephritis

This is one of the commonest types of glomerulonephritis in the adult; there are two peaks of disease (patients in their mid-20s and those aged 60–70 years). The clinical presentation may be nephrotic syndrome, asymptomatic proteinuria or CRF.

- Renal histology is characterised by granular IgG and complement deposition on the glomerular basement membrane; immune complexes are sub-epithelial (outer aspect of basement membrane) and appear as 'spikes' with silver stain.
- A third of patients progress through CRF to ESRD, a third respond to immunosuppressive therapy (eg cytotoxic regimes such as the Ponticelli regime: chlorambucil alternating with corticosteroids), and the disease remits spontaneously in a similar proportion of patients.
- In patients with persistent proteinuria (which can sometimes be in the nephrotic range) the mainstay of treatment is blood pressure control and limitation of proteinuria with ACE inhibitors and/or AIIRBs.
- Renal vein thrombosis may occur in up to 5% of patients. Patients at greatest risk are those with serum albumin <20 g/l, and these should receive prophylactic-dose heparin. Unfractionated heparin is generally safe, but note that there have been reports of serious haemorrhagic complications in patients with renal failure who have been treated with 'normal' doses of low molecular weight heparin (enoxaparin at reduced dose can be safely used).
- Membranous glomerulonephritis may be idiopathic, or secondary to other conditions (see below).
- As stated before, the condition can recur in renal transplants.

Secondary causes of membranous glomerulonephritis

- **Malignancy**
  Bronchus, stomach, colon, lymphoma, chronic lymphoid leukaemia (CLL) (high suspicion of these in elderly patients)
- **Connective tissue disease**
  SLE, rheumatoid arthritis, Sjögren's syndrome, mixed connective tissue disease
- **Chronic infections**
  (eg hepatitis B or C, malaria, syphilis)
- **Drugs**
  Gold, penicillamine, captopril, NSAIDs
- **Others**
  Sarcoidosis, Guillain–Barré syndrome, primary biliary cirrhosis (all rare)

Causes of renal vein thrombosis

- **Acute thrombosis**
  Infantile gastroenteritis
  Acute pyelonephritis (high mortality)
  Renal cell carcinoma (with renal vein invasion)
- **Chronic thrombosis**
  Amyloidosis
  Nephrotic syndrome due to glomerulonephritis (particularly membranous glomerulonephritis)

Focal segmental glomerulosclerosis (FSGS)

The **primary** form of FSGS accounts for <10% of nephrotic syndrome in children and the elderly, but up to 20% in young adults. It can also frequently present with proteinuria and/or CRF. When occurring in childhood, the clinical pattern is often identical to minimal change disease, and it may be misdiagnosed as such. There are also familial forms of FSGS. Focal glomerular deposits of IgM are seen at biopsy.

- **Secondary FSGS**: this can be seen in patients with heroin abuse, those with HIV infections and AIDS, and it is frequently seen in patients with obesity or when the functioning renal mass is reduced (eg after nephrectomy). In the latter cases, the glomerulosclerosis probably occurs as a result of haemodynamic stress and/or ischaemic changes within the glomeruli, which also explains why it has been associated with renovascular disease.

Treatment of primary FSGS: it is important to distinguish this clinically from secondary FSGS, as patients with the latter should not be treated with immunosuppression, but with optimal blood pressure control with ACE inhibitors/AIIRBs. In nephrotic patients with primary disease >40% will respond to moderate-dose steroids given for 3–6 months. Frequent-relapsers are treated in a similar way to those with minimal change nephropathy.

Outcome of FSGS: a rapidly deteriorating clinical course is seen in 2%, whereas 25% of all patients will eventually progress to ESRD. There is a high rate of recurrence in transplants.

Mesangioproliferative glomerulonephritis (IgA nephropathy or Berger's disease)

This is a very frequent condition, the commonest primary glomerulonephritis in adults. It typically affects young adults, presenting with microscopic or recurrent macroscopic haematuria. The haematuric episodes are usually 'synpharyngitic' (ie occurring 0–3 days after upper respiratory tract infection (URTI)). Many cases are probably undiagnosed as most physicians only occasionally biopsy the kidneys of patients with isolated microscopic haematuria. There is a marked increased incidence in the Far East (associated with HLA DQW7). The serum IgA is increased in 50% of patients; the condition is considered to be autoimmune, perhaps due to dysregulation of IgA metabolism. Other features of IgA nephropathy are:

- IgA nephropathy can be associated with cirrhosis, dermatitis herpetiformis, coeliac disease and mycosis fungoides. It occurs in the Wiskott–Aldrich syndrome.
- Renal biopsy features show proliferation of mesangial areas of the glomerulus; immunological staining is strongly positive for IgA in these areas. A similar histological picture may be seen in **Henoch–Schönlein nephritis**, and the pathogenesis is thought to be similar in the two conditions. Crescents may be present during haematuric episodes.

Treatment of IgA nephropathy: nephrotic presentations should be treated as for minimal change nephropathy. Patients with CRF and low-grade proteinuria may show stabilisation of renal function with a 6-month regime of alternate day steroids. The possible beneficial effects of fish oil (ω-3 fatty acids) remain uncertain. Otherwise the mainstay of treatment is optimal blood pressure control with ACE inhibitors/AIIRBs, as for other chronic nephropathies.

Outcome of IgA nephropathy: 25% of patients will progress to ESRD by 20 years after disease onset; however, the overall prognosis is certain to be better than this as the mildest cases are likely to remain undiagnosed. Clinical criteria help identify patients with better prognosis – those with proteinuria <1 g/24 h at presentation have 98% renal survival at 15 years, compared to 65% of patients with proteinuria >1 g/24 h. The disease frequently recurs in transplants.

Mesangiocapillary glomerulonephritis (MCGN)

There are three forms of mesangiocapillary (or membranoproliferative) glomerulonephritis:

- Type I: immune deposits in the subendothelial space and mesangium. This can occur in association with or without mixed **cryoglobulinaemias**, and **hepatitis C** may underlie the problem in 70–90%; other causes are hepatitis B, subacute bacterial endocarditis (SBE), shunt nephritis, malaria, SLE, Sjögren's syndrome, sickle cell disease, α-antitrypsin deficiency, hereditary complement deficiencies and malignancy (CLL, non-Hodgkin's lymphoma).
- Type II: dense deposits in the mesangium ('dense deposit' disease) leading to characteristic double-contouring of the basement membrane on renal biopsy. This is usually familial, and associated with partial lipodystrophy or factor H deficiency. Patients have reduced serum complement and the presence of circulating C_3 nephritic factor. The latter binds to the alternative pathway C3 convertase preventing its inactivation by factor H; continued complement activation results.
- Type III: immune deposits diffusely present in subendothelial space and mesangium. Often associated with hepatitis C or B infections (and the secondary causes as for type I MCGN).

Patients usually present with microscopic haematuria and low-grade proteinuria, nephrotic syndrome (35%), CRF or with rapidly deteriorating renal function (10%). The overall prognosis is fairly poor with 50% progressing to ESRD; steroids are only occasionally effective, but are used in childhood nephrotic presentations. There is a high rate of recurrence of MCGN in transplants.

Diffuse proliferative glomerulonephritis

This is the histological pattern of the classic post-streptococcal glomerulonephritis which usually presents with the nephritic syndrome or ARF; children and young adults are most often affected. The disorder is typically preceded (by 10–21 days) by a sore throat, or (most often in Third World countries) skin disease (impetigo).

- Serum C_3 is low and there is diffuse proliferation within glomeruli at biopsy.
- Post-infective cases usually recover spontaneously with restoration of full renal function.
- The same histological picture may be seen in patients with Goodpasture's syndrome and SLE nephritis.

Rapidly progressive glomerulonephritis (RPGN) – including Goodpasture's syndrome

The term 'rapidly progressive' glomerulonephritis is a clinical description of rapidly deteriorating renal function due to an underlying glomerulonephritis. The histological counterpart is a **crescentic glomerulonephritis**, and so the two terms are (sometimes incorrectly) used interchangeably. They refer to the renal lesions which excite great interest from the nephrologist, not least because patients are often very sick with hypercatabolic ARF and possibly associated systemic disease (eg pulmonary haemorrhage), but also because the underlying disease processes are potentially treatable provided that investigation and therapy are expedient. All age groups may be affected and the presentation is usually ARF or nephritic syndrome.

- Causes of RPGN include Goodpasture's syndrome, ANCA +ve vasculitis, lupus nephritis and, as described above, MCGN and occasionally FSGS.
- Crescentic nephritis may be 'idiopathic' but is more often associated with Goodpasture's syndrome, ANCA +ve vasculitis or SLE.

ANCA +ve vasculitis and lupus nephritis are both considered in detail in Section 12, Systemic disorders and the kidney, and hence the remainder of this section will concentrate on Goodpasture's syndrome and its treatment, which is similar to that for the former conditions.

Goodpasture's syndrome

This is characterised by the presence of circulating anti-GBM antibodies (the GBM antigen is a component of type 4 collagen), which localise to the glomerular and pulmonary capillary basement membranes. The condition is rare (<1 case/million per year), tends to affect the elderly or patients in their 20–30s, and may be triggered by inhaled hydrocarbons.

- **Pulmonary haemorrhage** occurs in 50% of patients with Goodpasture's; the most vulnerable are young male smokers. It is also seen in ANCA +ve disease (Wegener's and microscopic polyangiitis), which is considered later. The occurrence of pulmonary haemorrhage confers a greater mortality and is a definitive indication for plasma exchange.
- Specific biopsy changes are seen in Goodpasture's syndrome, with IgG deposited on the glomerular basement membrane in a linear pattern. The glomerulonephritis is of the diffuse proliferative type, and typically there is extensive crescent formation (epithelial cell proliferation arising from Bowman's capsule).
- **Prognosis**: Renal functional recovery is rarely seen if the patient presents with advanced ARF (eg creatinine >600 μmol/l) and/or anuria. Overall mortality is >20%. Elderly patients are at particular risk from infective complications after immunosuppression; patients who have pulmonary haemorrhage are at greatest risk of mortality. Transplantation is possible once the patient is rendered autoantibody negative.

Treatment of RPGN and crescentic nephritis

The following is applicable to most diseases causing RPGN and/or crescentic glomerulonephritis. Treatment is with aggressive immunosuppressive therapy with or without **plasma exchange**. The latter is essential for patients with pulmonary haemorrhage who have a circulating autoantibody (ie anti-GBM or ANCA) in high titre, and it is used in most cases of Goodpasture's syndrome. The aim of plasma exchange is to rapidly remove the autoantibodies, allowing time for the immunosuppressive drugs to act to reduce their formation (indications for plasma exchange in renal disease are shown below). A typical regime for Goodpasture's syndrome would be:

- **Induction therapy**: high-dose steroids (iv methylprednisolone 1 g on three consecutive days, followed by prednisolone 1 mg/kg) with 7 × 4-litre plasma exchanges within the first 10–14 days. Pulsed iv cyclophosphamide (0.5–1 g each month) is given for the first 6 months, by which stage the steroid dose will have been tapered to around 10–20 mg/day.
- **Maintenance therapy**: low-dose steroid and azathioprine are continued for a further 12–18 months (or even longer in some cases of cANCA +ve vasculitis (see later), or Goodpasture's with persistence of anti-GBM antibody).

Plasma exchange in renal disease

- **Agreed benefit**
  Goodpasture's syndrome
  ANCA +ve diseases: especially with pulmonary–renal presentation (mandatory with severe pulmonary haemorrhage); also for dialysis-requiring ARF
  Idiopathic crescentic glomerulonephritis
  Cryoglobulinaemias
  Myeloma: cases with hyperviscosity
  HUS and TPP
- **Uncertain benefit**
  SLE nephritis: severe lupus ARF
  Henoch–Schönlein nephritis: with crescentic forms and ARF
  Myeloma: with ARF due to cast nephropathy (see later)

Hypocomplementaemia and glomerulonephritis

The following disorders are often associated with glomerulonephritis coupled with *low serum complement* (C_3).

- **SLE**
  Membranous, proliferative or crescentic glomerulonephritis
- **Shunt nephritis**
  Focal segmental proliferative glomerulonephritis (or MCGN); classically associated with coagulase-negative staphylococcal infection of ventriculo-atrial shunts
- **Primary complement deficiency (eg C1q, C2 or C4 deficiency)**
  Associated with lupus-like syndromes, glomerulonephritis (usually mesangiocapillary type) and increased risk of bacterial infection
- **Endocarditis**
  Focal segmental proliferative glomerulonephritis
- **Post-streptococcal glomerulonephritis**
- **Mesangiocapillary glomerulonephritis**
  (See earlier section)
- **Cryoglobulinaemia**
  Especially type II (see below)

Cryoglobulinaemia

Immunoglobulins which precipitate on cooling may be monoclonal or polyclonal (for classification *see* Chapter 10, Immunology). They can induce a small vessel vasculitis, particularly affecting skin and kidneys. Type II (mixed monoclonal) and type III (polyclonal) cryoglobulinaemias are associated with glomerulonephritis (mesangiocapillary or membranoproliferative).

7. INHERITED RENAL DISEASE

The commonest inherited renal diseases are polycystic kidney disease and Alport's syndrome. Rarer disorders include other renal cystic disease, disorders of amino acids and familial glomerulonephritis; the latter conditions are encountered much more often in paediatric nephrology.

7.1 Autosomal dominant polycystic kidney disease (ADPKD)

Autosomal dominant polycystic kidney disease (ADPKD) is the most common inherited renal condition, and the genes have now been identified:

- **PKD1**: chromosome 16 in 86% of PKD patients (mean age of ESRD: 57 years)
- **PKD2**: chromosome 4 in 10% (ESRD mean age: 69 years).

The diagnosis is usually made by ultrasound; cysts usually develop during the teenage years so that first-degree relatives aged >20 years, with a normal scan, can be >90% confident of being disease-free; the confidence level rises to 98% at 30 years of age. Cysts develop from all segments of the nephron. The prevalence of ADPKD is 1 in 1000; the condition accounts for about 10% of RRT patients in the UK.

Diagnostic criteria for ADPKD

In a patient known to be at 50% risk because of family history, diagnosis would be suggested by the following ultrasound findings:

- two cysts, either unilateral or bilateral, if aged < 30 years
- two cysts in each kidney in patients aged 30–59 years
- four cysts in each kidney in patients > 60 years.

Sporadic cases (no family history) are also commonly seen.

Clinical features

Patients may present with abdominal pain or mass, hypertension, urinary tract infection (UTI), renal calculi (10%), macroscopic haematuria or CRF.

- The age of onset of CRF varies widely (eg 25–60 years); not all patients develop ESRD.
- In established patients, intermittent presentation with severe abdominal pain is common, but, other than for UTI and calculi, the exact cause may be difficult to identify (cyst expansion, cyst rupture, intra-cystic haemorrhage).
- **Treatment** of the progressive CRF in ADPKD is as for other chronic nephropathies (ie hypertension control, ACE inhibitors/AIIRB therapy, etc).

Associations of ADPKD*

- Liver cysts: 70%
- Berry aneurysms: 8% (see below)
- Pancreatic cysts: 10%
- Mitral valve prolapse or aortic incompetence
- Hepatic fibrosis (rare)
- Diverticular disease

*There is no increased incidence of renal malignancy in ADPKD (see von Hippel–Lindau syndrome overleaf)

Intra-cranial aneurysms in ADPKD

There is familial clustering (ie if family history of aneurysms, then >20% of patients with ADPKD will be found to have them, compared to 5% if no family history). The majority are asymptomatic; the risk of rupture increases with aneurysm size (eg 4% per year if >10 mm). Rupture is associated with a 30–50% chance of severe morbidity/mortality. Most patients have normal renal function at the time of rupture. There is currently some debate as to the value of screening (with MR angiography) for intra-cranial aneurysms in ADPKD.

7.2 Other renal cystic disorders

- **Autosomal recessive PKD**: rare (1/10, 000 births). The gene is localised to chromosome 6. ESRD develops early in childhood; 100% have hepatic fibrosis. The prognosis is poor.
- **von Hippel–Lindau (VHL) syndrome**: autosomal dominant, the gene is localised on chromosome 3. Renal cysts are pre-malignant (>50%) and bilateral nephrectomy is often necessary. It is likely that patients previously thought to have renal malignancy in association with ADPKD actually had VHL. Patients are also at risk of spinocerebellar haemangioblastoma, retinal angiomas, pancreatic cysts, islet cell tumours and phaeochromocytoma.
- **Tuberous sclerosis**: dominantly inherited (either chromosome 9 or 16), and affects 1 in 10, 000 individuals; patients develop epilepsy (80%), mental retardation (50%), hamartomas, renal cysts and angiomyolipomas. Skin lesions include shagreen patches, ash-leaf spots and adenoma sebaceum.
- **Juvenile nephronophthisis-medullary cystic disease complex**: two different terms are used for two similar diseases which differ only in their age of onset and mode of transmission. Cysts occur in the renal medulla, and patients have chronic tubulointerstitial nephritis, salt-wasting and progressive CRF. **Juvenile nephronophthisis (NPH)** occurs in children, is autosomal recessive, and accounts for up to 15% of childhood ESRD; 10–15% of children have retinal abnormalities (a form of retinitis pigmentosa). In adults a histopathologically identical disease, **autosomal dominant medullary cystic disease**, leads to ESRD in the third and fourth decades; it is uncommon and is not associated with extra-renal abnormalities.
- **Medullary sponge kidney (MSK)**: sporadic; the cysts develop from ectatic collecting ducts. These may calcify, leading to the classical nephrocalcinosis associated with MSK. Patients have a benign course except that renal calculi and upper urinary tract infections are commonly associated.
- **Acquired cystic disease**: cystic change is common in the rudimentary kidneys of dialysis patients, and especially in scarred kidneys; most cysts develop from proximal tubules. They are present in >5% of patients at the onset of RRT, and in >80% after 10 years of dialysis. Malignant change is thought to occur with an annual incidence of about 1%.
- **Simple cysts**: fluid-filled, solitary or multiple, these are usually harmless, incidental findings at ultrasound or IVU. The cysts may grow to considerable size (eg >10 cm). They occasionally require percutaneous drainage because of persistent loin pain. Simple cysts are very common affecting 2% of patients aged <50 years, 11% aged 50–70 years and >20% of the elderly.

7.3 Alport's syndrome

The prevalence of Alport's syndrome is 1/5000 individuals; 85% have X-linked dominant inheritance, but other families may show dominant or recessive inheritance. The primary defect is an abnormal GBM (seen at electron microscopy) with variable thickness and splitting ('basket weave' appearance); the Goodpasture antigen is absent in the GBM (hence the predisposition of patients to anti-GBM glomerulonephritis after transplantation).

- Clinical presentation is with deafness, persistent microscopic haematuria, proteinuria and CRF; 30% develop nephrotic syndrome.
- Renal failure develops in all affected males; the rate of progression is heterogeneous between families (ie ESRD before 30 years in some, yet only by 60 years in others).
- Carrier females may have urinary abnormalities (haematuria, proteinuria), and usually do not develop renal failure.
- **Bilateral sensorineural deafness** is characteristic, but the hearing loss may only be mild; familial progressive nephritis may occasionally occur without deafness.
- Other extra-renal manifestations are: ocular abnormalities occur in 40% (**lenticonus** – conical or spherical protrusion of the surface of the lens into the anterior chamber, retinal flecks or cataracts); macrothrombocytopenia; leiomyomata (rare).
- The molecular defect involves the gene encoding for the α5-chain of type IV collagen; alteration of this chain is thought to prevent integration of the α3-chain into the GBM.

7.4 Benign familial haematuria (BFH) and thin membrane nephropathy

Up to 25% of patients referred to a nephrologist for investigation of microscopic haematuria have this condition. It is common in families, when it is termed '**Benign familial haematuria**'; the inheritance pattern is dominant although the gene has not been identified. Sporadic cases are designated as '**thin membrane nephropathy**'. The normal thickness of the GBM is around 450 nm; patients with BFH/thin membrane nephropathy have an average GBM thickness of <250 nm. Patients usually have normal blood pressure and renal function; long-term follow-up is recommended as there appears to be a very small risk of renal failure (perhaps because some patients represent variants of Alport's syndrome, or IgA nephropathy may co-exist).

7.5 Other inherited disorders associated with renal disease

The list is far from comprehensive as many rare disorders have been described.

- **Conditions associated with renal structural disorders**
  Cystic renal diseases (see above)
  Brachio-oto-renal syndrome (AD)
  Dandy–Walker syndrome (polycystic kidneys: (AR))
- **Inherited conditions with glomerular disease**
  Alport's syndrome and variants (see above)
  Congenital nephrotic syndrome (eg Finnish-type (AR))
  Nail–Patella syndrome (AD)
  Familial glomerulonephritis (eg some forms of FSGS or IgA nephropathy; Wiskott–Aldrich syndrome (XL))
  Inherited complement deficiency
  Charcot–Marie–Tooth disease (?AD)
- **Metabolic disorders with renal involvement**
  Fabry's disease (XL)
  Primary amyloidosis (AD)
  Familial Mediterranean fever (AR)
  Cystinosis (AR)
  Primary oxalosis (AR)
- **Inherited tubular disorders**
  Cystinuria (AR)
  Swachman's syndrome (AR)
  Marble brain disease (AR)
  Hypophosphatasia (AR)
- **Renal diseases which have genetic influence**
  Benign familial haematuria (AD)
  Reflux nephropathy

AD = autosomal dominant; AR = autosomal recessive; XL = X-linked

8. RENAL INTERSTITIAL DISORDERS

8.1 Interstitial nephritis

Inflammation of the renal tubulointerstitium may be acute or chronic; a recognised precipitating cause can be found in the majority of patients.

Acute interstitial nephritis (AIN)

AIN accounts for about 2% of all ARF cases, but for 25% of all drug-induced ARF. Most cases are due to an immunologically induced hypersensitivity reaction to an antigen – classically a drug or an infectious agent. The presentation is usually with mild renal impairment and hypertension or, in more severe cases, ARF which is often non-oliguric. Systemic manifestations of hypersensitivity may occur and include fever, arthralgia, rash, eosinophilia and raised IgE.

- **Diagnosis**: urinalysis may be unremarkable (eg minor proteinuria), although urinary eosinophils may be present. If >1% of urinary white cells are eosinophils, then this suggests the diagnosis. Renal biopsy shows oedema of the interstitium with infiltration of plasma cells, lymphocytes and eosinophils; there is often ATN with variable tubular dilatation. Occasionally there is a granulomatous reaction (sarcoidosis can cause AIN). Note that AIN may need to be distinguished from acute pyelonephritis, in which condition most of the inflammatory infiltrate will be composed of neutrophils.
- **Treatment**: cessation of precipitating cause (eg drugs). Most cases will improve without further treatment, but studies show that moderate-dose oral steroids (eg 1 mg/kg, tapered over 1 month) can hasten recovery of renal function. Most patients make a near-complete renal functional recovery.

Causes of acute interstitial nephritis

- **Idiopathic** (rare – can be associated with anterior uveitis)
- **Infections**
  Viral (eg Hanta virus), bacterial (eg leptospirosis), mycobacterial
- **Drugs**
  eg rifampicin, allopurinol, **methicillin**, penicillin, cephalosporins, sulphonamides, furosemide, thiazide diuretics, cimetidine, amphotericin, aspirin, **NSAIDs**
- **Other:** sarcoidosis

Chronic tubulointerstitial nephritis (TIN)

Many diverse systemic and local renal conditions can result in chronic inflammation within the tubulointerstitium. Patients present with CRF or ESRD; some patients may also manifest RTA (usually type 1), nephrogenic diabetes insipidus (DI) or salt-wasting states. Renal biopsy findings involve a chronic inflammatory infiltrate within the interstitium (granulomatous in sarcoid and TB), often with extensive scarring and tubular loss; the latter indicates that renal function can never be fully recovered.

Certain common causes of CRF are associated with TIN and macroscopically abnormal kidneys – eg reflux nephropathy, analgesic nephropathy, obstructive and cystic renal disease. However, **TIN with macroscopically normal kidneys** accounts for about 3% of all ESRD, and the more common causes include sarcoidosis, Sjögren's syndrome, lithium toxicity, urate nephropathy, heavy metal nephropathy and Balkan nephropathy (see box overleaf).

Causes of chronic interstitial nephritis

- **Immunological diseases**
  eg SLE, Sjögren's syndrome, rheumatoid arthritis, systemic sclerosis
- **Haematological disorders**
  Myeloma, light-chain nephropathy, sickle-cell disease
- **Heavy metals (and other toxins)**
  eg lead, cadmium, Chinese herb nephropathy (*see* Section 13.3 Toxic nephropathy)
- **Metabolic disorders**
  eg hypercalcaemia, hypokalaemia, hyperuricaemia
- **Other**
  Irradiation, chronic transplant rejection
- **Granulomatous disease**
  Wegener's, TB, sarcoidosis
- **Drugs**
  Ciclosporin A, cisplatin, lithium, iron, analgesics (see Analgesic nephropathy, opposite)
- **Chronic infections**
  Chronic pyelonephritis (TB)
- **Hereditary disorders**
  eg nephronophthisis, Alport's
- **Endemic disease**
  Balkan nephropathy (see below)

Treatment of TIN

This is of the underlying condition (or drug/toxin withdrawal); steroids may be beneficial in some autoimmune or inflammatory disorders. The progressive CRF is treated as for other chronic nephropathies.

Balkan nephropathy

A chronic interstitial renal disease endemic in villages along the tributaries of the river Danube (eg Romania, Bulgaria, Bosnia, Croatia). There is extensive scarring, and patients progress to ESRD.

- Urothelial malignancy is increased 200-fold.
- Patients have coppery yellow pigmentation of palms and soles.
- **Aetiology**: initially thought to be a chronic toxic nephropathy (eg trace metals in water) or viral infection. Although recent evidence has suggested that chronic exposure to a fungal toxin (eg ochratoxins, products of the fungus *Penicillium*, which may grow in stored maize) may be important, genetic studies suggest an underlying dominant inheritance pattern, with a marker on chromosome 3. It is suspected that the environmental factors modify the expression of the genetic predisposition.

8.2 Analgesic nephropathy and papillary necrosis

Analgesic nephropathy

In the 1950s to 1970s analgesic nephropathy was the most common cause of both ARF and CRF in parts of Europe and Australia (eg 25% of ESRD in Australia). The condition is now in decline, especially since the withdrawal of Phenacetin from the pharmaceutical market; aspirin and NSAIDs are now the most common causative agents. The hallmarks of the condition are the history of chronic analgesic usage (eg for backache, pelvic inflammatory disease, headache) and of addictive or dependent personality traits, renal pain (due to papillary necrosis) and CRF. There is a classical radiological appearance on IVU – 'cup & spill' calyces due to papillary necrosis, with renal scarring.

- Renal biopsy is of no diagnostic value.
- Women are affected more often than men (4:1).
- As with other TIN, nephrogenic DI, salt-wasting and distal RTA can be associated.
- Increased risk of urothelial malignancy (there may be multiple synchronous lesions).
- Patients are at threefold increased risk of CVS disease (contributed to by hypertension, hyperlipidaemia, smoking and Phenacetin-induced formation of atherogenic oxidised LDL).

Causes of renal papillary necrosis

- **Toxic**
  Classical analgesic nephropathy
  TB
- **Ischaemic**
  Sickle cell disease
  Acute pyelonephritis
  Accelerated hypertension
  Profound shock
  Diabetes mellitus
  Urinary tract obstruction
  Hyperviscosity syndromes
  NSAID-induced

9. REFLUX NEPHROPATHY AND URINARY TRACT INFECTIONS

9.1 Vesico-ureteric reflux and reflux nephropathy

Reflux nephropathy is the term applied when small and irregularly scarred kidneys (**chronic pyelonephritis, CPN**) are associated with **vesico-ureteric reflux** (**VUR**). It is the commonest cause of CPN, but there are other causes (eg obstructive injury, analgesic nephropathy). Scarring is necessary for the development of reflux nephropathy and this almost only occurs during the first five years of life. The end result of reflux nephropathy is hypertension, proteinuria, CRF and, eventually, ESRD; reflux nephropathy still accounts for at least 10% of adult patients entering RRT programmes, and is the commonest cause of ESRD in children.

- **Epidemiology**: VUR is very common in utero, and 0.5% of all neonates are affected. Around 1% of children will have VUR, but this disappears in 40% by the age of 2 years. In young children VUR usually presents with a complicating urinary tract infection (UTI). About 30% of children with UTI will have some degree of VUR and 10% will have evidence of reflux nephropathy. Five per cent of women with symptomatic UTI will have reflux nephropathy; however, documented UTI occurs in <50% of adults with the nephropathy.
- **Grading**: reflux can be graded: from grade I (involving reflux into ureter only) to grade V (gross dilatation and tortuosity of ureter, renal pelvis and calyces) – see Figure 2.
- **Diagnosis** is by micturating cystography (radionuclides can be used in children); scarring can be demonstrated by ultrasound and DMSA.
- **Pathogenesis of renal scarring**: scars will only form if there is intra-renal reflux accompanied by urinary infection. The scars form at the sites of the intra-renal reflux; severity of scarring is proportional to the degree of VUR. Note that there is no evidence that UTI occurring without VUR will lead to scarring.
- **Genetic predisposition**: first-degree relatives of patients with reflux have a greatly increased chance of VUR; it is recommended that offspring or siblings (if a child) of affected patients undergo screening. The gene is thought to be dominant but its effect is modified by environmental factors; the gene frequency has been estimated to be 1:600.

Management of VUR and reflux nephropathy

All children with UTI should be investigated for VUR. The aim of treatment for patients with VUR is to prevent renal scars. As these occur early in life there is no place for anti-reflux surgery to prevent renal scars in adults who have VUR. Few surgeons operate on children with grades I–III reflux as these tend to resolve spontaneously; those with grade II or worse reflux should receive prophylactic antibiotic therapy (eg low-dose nitrofurantoin, trimethoprim or cotrimoxazole, or cefalexin in those with CRF) until puberty in order to minimise UTI.

There is now debate as to the best management of patients with grades IV and V VUR. Surgery (eg endoscopic injection of collagen behind the intra-vesical ureter, lengthening of the submucosal ureteric tunnel and ureteric re-implantation) has its protagonists. However, other clinicians would advocate long-term antibiotics (as above). Whichever the approach, UTI should be treated promptly and, as with all forms of chronic, potentially progressive renal disorders, hypertension must be controlled properly (with use of ACE inhibitors/AIIRBs). Note that patients with reflux nephropathy have an increased incidence of renal calculi.

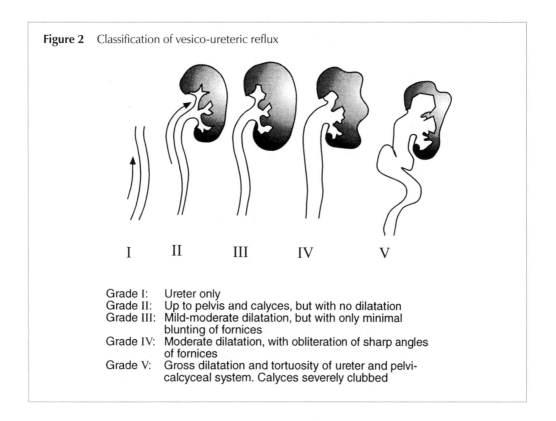

Figure 2 Classification of vesico-ureteric reflux

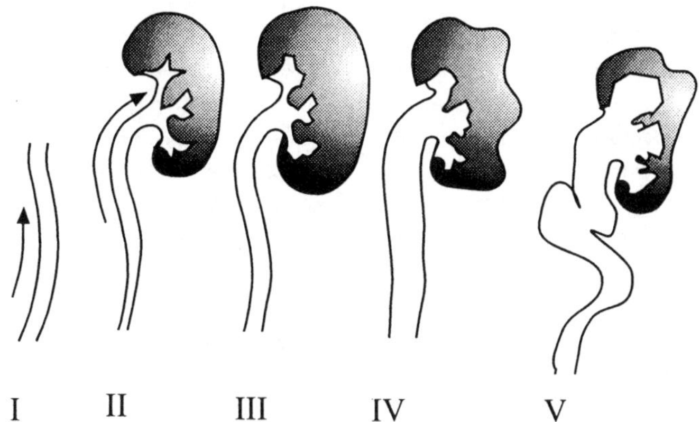

Grade I: Ureter only
Grade II: Up to pelvis and calyces, but with no dilatation
Grade III: Mild-moderate dilatation, but with only minimal blunting of fornices
Grade IV: Moderate dilatation, with obliteration of sharp angles of fornices
Grade V: Gross dilatation and tortuosity of ureter and pelvi-calcyceal system. Calyces severely clubbed

9.2 Urinary tract infection (UTI)

Apart from the outer one-third of the female urethra, the urinary tract is normally sterile. UTIs are the commonest bacterial infections managed in general practice; they predominantly affect women (except in infants, patients aged >60 years, and those with co-morbid diseases). Coliforms are by far the most common pathogens. Several important definitions are applied:

- **Acute uncomplicated UTI**: **acute cystitis** and **acute pyelonephritis**. The incidence of cystitis is 0.5% per year in sexually active women. It may recur in 40% of healthy women, even when their urinary tracts are normal. Three-day antibiotic treatment regimes are recommended for acute cystitis because of cost, compliance and efficacy. In those with recurrent cystitis, attention to hygiene, post-coital micturition and fluid intake are recommended; in post-menopausal women, intra-vaginal oestrogen pessaries may be beneficial, probably by altering the vaginal flora.
- **Complicated UTI**: these occur in patients with abnormal urinary tracts (eg stones, obstruction, ileal conduits, VUR, neuropathic bladder) and very commonly in patients with urinary catheters (see overleaf). The definition also incorporates UTI in patients with CRF and renal transplants.

- **Asymptomatic bacteriuria**: two separate urinary specimens showing bacterial colony counts of $>10^5$/ml of the same organism in an asymptomatic patient. The prevalence may be 3–5% in adult women (and 0.5% in men); it increases greatly in the elderly (eg 50% of women) and in institutionalised patients. It should always be treated if detected in pregnant women, as 15–20% of patients will otherwise develop acute pyelonephritis (*see* Chapter 12, Maternal Medicine).
- **Urethral syndrome**: patients have 'abacterial' cystitis. Causes include true recurrent UTI (but with low bacterial counts), and genital (eg *Chlamydia*), vaginal (eg *Trichomonas* or *Candida*) or fastidious organisms (eg *Ureaplasma, Lactobacillus*) infections. Postmenopausal women may develop the syndrome because of atrophic vaginitis due to oestrogen deficiency.

Long-term antibiotic treatment regimes: these may be appropriate for patients prone to recurrent UTI, and especially in those with an underlying predisposition (except those with urinary catheters). The regimes may involve rotating monthly antibiotic courses (eg amoxicillin, a quinolone and a cephalosporin) or low-dose, once-daily, long-term nitrofurantoin or trimethoprim.

Predispositions to urinary tract infection

- **Abnormal urinary tract**
  eg calculi, VUR, reflux nephropathy, analgesic nephropathy, obstruction, atonic bladder, ileal conduit, in-dwelling catheter, **pregnancy** (where the urinary tract abnormality is temporary)
- **Impaired host defences**
  Immunosuppressive therapy (including transplanted patients), diabetes mellitus, atrophic vaginitis
- **Virulent organisms**
  (eg urease-producing *Proteus*)

Other specific forms of UTI

- **Urinary-catheter-associated infection**: up to 5% of all hospital admissions may be due to nosocomial UTI, and the majority of these occur in patients with long-term in-dwelling catheters. The incidence of bacteriuria is 3–10% per day of catheterisation, and so the duration of catheterisation is the greatest risk factor. Most infections are asymptomatic, but catheter-associated infections are the commonest source of Gram –ve septicaemia in hospitalised patients. Most cases of 'infection' do not require treatment; if lower urinary tract symptoms occur, a single antibiotic dose may be as effective as a full course of therapy (which predisposes to bacterial resistance); it may also be appropriate to change the catheter (if needed long-term) as organisms are harboured within the bio-film lining of the catheter.
- **Prostatitis**: prostatitic symptoms are experienced by 50% of men, but are caused by bacteria in only a minority. **Acute bacterial prostatitis** is rare; patients present with symptoms of cystitis and the prostate is swollen and tender. There will be pyuria and a positive urine culture. The commonest pathogens are the Gram –ve bacilli, *E. coli*, *Proteus*

and *Klebsiella*. Antibiotic treatment is needed for 1 month. **Chronic prostatitis** is manifest by recurrent UTI with the same organism. It is characterised by a qualitative difference in the first voided urine (no pyuria), compared to that passed after prostatic massage (>10 white blood cells per high-power field, bacterial colony count 10-fold greater). Treatment is with quinolone antibiotics for 1–3 months.

- **Renal abscess**: usually due to *Staphylococcus aureus* after haematogenous spread to the kidney. May present as a renal mass but renal abscesses are often insidious and non-specific. CT is needed for diagnosis. Treatment is with antibiotics, percutaneous drainage for larger abscesses and sometimes nephrectomy.
- **Emphysematous pyelonephritis**: this is a necrotising, life-threatening form of acute pyelonephritis caused by gas-forming organisms (including *E. coli*, *Pseudomonas*, *Klebsiella* and *Proteus*). Ninety per cent of cases occur in diabetics. Plain X-ray will demonstrate the gas, but CT will localise this better. Emergency nephrectomy and broad-spectrum antibiotics are required, but even then mortality is 20%.
- **Xanthogranulomatous pyelonephritis**: this is a rare chronic renal infection that is associated with obstruction. Renal tissue is replaced with lipid-laden infiltrating macrophages (foam cells); the xanthomatous tissue may extend beyond the renal capsule into neighbouring structures. Patients are usually middle-aged women with flank pain, fever, a palpable renal mass and +ve MSU. Nephrectomy provides the only chance of cure.

9.3 Tuberculosis of the urinary tract

TB reaches the urinary tract via haematogenous spread. Most patients are 20–40 years of age, with men affected twice as commonly as women. Twenty-five per cent of patients are asymptomatic; a further 25% have asymptomatic pyuria or microscopic haematuria, and painless macrohaematuria is common. Hypertension is unusual, but genital involvement (epididymitis and prostatitis in men, salpingitis and pelvic pain in women) is commonly associated.

- The renal medullary regions are most commonly affected. In the early stages, ulcerating lesions and granulomas are seen in the renal pyramids and collecting systems; renal histology shows chronic interstitial nephritis with granulomas.
- As the disease progresses scarring occurs with ureteric strictures, hydronephrosis, subcapsular collections, perinephric abscesses or renal atrophy. The bladder may be fibrotic and small. The caseating material may eventually calcify.
- **Treatment**: standard anti-tuberculous therapy is recommended. Surgery may be indicated for obstruction and strictures. Nephrectomy for non-functioning kidneys is no longer routine as prolonged anti-TB therapy can render the calcified, caseous masses ('cement kidney') sterile.

10. RENAL CALCULI AND NEPHROCALCINOSIS

10.1 Renal calculi (nephrolithiasis)

Renal stones are common, with an annual incidence of approximately 2 per 1000 and a prevalence of 3% in the UK. Calcium-containing stones are commonest.

Stone composition

- Calcium oxalate: 25%
- Mixed calcium oxalate/phosphate: 40%
- Calcium phosphate: 5%
- Urate: 10% (radiolucent)
- Cystine: 2%
- Xanthine: 1% (radiolucent)
- Staghorns ('struvite' containing magnesium ammonium phosphate and sometimes calcium): 20%; associated with infection with urease-producing bacteria (eg *Proteus* spp.)

- **Basic investigation**: this should include stone analysis, MSU, assessment of renal function, serum calcium and phosphate, and a qualitative test for urinary cystine. The 24-hour urinary excretion of oxalate, calcium (should be >7.5 mmol/day), creatinine and uric acid may also be helpful, and RTA should be excluded (urine pH).

Conditions predisposing to urolithiasis

- **Metabolic abnormalities**
  Idiopathic hypercalciuria (most common)
  Primary hyperparathyroidism (and other causes of hypercalcaemia)
  Renal tubular acidosis
  Cystinuria
  Hyperoxaluria (primary or secondary)
  High dietary oxalate intake (eg glutinous rice or leafy vegetables in Thailand)
  Uric aciduria
  Hypocitraturia (eg chronic diarrhoea, excess laxative and diuretic use)
- **Renal structural abnormalities**
  Polycystic kidney disease
  Medullary sponge kidney
  Reflux nephropathy
  Nephrocalcinosis (see opposite)
- **Other causes**
  Chronic dehydration (common, eg chronic diarrhoea, warm climates)
  Triamterene
  Industrial exposure to cadmium or beryllium

Treatment

General measures: large fluid intake and low protein diet. Associated urinary infection should be eradicated where possible (very difficult with staghorn calculi). Treat other underlying causes (eg allopurinol for urate stones, surgery for hyperparathyroidism).

Thiazide diuretics (eg chlortalidone): increase tubular absorption of calcium in patients with hypercalciuria, and will therefore reduce the likelihood of super-saturation of calcium products within the urine. Citrate may be beneficial for calcium oxalate stones.

The specific treatment of patients with **cystinuria** is described in Chapter 13, Metabolic Diseases.

Stone removal: ureteric calculi <0.5 cm may be passed spontaneously. Lithotripsy alone may be used for larger ureteric stones and for pelvi-calyceal stones <4 cm (obstruction being prevented by double J-stent insertion); larger calculi can be 'debulked' by this technique before surgical extraction.

10.2 Nephrocalcinosis

This is defined as the deposition of calcium salts within the renal parenchyma; it may be associated with urinary calculi.

Causes

- **Cortical nephrocalcinosis**
  Cortical necrosis (see 'tram-line' calcification)
  Chronic glomerulonephritis
- **Medullary nephrocalcinosis**
  Hypercalcaemia (eg primary hyperparathyroidism, sarcoidosis, hypervitaminosis D, milk–alkali syndrome)
  Idiopathic hypercalciuria
  Renal tubular acidosis
  Primary hyperoxaluria
  Berylliosis
  Thyrotoxicosis
  Sulphonamides
  Medullary sponge kidney
  Tuberculosis

11. URINARY TRACT OBSTRUCTION AND TUMOURS

11.1 Urinary tract obstruction

Chronic urinary tract obstruction (most often due to prostatic disease, calculi and bladder lesions) is a common cause of CRF; obstruction must also be excluded in every case of ARF. The causes of renal tract obstruction are shown in the box opposite. The term **obstructive nephropathy** refers to pathological renal damage resulting from obstruction.

Acute obstruction

This is often painful due to distension of the bladder, ureter(s) or pelvi-calyceal systems. Complete obstruction will result in anuria and ARF; anuria may also occur even when obstruction is unilateral, due to the intense afferent arteriolar vasoconstriction (similar to that seen in ischaemic ARF) which is also contributory to the ARF.

- **Diagnosis**: obstruction is one of the few truly reversible causes of renal failure, but diagnosis and treatment need to be expedient in order to allow renal functional recovery. Ultrasound is the chief mode of diagnosis, but it may only show minimal pelvi-calyceal dilatation in the early stages of acute obstruction.
- **Treatment and prognosis**: temporary drainage can often be achieved by percutaneous nephrostomy or by endoscopic ureteric stenting, pending definitive surgical correction. Relief of obstruction may be followed by massive diuresis (temporary nephrogenic DI), but if the obstruction has been relieved within 2 weeks then full renal functional recovery is likely, unless there is complicating pyonephrosis.

Chronic obstructive nephropathy

This is usually associated with CRF or ESRD and it is often complicated by chronic UTI. Obstruction accounts for 5% of all cases of ESRD. Salt-wasting nephropathy and chronic metabolic acidosis are common, the latter contributing to the advanced renal bone disease recognised in some patients.

- **Differential diagnosis**: there may be diagnostic uncertainty when the upper tracts are dilated (but non-obstructed). This is seen in VUR, post-obstructive atrophy, congenital mega-calyces and mega-ureters and in some cases of CPN. In such cases diuresis renography or retrograde pyelography will exclude obstruction. Occasionally, the Whitaker test, which involves puncture of the collecting system followed by pressure flow studies, is necessary to diagnose obstruction.
- **Pathology and outcome**: there is permanent renal histopathological damage that results from a combination of parenchymal compression, renal ischaemia and perhaps infection. In severe cases severe tubular loss, interstitial fibrosis and cortical atrophy are observed. If the obstruction is relieved (eg in < 12 weeks), renal functional decline can stabilise and dialysis may be prevented.

Causes of urinary tract obstruction

- **Within the lumen**
  Tumour (eg urothelial lesions of bladder, ureter or renal pelvis)
  Renal calculi
  Papillary necrosis (sloughed papilla)
  Blood clot

- **External compression**
  Malignancy: retro-peritoneal neoplasia including para-aortic lymphadenopathy and pelvic cancer (eg cervical or prostatic carcinoma)
  Other 'tumours': aortic aneurysm; pregnancy (hydronephrosis of pregnancy is very common, is usually asymptomatic, and resolves fully after delivery); haematomas
  Aberrant arteries (PUJ obstruction)
  Retro-peritoneal fibrosis (eg malignant, idiopathic, peri-aortitis, drugs (see below))
  Prostatic disease: benign hypertrophy or malignancy
  Inflammatory disorders (eg diverticulitis, Crohn's disease, pancreatitis)
  Iatrogenic: surgical ligation of ureter

- **Within the wall of urinary tract structures**
  Neuromuscular dysfunction (eg pelvi-ureteric junction (PUJ) obstruction, neuropathic bladder (spina bifida, spinal trauma – see below))
  Ureteric or vesico-ureteric stricture: TB, schistosomiasis, previous calculi, after surgery, congenital, irradiation (eg for seminoma of testis), malignancy, ureterocele
  Urethral stricture (eg gonococcal) following instrumentation
  Posterior urethral valves (see overleaf)
  Congenital bladder neck obstruction

Neuropathic bladder

In childhood**, spina bifida** with myelomeningocele is by far the commonest cause of a neuropathic bladder. Spina bifida has an incidence of around 1–5 per 1000 births; siblings of affected individuals have a 10- to 20-fold chance of having the condition. Urinary tract complications are present at birth in 15%, and will develop in 50%, often over many years. Most of these patients have incomplete bladder emptying due to urethral sphincter dyssynergia, but those with the least neurologic lesion are paradoxically able to generate very high pressures within the bladder, with greatest risk of renal damage.

- The main urinary tract abnormalities are incontinence, infection and reflux with upper tract dilatation, the latter leading to CRF and ESRD.
- Patients usually have associated bowel dysfunction.

- **Treatment**: is with anticholinergic drugs, intermittent self-catheterisation and, in more severe cases, urinary tract diversion into an ileal conduit. Note that chronically infected urinary tracts will need to be removed prior to renal transplantation.

Posterior urethral valves (PUV)

These occur in male infants and account for 10% of childhood hydronephrosis; the valves are mucosal diaphragms in the posterior urethra at the level of the prostate. PUV can now be detected ante-natally with ultrasound. Fifty per cent of patients present before the first year of life with poor stream, distended bladder and failure to thrive (due to renal failure). Most have VUR and dilated upper tracts.

- **Treatment**: urinary diversion should be avoided; self-catheterisation is usually necessary. Approximately 20% of affected individuals will progress to ESRD, largely because of late initial presentation.

11.2 Retroperitoneal fibrosis (RPF)

An uncommon, progressive condition in which the ureters become embedded in dense fibrous tissue (the ureters are drawn medially) often at the junction of the middle and lower thirds of the ureter, leading to obstruction. The majority of cases are thought to result from an immunologically mediated peri-aortitis, and steroids are of benefit in these 'idiopathic' forms of RPF.

- **Other associations**: retroperitoneal malignancy (eg colonic, bladder or prostatic cancer, lymphoma), previous irradiation, inflammatory abdominal aortic aneurysm, other fibrosing conditions (eg mediastinal fibrosis, sclerosing cholangitis), drugs (eg methysergide and some β-blockers) and granulomatous disease (TB or sarcoidosis).
- **Investigation**: ESR is often very high, IVU shows medial deviation of the ureters and a peri-aortic mass may be seen at CT scan.
- **Treatment**: ureterolysis (with tissue biopsy) with long-term steroid therapy (as relapse is common). Malignant RPF can be palliated with ureteric stenting, or with percutaneous nephrostomy.

11.3 Urinary tract tumours

Benign renal tumours: include adenomata, which are very common (however, just as with thyroid adenoma and carcinoma, their histological differentiation from malignant lesions can be difficult), hamartomas and renin-secreting (juxta-glomerular cell) tumours.

Renal cell carcinoma (hypernephroma): arise from the tubular epithelium; they are more likely in smokers, and at least 50% of patients with von Hippel–Lindau syndrome will develop them (usually multiple and bilateral). As mentioned previously, **acquired cystic kidney disease** in patients with renal failure is a major risk factor; the cumulative incidence of malignant change is about 1%, and accounts for 80% of renal cell carcinomas in dialysis patients.

- The hallmark of renal cell carcinoma is its propensity to invade the renal veins, with passage of tumour emboli to lung.
- Other unusual clinical features include PUO, left varicocele (renal vein invasion leads to left testicular vein occlusion), and endocrine effects (secretion of erythropoietic factor resulting in polycythaemia (3%), PTH-like substance, renin and ACTH). Five-year survival is about 50%.

Wilm's tumour (nephroblastoma): these are tumours of early childhood, and are derived from embryonic renal tissue (so containing combinations of poorly differentiated epithelium and connective tissues). They become enormous and metastasise early. Treatment is with nephrectomy and actinomycin D, providing a three-year survival rate of 65%.

Urothelial tumours: very common and usually derived from transitional epithelium, although squamous carcinoma (far worse prognosis) is recognised. The usual presentation is with bleeding or urinary tract obstruction. Tumours are often multiple, and so investigation of the complete urinary tract is indicated.

- Several carcinogens (eg smoking, rubber and aniline dye exposure, analgesic nephropathy) have been aetiologically linked to this type of malignancy.
- Other risk factors include renal calculi, cystic kidney disease, chronic cystitis and *Schistosoma haematobium* infection (NB *Schistosoma mansoni* is associated with glomerulonephritis).
- Nephro-ureterectomy is indicated for lesions of ureter or renal pelvis, and cystectomy with resection of urethral mucosa for advanced bladder cancer; surgery combined with radiotherapy provides a five-year survival of 50%.

Metastatic disease (involving the kidney): most commonly from breast, lung, stomach, lymphoma or melanoma.

12. SYSTEMIC DISORDERS AND THE KIDNEY

12.1 Amyloidosis

Amyloidosis is due to over-production of proteinaceous material which deposits in an organised formation within tissues. Kidney involvement leads to presentation with proteinuria, nephrotic syndrome or CRF; biopsy demonstrates characteristic Congo-red-staining extracellular fibrillar material within the mesangium, interstitium and vessel walls. SAP scan (labelled amyloid fibrils which localise to amyloid deposits after injection) may be useful to demonstrate the full extent of disease in all organs. Amyloid is classified according to the amyloid proteins involved, as well as the underlying disease process.

Immunologlobulinic amyloid (AL-amyloidosis)

The incidence of AL-amyloidosis is 9 per million/year. Free immunoglobulin light chains (hence the 'L') are secreted by a clone of B-cells; 25% of patients have an underlying immunoproliferative disease (usually myeloma), but many more probably have a monoclonal gammopathy (MGUS). Median age of presentation is above 60 years.

- Nephrotic syndrome, postural hypotension and peripheral neuropathy are more likely in cases without myeloma.
- AL-amyloid may infiltrate any organ other than the brain – eg heart (restrictive cardiomyopathy in 30%, sick-sinus syndrome and arrhythmias), macroglossia, GI tract (motility disturbance, malabsorption, haemorrhage), neuropathy (peripheral and autonomic) and bleeding diathesis.
- **Treatment**: cases associated with myeloma receive conventional therapy. In 'primary amyloid', regimes involving prednisolone with either melphalan or colchicine have been shown to extend survival duration by only 50% (see below). Autologous bone marrow transplantation (after high-dose chemotherapy) provides the only prospect of cure.
- **Prognosis**: is poor, with median survival of 12 months, and only 25% alive at 3 years. Survival is shorter in those with myeloma, heart disease and autonomic neuropathy. Cardiac involvement accounts for half of deaths.

AA-amyloidosis

Chronic infections (eg TB, empyema) now account for fewer cases than previously; 70% of cases are due to autoimmune inflammatory conditions. In AA-amyloidosis the kidney is the main target organ – cardiac involvement and neuropathy are uncommon. Prognosis is consequently better than for AL-amyloidosis with median survival of 25 months, and 40% 3-year survival.

Treatment: the underlying inflammatory or infective disorder should be treated. Although previously there has been little apparent benefit from specific drug therapy, colchicine has been shown to prevent disease progression in **familial Mediterranean fever** (another form of AA-amyloidosis), which is encouraging. It has been trialled in patients with rheumatoid arthritis with some success. A few patients with AA-amyloidosis have received renal transplants; recurrent amyloid is seen in >10%.

Classification of amyloidosis

Primary amyloid
AL type, which is serum amyloid protein A coupled with immunoglobulin light chains

Hereditary amyloid
(eg familial Mediterranean fever)
Fibrils are formed from other proteins (lysosomes, apolipoproteins, fibrinogen); the amyloid is of **AA type**

Secondary amyloid
This is usually **AA type** (fibrils composed of acute phase protein)

- **Secondary to chronic suppurative disorders**
  Tuberculosis, osteomyelitis, empyema, bronchiectasis, syphilis, leprosy
- **Secondary to chronic inflammatory disorders**
  Rheumatological conditions – rheumatoid arthritis, psoriatic arthritis, ankylosing spondylitis, Still's disease, Reiter's syndrome, Sjögren's syndrome, Behçet's disease
  Gastrointestinal conditions – Whipple's disease, inflammatory bowel disease
  Paraprotein-related conditions – myeloma (AL type), benign monoclonal gammopathy (AL type)
- **Other secondary amyloid**
  Heroin abuse, paraplegia, renal cell carcinoma
- **Dialysis-related amyloid**
  This does not deposit in the kidneys, as it is a complication of long-term dialysis. It is due to failure of clearance of β_2-microglobulin (see Section 5.4)

12.2 Renovascular disease

Atherosclerotic renovascular disease (ARVD)

ARVD accounts for 99% of all renovascular disease. It is increased with ageing, is associated with common atherogenic risk factors (ie hypertension, hyper-cholesterolaemia, smoking, diabetes, etc) as well as with the presence of generalised vascular disease – it can be demonstrated in 30% of patients undergoing coronary angiography, >50% with peripheral vascular disease and it affects 30% of patients with CCF aged >70 years. As older patients are now readily admitted to RRT programmes, ARVD is found to be increasingly associated with ESRD (15–20%), although it probably only accounts for the renal failure in the minority (see below).

Clinical presentation is with hypertension, CRF or ESRD, 'flash' pulmonary oedema (10%), and ARF due to acute arterial occlusion or related to ACE-I. Prognosis is poor (5-year survival <20%) due to co-morbid vascular events. Many cases of ARVD are thought to be incidental, occurring as a result of hypertension and CRF (pro-atherogenic state), rather than being the cause of them.

- **Flash pulmonary oedema**: mechanism probably involves reduced natriuretic capability, coupled with left ventricular hypertrophy and severe hypertension, in patients who usually have severe bilateral disease. Patients are particularly prone to developing the episode of pulmonary oedema at night, largely because of posture-related redistribution of fluid, but possibly also because of diurnal variations in vasoactive peptides.
- **Pathogenesis of CRF**: the correlation between severity of proximal lesions (ie degree of renal artery stenosis (RAS) or occlusion) and renal function is poor; this explains why revascularisation procedures are only variably successful. Parenchymal disease, manifest by intra-renal atheroma, ischaemic change and cholesterol embolisation ('ischaemic nephropathy'), is now being recognised as a major determinant of renal functional outcome.
- **Radiological diagnosis**: **MR angiography** is now the optimum non-invasive screening test for ARVD diagnosis. It is indicated in patients with vascular bruits or asymmetrical kidneys on ultrasound, and in cases of unexplained CRF or severe hypertension. **CT angiography** is also increasingly used, but can be complicated by radio-contrast nephropathy in patients with CRF (*N*-acetyl cysteine may help prevent this). Captopril renography (low sensitivity in patients with CRF) is now rarely used. **Doppler ultrasound** is time-consuming and highly observer-dependent. **Conventional i.a. angiography** is now largely reserved for patients with complex anatomy, and when confirming renal arterial anatomy prior to revascularisation. Ninety per cent of RAS lesions are 'ostial' (occurring within the first 1 cm of the renal artery origin).
- **Revascularisation procedures**: renal angioplasty with or without stenting accounts for >95% of all revascularisation (the remainder being surgical reconstructions – especially indicated with complicated lesions, eg related to aortic aneurysm). Improved hypertension control can be anticipated, but cure (ie no need for antihypertensive agents) is unusual. Improvement in renal dysfunction is variable, and this is explained by the fact that many cases of ARVD are incidental, and of little pathogenetic significance. Patients should also receive aspirin and cholesterol-lowering therapy for their general atherosclerotic risk.

Fibromuscular dysplasia (FMD)

FMD accounts for 1% of all renovascular disease; it occurs in the young (20–35 years), and the majority of patients are female. The stenoses may be long and can be distal in the renal artery; they appear as a 'string of beads' at angiography. Patients usually present with severe hypertension, but renal failure is unusual. As the kidney beyond a fibromuscular stenosis is usually healthy, revascularisation may cure the hypertension, and it often restores renal function completely in the sub-group of patients with renal impairment. FMD is associated with other arterial lesions (eg carotid stenosis in 10%, stenosis of the middle of the abdominal aorta).

12.3 Connective tissue disorders and the kidney

Most of the connective tissue disorders have the propensity to cause renal disease, and characteristic features are described below (*see also* Chapter 20, Rheumatology); lupus nephritis and systemic sclerosis merit more detailed coverage.

- **Mixed connective tissue disease**: membranous or diffuse proliferative glomerulonephritis (uncommon).
- **Sjögren's syndrome**: renal involvement is most often manifest by renal tubular dysfunction (RTA1 or 2) with interstitial nephritis; cryoglobulinaemia and membranous or focal proliferative glomerulonephritis are less common.
- **Rheumatoid arthritis**: renal disease is common, and usually due to amyloid or less often the effects of drug therapy. Rheumatoid-related membranous or mesangioproliferative glomerulonephritis is fairly common and is manifest by microscopic haematuria and mild proteinuria. Membranous glomerulonephritis is also recognised (not just an association with gold or penicillamine therapy) and is increased in patients with HLA-DR3.
- **Seronegative spondylarthropathies**: ankylosing spondylitis and Reiter's syndrome can be associated with IgA nephropathy.
- **Relapsing polychondritis**: this disorder is associated with cartilage inflammation leading to destruction and deformity (eg saddle nose, floppy ears). Crescentic, mesangioproliferative or membranous glomerulonephritis may occur.

SLE nephritis

Over 5% of patients with SLE have renal involvement at presentation, and around 60% of patients will develop overt renal disease at some stage. Lupus nephritis is commoner in black patients and in women (10-fold greater than in men), and 90% will have ANF antibodies. Renal disease can be manifest by any syndromal picture (eg proteinuria, nephrotic syndrome, rapidly progressive glomerulonephritis with ARF, CRF) but proteinuria is present in almost all patients with nephritis. Similarly, many different patterns of glomerular disease are recognised (the histological picture may even change, over time, within the same individual). Note that drug-induced SLE only rarely affects the kidneys. Although lupus nephritis can present with marked patient morbidity, the results of prompt immunosuppressive treatment are now gratifying.

Renal histology – WHO classification: the pattern has previously been thought to be of prognostic value, with focal proliferative and membranous lesions providing a favourable renal outcome; diffuse proliferative or crescentic glomerulonephritis predicts the worst renal prognosis. 'Wire loop' lesions (thickened capillary walls – EM shows electron-dense deposits) are characteristic; immunofluorescence is positive for most immunoglobulins (IgG, IgM, IgA) and complement components (C_3, C_4, C_{1q}). A synopsis of the WHO classification is:

- class I: mild changes
- class II: mesangioproliferative changes
- class III: focal proliferative glomerulonephritis (variable severity)
- class IV: severe diffuse proliferative glomerulonephritis
- class V: membranous glomerulonephritis.

Treatment: Patients with mild disease (eg WHO classes I and II) usually require no treatment. However, irrespective of the WHO class, most patients with significant proteinuria are likely to receive at least prednisolone and ACE inhibitor therapy. Acute SLE with ARF (classes III and IV – usually diffuse, crescentic or severe focal proliferative glomerulonephritis) should be treated as for 'RPGN/crescentic nephritis' (*see* Section 6, Glomerulonephritis and associated syndromes), with an intense induction regime (high-dose steroid, and usually pulsed iv cyclophosphamide) followed by maintenance therapy. Patients with class V histology who present with the nephrotic syndrome are treated similarly, although there is less evidence of conclusive benefit. Although plasma exchange has been used in patients with crescentic disease, and in those with severe extra-renal manifestations of SLE, there is again little evidence of improved outcome.

- Recent trials have shown a benefit with treatment regimes involving mycophenolate mofetil (MMF).
- In many patients the immunosuppression can be tapered, and withdrawn by 5 years, even in those presenting with severe ARF.

Prognosis of renal lupus: <10% of cases with nephritis now progress to ESRD (historically, renal disease used to be the commonest cause of death in SLE). The SLE syndrome often becomes quiescent once the patients reach RRT. Lupus nephritis rarely recurs in renal transplants.

Systemic sclerosis

Renal disease is always accompanied by hypertension; the hallmark presentation is 'scleroderma renal crisis' with accelerated hypertension, microangiopathic haemolytic anaemia and ARF. Prominent pathological changes are seen in the interlobular arteries (severe intimal proliferation with deposition of mucopolysaccharides – so-called 'onion skin' appearance); fibrinoid necrosis of afferent arterioles and secondary glomerular ischaemia are common. The essential treatment is with ACE inhibitors for hypertension control; many patients progress to ESRD, but renal function has been known to recover after many months of dialysis, particularly in those patients who presented with renal crisis. The overall prognosis is poor because of other organ involvement (especially restrictive cardiomyopathy and pulmonary fibrosis).

12.4 Diabetic nephropathy

Diabetic nephropathy is now the most common cause of ESRD in the UK, accounting for 25% of patients. In recent years there have been advances in the understanding of the natural history, pathogenesis and treatment of diabetic nephropathy, but the mortality of this group remains high, largely because of associated CVS disease.

Epidemiology

Nephropathy, defined as persistent albuminuria (>300 mg/24 h, which equates to >500 mg/24 h of total proteinuria) occurs with a cumulative incidence of 30% after 40 years in type I diabetics. In type II diabetics, nephropathy is already prevalent in 10% at the time of diabetes diagnosis (reflecting previous 'sub-clinical' hyperglycaemia), and there is a 25% 20-year cumulative incidence of nephropathy. About one-fifth of these latter patients will develop CRF and be at risk of ESRD (ie 5 % of all type II diabetics) – the remainder succumb to other complications of diabetes before they develop significant CRF. As type II diabetes is 10–15 times more common than type I in Western populations, the prevalence of patients with nephropathy in type II diabetes is substantially higher than in those with type I diabetes. In a UK diabetic clinic, the prevalence of nephropathy is about 5% at any time.

- Genetic influence: diabetics in certain racial groups have a far greater risk of developing nephropathy (eg Asians, Pima Indians). In the UK, the likelihood of ESRD is 3-fold greater in Asian and Afro-Caribbean diabetics than in Caucasians.
- Nephropathy is usually associated with retinopathy (common basement membrane pathology); renovascular disease and other arterial pathology are common.

Natural history of nephropathy

In type I diabetes the stages of development of nephropathy have been well characterised:

- **Stage 1**: at the time of diabetes diagnosis the GFR is elevated by >20% compared to age-matched controls. Urinary albumin excretion rate (UAER) is also increased; both are reduced by commencement of insulin.
- **Stage 2**: GFR remains elevated (due to hyperfiltration) and kidneys are hypertrophied but blood pressure and UAER are normal. The GFR appears to be linked to glycaemic control, with greatest hyperfiltration associated with worse control (up to a plasma glucose of 14 mmol/l). There are early histologic changes with thickening of glomerular basement membranes and mesangial expansion. This stage typically lasts for 5–15 years after diabetes diagnosis.
- **Stage 3**: microalbuminuria (or 'incipient nephropathy') is present (UAER 30–300 mg/day, or 20–200 μg/min). The GFR remains elevated or returns to the normal range. Blood pressure starts to rise (in 60%). Microalbuminuria occurs in 30–50% of patients at 5–10 years after diabetes onset, and 80% of these patients go on to develop overt nephropathy (stage 4) over 10–15 years. Histologic changes progress from those seen in stage 2.
- **Stage 4**: 'established' or 'overt' nephropathy is associated with increasing macro-proteinuria ('persistent proteinuria'), which may become nephrotic in 30%, and declining GFR (eg average 10 ml/min per year) in all patients. Hypertension is present in most (80%) and is correlated with the rate of decline of GFR. Renal histology typically shows diffuse glomerular sclerosing lesions (all patients) and vascular changes; 10% have Kimmelstiel–Wilson nodules (focal glomerular sclerosis).
- **Stage 5**: development of ESRD occurs at an average of 7 years from onset of stage 4.

It is thought that the development of nephropathy occurs in a similar fashion in type II diabetes.

Screening and prevention

Patients should be **screened** for microalbuminuria in the diabetic clinic; the albumin:creatinine ratio (ACR – *see* Section 2.1 Urinalysis) in an early morning specimen is more practical than obtaining timed urine collections. An ACR of >2.5 is generally taken as the cut-off for microalbuminuria (equivalent to an UAER of > 35 μg/min, or 45 mg/24 h).

- Studies in type I diabetics have shown that tight glycaemic control can reduce the likelihood of patients developing microalbuminuria (by 40%), and there is emerging evidence that intensive insulin regimes may prevent some microalbuminuric patients progressing to overt nephropathy.
- However, the latter has been clearly shown with trials using ACE inhibitors in type I diabetes, and with AIIRBs in type II. These agents also slow the time of doubling of serum creatinine and the time to ESRD in patients with established nephropathy; comparisons with other antihypertensive agents suggest that their renoprotective effects are partly independent of hypertension control.
- It is now accepted that blood pressure should be targeted to 125/75 mmHg in patients with stage 4 nephropathy – this will slow, but not prevent, the inexorable decline of GFR in patients with overt nephropathy.

Outcome

The mortality of these patients is very high (eg patients with insulin-dependent diabetes mellitus have a 20-fold greater mortality than the general population) and this relative risk may be magnified a further 25-fold in those with proteinuria (eg 2-year mortality of 30% in patients with ESRD), largely due to co-morbid cardiovascular disease. Many patients with stage 4 nephropathy in type II diabetes will die before they reach ESRD.

- Microalbuminuria confers an excess risk of mortality compared to patients with normalbuminuria – eg 4-year mortality 28% in type II diabetics with microalbuminuria, compared to 4% in those without. It is thought that microalbuminuria represents the renal manifestation of a generalised vascular endothelial dysfunction.
- All patients who reach ESRD are considered for RRT. Most patients require screening for coronary artery disease before listing for transplantation; combined renal and pancreatic transplantation is now feasible in selected patients (*see in* Section 5.5 Renal transplantation). Five-year survival of transplanted diabetics is 45–75%.

12.5 Thrombotic microangiopathies

Haemolytic–uraemic syndrome and **thrombotic thrombocytopenic purpura** share similar renal histologic features and pathophysiology (*see also* Chapter 9, Haematology). In both conditions there is a microangiopathic haemolytic anaemia (MAHA), with anaemia, RBC fragments and schistocytes. Platelet clumping occurs within the intra-vascular thrombi, and hence thrombocytopaenia is a major feature. The typical renal histological lesions include intraglomerular thrombi with ischaemia and arteriolar lesions.

Haemolytic–uraemic syndrome (HUS)

HUS is the commonest cause of ARF in children (because ARF is rare in children), but it is also seen in adults (5 cases per million/year). Children aged <4 years account for 90% of cases. Two main forms of HUS are recognised:

Typical or diarrhoea-associated (D^+) HUS: the onset is explosive, with ARF, and epidemics of the disease occur. A third of UK cases are due to verotoxin-producing *E. coli* O157:H7 (VTEC); the toxin damages vascular endothelium, predisposing to the micro-angiopathy. *Shigella dysenteriae* can also be associated. The intra-vascular abnormalities are largely confined to the kidneys. Ninety per cent of patients with D^+HUS make a good recovery, but 5% die during the acute illness; up to 40% of patients have decreased GFR at long-term follow-up.

Atypical HUS: tends to affect older children and adults; most patients have no diarrhoea (D^-HUS). Many D^-HUS cases are thought to be familial, and there is progressive renal dysfunction with neurologic episodes that can resemble TTP. **Familial forms** of HUS/TTP can be associated with factor H deficiency (which may limit cleavage of unusually large von Willebrand factors, leading to continued platelet activation and hence the pathogenesis of HUS or TTP). These forms have a poorer prognosis, with ESRD or death occurring in >50% of patients.

- **Monitoring of disease**: in typical HUS red cell fragmentation and the platelet count are the best means of monitoring disease activity. LDH levels are high (due to haemolysis), but this may also represent tissue infarction.
- **Treatment**: the mainstay of therapy is infusion of fresh frozen plasma (FFP) and plasma exchange. The latter are more effective in adult D^+HUS than in childhood forms; prostacyclin infusion may also be of benefit in D^+HUS. In atypical HUS, FFP and plasma exchange may lower the risk of ESRD and mortality.

Thrombotic thrombocytopenic purpura (TTP)

In TTP, explosive ARF is less prominent, but neurological abnormalities are usual (due to formation and release of microthrombi within the brain vasculature). Again two main forms are recognised:

- **Acute TTP**: 90% of patients with TTP present with abrupt onset with neurologic signs, fever and purpura. Plasma exchange and FFP infusion are indicated for this condition. Previously invariably fatal, survival now approaches 90%.
- **Relapsing TTP**: adults are usually affected and chronic disease is more likely – the condition can appear similar to atypical HUS. Some of these cases are probably familial HUS/TTP.

Secondary causes of HUS and TTP

These include:

- pregnancy-associated thrombotic microangiopathy (see Chapter 12, Maternal Medicine).
  –TTP
  –HELLP syndrome
  –Post-partum HUS
- HIV-associated thrombotic microangiopathy
- cancer-associated thrombotic microangiopathy
- drugs (eg ciclosporin).

12.6 Hypertension and the kidney

A detailed description of hypertension is beyond the scope of this chapter; but see also Chapter 1, Cardiology. The kidney is often damaged by essential hypertension, or it can be central to the pathogenesis of many cases of secondary hypertension.

Primary (essential) hypertension and renal damage

End-organ renal damage is common and is usually manifest with asymptomatic proteinuria and/or CRF (**hypertensive nephrosclerosis**). Microalbuminuria develops in 20–40% of patients with essential hypertension, and persistent proteinuria (occasionally nephrotic) in a smaller proportion. Typical histological lesions include vascular wall thickening and luminal obliteration, with widespread interstitial fibrosis and glomerulosclerosis.

- Elevated creatinine develops in 10–20% of patients; the risk is greater in African-Americans, the elderly and those with higher systolic blood pressure.
- Progression to ESRD occurs in 2–5% over 10–15 years. Hypertension accounts for about 30% of all ESRD in the USA and 15% in the UK.
- It is thought that many patients who present with ESRD of unknown aetiology, especially with small, smooth kidneys visible at ultrasound, actually have long-standing hypertensive renal disease.

Treatment and targets: all patients should have their blood pressure controlled to <140/85 mmHg. In those with proteinuria and/or renal impairment, a target blood pressure of <130/80 mmHg should be sought. ACE inhibitors and AIIRBs are specifically indicated for the reasons described earlier in the chapter.

'Malignant' or accelerated hypertension: this refers to presentation with severe diastolic hypertension (eg DBP > 120 mmHg) with grade 3 or 4 retinopathy (haemorrhages and/or exudates (grade 3) with/without papilloedema). Patients may have ARF, significant proteinuria and non-renal complications such as encephalopathy or cardiac failure. The condition constitutes a medical emergency. Typical histological lesions include arterial fibrinoid necrosis (which also accounts for the retinal abnormalities) coupled with severe tubular and glomerular ischaemia.

Secondary hypertension

Over 90% of hypertension is idiopathic, approximately 5% is due to renal disease, 2–3% due to primary hyperaldosteronism, and <1% has either an alternative rare endocrine or other cause.

Hypertension due to renal disease

Renal disease accounts for the majority of cases of secondary hypertension. The pathogenesis involves stimulation of renin release with activation of the RAA, reduced natriuretic capacity, and disorganisation of intra-renal vascular structures. The majority of patients with CRF are hypertensive, and it is evident in at least 90% of the dialysis population and over 60% of transplant patients. It is the chief contributor to the LVH and associated high cardiovascular mortality of these patients.

- Most forms of renal disease are complicated by hypertension, but exceptions are some patients with chronic pyelonephritis who have salt-wasting (normotensive).
- Although ARVD is invariably associated with hypertension it may only be pathogenetically significant in the minority.
- **Coarctation of the aorta**: hypertension is seen in the upper limbs only. Rib-notching may be seen on X-ray.
- **Endocrine**: Cushing's syndrome, phaeochromocytoma, acromegaly and apparent mineralocorticoid excess (*see* Section 3.4 Hypokalaemia) are all rare causes. It is now believed that **primary hyperaldosteronism** (associated with bilateral or unilateral adrenal hyperplasia) may account for about 3% of all hypertension (*see* Chapter 1, Cardiology and Chapter 4, Endocrinology).
- **Other secondary hypertension**: alcohol, obesity.

12.7 Myeloma and the kidney

Myeloma occurs with an incidence of 30–40 cases/million, and at a median age of 70–80 years. Renal involvement may present with ARF, CRF and/or proteinuria. Note that Bence–Jones proteinuria is not detected by standard urinary dipsticks.

Renal failure due to myeloma

ARF: some degree of renal impairment is observed in 50% of patients with myeloma; this is reversible in the majority (in those where it is secondary to hypercalcaemia, hypovolaemia, infection of nephrotoxic drugs), but 10% of patients may need dialysis. The latter cases are usually due to **light chain or 'cast' nephropathy**.

CRF: due to amyloidosis (see above), and cast nephropathy associated with chronic interstitial nephritis (see overleaf).

Cast nephropathy

In this, free kappa (the most nephrotoxic) and lambda light chains excreted in the urine damage the tubules by direct nephrotoxicity and by cast formation. The intra-tubular casts are composed of hard, needle-shaped crystals and excite an interstitial infiltrate, often with multinucleate giant cells. ATN and tubular atrophy occur, and hence the potential for some recovery from an ARF episode.

- Patients with light-chain-only myeloma are more likely to have renal involvement.
- Cast nephropathy may also be seen in patients with MGUS (see below).

Treatment: is with rehydration (no evidence that alkaline solutions are beneficial) and supportive therapy. Hypercalcaemia should be treated with iv diphosphonates. ARF may improve with plasma exchange – a clinical trial is currently on-going. The myeloma should be treated with conventional regimes (eg dexamethasone and melphalan if the prognosis is >6 months; in younger patients, and those with lower tumour bulk and complications, VAD regimes are used, and patients may be considered for autologous stem cell transplantation).

Prognosis: renal recovery is only seen in about 15–20% of patients with cast nephropathy who require dialysis. The remainder need RRT – the prevalence of myeloma patients on dialysis programmes is about 2%. Renal transplantation is not appropriate. Patients with myeloma and ESRD have poor survival (< 50% at 1 year). Those with the greatest tumour mass have the worst prognosis.

Benign monoclonal gammopathy (MGUS)

(See *also* Chapter 9, Haematology.) This may be associated with light chain nephropathy, interstitial nephritis, amyloid and also mesangio-capillary glomerulonephritis. A significant proportion of patients with MGUS will develop myeloma during long-term follow-up.

12.8 Renal vasculitis

The kidney is often involved in systemic vasculitic illness. Several disorders are recognised, and these are classified and described more fully in Chapter 20, Rheumatology.

Small vessel pauci-immune vasculitis

These conditions affect small vessels (arterioles and veins) and are associated with glomerulonephritis, and pulmonary and skin vasculitis. They are usually associated with +ve serum ANCA (*see* Chapter 10, Immunology). Incidence is 10–20 cases/million each year. The major conditions are defined as:

- **Wegener's granulomatosis**: respiratory tract disease is characteristic and this involves necrotising granulomata within the upper respiratory tract (leading to sinusitis and nasal discharge, as well as damage to the nasal septum) and lungs (with haemoptysis). About 70% of patients are cANCA +ve, and 25% pANCA +ve.

- **Churg–Strauss syndrome**: vasculitis that is associated with asthma, eosinophilia and necrotising inflammation. Sixty per cent have +ve pANCA; 30% are ANCA –ve.
- **Microscopic polyangiitis (MPA)**: vasculitis occurring in the absence of evidence for the above two conditions (ie asthma, eosinophilia or necrotising granulomatous inflammation). Fifty per cent are pANCA +ve, and 40% cANCA +ve.

In all conditions, **ARF** is the usual renal presentation; renal histology shows necrotising glomerulitis typically associated with focal proliferative and/or crescentic glomerulonephritis (see Section 6.2 on 'RPGN/crescentic glomerulonephritis'). Pulmonary involvement is common, but blood pressure may be normal. A purpuric vasculitic skin rash is often seen.

Treatment: all of the above three conditions normally merit aggressive immunosuppressive therapy; typical regimes are described in Section 6.2 on 'RPGN/crescentic glomerulonephritis'. Patients with cANCA +ve disease are more likely to relapse after the cessation of maintenance therapy. In such cases, immunosuppression is continued for several further years.

Prognosis: 1-year renal and patient survival is >80%. Poorer renal prognosis is seen in patients with highest creatinine and/or oligo-anuria at presentation. Mortality is increased in patients with pulmonary haemorrhage. The risk of vasculitic relapse in transplanted patients is 20%.

Polyarteritis nodosa (PAN)

PAN is a rare, medium-sized arterial vasculitis which results in microaneurysm formation; hypertension is usually severe, and renal infarcts rather than glomerulonephritis are characteristic. Patients are usually ANCA –ve (unless there is also small vessel involvement, ie PAN-MPA overlap). Pulmonary (infiltrates and haemorrhage), GI tract (infarcts), neurological (mononeuritis multiplex) and systemic features (myalgia, PUO) are recognised, but the condition is notoriously difficult to confirm. A few cases are associated with hepatitis B infection. **Treatment** is as for small vessel vasculitis/crescentic nephritis.

Other vasculitides that can affect the kidney

- **Henoch–Schönlein nephritis**: in addition to the typical systemic features of this condition, some patients develop renal disease as a result of small vessel (typically post-capillary venulitis with IgA deposition) vasculitis. Glomerular lesions range from mild mesangial hypercellularity (similar to idiopathic IgA nephropathy) through to crescentic nephritis.
- **Kawasaki disease**: acute febrile illness, usually in children, associated with a desquamating erythematous rash and necrotising arteritis in some patients. It is the commonest cause of myocardial infarction in childhood, but significant renal disease is uncommon.
- Takayasu arteritis: this can be associated with RAS and renovascular hypertension.
- **Giant cell arteritis**: has been associated with rapidly progressive glomerulonephritis (RPGN), but such cases may represent Wegener's granulomatosis with temporal artery involvement.

12.9 Sarcoidosis and the kidney

Sarcoidosis (*see* Section 8.1 Interstitial nephritis) can be associated with:

- **ARF**: due to AIN. Ninety per cent of patients have systemic manifestations of sarcoidosis (eg hepato-splenomegaly, hypercalcaemia).
- **CRF**: associated with CIN and hypercalcaemia. Glomerular disease (membranous or proliferative glomerulonephritis) may rarely occur, and are associated with microscopic haematuria and significant proteinuria.

Treatment: most patients respond promptly to oral steroids, which can be tapered at 3–6 months. Relapses occur, but are usually steroid-responsive. Serum ACE may be useful for monitoring disease activity and predicting likelihood of relapses.

13. DRUGS AND THE KIDNEY AND TOXIC NEPHROPATHY

(*See also* Chapter 2, Clinical Pharmacology, Toxicology and Poisoning.)

13.1 Renal elimination of drugs

Drugs may be eliminated via the kidneys by two main mechanisms:

- **Glomerular filtration**: a passive process; such drugs will be water-soluble.
- **Active tubular secretion**: drugs act as substrates for secretory processes that are designed to eliminate endogenous molecules; the tubular pathways are different for organic anions (basolateral tubular membrane) and cations (located on the luminal brush border).

Examples of drugs which are secreted by the tubule

- **Anionic drugs**
  Acetazolamide
  Cephalosporins
  Penicillin
  Loop diuretics
  Thiazide diuretics
  Probenecid
  Salicylates
- **Cationic drugs**
  Amiloride
  Cimetidine
  Ranitidine
  Metformin
  Morphine
  Quinine

13.2 Drug nephrotoxicity

Drugs can lead to renal damage in a number of different ways, and examples are given below.

Alterations in renal blood flow

- **NSAIDs**: alteration in prostaglandin metabolism can lead to a critical reduction in glomerular perfusion (particularly when there is reduced renal reserve or CRF). Interstitial nephritis may also result from NSAIDs.
- **ACE inhibitors (and angiotensin II receptor blockers)**: ARF or renal impairment occurring in patients who are critically dependent upon the RAA system (those with reduced renal perfusion (eg CCF, loop diuretics, hypovolaemia and severe renovascular disease)) is well recognised with these agents.
- **Ciclosporin A**: toxicity can be acute (due to renal vasoconstriction) or chronic. The latter is a common cause of transplant dysfunction, and is associated with arterial damage (intimal proliferation and hyaline degeneration of the vascular media), tubular vacuolation and atrophy and interstitial fibrosis.

Direct tubular toxicity

- **Aminoglycosides**: disturbance of renal function is seen in up to a third of patients receiving aminoglycosides. Five per cent of filtered gentamicin is actively reabsorbed by proximal tubular cells, within which the drug is concentrated; binding to phospholipid results in disturbed intracellular regulation with inhibition of microsomal protein synthesis and, eventually, ATN.
- **Cisplatin**: selectively toxic to proximal tubules, by inhibiting nuclear DNA synthesis; ATN results. The platinum component may not be the major damaging influence as carboplatin is less nephrotoxic.
- **Amphotericin**: this is toxic to distal tubular cells in a dose-dependent manner; ATN results, and is accompanied by non-oliguric ARF. Liposomal formulations minimise the nephrotoxic risk.

Glomerulonephritis

- **Gold**: proteinuria occurs (usually within 6 months of the start of therapy) in about 5% of patients receiving gold, and this is not dose-related. Therapy should be stopped if it exceeds 1 g/24 h; resolution is then usual by 6 months. Gold is found in the mesangial cells at renal biopsy; it is believed to induce an immune-complex glomerulonephritis (usually membranous, but occasionally minimal change nephropathy).
- **Penicillamine**: the risk of membranous glomerulonephritis is greater than with gold; it is dose-related, and the onset of proteinuria may be delayed to 18 months after the start of treatment.

Other nephrotoxic effects of drugs

Interstitial nephritis and retro-peritoneal fibrosis are covered in earlier sections, and drug-induced SLE syndromes in Chapter 20, Rheumatology. Nephrogenic DI is the commonest renal complication of **lithium** therapy; interstitial fibrosis and CRF are rare.

13.3 Toxic nephropathy

This refers to renal damage resulting from drugs (as above) or radio-contrast media (see Section 4.3) or environmental toxins (eg heavy metals) and poisons (eg Paraquat).

Causes of environmental and occupational toxic nephropathy

- **Heavy metals**
  Mercury
  ARF, proteinuria and nephrotic syndrome (minimal change or membranous nephropathy)
  Lead
  Acute poisoning leads to ARF with ATN; chronic interstitial nephritis and Fanconi syndrome are seen with chronic exposure
  Cadmium
  Similar renal pathology and clinical presentation as for lead
  Arsenic
  Acute poisoning causes ARF with ATN and cortical necrosis; interstitial fibrosis leads to CRF with chronic exposure
  Bismuth
  Proteinuria, Fanconi syndrome and ARF have been described
- **Hydrocarbons and organic solvents**
  Carbon tetrachloride
  ARF
  Ethylene glycol
  This is rapidly metabolised to oxalic acid which crystallises within the renal tubules; ATN results
  Petroleum-based hydrocarbons
  These can predispose to glomerulonephritis (eg Goodpasture's syndrome or membranous glomerulonephritis)
  Paraquat
  ARF, usually lethal due to irremediable pulmonary disease
- **Plant and animal toxins**
  Snake, spider and hornet venoms
  Directly nephrotoxic, or induce ATN, cortical necrosis (often associated with DIC), or muscle necrosis and rhabdomyolysis
  Bee sting
  Rare cause of nephrotic syndrome
  Mushroom poisoning
  ARF
  Poison ivy or oak
  Rare causes of nephrotic syndrome

Chapter 16
Neurology

CONTENTS

Neurology

1. CEREBRAL CORTEX

1.1 Cortical localisation

Figure 1 Lateral surface of the human brain

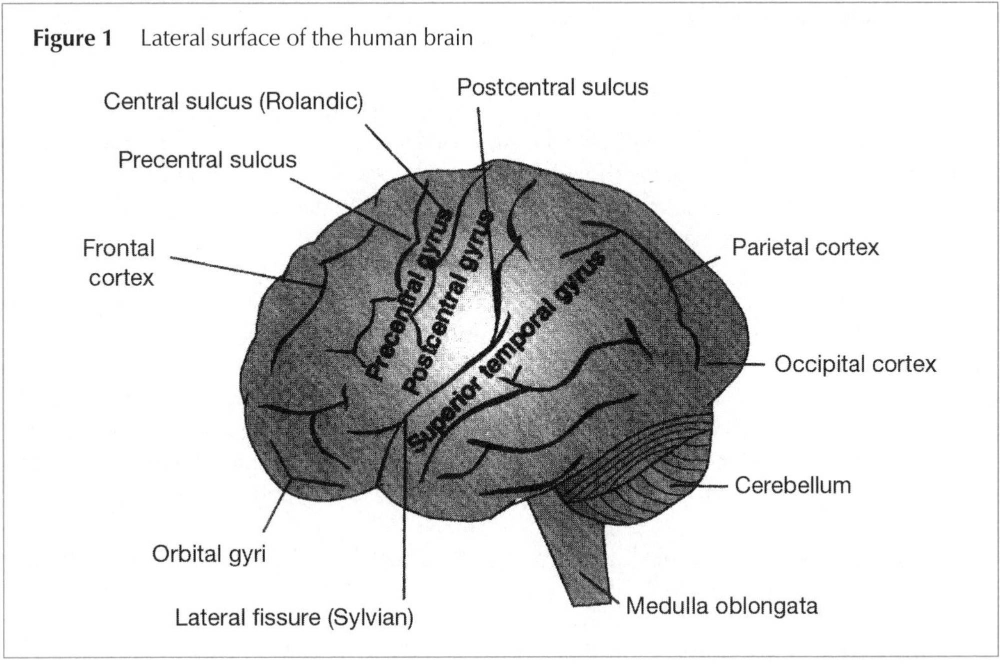

The cortical surface is divided into frontal, parietal, temporal and occipital lobes. Primary motor and sensory cortices are located as follows.

- **Motor**
  Precentral gyrus (frontal lobe)
- **Somatosensory**
  Postcentral gyrus
- **Auditory**
  Superior temporal lobe (Heschl's gyrus)
- **Visual**
  Occipital cortex (calcarine sulcus)
- **Olfactory**
  Frontal lobe (orbitofrontal cortex)

In general, primary sensory cortices receive input from subcortical structures. Signals reach the somatosensory cortex via the posterior limb of the internal capsule (the anterior limb carries descending motor output in the form of the corticospinal tracts). Auditory signals reach the temporal cortex via the medial geniculate nucleus of the thalamus. Visual signals reach the calcarine sulcus (V1) from the lateral geniculate nucleus.

After processing in primary sensory areas, corticocortical connections carry signals into secondary association cortices. The pattern of connections of the visual cortex is best understood in the following way. From primary visual cortex (V1), parallel pathways carry signals outward, with different types of processing being carried out in different functionally specialised areas. One way of thinking about visual processing is to contrast a dorsal 'where' stream, passing dorsally into the parietal cortex and concerned with object localisation, with a ventral 'what' stream passing into the temporal cortex and concerned with object identity.

A distributed network of cortical areas in the dominant hemisphere subserves **language function**. Two areas are especially important.

- **Broca's area**: in the dominant frontal lobe, which is concerned with speech output.
- **Wernicke's area**: in the dominant posterior superior temporal gyrus, which is concerned with word comprehension.

Frontal lobe lesions may cause:

- anosmia
- abnormal affective reactions
- difficulties with planning tasks or those requiring motivation
- primitive release reflexes (eg grasp, pout, rooting)
- Broca's aphasia ('telegraphic' output aphasia)
- perseveration
- personality change (apathetic versus disinhibited).

Parietal lobe lesions tend to cause disorders of spatial representation or apraxias (disorders of learned movement unrelated to muscular weakness) such as those shown below. Parietal lobe lesions may also cause visual field defects, usually a homonymous inferior quadrantanopia, as the upper loop of the optic radiation (*see* Section 3 on neuro-ophthalmology) runs through the parietal lobe.

Parietal lobe lesions may cause:

- visuospatial neglect or extinction (both usually associated with right parietal lobe lesions)
- astereognosis (failure to recognise common objects by feeling them)
- Gerstmann's syndrome (dominant parietal) consisting of alexia (inability to read), agraphia (inability to write), right/left confusion and finger agnosia (inability to identify fingers by name)
- apraxia (dominant)
- acalculia (inability to perform mental arithmetic; dominant)
- agraphia (dominant)
- dressing apraxia (dominant)
- constructional apraxia (non-dominant)
- anosognosia (denial of illness; non-dominant).

Occipital lesions may cause:

- cortical blindness
- homonymous hemianopia
- visual agnosia (inability to comprehend the meaning of objects despite intact primary visual perception)
- specific visual processing defects, eg akinetopsia (impaired perception of visual motion), achromatopsia (impaired perception of colour).

Temporal lobe lesions may cause:

- Wernicke's aphasia
- impaired musical perception
- auditory agnosia
- memory impairment (eg bilateral hippocampal pathology)
- cortical deafness (bilateral lesions of auditory cortex)
- emotional disturbance with damage to limbic cortex.

Temporal lobe lesions may also cause visual field defects, usually a homonymous superior quadrantanopia, as the lower loop of the optic radiation (*see* Section 3 on neuro-ophthalmology) runs through the temporal lobe.

1.2 Dementia

Dementia is an acquired, progressive loss of cognitive function associated with an abnormal brain condition. It is not a feature of normal ageing.

Other disorders may masquerade as dementia, including depression, postictal states, acute confusional states (including drug-induced) and psychotic illnesses of old age.

By far the commonest cause of dementia is **Alzheimer's disease**. Other important dementias include:

- Lewy body dementia
- multi-infarct dementia.

Rarer causes of dementia include:

- fronto-temporal dementia (Pick's disease)
- Creutzfeldt–Jacob disease
- progressive supranuclear palsy
- AIDS-associated dementia
- Huntington's disease.

Treatable causes of cognitive impairment (which can masquerade as dementia)

- Intracranial tumour
- Normal pressure hydrocephalus
- Thiamine (vitamin B_1) deficiency
- Vitamin B_{12} deficiency
- Hypothyroidism
- Acute confusional state
- Depression
- Chronic drug intoxication

Alzheimer's disease

The earliest symptom of Alzheimer's disease (AD) is typically forgetfulness for newly acquired information. The disease progresses to disorientation, progressive cognitive decline with multiple cognitive impairments and disintegration of personality.

The neuropathology consists of:

- **Macroscopically**: the brain is atrophied with enlarged ventricles. Hippocampal atrophy is particularly prominent and can be one of the first signs of AD.
- **Microscopically**: there is neuronal loss throughout the cortex and two distinctive pathological features; namely, **plaques** (which contain a core of β-amyloid) and **neurofibrillary tangles** (which contain hyperphosphorylated tau protein). Tangles and plaques occur throughout the cortex in overlapping but separate distributions. The density of tangles **can** correlate with dementia severity.

- **Neurotransmitter changes**: there is a loss of cholinergic neurones and a loss of choline acetyl transferase activity throughout the cortex, although other neurotransmitter systems are also affected.

Genetic abnormalities associated with Alzheimer's disease

Fewer than 5% of AD cases are familial (typically autosomal dominant) and three main mutations are described. A point mutation to the presenilin-1 gene (chromosome 14) accounts for up to 50% of familial AD. Less common are mutations to the β-amyloid precursor protein (APP) gene (chromosome 21) or the presenilin-2 gene (chromosome 1).

- **Down's** syndrome (trisomy 21) is associated with mental retardation and the formation of senile plaques and neurofibrillary tangles in the same brain regions commonly affected by AD. Clinically, Down's syndrome patients develop progressive cognitive impairment from their fifth or sixth decade. The gene coding for amyloid precursor protein is located on chromosome 21 and it is thought that there is overproduction of β-amyloid in these individuals.
- **Apolipoprotein E** (ApoE) is a protein synthesised in the liver that serves as a cholesterol transporter. There are three major forms of ApoE that are specified by different alleles of the ApoE gene on chromosome 19 (ε2, ε3, ε4). The ε4 allele has a greatly increased frequency (around 50%) in patients with AD. The effect of this allele is to decrease the age of onset of AD. After the effect of age, ApoE4 is the most significant risk factor for AD.

Pick's disease

Pick's disease is also known as focal lobar atrophy, and is an example of a focal dementia predominantly affecting frontotemporal function. Atrophy is circumscribed affecting most often the frontal and/or temporal lobes. Pick bodies are seen within the cellular cytoplasm on light microscopy. Clinically, patients present with progressive language disturbance, often affecting output rather than comprehension, and behavioural changes. Frontal lobe features are prominent.

Creutzfeldt–Jakob disease

Creutzfeldt–Jakob disease (CJD) is clinically characterised by:

- rapidly progressive dementia
- myoclonus
- young age of onset.

CSF examination is usually normal, though CSF protein may be mildly elevated. There is a **characteristic EEG** with biphasic high-amplitude sharp waves.

The most common cause is sporadic, but there are familial forms. A **new variant CJD** (nvCJD) has recently been reported with a neurobehavioural presentation (often depression) in people aged under 40; this form is thought to be associated with interspecies transmission of the bovine spongiform encephalopathy (BSE) agent.

Invasive brain biopsy is currently the only definitive way of diagnosing CJD ante-mortem, though serological tests show some promise. The disease is rapidly progressive and most patients die within a year of diagnosis.

CJD is a **prion** disease.

- prion protein is a normal product of a gene found in many organisms
- it is membrane bound
- infectious agent is resistant to heat, irradiation and autoclaving
- an abnormal isoform accumulates in the spongiform encephalopathies, and this abnormal isoform is thought to be the infectious agent.

See also Chapter 9, Haematology (transfusion transmitted infection) and Chapter 14, Molecular Medicine, which contain further discussion of prion diseases.

Normal pressure hydrocephalus

This should be considered in the differential diagnosis of dementia and consists of the triad of dementia, gait abnormality and urinary incontinence. Urinary symptoms are initially of urgency and frequency, and progress to frontal lobe incontinence (patients indifferent to their incontinence). Gait and posture may mimic Parkinson's disease.

The syndrome appears to be due to a defect in absorption of CSF due to thickening of the basal meninges, or in the cortical channels over the convexity and near to the arachnoid villi. The aetiology may be secondary to meningitis, head injury or subarachnoid haemorrhage. The ventricles are dilated and radiologically hydrocephalus is found, but the pressure is only intermittently high.

Headaches are not usually a complaint and papilloedema is **not** found. Treatment with a ventriculoperitoneal shunt may improve symptomatology.

1.3 Multiple sclerosis (MS)

Clinical presentation of MS

Multiple sclerosis (MS) is thought to be a cell-mediated autoimmune disease associated with immune activity directed against central nervous system (CNS) antigens, principally myelin. Clinical consensus identifies four different subtypes of MS, which may possibly reflect different immunological subtypes:

- **Relapsing/remitting disease** is the most common form of MS (80–85% of patients). Short-lasting acute attacks (4–8 weeks) are followed by remission and a steady baseline state between relapses. The average number of relapses is around 0.8/year.
- **Secondary progressive disease**: about 30–50% of patients with relapsing/remitting disease will subsequently show progressive deterioration with relapses becoming less prominent within about 10 years of MS disease onset.

- **Primary progressive disease**: 10–15% of patients show progressive deterioration from onset without any superimposed relapses. Age of onset is typically later than for relapsing/remitting disease.
- **Progressive-relapsing disease**: a small number of patients with primary progressive disease also experience superimposed relapses associated with gradual disease progression.

Good prognostic factors are:

- relapsing-remitting course
- female sex
- early age at onset
- presence of sensory symptoms.

The aetiology of MS is still unclear but there is undoubtedly a genetic component, with an increased relative risk (20–40%) in siblings compared to the general population. However, as the concordance rate in monozygotic twins is only 25%, there appears to be a substantial environmental component as well.

Optic neuritis is a common presentation of MS:

- isolated optic neuritis: 40–60% chance of subsequent MS
- a cause of painful visual loss
- treat with methylprednisolone
- colour vision is affected early and residual abnormality may persist after recovery.

Diagnosis of MS

This typically requires the demonstration of brain or spinal cord lesions that are disseminated in time and anatomical location. A definitive diagnosis, therefore, is hard to make at the time of the first neurological episode, although if MRI reveals typical lesions this is highly suggestive. Supportive investigations may include:

- T2-weighted MRI showing demyelinating plaques. The presence of gadolinium enhancing lesions is the most predictive MRI parameter, although these are not always present
- delayed visual evoked response potentials (VEPs)
- oligoclonal bands in the CSF (but not the serum – see below).

Diagnosis of primary progressive disease is often hardest, as clear evidence for lesions disseminated in time and (anatomical) space is often obscured by the progressive course of the disease. Brain MRI may be normal in this form of MS, although multiple lesions may be visible in the spinal cord.

Oligoclonal bands in the CSF

Oligoclonal bands in the CSF indicate intrathecal immunoglobulin synthesis. These are not specific to MS and other causes include neurosarcoidosis, CNS lymphoma, SLE, neurosyphilis, subarachnoid haemorrhage (rare), subacute sclerosing panencephalitis (SSPE) – a rate, late complication of measles – and Guillain–Barré syndrome.

Treatments available for MS

Significant advances have been made in the treatment of MS in recent years, principally in the use of interferon preparations for relapsing-remitting MS.

Steroids

NICE guidelines suggest that individuals suffering an acute relapse should be treated with methylprednisolone, either orally (500 mg to 2 g daily) or intravenously (500 mg to 1 g daily) for three to five days. Steroids have no effect on the incidence of relapses, and are not useful other than for treatment of acute attacks.

Interferon β

The 'Association of British Neurologists' guidelines suggest that interferon β should be offered to patients (aged 18 years or older), who have no contraindications to therapy, in the following clinical situations:

Relapsing-remitting MS: patients should be able to walk independently (at least 100 m without assistance) and will have had two clinically significant relapses in the previous two years.

In patients with relapsing **secondary progressive MS**, treatment should only be considered when relapses are the dominant cause of the increasing disability. The following criteria should be fulfilled:

- able to walk at least 10 m (with or without assistance)
- at least two disabling relapses in the previous two years
- minimal increase in disability due to slow progression over the previous two years.

Interferons are not currently recommended for primary progressive MS, or in secondary progressive MS without relapses. There are two main forms of interferon (IFN) available:

- IFNβ-1b (Betaferon) is produced in a bacterial system and differs slightly from natural human IFNβ
- IFNβ-1a (Avonex and Rebif) is produced in mammalian cells and is thought to be similar to natural human IFNβ.

All IFNβ preparations reduce the frequency and severity of relapses in relapsing-remitting MS (by about one-third) and delay progression to disability. The accumulation of brain lesions on MRI is reduced. IFNβ also inhibits the progression of disability in secondary progressive MS, but its effect on primary progressive MS is presently unknown.

Treatment with IFNβ is by subcutaneous injection and is generally well tolerated. Common side-effects are 'flu-like symptoms (fever, chills, myalgia, headache) and local reactions at the injection site. IFNβ is contraindicated in pregnancy. The mechanism of action of IFNβ in MS is not fully understood, but it may act by preventing activated T-lymphocytes from crossing the blood-brain barrier.

The effects of IFNβ are sustained for at least five years after commencement of therapy, but the optimum duration of therapy is not known. Neutralising antibodies can develop to both IFNβ-1b (40% of patients) and IFNβ-1a (20% of patients). These antibodies are associated with a reduction in the drug effects on relapse rate and also MRI lesions; in some patients the antibodies disappear subsequently, but in others they persist. It is unclear whether neutralising antibodies influence progression of disability in any way.

Other immunomodulatory agents for MS treatment

- **Copolymer 1** (glatiramer acetate) and **IV immunoglobulin** therapy both significantly reduce the frequency of attacks of relapsing-remitting MS.
- **Oral low-dose methotrexate** therapy also slows down the progression of disability in secondary progressive MS (and possibly in primary progressive MS).

1.4 Epilepsy

An epileptic seizure is a paroxysmal discharge of neurones sufficient to cause clinically detectable events apparent either to the subject or an observer. Epilepsy is a disorder where more than one such seizure (not including febrile seizures) has occurred. The prevalence of epilepsy is relatively constant at different ages and is around 0.7%, whereas the incidence follows a U-shaped curve with the highest incidence in the young and elderly.

A simplified classification of epilepsy

- **Generalised seizures**
  Tonic-clonic
  Absences (3 Hz spike-and-wave activity in ictal EEG)
  Partial seizures secondarily generalised
- **Partial seizures**
  Simple partial seizures
  Complex partial seizures
- **Others**
  eg myoclonic or atonic

- A typical **tonic-clonic** seizure begins without warning. After loss of consciousness and a short tonic phase, the patient falls to the ground with generalised clonic movements. There may be incontinence and there is post-ictal confusion.
- **Simple partial seizures** may affect any area of the brain, but consciousness is not impaired and the ictal EEG shows a local discharge starting over the corresponding cortical area. Any simple seizure may progress (for example, motor seizures may show a Jacksonian march) and become secondarily generalised with a supervening tonic-clonic seizure.

- Consciousness is impaired by **complex partial seizures** that typically have a medial temporal (often hippocampal) focus. An aura (sense of *déjà vu*, strong smell or rising sensation in the abdomen) may precede the seizure, followed by loss of consciousness. There may be automatisms (repetitive stereotyped semi-purposeful movements).

Imaging is usually carried out in most if not all patients with seizures; focal seizures usually imply a focal pathology and imaging is mandatory in such circumstances.

Anticonvulsant agents are discussed in Chapter 2, Clinical Pharmacology, Toxicology and Poisoning.

Treatment of epilepsy

Patients presenting with a first seizure have an overall risk of recurrence of about 35% at two years. Most neurologists do not therefore advocate routine treatment for a first seizure. However, some groups have a higher recurrence risk (eg 65% at two years for patients with a remote neurological insult and an EEG with epileptiform features) and in these sub-groups treatment may be considered.

- After the second or subsequent seizures, drug treatment is routinely advised as the recurrence risk is much higher.
- Carbamazepine and sodium valproate are widely accepted as drugs of first choice for partial and generalised seizures, respectively.
- Note that 40% of patients with epilepsy will be women of child-bearing age. As valproate is associated with a higher incidence of neural tube defects than other agents, the choice of monotherapy may need to be reviewed (*see* Chapter 2, Clinical Pharmacology, Toxicology and Poisoning).

Any anti-epileptic should be introduced at a low dose and the clinician must be vigilant for idiosyncratic reactions. The dosage can then be escalated until either control is achieved or the maximum allowed dose is reached. If control is not achieved with monotherapy, then at least one additional trial of monotherapy is recommended before combination therapy is considered.

Epilepsy and driving

Current regulations are such that following a first seizure (whether diagnosed as epilepsy or not), driving is not permitted for one year with a medical review before restarting driving. Loss of consciousness in which investigations have not revealed a cause is treated in the same way as for a solitary fit.

Patients with epilepsy may be allowed to drive if they have been free from any epileptic attack for one year, or if they have had an epileptic attack whilst asleep more than three years ago and attacks subsequently only when asleep.

To obtain a vocational (HGV, etc) driving licence patients should have been free of epileptic attacks AND off all anti-epileptic medication AND free from a continuing liability to epileptic seizures (eg structural intracranial lesion) for 10 years.

Epilepsy and pregnancy

Seizure rate in pregnancy is predicted by seizure rate prior to pregnancy. All epileptic drugs have teratogenic effects including:

- cleft-lip/palate
- congenital heart defects
- urogenital defects
- neural tube defects (especially valproate).

Teratogenic effects are more likely if more than one drug is used. Nevertheless, anti-epileptic drugs are not contraindicated in pregnancy, as the effects of uncontrolled epilepsy may be more risky.

There is no increase in infant mortality for epileptic mothers. Folic acid supplementation decreases the incidence of malformations.

2. MOVEMENT DISORDERS

2.1 Tremors, myoclonus, dystonia and chorea

Essential tremor is a postural tremor of the hands in the absence of any identifiable cause such as drugs.

- Autosomal dominant with incomplete penetrance (35% will have no family history).
- Propranolol is the most effective medication.
- Stress will worsen the tremor.
- Alcohol will improve the tremor.

Resting tremor is seen when the limbs are completely supported and relaxed, and is typical of Parkinsonism ('pill-rolling').

An **action tremor** is typically caused by an ipsilateral cerebellar hemisphere lesion. **Myoclonus** is characterised by the occurrence of sudden involuntary jerks ('fragmentary epilepsy').

Causes of myoclonus

- Physiological (normal) hypnic jerks whilst falling asleep
- Drug-induced (eg amitriptyline)
- Alzheimer's disease
- Juvenile myoclonic epilepsy
- Inherited as part of other myoclonic epilepsies (eg Lennox–Gastaut syndrome)
- Metabolic (liver or renal failure)
- Creutzfeldt–Jakob disease
- Following anoxic cerebral injury (eg cardiac arrest)
- As part of a progressive myoclonic encephalopathy (eg Gaucher's disease)

Dystonia is characterised by prolonged spasms of muscle contraction; focal dystonias include spasmodic torticollis, writer's cramp and blepharospasm. Myotonic dystrophy is discussed in Section 9.1.

Chorea is a continuous flow of small, jerky movements from limb to limb.

Causes of chorea

- Huntington's disease
- Rheumatic (Sydenham's) chorea
- SLE
- Polycythaemia rubra vera
- Neuroacanthocytosis
- Chorea gravidarum (during pregnancy)
- Thyrotoxicosis
- Drug-induced (eg oral contraceptives, phenytoin, neuroleptics)

Athetosis is a slow sinuous movement of the limbs, and is often seen after severe perinatal brain injury. In the past, athetosis was also used to describe movements that would now be called dystonic.

2.2 Parkinsonism

Parkinsonism refers to a triad of symptoms:

- resting tremor
- bradykinesia
- rigidity.

This pattern of symptoms comprises an akinetic-rigid syndrome.

Causes of an akinetic-rigid syndrome

- Idiopathic Parkinson's disease
- Drug-induced Parkinsonism
- Normal pressure hydrocephalus
- Progressive supranuclear palsy (PSP)
- Diffuse Lewy body disease
- Dementia pugilistica (secondary to boxing or chronic minor head injury)
- Post-encephalitic Parkinsonism
- Depression with psychomotor retardation
- Parkinson's Plus syndromes
- Multiple system atrophy (eg Shy–Drager syndrome, olivopontocerebellar atrophy)
- Intoxications (eg carbon monoxide, MPTP, illegal narcotic, manganese)

The diagnosis of idiopathic Parkinson's disease is often inaccurate and there is no single diagnostic test.

Pointers include:

- an asymmetric onset
- persistent asymmetry
- good therapeutic response to L-dopa initially (over 90% will improve symptomatically).

Treatment of Parkinson's disease

Levodopa has been the mainstay of symptomatic treatment of Parkinson's disease since the 1970s. However, in recent years levodopa has been used less frequently as a first-line treatment, particularly for young patients, because of its involvement in the generation of long-term motor complications (eg end of dose wearing-off effect, unpredictable on/off switching). Such complications affect 10% of patients for every year of levodopa treatment.

- Modified-released levodopa has a similar rate of long-term motor complications.
- **Selegiline** was commonly added to levodopa in later disease as initial studies suggest that it might have neuroprotective effects. However, this was not confirmed in subsequent trials and indeed one trial found increased mortality with selegiline (although this was not confirmed at follow-up).
- **Anticholinergics** (eg benzhexol) are frequently used for the control of tremor, but they are probably less efficacious than levodopa in respective of other motor symptoms (and they have a worse side-effect profile).

More recently, modern **dopamine agonists** (eg ropinirole, pramipexole, cabergoline and pergolide) have been introduced. Initial trial results suggest that monotherapy with these agents may be marginally less efficacious than with levodopa, but these agents generate fewer long-term motor complications. Many neurologists would now recommend that Parkinson's disease is initially treated with such dopamine agonist monotherapy, particularly for young patients, with small amounts of levodopa added as the disease progresses.

However, there is no absolute consensus on treatment of Parkinson's disease and the outcome of several therapeutic trials, which are in progress, is awaited.

In the differential diagnosis of Parkinsonism, two groups of Parkinsons Plus syndromes are of particular importance: progressive supranuclear palsy and the multiple system atrophies.

Progressive supranuclear palsy (PSP)

Also known as Steele–Richardson syndrome, this presents in the seventh decade with Parkinsonism, characteristic ophthalmoplegia and dementia.

The ophthalmoplegia is described in Section 3.3.

Other features of PSP may include pseudobulbar palsy, and dementia late in the course of the illness.

Multiple system atrophies

A number of disorders fall into this category, including Shy–Drager syndrome and olivopontocerebellar atrophy. They are clinically characterised by:

- parkinsonism
- autonomic failure
- cerebellar and pyramidal features (olivopontocerebellar atrophy).

2.3 Huntington's disease (Huntington's chorea)

Huntington's chorea is inherited as an autosomal dominant disorder that normally begins in the third or fourth decade and which is clinically characterised by the triad of:

- chorea (which patients can temporarily suppress)
- cognitive decline
- positive family history.

Other motor symptoms include dysarthria, dysphagia, ataxia, myoclonus and dystonia. Childhood onset is atypical and may be associated with rigidity.

Genetics of Huntington's chorea

- Autosomal dominant with complete penetrance
- There is expansion of the CAG trinucleotide repeat within this gene (see Chapter 14, Molecular Medicine)
- Gene is on chromosome 4 and codes for a protein, huntingtin
- Genetic testing in asymptomatic individuals is now available

Neuropathologically the disease causes neuronal loss in cortex and striatum, especially the caudate. Treatment is unsatisfactory and relies on neuroleptics, which partially relieve chorea through interfering with dopaminergic transmission.

Other causes of chorea

- Levodopa-induced chorea in Parkinsonism
- SLE
- Antiphospholipid syndrome
- Wilson's disease
- Sydenham's chorea (autoimmune, preceded by group A Streptococcus infection)
- Neuroacanthocytosis

2.4 Wilson's disease

This is an autosomal recessive condition. The responsible gene is ATP7B, located on chromosome 13. The gene sequence is similar to sections of the gene ATP7A, which is defective in Menke's disease (another disease caused by defects in copper transport). The similar sequences code for copper-binding regions, part of a P-type ATPase transmembrane protein. Clinically, the disease is characterised by abnormal copper deposition in the basal ganglia, as well as elsewhere in the brain, the eye and in the liver. This disorder should be considered in any young person presenting with an extrapyramidal syndrome. Psychiatric symptoms are particularly common in adults. (*See also* Chapter 13, Metabolic Diseases and Chapter 6, Gastroenterology).

3. NEURO-OPHTHALMOLOGY

This section should be read in conjunction with Chapter 17, Ophthalmology.

3.1 Visual fields

The optic pathways, and the visual defects resulting from various lesions at different sites are illustrated in the following figure.

Figure 2 Optic pathway abnormalities and associated defects

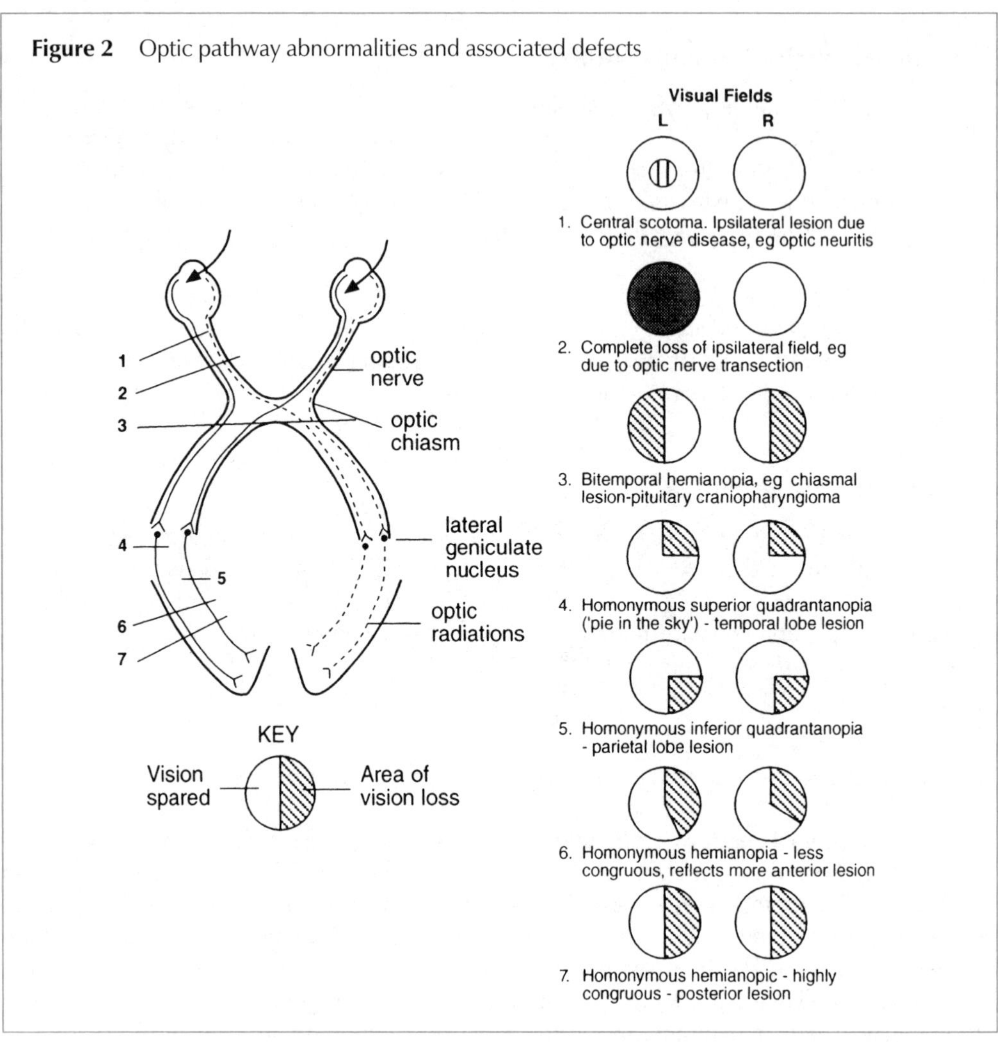

Optic nerve fibres leave the retina, and travel in the optic nerve to the optic chiasm. Lesions of the retina and optic nerve produce field defects in the **ipsilateral eye alone**. Lesions at the optic chiasm typically produce **bitemporal hemianopia**. Causes include:

- pituitary tumour (compression from below)
- craniopharyngioma
- intracranial aneurysm
- meningioma
- dilated third ventricle.

From the optic chiasm fibres run in the optic tract to the lateral geniculate nucleus (thalamus). **Retrochiasmal** lesions produce **homonymous** field defects, the degree of congruity increases with more posterior lesions. From the lateral geniculate nucleus fibres pass in the optic radiation to the primary visual cortex, located in the occipital cortex. The fibres from the lower and upper quadrants of the retina diverge, the upper fibres (lower half of the visual field) passing though the parietal lobes, the lower fibres (upper half of the visual field) through the temporal lobes. Hence:

- temporal lobe lesions may cause superior quadrant homonymous hemianopia
- parietal lobe lesions may cause inferior quadrant homonymous hemianopia.

Note that the decussation of fibres at the optic chiasm means that the right visual field is represented in the left occipital cortex and vice versa.

- Within the **calcarine sulcus**, there is a topographic representation of the visual field with more peripheral regions represented anteriorly, and more central (foveal) regions located posteriorly.
- At the very tip of the occipital lobe, the representation of the fovea (macula) is a vascular watershed, supplied by the posterior and middle cerebral arteries. Sparing of this area ('foveal sparing') may therefore occur with a posterior cerebral artery CVA.

Cortical blindness

This is usually due to bilateral occipital infarcts and it results in severe or complete loss of vision. Other features:

- Pupillary responses are preserved.
- The patient may deny that they have visual loss (Anton's syndrome).
- Macular sparing may occur and the patient may have a tiny island of preserved central field which will allow some useful reading vision. However, this central field may be so small as to be useless for distance vision.

3.2 Pupils

Pupil size depends on both pupillodilator (sympathetic) and pupilloconstrictor (parasympathetic) fibres. Pupilloconstrictor fibres travel from the Edinger–Westphal nucleus in the midbrain to the orbit on the third nerve. The path of sympathetic fibres is described below.

The pupillary light reflex pathway has two parts:

- **afferent**: retina, optic nerve, lateral geniculate body, midbrain
- **efferent**: Edinger–Westphal nucleus (midbrain) to third nerve.

Afferent pupillary defect

This is detected by the 'swinging flashlight' test. If the amount of light information carried by one eye is less than that from the contralateral side when the light is swung from the normal to the abnormal side, pupil dilatation is observed. This is also known as a Marcus Gunn pupil.

An afferent pupillary defect is a sign of **asymmetrical disease anterior to the chiasm**.

Causes:

- retinal disease (eg vascular occlusion, detachment)
- optic nerve disease (eg optic neuritis, glaucoma) with asymmetric nerve damage.

Causes of a small pupil (miosis)

Miosis can be caused by:

- **senile miosis**
- **pontine haemorrhage**
- **Horner's syndrome**: see below
- **Argyll Robertson pupil**: bilateral (may be asymmetrical) small irregular pupils which do not react to light but accommodate normally. They dilate poorly in the dark and in response to mydriatics. Lesion is in the rostral midbrain near the Sylvian aqueduct, such that the light reaction fibres are interfered with, but the more ventral near fibres are spared
- **drugs**: systemic (opiates); topical (pilocarpine)
- **myotonic dystrophy**.

Horner's syndrome

Horner's syndrome is caused by interruption of sympathetic pupillomotor fibres (see the box below), and is one of the causes of a small pupil (miosis).

Causes of Horner's syndrome

Anatomical structures	Causes
Brainstem or spinal cord First-order neurone	Vascular, trauma, neoplastic demyelation, syringomyelia, ependymoma
Pre-ganglionic lesion Second-order neurone: anterior roots (C8-T3), sympathetic chain	**Chest lesion**: apical carcinoma, cervical rib, mediastinal mass **Cervical lesion**: lymphadenopathy, trauma, thyroid neoplasm **Surgical**: thyroidectomy, carotid angiography, endarterectomy
Post-ganglionic lesion Third-order neurone: stellate ganglion carotid sympathetic plexus, fibres to eyelid in branch of III, fibres to pupil in ciliary nerve	Internal carotid artery dissection, cavernous sinus lesions, orbital apex disease

Clinical characteristics of Horner's syndrome

- **Miosis**: hydroxyamphetamine differentiates between pre- and post-ganglionic (miosis more evident in dim light 'dilation lag').
- **Enophthalmos**: apparent, due to narrowing of the palpebral aperture by ptosis and elevation of the lower lid.
- **Ptosis**: partial – levator palpebrae is 30% supplied by sympathetic.
- **Anhidrosis**: whole face means lesion proximal to common carotid artery.
- **Vasodilatation**.

Congenital Horner's syndrome is associated with difference in iris colour (heterochromia).

Causes of a large pupil (mydriasis)

Mydriasis can be due to:

- **Adie's (tonic) pupil**: idiopathic dilated pupil with poor reaction to light and slow constriction to prolonged near effort. Seventy per cent female, 80% initially unilateral, 4% per year becoming bilateral. Associated with decreased deep tendon reflexes (Holmes Adie syndrome).
- **Third nerve palsy**: see later.
- **Drugs**: systemic (eg antidepressants, amphetamines); mydriatrics (eg tropicamide, atropine).
- **Trauma**: sphincter pupillae rupture.

3.3 The oculomotor system and its disorders

A mnemonic to remember oculomotor innervation is: $\mathbf{LR_6(SO_4)_3}$

The sixth nerve supplies lateral rectus, the fourth supplies superior oblique and the third nerve innervates the others.

Disorders of conjugate gaze

Symmetrical and synchronous movements of the two eyes together are known as **conjugate eye movements**.

Causes of oculomotor palsies

- Ischaemic infarction of a nerve
- Intracerebral aneurysm
- Head trauma
- Neurosarcoidosis
- Myasthenia gravis
- Tumours at the base of the brain (eg glioma, metastasis, carcinomatous meningitis)
- Ophthalmoplegic migraine
- Arterides
- Meningitides (eg syphilitic or tuberculous)
- Orbital lymphoma
- Orbital cellulitis

Causes of bilateral ophthalmoplegia

- Dysthyroid disease
- Myasthenia gravis
- Myositis
- Midbrain tumour or infarction
- Guillain–Barré syndrome
- Basal meningitides (eg tuberculous)
- Wernicke's encephalopathy

The effects of paresis on diplopia are predicted by three rules.

1. Paresis of horizontally acting muscles tends to cause horizontal diplopia, and vertical paresis leads to vertical diplopia.
2. The direction of gaze in which the separation of the images is maximum is the direction of action of the paretic muscles.
3. The image seen furthest from the centre of gaze (the **false** image) usually belongs to the paretic eye, so when covering the paretic eye, this image will disappear.

Third nerve

The third nerve nucleus is a large nucleus located in the midbrain at the level of the superior colliculus. Fibres pass through the red nucleus and the pyramidal tract in the cerebral peduncle. The nerve then passes between the posterior cerebral and superior cerebellar arteries, through the cavernous sinus and into the orbit via the superior orbital fissure. The large nuclear size of the third nerve means that it is rarely entirely damaged by lesions and complete third nerve palsies tend to be caused by **peripheral lesions**. Complete third nerve palsy causes:

- ptosis
- eye deviated down (preserved superior oblique) and out (preserved lateral rectus)
- all other movements reduced or absent, dependent on whether partial or complete
- pupil fixed and dilated.

Lateral gaze is intact and attempted downward gaze causes intorsion (inwards rotation of the eye); normal down gaze requires not only superior oblique but also inferior rectus.

The pupil may be normal (pupil-sparing or 'medical' third) or dilated and fixed to light (so-called 'surgical' third). This is because parasympathetic pupilloconstrictor fibres run on the surface of the nerve; these are fed by the pial vessels and are therefore spared in palsies of vascular aetiology. However, they are affected early by a compressive lesion (when the pupil is involved in 95% of cases).

Causes of a third nerve palsy

- Posterior communicating artery aneurysm (usually but not always painful)
- Diabetes, usually pupil-sparing (75%)
- Arteriosclerotic
- Cavernous sinus pathology (eg thrombosis, aneurysm, fistula, pituitary mass). Frequently associated with lesions of cranial nerves IV, V and VI (see Section 3.5)
- Orbital apex disease, such as tumours, thyroid disease, orbital cellulitis, granulomatous disease; often associated with palsies of cranial nerves IV–VI and optic nerve dysfunction
- Trauma
- Uncal herniation; the third nerve travels anteriorly on the edge of the cerebellar tentorium and may be compressed by the uncal portion of the temporal lobe with increased intracranial pressure due to a supratentorial cause

Fourth nerve

The fourth nerve nucleus lies in the midbrain at the level of the inferior colliculus. The fourth nerve has the longest intracranial course; passing between the posterior cerebral and superior cerebellar arteries, lateral to the third nerve and into the orbit through the cavernous sinus and superior orbital fissure. It is the only nerve to exit the dorsal aspect of the brainstem. A fourth nerve lesion is the commonest cause of vertical diplopia. Looking down and in is most difficult and classically the patient notices diplopia descending stairs or reading.

Causes of a fourth nerve palsy

- Vascular (20%)
- Diabetes
- Vasculitis
- Cavernous sinus syndrome
- Congenital (decompensation causes symptoms) (30%)
- Trauma (susceptible to contrecoup injury, for example whiplash because of dorsal brainstem exit) (30%)
- Orbital apex syndrome

Sixth nerve

The sixth nerve nucleus lies in the mid-pons inferior to the IVth ventricle, and is motor to the lateral rectus. A sixth nerve palsy causes convergence of the eyes in primary position and diplopia maximal on lateral gaze towards the side of the lesion. The affected eye **deviates medially** due to the unopposed action of medial rectus.

Causes of a sixth nerve palsy

- Vascular
- Trauma
- Cavernous sinus syndrome
- Orbital apex syndrome
- Increased intracranial pressure (false localising sign due to stretching of the nerve)

Other disorders of conjugate gaze

Internuclear ophthalmoplegia is a disorder of horizontal eye movement due to a lesion in the medial longitudinal fasciculus which connects the IIIrd and VIth cranial nerve nuclei in the pons (see accompanying figure).

Figure 3 Pathology of internuclear ophthalmoplegia

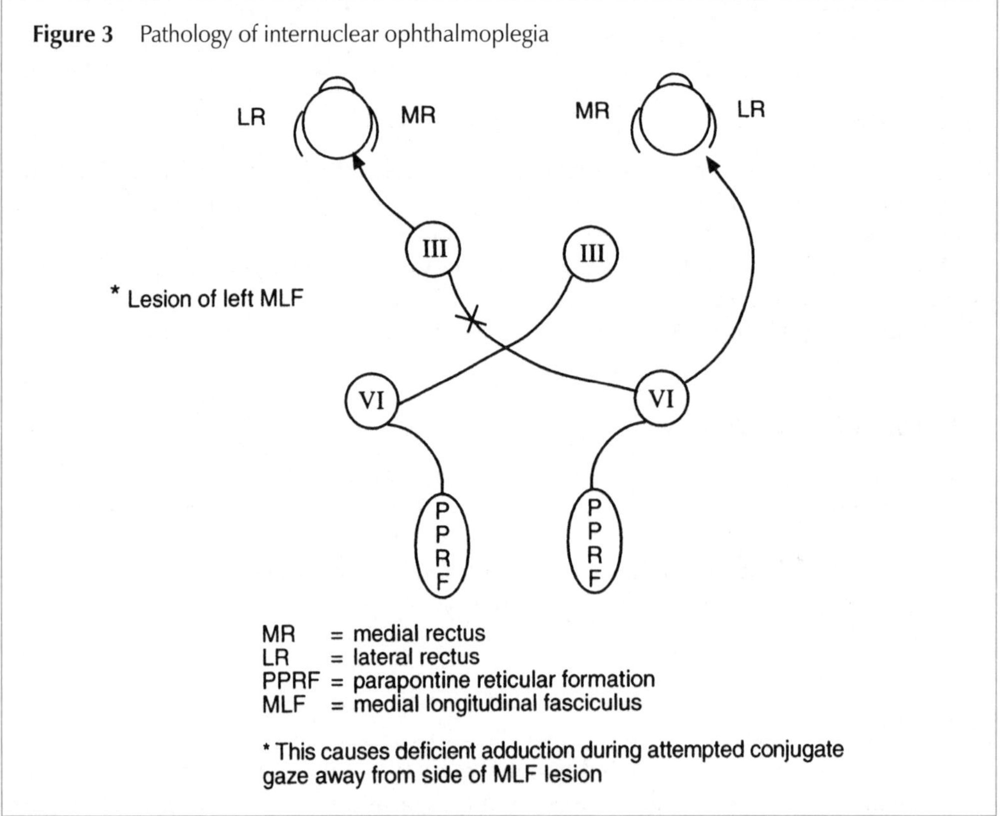

Features of internuclear ophthalmoplegia

- Impaired adduction of the eye ipsilateral to the lesion (complete paralysis – minor slowing)
- Horizontal nystagmus in the abducting eye contralateral to the lesion
- Convergence normal (this differentiates from a medial rectus lesion)
- Vertical gaze nystagmus occasionally present.

Bilateral internuclear ophthalmoplegia results in defective adduction (bilaterally), with nystagmus in the abducting eye.

Causes of internuclear ophthalmoplegia

- Multiple sclerosis (most common: may be bilateral in younger adults)
- Vascular
- Trauma
- Occlusion of the basilar artery
- SLE
- Miller–Fisher syndrome
- Drug overdose (barbiturates, phenytoin or amitriptyline)
- Wernicke's encephalopathy

Causes of **impaired vertical conjugate gaze** include progressive supranuclear palsy, Parinaud's syndrome and thalamic or midbrain pathology.

Progressive supranuclear palsy (Steele–Richardson syndrome): the ophthalmoplegia is a paresis of vertical conjugate gaze which is supranuclear; down gaze cannot be elicited voluntarily but if the patient is allowed to fixate whilst the head is moved passively, the eyes have a full range of movements (Doll's head movement). This pattern implies that while the oculomotor nuclei are intact, in that the eyes can be driven into eccentric positions within the orbit, the supranuclear descending control of voluntary eye movements is impaired.

Parinaud's syndrome is also known as the dorsal midbrain syndrome, with damage to the midbrain and superior colliculus. It leads to:

- impaired upgaze and accommodation
- retraction of the eyelids
- loss of light reflex with preserved convergence reflex
- convergence retraction nystagmus
- relative mydriasis.

Possible causes include pineal tumour, stroke or haemorrhage, hydrocephalus or demyelinating disease.

Other causes of upgaze palsy

- Progressive supranuclear palsy
- Parinaud's syndrome
- Myasthenia gravis
- Miller–Fisher syndrome
- Thyroid eye disease – mimics upgaze weakness by causing fibrosis of inferior recti

3.4 Nystagmus

Nystagmus is a defect of control of ocular position that leads to a rhythmic involuntary to-and-fro oscillation of the eyes. There are three types:

- **pendular**: no distinct fast and slow phases, both being of equal velocity
- **jerk**: distinct fast and slow phases; the amplitude usually increases with gaze towards the direction of the fast phase
- **rotatory**: combination of vertical and horizontal nystagmus.

Causes of congenital nystagmus

- X-linked or autosomal dominant; usually horizontal
- Secondary to poor vision (eg Albinism, untreated congenital cataract, congenital optic atrophy).

Causes of acquired nystagmus

- **Vestibular lesions**: the lesion may be in the VIIIth nerve, inner ear, brainstem or vestibular pathway; jerky nystagmus with fast phase away from the side of the lesion and made worse by gaze in that direction; typically improves with visual fixation
- **Cerebellar lesions**: fast phase towards the side of the lesion
- **Drug-induced** (eg alcohol, barbiturates, phenytoin).

Downbeat nystagmus (where the fast phase is down) is associated with foramen magnum lesions (eg Arnold–Chiari malformation, spinocerebellar degeneration, syringobulbia, platybasia), whereas upbeat nystagmus is typically due to intrinsic brainstem disease, or rarely cerebellar vermis lesions or organophosphates.

3.5 Cavernous sinus syndrome

The major structures passing through the cavernous sinus are the IIIrd, IVth and VIth cranial nerves, the ophthalmic division of the Vth nerve, the sympathetic carotid plexus and the intracavernous carotid artery (see figure 4). Lesions in this region may therefore produce a total internal and external ophthalmoplegia. The main causes of cavernous sinus are:

- **trauma**
- **vascular**: aneurysm of intracavernous carotid artery or the posterior communicating artery; cavernous sinus thrombosis; carotico-cavernous fistula
- **neoplastic**: primary intracranial tumours, direct spread from nasopharyngeal tumours or metastatic
- **inflammatory**: due to infection (eg sinusitis, tuberculosis, or inflammatory disease such as Wegener's granulomatosis).

Figure 4 Main structures passing through the cavernous sinus

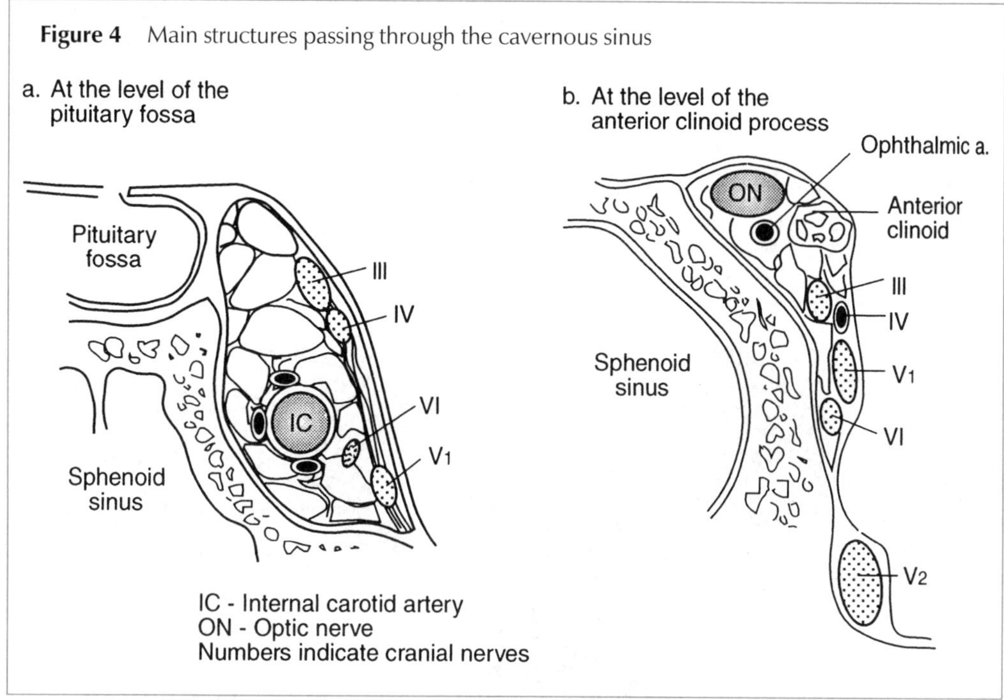

Carotico-cavernous fistula

This may be either a high or low pressure shunt.

- **High pressure, high flow**: shunt due to a fistula between the cavernous sinus and the intracavernous carotid artery. Usually traumatic in origin, producing marked proptosis which may be pulsatile, palsies of the IIIN, IVN and VIN, an orbital bruit with an injected chemotic eye and elevated intra-ocular pressure secondary to raised episcleral venous pressure.
- **Low pressure, low flow**: shunt occurs because of communication between the dural branches of the internal or external carotid arteries and the cavernous sinus. This type is more common in elderly patients, often occurring spontaneously in arterio-sclerotic individuals, and results in a milder clinical picture.

4. OTHER BRAINSTEM AND CRANIAL NERVE DISORDERS

The brainstem and locations of the principal cranial nerve nuclei are illustrated below.

Figure 5 Locations of the principal cranial nerve nuclei within the brainstem

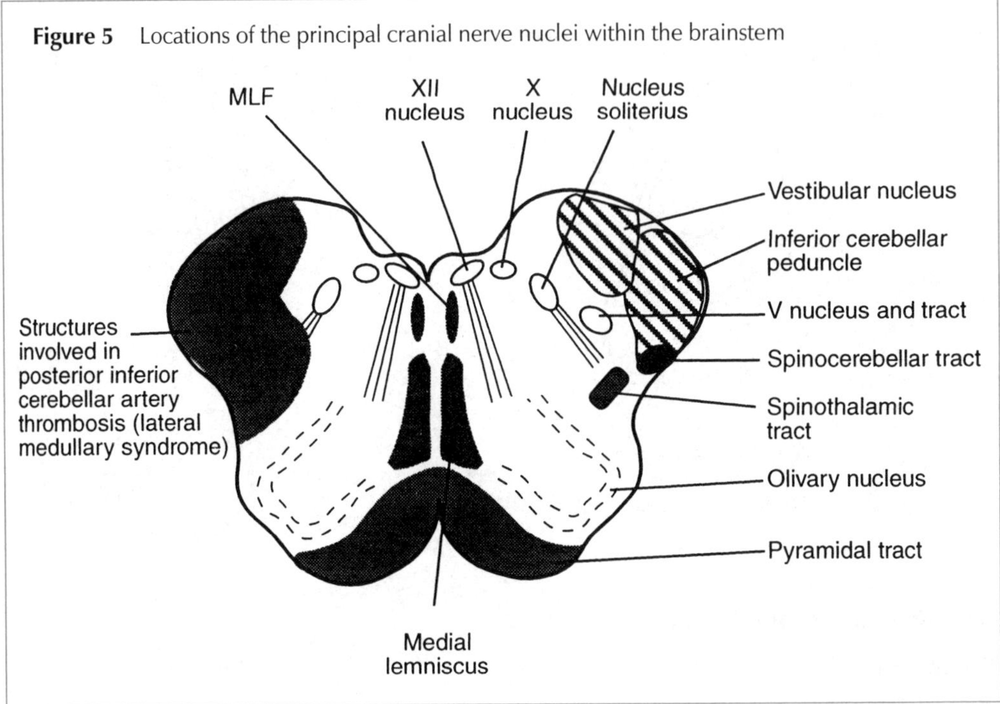

4.1 Facial nerve

The facial nerve has the following functions:

- motor to the muscles of facial expression
- taste fibres from the anterior two-thirds of the tongue (in the chorda tympani)
- taste from the palate (nerve of the pterygoid canal)
- secretomotor parasympathetic fibres to parotid, submandibular and sublingual glands
- nerve to stapedius.

Taste fibres, nerve to stapedius and to the facial muscles leave the nerve **below** the geniculate ganglion.

Causes of a facial nerve palsy

- Brainstem tumour
- Neurosarcoidosis
- Cerebello-pontine angle lesions (eg acoustic neuroma)
- Cholesteatoma
- Lyme disease
- Stroke
- Multiple sclerosis
- Otitis media
- Ramsay–Hunt syndrome
- Diabetes
- Guillain–Barré syndrome

If the palsy is bilateral, exclude myasthenia gravis, facial myopathy (look for ptosis) and neurosarcoidosis. Weakness of frontalis (forehead) indicates a nuclear or intranuclear (LMN) lesion.

Bell's palsy

An isolated facial nerve palsy of acute onset, thought secondary to viral infection.

- Unilateral facial weakness
- Pain behind ear
- Absent taste sensation on anterior two-thirds of tongue

Usually recovery begins by two weeks but the palsy may be prolonged and 10% have residual weakness. Electrophysiological tests can help predict the outcome and tapering dose of steroids (given from onset) improves the outcome. Tarsorrhaphy may be needed to prevent corneal damage

Ramsay–Hunt syndrome

Features include Herpes zoster, affecting the geniculate ganglion, and facial palsy with herpetic vesicles in the auditory meatus. Deafness is a complication.

4.2 Trigeminal neuralgia

This is characterised by brief lancinating pain in the distribution of one of the divisions of the trigeminal nerve. It is more common in patients over the age of 50 and in women. Maxillary and mandibular divisions are most often affected, it is almost always unilateral and trigger points are common. It may be a presenting symptom of MS in younger patients.

Treatment includes:

- carbamazepine/phenytoin
- clonazepam
- baclofen
- thermocoagulation of trigeminal ganglion
- surgical section of nerve root.

4.3 Vestibulocochlear nerve

Damage to the eighth cranial nerve may result in deafness or vertigo (see below). At the bedside, sensorineural and conductive deafness are distinguished by Rinne's and Weber's tests.

Rinne's test

- Air>bone conduction normally
- Hearing decrease and bone<air conduction in conduction deafness
- Hearing decreased and air>bone conduction in sensorineural deafness.

Weber's test

- Central normally
- Lateralises to normal side in sensorineural deafness
- Lateralises to deaf side in conduction deafness.

Causes of deafness

Conduction	Sensorineural
Ear wax	Acoustic neuroma
Otosclerosis	Paget's disease
Middle ear infection	Central lesions (MS/CVA/glioma)
	Congenital (maternal infections, congenital syndromes)
	Ménière's disease
	Head trauma
	Drugs and toxins (aminoglycoside antibiotics, frusemide, lead)

Several drugs may cause tinnitus, including aspirin, frusemide and aminoglycosides.

Vertigo

Neurological disorders causing vertigo are typically due to pathology of the labyrinthine structures of the middle ear, the brainstem vestibular nuclei, or the vestibulocochlear nerve that connects the two.

Common causes of vertigo

Labyrinthine (peripheral)	Brainstem (central)
Trauma (including barotrauma)	Acute vestibular neuronitis
Ménière's disease	Vascular disease
Acute viral infections	MS
Chronic bacterial otitis media	Space-occupying lesions (eg brainstem glioma)
Occlusion of the internal auditory artery	Toxic causes (eg alcohol, drugs)
	Hypoglycaemia

Acoustic neuroma

Acoustic neuroma is a benign tumour arising on the eighth cranial nerve as it emerges from the brainstem in the cerebellopontine angle. It is a common cause of a **cerebellopontine angle syndrome:**

- Cranial nerve VIII is affected early, but the patient may not report hearing loss, tinnitus and vertigo
- Corneal reflex (cranial nerve V) is absent
- Facial sensation is abnormal (V nerve)
- The facial nerve is affected late

Investigation is by use of MRI or high-resolution CT scanning, and treatment is surgical removal.

4.4 Lateral medullary syndrome

The lateral medullary (Wallenberg's) syndrome is usually due to vertebral artery or posterior inferior cerebellar artery occlusion, that damages the dorsolateral medulla and inferior cerebellar peduncle (see figure 5 at the start of Section 4, page 566).

Features of the lateral medullary syndrome

- Ipsilateral loss of pain and temperature sensation on the face (V)
- Ipsilateral paralysis of palate, pharynx and vocal cords (IX, X)
- Ipsilateral ataxia (inferior cerebellar peduncle)
- Contralateral loss of pain and temperature sensation on the body (spinothalamic tract)
- Ipsilateral Horner's syndrome (descending sympathetic outflow)
- Vertigo, nausea and vomiting, nystagmus (vestibular nuclei)

4.5 Other causes of cranial nerve palsies

The cranial nerves may commonly be involved in the following neuropathies:

- **diabetes mellitus**: CNIII or other oculomotor
- **Guillain–Barré/Miller–Fisher**: CN VII, oculomotor
- **diphtheria**: classically CN IX
- **neurosarcoidosis**: CN VII and bilateral VII.

5. SPINAL CORD DISORDERS

5.1 Neuroanatomy

The spinal cord ends at the lower border of L2. There is one principal descending pathway, the corticospinal tract, which crosses in the midbrain. The two principal ascending sensory pathways are the dorsal columns and spinothalamic tracts (see below).

Ascending sensory pathways

Dorsal (posterior) columns	Spinothalamic tracts
Joint position sense and vibration	Pain and temperature
Carry sensation from the same side of the body (ipsilateral – uncrossed)	Incoming fibres cross immediately or within a few segments
Synapse in the brainstem at the cuneate and gracilis nuclei, then decussate	Crossed tract results in **lamination** with fibres from legs outside fibres from the arms

5.2 Brown–Séquard syndrome

This clinical syndrome is caused by lateral hemisection of the spinal cord resulting in:

- ipsilateral upper motor neurone (UMN) weakness below the lesion (severed descending corticospinal tract fibres)
- ipsilateral loss of joint position sense and vibration (severed ascending dorsal column fibres)
- contralateral loss of pain and temperature sensation (severed crossed ascending spinothalamic tract fibres).

Light touch sensation is often clinically normal below the lesion, and the clinical syndrome is most commonly (but not exclusively) caused by multiple sclerosis.

5.3 Motor neurone disease (MND)

Motor neurone disease (MND) is a degenerative disorder affecting both lower motor neurones (LMN) and upper motor neurones (UMN) supplying limb and bulbar muscles. There is no involvement of sensory nerves, and the aetiology is unknown. There are three principal types.

- **Progressive muscular atrophy**: typically presents with LMN signs affecting a single limb that then progresses. Best prognosis (still poor).
- **Amyotrophic lateral sclerosis**: both LMN and UMN are involved; typical clinical picture would be LMN signs in the arms and bilateral UMN signs in the legs. Intermediate prognosis.
- **Progressive bulbar palsy**: bulbar musculature affected with poor prognosis.

Examination may initially show only fasciculation but progresses to widespread wasting and weakness, spastic dysarthria and exaggerated reflexes.

Diagnosis of MND

Diagnosis is largely clinical but confirmatory investigations include nerve conduction studies and EMG, which show evidence of chronic partial denervation and widespread fasciculation with normal sensory nerves and preserved motor nerve conduction velocity (these latter features distinguish the disorder from peripheral neuropathies). CSF protein concentration may be slightly increased. Prognosis is poor with death within five years typical.

Treatment of motor neurone disease

Riluzole is a drug which affects glutamate neurotransmission in a complex fashion. It is usually well tolerated, is associated with a modest improvement in survival (about 2–3 months at 18 months) and is NICE-approved for treatment of probable or definite MND. However, its effects upon quality of life remain unknown and it should be emphasised that the mainstay of treatment of MND remains symptomatic, with a multidisciplinary approach to problems such as nutrition and ventilation.

5.4 Absent knee jerks and extensor plantars

The causative lesion typically produces both LMN (diminished reflexes) and UMN (extensor plantars) signs.

Causes include:

- Friedreich's ataxia
- subacute combined degeneration of the cord
- motor neurone disease
- taboparesis
- conus medullaris compression (the conus represents the transition between spinal cord proper and the filum terminale at the lower end of the cord). Compression can cause UMN signs from cord compression and LMN signs from filum terminale (nerve root compression).

6. VASCULAR DISORDERS, CEREBRAL TUMOURS AND OTHER CNS PATHOLOGIES

This section considers vascular disorders of the CNS, the important causes of headache, cerebral tumours and a number of metabolic disorders affecting the CNS.

6.1 Transient ischaemic attacks

A transient ischaemic attack (TIA) is a focal CNS disturbance developing and fading over minutes or hours to give full recovery within 24 hours. Most TIAs are caused by embolism.

Differential diagnosis of TIA

- Migraine
- Malignant hypertension
- MS (unusual)
- Epilepsy
- Hypoglycaemia

Modifiable risk factors for TIA include hypertension, diabetes mellitus, cigarette smoking, drug use (drugs of abuse, oral contraceptive pill, alcohol), elevated haematocrit and carotid stenosis. Medical management with oral aspirin significantly decreases the chance of subsequent TIA or stroke.

Carotid arterial stenosis

If a severe (70–99%) carotid stenosis is present then the existing evidence suggests that carotid endarterectomy (by an experienced surgeon) should be undertaken. Carotid endarterectomy carries a relatively high (about 8%) risk of perioperative stroke, so the patient trades a short-term increased risk of stroke for a significant long-term reduction in subsequent risk.

6.2 Stroke

A completed stroke is a focal CNS disturbance due to a vascular cause where the deficit persists. The aetiology may be embolic, thrombotic or haemorrhagic. The presenting symptoms depend on the vascular territory involved.

Lacunar strokes

Lacunar infarctions occur where small intracerebral arteries are occluded by atheroma or thrombosis. Typically small low-density subcortical lesions are seen in the area of the internal capsule.

- Lacunar syndromes cause a pure motor, sensorimotor or pure sensory stroke, with no involvement of higher cortical functions.
- Lacunar infarcts have a low mortality and relatively good prognosis for recovery; they are primarily associated with hypertension.

Other types of stroke involve either the anterior or posterior cerebral circulation. **Intracerebral haemorrhage** is primarily associated with the rupture of micro-aneurysms situated in the basal ganglion or brainstem.

Risk factors for stroke

- Diabetes
- Hypertension
- Smoking
- Cocaine abuse
- Previous TIA or stroke
- Male sex
- Increased Hb, haemoglobinopathy
- Family history

Diagnosis of stroke is on clinical grounds supported by neuroimaging. (CT is commonly used initially in order to distinguish between haemorrhage and ischaemic causes; however, note that up to 50% of early CT scans will be normal in acute ischaemic stroke.) Management of stroke is initially conservative, though patients with expanding cerebellar or cerebral haematoma may need surgical treatment. Aspirin is effective in secondary prevention. Mortality from stroke is between 20 and 30%, with poorer prognosis in old patients with depressed level of consciousness.

Factors associated with a poor prognosis in stroke

- Complete paralysis of a limb (MRC grade 0 or 1)
- Loss of consciousness at onset of stroke
- Higher cerebral dysfunction
- Coma or drowsiness at 24 hours
- Old age

6.3 Subarachnoid haemorrhage

Around 5–10% of all strokes are due to subarachnoid haemorrhage (SAH). Causes include:

- ruptured arterial aneurysm
- trauma
- ruptured arteriovenous malformation
- cocaine or amphetamine abuse
- hypertension.

Eighty per cent of intracranial aneurysms are located in the anterior circulation, most on the anterior communicating artery, and 15% are bilateral.

Investigation of subarachnoid haemorrhage

SAH is typically investigated with CT and lumbar puncture (LP).

- CT may be negative in up to 20% of suspected SAH, so a normal CT does not exclude the diagnosis.
- LP shows xanthochromia (due to red cell breakdown products, only visible >4 hours after haemorrhage).
- Other recognised findings include transient glycosuria, low CSF glucose or lengthening of the QT interval (leading to tachyarrhythmias or torsades des pointes).

Treatment of SAH

The management of SAH depends upon making the diagnosis, locating the underlying aneurysm and occluding it. About a quarter of patients will die within a day of presentation, and a third of those that survive the first day will subsequently die of complications or rebleeding. At presentation, several factors have prognostic value for poor outcome, the most important of which are decreased level of consciousness, increasing age and amount of blood visible on CT scan.

- All patients are typically treated with oral nimodipine, which reduces intracranial vasospasm and so can prevent delayed cerebral ischaemia. It probably reduces the risk of poor outcome by about a third.
- Early operative intervention to occlude the causative aneurysm is now usual practice for most patients in reasonable condition, but this is not supported by randomised controlled trial evidence.

Complications of subarachnoid haemorrhage

Neurological
- Rebleeding
- Hydrocephalus
- Focal ischaemic injury from cerebral vasospasm

Systemic
- Fever
- Tachyarrhythmias secondary to catecholamine release
- Neurogenic pulmonary oedema (rarely)
- Hyponatraemia secondary to syndrome of inappropriate antidiuretic hormone

Intracranial aneurysms are associated with:

- polycystic kidney disease
- Ehlers–Danlos syndrome
- fibromuscular dysplasia causing renal artery stenosis
- medium vessel arteritides (eg polyarteritis nodosa)
- coarctation of the aorta.

6.4 Headache

Headache is an extremely common symptom that has a multiplicity of causes. Leaving aside acute unexpected headaches caused by, for example, subarachnoid haemorrhage, important causes of chronic recurrent headache include:

- tension headache
- classical (accompanied by focal neurological symptoms) or common migraine
- cluster headache
- headaches in association with raised intracranial pressure.

Migraine

Migraine is classically preceded by a visual aura followed by a unilateral throbbing headache with photophobia and nausea.

Features of migraine

- EEG and neurovascular abnormalities associated with the headache
- Rarely may result in stroke
- May have unilateral lacrimation
- Can be associated with (reversible) neurological signs (eg hemiplegic migraine)

The neurological symptoms suggest a vascular origin, and a popular hypothesis is that of 'spreading depression' of cortical blood flow. However, whilst changes in cerebral perfusion undoubtedly occur, it is presently not clear whether these are primary or whether brainstem neuroregulatory abnormalities of serotonergic or noradrenergic neurotransmitters are more important. Therapy is aimed at stopping an attack (abortive) or if the frequency of attacks is high enough, regular medication is given as a prophylactic agent.

Migraine therapy

Abortive	Prophylactic
Paracetamol	Propranolol
Codeine ± antiemetic	Pizotifen
Ergotamine*	Amitriptyline
Sumatriptan ($5HT_1$ agonist)	Methysergide

* Ergotamine is contraindicated with cardiovascular/peripheral vascular disease as it is a vasoconstrictor; also in pregnancy, Raynaud's or with renal impairment

Cluster headache

Cluster headache has a distinct pattern, with attacks occurring in clusters lasting days or weeks and remissions lasting months. Males are more often affected than females, and onset of attacks is typically between 25 and 50 years.

Typical features of cluster headache

- Unilateral severe headache lasting up to an hour
- Lacrimation
- Partial Horner's may occur
- Pain may be retro-orbital
- Redness of ipsilateral eye
- Nasal stuffiness

The aetiology is not known and treatment is difficult. Management of the acute attack includes inhaled oxygen (face mask), ergotamine and sumatriptan. Steroids may be helpful. Lithium treatment is used for prophylaxis.

6.5 Benign intracranial hypertension (BIH)

This term refers to a group of patients who present with headaches and profound papilloedema, yet have no focal neurological signs or intracranial lesion on imaging. The most common presentation is in overweight young women and comprises:

- headache
- blurred vision
- dizziness
- transient visual obscurations
- horizontal diplopia.

Papilloedema is found on examination, with peripheral constriction of the visual fields and enlarged blind spot. The CSF pressure is elevated.

Iatrogenic (drug-induced) causes include:

- oral contraceptive pill
- steroids
- tetracycline
- vitamin A
- nitrofurantoin
- nalidixic acid.

Treatment of BIH

This consists of weight loss, acetazolamide and repeated lumbar puncture to reduce the CSF pressure. In more resistant cases or those associated with regular recurrence, **ventriculo-peritoneal shunt** may be necessary. **Optic nerve sheath fenestration** can be performed in patients whose sight is threatened.

6.6 Wernicke's encephalopathy

This is a neurological syndrome of acute onset characterised by:

- ataxia
- ophthalmoplegia
- nystagmus
- global confusional state
- polyneuropathy (in some cases).

It may evolve into Korsakoff's syndrome, with a dense amnesia and confabulation. The syndrome is commonly associated with alcoholism and may be precipitated by a sudden glucose load, but may also be caused by prolonged vomiting (eg hyperemesis gravidarum), dialysis or gastrointestinal cancer.

Red cell transketolase activity is reduced. Neuropathologically it is characterised by periaqueductal punctate haemorrhage. Treatment with thiamine should lead to rapid reversal of the neurological symptoms, though the memory disorder may endure. (*See* Chapter 18, Psychiatry, for further discussion.)

6.7 Cerebral tumours

Primary and secondary intracranial neoplasms have an approximately equal incidence. Both produce presenting symptoms through local neural damage giving rise to focal neurological symptoms, epilepsy or symptoms of raised intracranial pressure, such as headache. The most common presenting symptoms of a glioma are epilepsy and headache.

Gliomas

Gliomas are the most common primary intracranial neoplasm. Most commonly gliomas are derived from the astrocyte cell line, though less commonly oligodendrogliomas, ependymomas and gangliogliomas may occur.

- **Treatment**: confirmation of diagnosis necessary by brain biopsy. If possible, surgical removal should be undertaken followed by radiotherapy. Adjuvant chemotherapy for high-grade gliomas is under evaluation.
- **Prognosis**: this is relatively poor. Even grades I and II astrocytomas have survival rates of 10–30% at five years, whereas glioblastoma multiforme (grade IV astrocytoma) is usually rapidly fatal within a year.

7. CNS INFECTIONS

CSF abnormalities in bacterial and viral meningitis are discussed in Section 10 of this chapter and causative organisms are listed in Chapter 11, Infectious Diseases. For HIV-related neurological disease *see* Chapter 8, Genito-urinary Medicine and AIDS.

7.1 Encephalitis

Acute viral encephalitis involves not simply the meninges (a viral meningitis) but also the cerebral substance. Confusion and altered consciousness are thus prominent, and seizures and focal neurological signs may occur. Viral encephalitis is often secondary to Herpes simplex, but may also be secondary to infection with mumps, zoster, EBV or Coxsackie and echoviruses. *See also* Chapter 11, Infectious Diseases.

Herpes simplex encephalitis

Clinical features of Herpes simplex encephalitis

- Fever
- Focal symptoms (eg musical hallucinations)
- Confusion
- Focal signs (eg right-sided weakness and aphasia)

Focal signs are related to anterior temporal lobe pathology, which may be visible on CT or MRI. Normal CSF findings are occasionally seen, but typically there is a lymphocytosis with red cells also present. In a minority (20%) of cases the CSF sugar may be low. Investigation with imaging or with EEG may confirm focal temporal lobe involvement, and definitive diagnosis can be made with polymerase chain reaction (PCR) to detect viral DNA in the CSF. Treatment with aciclovir should be started on suspicion of the diagnosis.

7.2 Lyme disease

Lyme disease is caused by a spirochaete, *Borrelia burgdorferi*, which is transmitted by ticks. The illness can be subacute or chronic and evolves in poorly defined stages. A ring-like erythematous lesion (erythema migrans) at the site of the tick bite is accompanied by influenza-like symptoms, with neurologic (or cardiac) symptoms appearing weeks to months later. Usually, neurological involvement appears as 'viral-like' meningitis with or without cranial mononeuropathies. Treatment is with oral doxycycline in the initial stages but the meningitis is usually treated with intravenous ceftriaxone.

Neurological abnormalities in Lyme disease

- Cranial neuropathies
- Bell's palsy
- Low-grade encephalitis
- Meningitis
- Cerebellar ataxia
- Mononeuritis multiplex

8. PERIPHERAL NERVE LESIONS

8.1 Mononeuropathies

A peripheral lesion of a single nerve is known as a mononeuropathy. Commonly mononeuropathies are associated with compressive lesions or have a vascular aetiology. Two of the most important mononeuropathies (other than oculomotor palsies) are carpal tunnel syndrome and common peroneal nerve palsy.

Carpal tunnel syndrome

The most common peripheral nerve entrapment syndrome. Symptoms are of numbness and dysaesthesia affecting median nerve (lateral three-and-a-half fingers), and weakness of median nerve innervated muscles (see below).

Conditions associated with carpal tunnel syndrome:

- pregnancy
- obesity
- hypothyroidism
- acromegaly
- amyloidosis
- rheumatoid arthritis.

Treatment is with wrist splints, occasionally diuretics or surgical decompression.

Common peroneal nerve palsy

This nerve is motor to tibialis anterior and the peronei muscles. Patients usually present with foot drop and weakness of:

- inversion (L4) of the foot
- dorsiflexion (L5; tibialis anterior)
- eversion (S1; peronei).

Sensory loss over the dorsum of the foot is usually present, but not prominent. Distinction from L5 root lesion is made by demonstrating that foot eversion is intact (for a root lesion).

Causes of common peroneal palsy

- Compression at the fibula neck, where the nerve winds round the bone (eg below-knee plasters)
- Connective tissue disease/vasculitis
- Weight loss
- Diabetes mellitus
- Polyarteritis nodosa
- Leprosy

Other causes of (unilateral) foot drop include diabetes mellitus (other than due to common peroneal nerve palsy), stroke, multiple sclerosis and prolapsed intervertebral disc.

Other mononeuropathies affecting the hand and arm

The **median nerve** supplies some of the muscles of the thenar eminence (abductor pollicis, flexor pollicis brevis and opponens pollicis) and the lateral two lumbricals.

The **ulnar nerve** supplies the muscles of the hypothenar eminence (abductor digiti minimi), the medial two lumbricals and all the interossei (remember dorsal abduct, palmar adduct – 'dab and pad').

The **radial nerve** does not supply muscles in the hand. It supplies primarily the extensor compartment of the forearm.

Causes of wasting of the small muscles of the hand

- Arthritis
- Motor neurone disease
- Other cervical cord pathology
- Syringomyelia
- Polyneuropathies
- Brachial plexus injury (eg trauma, Pancoast's tumour)

8.2 Polyneuropathies

Polyneuropathies have a heterogeneous set of causes. Typically peripheral nerves are affected in a diffuse symmetrical fashion; symptoms and signs are most prominent in the extremities. Different aetiologies may be associated with involvement of mainly motor, mainly sensory or mainly autonomic fibres.

Causes of polyneuropathy

Mainly sensory neuropathies
Diabetes mellitus
Leprosy
Amyloidosis
Vitamin B_{12} deficiency
Carcinomatous neuropathy
Uraemic neuropathy

Mainly motor neuropathies
Guillain–Barré syndrome (see overleaf)
Porphyria
Lead poisoning
Diphtheria
Hereditary sensory and motor neuropathy (HSMN) types I and II
Chronic inflammatory demyelinating polyneuropathy (CIDP)

Motor neuropathies cause partial denervation of muscle. An important sign of denervation is fasciculation, which is particularly prominent in disorders of the anterior horn cell in addition to the motor neuropathies described above.

Causes of fasciculation

- Motor neurone disease
- Thyrotoxicosis
- Cervical spondylosis
- Syringomyelia
- Acute poliomyelitis
- Metabolic – severe hyponatraemia, hypomagnesaemia
- Drugs (clofibrate, lithium, anticholinesterase, salbutamol)

Autonomic neuropathies

Autonomic neuropathy may present with:

- postural hypotension
- abnormal sweating
- diarrhoea or constipation
- urinary incontinence
- absence of cardiovascular responses (eg to Valsalva's manoeuvre)
- impotence.

Principal causes of autonomic neuropathy

- Diabetes mellitus
- Amyloidosis
- Chronic hepatic failure
- Guillain–Barré syndrome
- Renal failure
- Multiple system atrophies (ie Shy–Drager syndrome/OPCA)

Palpable peripheral nerves are recognised in the following polyneuropathies:

- Charcot–Marie–Tooth (HMSN II)
- amyloidosis
- lepromatous leprosy
- acromegaly.

Guillain–Barré syndrome

Guillain–Barré syndrome (GBS) is an uncommon acute post-infective polyneuropathy. A progressive ascending symmetric muscle weakness (ascending polyradiculopathy) leads to paralysis, maximal by one week in more than half of patients. Symptoms frequently begin after a respiratory or gastrointestinal infection; *Campylobacter jejuni* infection is associated with a worse prognosis.

Sensory symptoms may be present but are typically not associated with objective sensory signs. Papilloedema may occur. The condition may be associated with urinary retention or cardiac arrhythmia (autonomic involvement). Some patients will require intubation and artificial ventilation.

Investigation typically reveals:

- elevated CSF protein (often very high)
- normal CSF white cell count
- slowing of nerve conduction velocity and denervation on EMG.

Poor prognostic features include:

- rapid onset of symptoms
- age
- axonal neuropathy on nerve conduction studies
- prior infection with *Campylobacter jejuni*.

Treatments include plasma exchange and intravenous immunoglobulin.

Miller–Fisher syndrome is a variant of Guillain–Barré syndrome and comprises ophthalmoplegia, ataxia and areflexia.

9. DISORDERS OF MUSCLE AND NEUROMUSCULAR JUNCTION

Disorders of muscle are known as myopathies. The most important feature is muscle weakness, variably accompanied by wasting, hypertrophy, pseudohypertrophy or other symptoms, such as myotonia. Signs are invariably symmetrical. Myopathies are usually painless (with the exception of inflammatory myopathies).

Note that fasciculations are signs of muscle denervation, and they indicate a disorder of motor nerves or the neuromuscular junction. They are not a feature of myopathy.

9.1 Myopathies

There are a number of different types of myopathies.

Classification of myopathies

- **Inflammatory** (eg polymyositis; *see* Chapter 20, Rheumatology)
- **Metabolic** (eg mitochondrial)
- **Drug-induced**
- **Inherited – dominant** (eg dystrophia myotonica; see overleaf); **recessive** (eg Duchenne; see below)
- **Secondary to endocrine disease** (principally thyrotoxicosis or hypothyroidism)

Muscular dystrophy

Duchenne muscular dystrophy is an X-linked disorder affecting about 1 in 3500 male births, though occasionally females may be affected (due to translocation of the short arm of the X chromosome, Xp21).

- The gene has now been isolated in this Xp21 region, and produces a protein named dystrophin that is normally present on the muscle sarcolemmal membrane. The pathogenesis is described in detail in Chapter 14, Molecular Medicine.
- In Duchenne dystrophy, the dystrophin protein is absent.
- Serum creatine kinase is elevated.

In Duchenne muscular dystrophy, weakness occurs progressively from about 3–4 years of age. Thirty per cent of sufferers show intellectual impairment with the overall IQ curve being shifted to the left. There is no effective treatment at present and death usually occurs from cardio-respiratory failure in the second or third decade of life.

In the milder **Becker dystrophy**, the dystrophic protein is seen but it is dysfunctional and present at a lower level than normal.

Distinguishing features in muscular dystrophy

	Duchenne	Becker
Immunofluorescent dystrophin on muscle biopsy	Undetectable	Reduced/abnormal
Wheelchair dependence	95% at <12 years	5% at <12 years
Mental handicap	20%	Rare

Dystrophia myotonica

An inherited myopathy (autosomal dominant) with onset in the third decade.

Features of dystrophia myotonica

- Myotonic facies
- Myotonia (delayed muscular relaxation after contraction)
- Wasting and weakness of the arms and legs
- Frontal baldness
- Testicular/ovarian atrophy
- Diabetes mellitus
- Cataract
- Cardiomyopathy
- Mild cognitive impairment

Diagnosis depends on the characteristic myotonic discharge on EMG in association with the clinical features listed above. Usually severe disability results within 10–20 years, and there is no treatment available though phenytoin may be used for symptomatic relief of myotonia.

9.2 Neuromuscular junction

Neuromuscular transmission is dependent on cholinergic transmission between the terminals of motor nerves and the motor end plate.

Myasthenia gravis

This is an antibody-mediated autoimmune disease affecting the neuromuscular junction; antibodies are produced to the acetylcholine receptors. It is a relatively rare disorder with a prevalence of about 1 in 20, 000. The pathogenesis is described in detail in Chapter 14, Molecular Medicine.

Most (but not all) patients have ptosis. Many have ophthalmoplegia, dysarthria and dysphagia, but any muscle may be affected. The pupil is never affected, but weakness of eye closure and ptosis is common. Quick lid retraction on refixation from down gaze is known as Cogan's sign.

Myasthenia gravis may mimic MND, mitochondrial myopathies, polymyositis, cranial nerve palsies or brainstem dysfunction.

Diagnosis of myasthenia gravis

- Tensilon test
- ACh receptor antibodies (present in 85–90%)
- Electrophysiology (repetitive stimulation gives rise to diminution in the amplitude of the evoked EMG response)
- Thyroid function tests (up to 10% have co-existent thyrotoxicosis)
- CT mediastinum

Treatment of myasthenia gravis

Primary treatment is with cholinesterase (ChE) inhibitors (eg pyridostigmine), and some patients will achieve control with these agents alone. The cause of the disease is usually modified with treatments directed at the **immune system**:

- **immunosuppression**: steroids, azathioprine, cyclophosphamide, ciclosporin A
- plasmapheresis
- intravenous immune globulin infusion.

In those with thymoma or hyperplasia of the thymus, up to 60% will improve or achieve remission after **thymectomy**. The benefits of surgery are greatest in patients aged less than 40 years.

Lambert–Eaton myasthenic syndrome (LEMS)

LEMS is commonly a paraneoplastic syndrome, most commonly associated with small cell carcinoma of the lung (also breast and ovarian cancer). However, in a variable proportion (up to 50%) of patients no cancer is found.

Clinical features of LEMS

- Fatigability
- Hyporeflexia
- Ocular and bulbar muscles rarely affected
- Autonomic symptoms (eg difficulty with micturition, dry mouth, impotence)

Unlike myasthenia gravis, ophthalmoplegia and ptosis are not features. Like myasthenia gravis, LEMS is an autoimmune disorder with antibodies produced to voltage-gated calcium channels in the muscle membrane. On examination, reflexes are absent but return **after** exercise (cf myasthenia gravis). EMG with repetitive stimulation shows an improvement in response.

10. INVESTIGATIONS USED IN NEUROLOGICAL DISEASE

10.1 Cerebrospinal fluid

Normal CSF findings

- **Pressure**
  60–150 mm of CSF (patient recumbent)
- **Protein**
  0.2–0.4 g/l
  Cell count
  Red cells 0, white cells <5/mm^3 (few monocytes or lymphocytes)
- **Glucose**
  More than 2/3 blood glucose

Abnormal CSF findings

Elevated protein

- Very high; >2 g/l
  Guillain–Barré syndrome
  Spinal block
  TB meningitis
  Fungal meningitis
- High
  Bacterial meningitis
  Viral encephalitis
  Cerebral abscess
  Neurosyphilis
  Subdural haematoma
  Cerebral malignancy

Low CSF glucose

- Bacterial meningitis
- TB meningitis
- Fungal meningitis
- Mumps meningitis (20%)
- Herpes simplex encephalitis (20%)
- Subarachnoid haemorrhage (occasionally)

Polymorphs

- Bacterial meningitis

Lymphocytes

- Viral encephalitis/meningitis
- Partially treated bacterial meningitis
- Behçet's syndrome
- CNS vasculitides
- HIV-associated
- Lymphoma
- Leukaemia
- Lyme disease
- Systemic lupus erythematosus

Oligoclonal bands in CSF

- Multiple sclerosis
- Neurosarcoidosis
- CNS lymphoma
- Systemic lupus erythematosus
- Subacute sclerosing panencephalitis rare, late complication of measles
- Subarachnoid haemorrhage (unusual)
- Neurosyphilis
- Guillain–Barré syndrome

10.2 Neuroradiology

CT and MR scanning of the brain and spinal cord are widely used in the investigation of neurological diseases. A comprehensive account is beyond the remit of this section.

Causes of intracranial calcification (on CT scan or skull X-ray)

- Oligodendroglioma
- Craniopharyngioma
- Pineal gland (may be normal finding)
- Sturge–Weber syndrome
- Aneurysm
- Meningioma
- Tuberculoma
- Tuberous sclerosis
- Toxoplasmosis
- Hypoparathyroidism (basal ganglia)

10.3 Electrophysiological investigations

EEG

The EEG is characteristically abnormal in the following conditions:

- **absence seizures**: 3 Hz spike-and-wave complexes
- **Creutzfeldt–Jakob**: periodic bursts of high-amplitude sharp waves.

Nerve conduction tests

Nerve conduction tests are used to investigate peripheral neuropathies. The technique involves stimulating a peripheral nerve (sensory or motor) and recording the action potential latency and amplitude further along the same nerve. This allows calculation of the conduction velocity of the nerve. These measures can be used to distinguish (amongst other things) between axonal and demyelinating neuropathies.

- **axonal**: reduced amplitude (loss of axons) but **preserved** conduction velocity
- **demyelinating**: preserved amplitude but **reduced** conduction velocity (loss of myelin).

Electromyography (EMG)

EMG is useful in disorders of the neuromuscular junction or investigation of myopathic processes. The technique involves stimulating the motor nerves while recording the compound action potential from muscles.

Characteristic abnormalities:

- **myasthenia gravis**: diminished response to repetitive stimulation
- **Lambert–Eaton syndrome**: enhanced response to repetitive stimulation
- **polymyositis**: fibrillation due to denervation hypersensitivity, reduced amplitude and duration of motor units
- **myotonic syndromes**: 'dive bomber' discharge (high-frequency action potentials).

Chapter 17
Ophthalmology

CONTENTS

Pupillary and eye movement disorders, nystagmus and visual field defects are all covered in the neuro-ophthalmology section of Chapter 16, Neurology.

Ophthalmology

Pupillary and eye movement disorders, nystagmus and visual field defects are all covered in the neuro-ophthalmology section of Chapter 16, Neurology.

1. BASIC ANATOMY OF THE EYE

1.1 Orbit

The orbit houses the globe, extraocular muscles, lacrimal gland, orbital fat and attendant arteries, veins and nerves.

1.2 Extraocular muscles

The four rectus muscles and the superior oblique arise at the orbital apex and pass forward to insert into the globe. The inferior oblique arises from the anteromedial orbital floor and runs along the lower surface of the globe to insert into its posterolateral aspect.

The innervation and primary action of each muscle are shown below – note all other movements are composite, ie due to the action of two muscles acting together.

Muscle	Nerve supply	Primary action
Superior rectus	III	Elevation in abduction
Inferior rectus	III	Depression in abduction
Medial rectus	III	Adduction
Lateral rectus	VI	Abduction
Inferior oblique	III	Elevation in adduction
Superior oblique	IV	Depression in adduction

1.3 The globe

Key features of the constituent parts are:

- **Cornea**: clarity maintained by avascularity, the regular structural array of component fibrils and its relative dehydrated state (maintained by endothelium).
- **Conjunctiva**: thin mucous membrane covering anterior sclera and lining eyelids.
- **Sclera**: tough fibroelastic coat.

- **Uveal tract**: anterior uvea comprises iris and ciliary body. Posterior uvea is the choroid, a vascular layer lining the sclera which nourishes outer retinal layers.
- **Retinal pigment epithelium**: cellular monolayer comprising the outermost layer of the retina.
- **Retina**: light-sensitive innermost layer of the globe. Converts light energy into electrical energy. It comprises: (i) rods – more plentiful in the peripheral retina, sensitive to low light and movement detection; and (ii) cones – concentrated within the macular region, particularly at the fovea, important for acuity and colour vision. Vascular supply is from the central retinal artery. Capillaries have non-fenestrated endothelium and tight junctions forming a blood–retinal barrier (analogous to the blood–brain barrier), preventing the passage of large molecules.
- **Lens**: positioned posterior to the iris and anterior to the vitreous, anchored by the zonules. It is enclosed by a capsule, the basement membrane of the lens epithelium. New lens fibres are continuously produced throughout life and the older fibres are compressed to form the lens nucleus. Reduced accommodation is found in later life because the lens is less deformable.

2. RETINAL DISORDERS

2.1 Retinal venous occlusion

Retinal vein occlusion probably occurs due to a dynamic change in blood flow at arteriovenous crossings and may affect the central retinal vein (CRVO) or one of its branches (BRVO).

Aetiology

- Systemic hypertension (most common)
- Increased intraocular pressure (central occlusion only)
- Diabetes mellitus
- Hyperviscosity states
- Vasculitides.

Clinical signs of retinal venous occlusion

- **Loss of vision**
  Variable extent depending on macular involvement and degree of retinal ischaemia produced
- **Relative afferent pupillary defect**
  With retinal ischaemia
- **Multiple retinal haemorrhages**
  Mainly superficial, in nerve fibre layer ('blood and thunder' appearance)
- **Retinal venous dilatation**
- **Cotton wool spots**
- **Vascular sheathing**
- **Neovascularisation**
  May occur in 20% CRVO and 1% BRVO due to ischaemia, ie similar pathogenesis to diabetic retinopathy. This may affect the anterior segment producing neovascular glaucoma, or the retina causing vitreous haemorrhage or retinal traction. Treatment is by retinal laser to abolish the ischaemic stimulus

2.2 Retinal arterial occlusion

As the central retinal artery is an end artery, occlusion of the central artery or one of its branches produces retinal infarction and visual loss in the area supplied.

Aetiology

- **Embolic**
- **Sudden rapid increase in intraocular pressure**
  To above central retinal arterial pressure
- **Arteritic**
  Most commonly giant cell arteritis (GCA). However, visual loss in GCA is only due to central retinal artery occlusion in 10% of cases; it usually affects vision by producing anterior ischaemic optic neuropathy, which damages the optic nerve head

Clinical signs of retinal arterial occlusion

- **Sudden, profound, painless loss of vision**
  (Corresponding sector field loss if branch occlusion)
- **Pale oedematous retina with cherry red spots at fovea (only lasts around 48 hours)**
  This is due to the choroidal reflex showing through at the fovea as the retina is thinner here
- **Relative afferent pupillary defect**
- **Neovascular complications (occur later)**
  Much rarer than with venous occlusions, probably because the retina is too severely damaged to produce angiogenic factor

Treatment is sometimes possible to dislodge the embolus if presentation occurs within a few hours of onset.

2.3 Hypertensive retinopathy

Retinal abnormalities represent the severity of hypertension and are characterised by:

- vascular constriction causing focal retinal ischaemia
- leakage leading to retinal oedema, haemorrhage and lipid deposition.

Arteriosclerotic changes reflect the duration of the hypertension. These include vessel wall thickening secondary to intimal hyalinisation, medial hypertrophy and endothelial hyperplasia.

Classification of hypertensive retinopathy

- **Grade 1**
  Arteriolar attenuation
- **Grade 2**
  Focal arteriolar attenuation (with 'arteriovenous nipping')
- **Grade 3**
  Haemorrhages, cotton wool spots (due to infarction of nerve fibre layer of retina)
- **Grade 4**
  Disc swelling – 'malignant' or 'accelerated' phase

Grades 3 and 4 are associated with severe target organ damage and high mortality (accelerated phase hypertension). Treatment is purely aimed towards the hypertension and any underlying cause.

2.4 Diabetic retinopathy

Diabetic retinopathy is related to the duration and control of the disease. It is the most common cause of blindness in patients aged 30–60 years. It is unusual in type I diabetes until 10 years after diagnosis, but eventually occurs in nearly all patients. It is present in 10% of type II patients at diagnosis, 50% after 10 years' disease and 80% after 20 years' disease.

Diabetic retinopathy is a **microvascular** disease. The following pathological changes are known to occur:

- **Loss of vascular pericytes**: thought to be responsible for the structural integrity of the vessel wall. A decrease therefore results in disruption of the blood–retinal barrier and leakage of plasma constituents into the retina.
- **Capillary endothelial cell** damage.
- **Basement membrane thickening** with carbohydrate and glycogen deposition.

Changes in red cell oxygen-carrying capabilities and increased platelet aggregation are also thought to contribute. The production of an angiogenic factor by ischaemic retina is the likely cause of neovascularisation. At all stages, good control of diabetes and of any coexisting hypertension and stopping smoking have been shown to reduce serious sequelae.

Figure 1 Consequences of retinal vascular leakage.

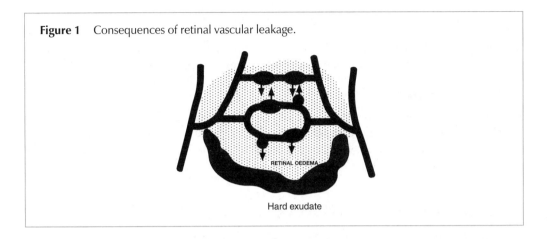

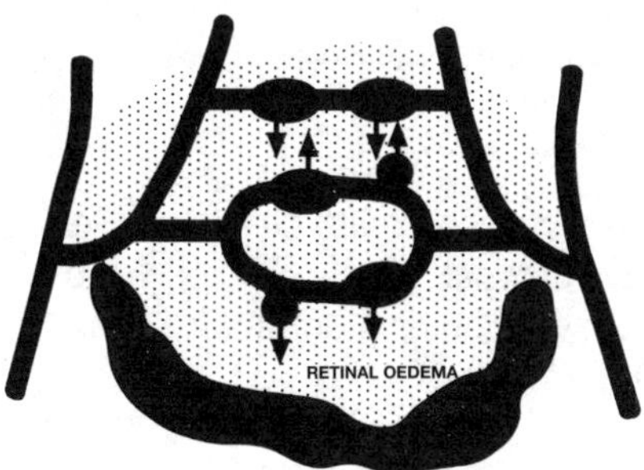

Classification of diabetic retinopathy

- **Background retinopathy**
  Does not affect visual acuity
  Microaneurysms – first clinical change, saccular pouch, either leaks or resolves due to thrombosis
  Haemorrhages – dot, blot and flame-shaped
  Exudates – leakage of lipid and lipoprotein
  No local treatment required; adequate control of diabetes only

- **Diabetic maculopathy**
  Most common cause of visual loss
  More common in type II diabetes
  Retinopathy within the macular region
  Oedematous retina may require laser treatment

- **Preproliferative retinopathy**
  Cotton wool spots – represent areas of axonal disruption secondary to ischaemia
  Venous changes – dilatation and beading
  Large deep haemorrhages
  Treatment controversial: some advocate prophylactic laser treatment, others recommend improving disease control and more frequent monitoring

- **Proliferative retinopathy**
  More common in type I diabetes
  Retinal neovascularisation: new vessels occur in thin-walled friable clumps on the venous side of the retinal circulation; new vessels on the disc are more ominous than those on the vascular arcades; vitreous haemorrhage, fibrosis and tractional retinal detachment may occur
  Iris neovascularisation: may be complicated by glaucoma
  Treatment with laser photocoagulation to retina is designed to abolish the production of angiogenic factor from ischaemic retina

Diabetic retinopathy may progress rapidly in some situations:

- pregnancy – 5% of patients with background changes develop proliferative retinopathy
- sudden improvement in control in previously poorly managed disease.

Diabetic papillopathy

Typically bilateral process in young type I diabetic patients. Associated with mild to moderate visual loss. Fundal examination reveals disc swelling, macular oedema with exudates and macular star. There is no specific management apart from control of the diabetes. Usually spontaneous recovery within 6 months.

Non-retinal eye disease in diabetics

The eye may be affected by diabetes in several other ways:

- **Visual changes**
  Secondary to osmotic lens changes with fluctuating glucose levels
- **Mononeuropathies**
  Leading to ophthalmoplegia
- **Snowflake cataract**
  Poorly controlled juvenile diabetes
- **Early-onset senile cataract**
- **Increased external eye infections**
  (eg conjunctivitis, styes)

2.5 Retinitis pigmentosa

Retinitis pigmentosa (RP) is a term describing a group of progressive inherited diseases affecting the photoreceptors and the retinal pigment epithelium. It is characterised by the triad of:

- **night blindness**: due to loss of rod function
- **tunnel vision**: loss of peripheral field also due to rod dysfunction; central visual acuity loss due to cone disease may also occur but tends to be a later feature
- **pigmented bony spicule**: fundal appearance with associated disc pallor and blood vessel attenuation.

There are three inheritance patterns: autosomal recessive, autosomal dominant and X-linked recessive.

Disease onset and progression vary between different groups and also between affected members within families. Autosomal recessive and X-linked recessive tend to be more severe.

Important systemic associations include the following:

- **Abetalipoproteinaemia (Bassen Kornzweig syndrome)**: autosomal recessive disease typically affecting Ashkenazi Jews. Treatment with high-dose vitamin E may help neurological and retinal disease. (See Chapter 13, Metabolic Diseases.)

- **Refsum's disease**: autosomal recessive disorder of phytanic acid metabolism leading to its accumulation in tissues, causing peripheral neuropathy, cerebellar ataxia, ichthyosis and deafness. Serum phytanic acid levels are elevated and examination of the CSF reveals elevated protein in the presence of a normal cell count. Refsum's disease is responsive to a phytanic-acid-free diet which excludes animal fats, dairy products and green leafy vegetables.
- **Usher's syndrome**: autosomal recessive condition with non-progressive sensorineural deafness.
- **Bardet–Biedl (Laurence–Moon–Biedl syndrome)**: autosomal recessive disease with mental retardation, obesity, hypogonadism, polydactyly, deafness and renal cystic disease.
- **Kearns Sayre syndrome**: disorder of mitochondrial inheritance with progressive external ophthalmoplegia, ptosis and heart block.

3. LENS ABNORMALITIES

3.1 Cataract

Cataract is an opacity of the lens. It is the most common cause of blindness worldwide. Many classifications exist according to type, aetiology and associations. Surgical intervention is indicated:

- when patient function is impaired because of decreased vision
- if the view of the fundus is impaired when monitoring or treating another condition (eg diabetes).

Causes of cataracts

- **Congenital**
  Autosomal dominant (25%)
  Maternal infection – rubella, toxoplasmosis, CMV, herpes simplex, varicella zoster
  Maternal drug ingestion – corticosteroids, thalidomide
  Metabolic – galactosaemia, hypocalcaemia, Lowe's syndrome, hypoglycaemia
  Chromosomal abnormalities (eg Down's syndrome, Turner's syndrome)
- **Toxic/drug-induced**
  (eg steroids, chlorpromazine, busulfan, gold, amiodarone)
- **Senile**
- **Secondary to ocular disease**
  (eg uveitis, high myopia)
- **Metabolic**
  Diabetes, hypoglycaemia, mannosidosis, Fabry's disease, Lowe's syndrome, Wilson's disease, hypocalcaemia, galactokinase deficiency
- **Traumatic**
  Penetrating or blunt injury, infra-red radiation, radiotherapy, electric shock
- **Miscellaneous**
  Myotonic dystrophy, progeria, atopic dermatitis

3.2 Lens dislocation

Lens dislocation results from disruption of the zonules that anchor it in position. Depending on the lens shift this may produce myopia or hypermetropia, or elevated intraocular pressure.

Causes of lens dislocation

- Marfan's syndrome: up and out
- Homocystinuria: down and in
- Ehlers–Danlos syndrome
- Autosomal recessive ectopia lentis
- Trauma
- Uveal tumours.

4. OPTIC NERVE DISORDERS

4.1 Optic neuritis

Inflammation of the optic nerve may affect the:

- **nerve head**: producing **papillitis** with optic disc swelling, hyperaemia and haemorrhages
- **retrobulbar portion of the nerve**: in which the nerve appears normal ('the patient sees nothing, the doctor sees nothing').

It is the presenting feature of 25% of patients with multiple sclerosis (MS); up to 70% of patients who have an attack of optic neuritis will develop MS (20% in the first two years).

Clinical signs of optic neuritis (in order of frequency of occurrence)

1. **Reduced visual acuity**
   Usually monocular (90%), progresses rapidly over a few days; improves over four to six weeks, achieving virtually normal vision in 90%, although RAPD usually persists
2. **Pain**
   Precedes visual loss by a few days, worsened by eye movements
3. **Red colour desaturation**
4. **Relative afferent pupillary defect**
5. **Paracentral or central scotoma**
6. **Visual evoked potential prolonged**
   Reflecting delayed conduction in optic pathway
7. **Variable degree of optic atrophy**

Causes of optic neuritis/papillitis

- **Demyelination**: (also post-viral syndromes)
- **Infections**: viral encephalitis (measles, mumps, chicken-pox), infectious mononucleosis, herpes zoster
- **Inflammatory**: contiguous with orbital inflammation, sinusitis or meningitis secondary to granulomatous optic nerve inflammation (eg TB, sarcoid, syphilis)
- **Other systemic disease**: (eg diabetes).

4.2 Causes of optic atrophy

Causes of optic atrophy

- **Congenital**
  Dominant or recessive
- **Secondary to optic nerve compression**
  (eg pituitary mass, meningioma, orbital cellulitis)
- **Drugs**
  Ethambutol, isoniazid, chloramphenicol, digitalis, chlorpropamide
- **Radiation neuropathy**
- **Carcinomatous**
  Due to microscopic infiltrates of the nerve and its sheath
- **Post-papilloedema**
- **Post-optic neuritis**
  See above
- **Post-trauma**
- **Toxic neuropathy**
  (eg tobacco (cyanide), arsenic, lead, methanol)
- **Nutritional**
  Vitamins B_1, B_2, B_6, B_{12}, folic acid and niacin deficiencies
  Tobacco–alcohol amblyopia may be toxic or nutritional with a good prognosis for recovery
- **Infiltrative neuropathy**
  (eg sarcoid, lymphoma, leukaemia)

4.3 The swollen optic nerve head

Papilloedema

Papilloedema means optic nerve head swelling **secondary to increased intracranial pressure**. This may be due to:

- space-occupying lesion
- hydrocephalus
- CO_2 retention
- idiopathic intracranial hypertension.

Papilloedema is usually bilateral. Features include:

- hyperaemia of the disc: due to capillary dilatation
- splinter haemorrhages of retina
- blurring of the disc margins: due to nerve fibre layer swelling
- exudates and cotton wool spots
- loss of spontaneous venous pulsation: absent in 20% of normal people
- loss of the cup is a late feature.

On clinical examination papilloedema produces an enlarged blind spot. **Transient visual obscurations**, with blacking out of vision lasting a few seconds, often due to positional change, also occur. Visual loss occurs late.

Foster–Kennedy syndrome is unilateral papilloedema with contralateral optic atrophy. It is due to a mass lesion compressing the optic nerve on one side causing ipsilateral atrophic changes and resulting in increased intracranial pressure and contralateral papilloedema.

Papillitis

This refers to inflammation of the optic nerve head (as distinct from retrobulbar neuritis) and is most frequently due to a demyelinative episode (see Section 4.1 above).

Anterior ischaemic optic neuropathy

Infarction of the anterior portion of the optic nerve results in acute severe visual loss which generally does not improve. This is the usual method by which giant cell arteritis affects vision (90%), retinal artery occlusion occurring in the other 10% of cases. It is essential to exclude this condition as it rapidly becomes bilateral. Giant cells and loss of the internal elastic lamina are evident histologically on temporal artery biopsy.

Ischaemic optic neuropathy is not always due to inflammatory arteritis; it may be due to arterio-sclerosis or to hypotensive events. If visual loss is incomplete an altitudinal (ie horizontal) field defect results.

Other causes of swelling of the optic nerve head

- Central retinal vein occlusion
- Orbital mass (eg optic nerve glioma, nerve sheath meningioma, thyroid eye disease and metastases)
- Accelerated phase hypertension (see above)
- Infiltrative neuropathy (eg lymphoma)
- Toxic neuropathy

5. UVEITIS AND SCLERITIS

5.1 Uveitis

Uveitis is inflammation of the uveal tract, which may affect the anterior and/or posterior uvea.

Anterior uveitis typically presents with pain, photophobia, a red eye, lacrimation and decreased vision.

Posterior uveitis presents with floaters (due to inflammatory debris in the vitreous) or impaired vision (secondary to choroiditis if the inflammatory lesion is within the macula).

Uveitis of any cause may be complicated by cataract or glaucoma. Anterior uveitis is most commonly idiopathic but there are also many associations with systemic diseases.

Systemic diseases associated with uveitis (in order of frequency of occurrence)

- **HLA-B27-associated uveitis**
- **Ankylosing spondylitis**
- **Sarcoidosis**
- **Inflammatory bowel disease**
- **Juvenile idiopathic arthritis**
  (Previously termed juvenile chronic arthritis)
- **Reiter's syndrome**
- **Infections**
  TB, syphilis, herpes simplex, herpes zoster, toxoplasmosis, toxocariasis, AIDS, leprosy
- **Behçet's disease**
- **Malignancy**
  Non-Hodgkin's lymphoma
  Leukaemia
  Retinoblastoma
  Ocular melanoma

Characteristics of uveitis associated with particular systemic diseases are:

- **HLA B27 genotype**: present in 50–60% of patients with anterior uveitis as compared to 6% of the population.
- **Ankylosing spondylitis**: recurrent anterior uveitis occurs in approximately 30% of patients with ankylosing spondylitis, and about 30% of males with unilateral uveitis will have ankylosing spondylitis. The uveitis may precede or follow the joint involvement and does not correlate with disease severity; 88% of those with uveitis have HLA B27.
- **Sarcoidosis**: acute or granulomatous. Anterior or posterior. Frequently bilateral and complicated. (*See* Section 8.4.)
- **Reiter's syndrome**: anterior uveitis occurs in 30% of patients. Other ocular features include conjunctivitis and keratitis; 85–95% of patients with ocular involvement have HLA B27.

- **Behçet's disease**: ocular disease occurs in 70% of patients. Anterior uveitis is often severe and bilateral. Conjunctivitis and episcleritis are seen and the retina is frequently affected by retinal vasculitis with infarction, secondary venous occlusion, retinal oedema, exudates and neovascularisation.
- **Juvenile idiopathic arthritis**: ocular involvement typically occurs in pauciarticular disease, particularly those patients who are ANA positive. Uveitic activity bears no relation to that of the arthropathy. The disease is usually bilateral and asymptomatic and therefore regular screening is required because of the high incidence of complications. These are cataract in 35% of patients, secondary glaucoma in 20% and band keratopathy in 40%.

Common causes of **posterior uveitis** (chorio-retinitis) are:

- **idiopathic**
- **inflammatory**: sarcoid
- **infections**: (see box on previous page) TB, syphilis (congenital and tertiary), leprosy, toxoplasmosis, toxocariasis and AIDS
- **malignancy**: leukaemia, lymphoma.

5.2 Scleritis

Inflammation of the sclera may be caused by

- Herpes zoster
- Ankylosing spondylitis
- Sarcoidosis
- Inflammatory bowel disease
- Gout
- Vasculitis: PAN, SLE, Wegener's, relapsing polychondritis, dermatomyositis, Behçet's

5.3 Causes of a painful red eye

- **Conjunctivitis** (bacterial is irritable, viral is painful)
- **Uveitis**
- **Scleritis** (causes listed above)
- **Corneal damage** (abrasion, keratitis (eg Herpes simplex and Herpes zoster))
- **Acute glaucoma** (due to angle closure or rubeosis).

6. SYSTEMIC DRUGS AND THE EYE

Blurred vision is very frequently reported as a side-effect of systemic medication. The following are common or sight-threatening complications. The list is not intended to be comprehensive of all ophthalmic side-effects.

- **Amiodarone**: causes vortex keratopathy in almost all patients. Epithelial deposits, which are reversible on cessation of drug, occur. These swirl out from a point below the pupil but are inconsequential to vision.
- **Chloroquine and hydroxychloroquine**: classically cause 'Bull's eye maculopathy'. There is central hyperpigmentation at the fovea surrounded by concentric rings of hypo and hyperpigmentation. Fundal changes occur after subjective visual loss. Baseline visual function (corrected near and distance acuity, colour vision, visual fields) should be established and these parameters monitored throughout treatment. Toxicity is rare with a cumulative chloroquine dose of less than 300 g, and it is much less likely to occur with hydroxychloroquine. Once visual loss occurs it may be progressive despite cessation of the drug.
- **Ethambutol**: causes optic neuropathy, more frequently when used in high doses or with renal impairment. The earliest feature is subjective reduction in visual acuity. Toxicity is usually reversible with early withdrawal of the drug. Visual acuity should be checked pre-treatment and during the course of drug usage.
- **Tamoxifen**: causes maculopathy and refractile opacities, which are associated with a mild reduction in vision.
- **Vigabatrin**: causes constriction of visual fields which may be severe. The onset is reported to occur from two months to five years after starting the drug. The field defect starts nasally and progresses to become concentric; the eyes are affected symmetrically. The aetiology is thought to be related to retinal toxicity, but this is not fully understood; the visual field defects usually persist on cessation of vigabatrin.
- **Drugs with anticholinergic effects** (eg tricyclics and anaesthetic agents such as atropine, glycopyrrolate and hyoscine): these can precipitate angle closure glaucoma in susceptible patients (usually those who are long-sighted).

7. INFECTIOUS AGENTS AND THE EYE

The following conditions may all be caused by infectious agents, as discussed in the previous section:

- congenital cataracts (maternal infection)
- optic neuritis/papillitis
- uveitis
- scleritis
- conjunctivitis.

7.1 Genito-urinary disease and the eye

All patients with genito-urinary disease affecting the eye warrant evaluation at a genito-urinary clinic for systemic investigation and treatment. Ophthalmic features of HIV/AIDS are covered in Chapter 8, Genito-urinary Medicine and AIDS.

Chlamydial conjunctivitis

This is sexually transmitted and most commonly found in young adults. It may be associated with non-specific urethritis or cervicitis. Typical features are as follows:

- It causes bilateral acute conjunctivitis which can persist for several weeks.
- This is often associated with pre-auricular lymphadenopathy.
- It may lead to **ophthalmia neonatorum**. Affected newborns will require systemic treatment.
- Diagnosis is by chlamydial culture or immunofluorescence.

Gonococcal conjunctivitis

There is typically a high hyperacute conjunctivitis with marked chemosis and lid swelling accompanied by copious discharge. This may be associated with corneal ulceration and the risk of perforation. A diagnostic swab may show Gram-negative diplococci, which may be grown on culture. Topical and systemic treatment are indicated.

Syphilis

The ophthalmic abnormalities are related to the particular stage of syphilis:
- **congenital**: interstitial keratitis (leads to clouding of the corneas in the second decade of life), iritis, chorioretinitis and optic atrophy
- **primary**: chancre may occur on the eyelid
- **secondary**: iritis occurs in 4% of patients with secondary syphilis and is usually bilateral; optic neuritis, chorioretinitis and scleritis are all associated
- **tertiary**: associated with optic atrophy, chorioretinitis, iritis, interstitial keratitis and the **Argyll Robertson pupil**.

7.2 Herpetic disease and the eye

Herpes simplex (HSV)

Most HSV infections are subclinical as 90% of the adult population are seropositive.

- **Primary infection with HSV**: this usually occurs in children and causes conjunctivitis with lid swelling. Lesions heal without scarring.
- **HSV reactivation**: this is associated with **epithelial keratitis**. The corneal ulceration may be 'dendritic', when lesions appear like the branch of tree, or 'geographic' when the lesions become much larger with an amoeboid shape. The corneal stroma may subsequently become involved. Treatment is with topical antiviral agents.

Herpes zoster

The painful acute vesicular rash follows a dermatomal pattern, and so disease affecting the fifth cranial nerve can affect the eye. If the rash is present on the tip of the nose (Hutchinson's sign) this indicates involvement of the nasociliary nerve and implies a higher risk of ophthalmic involvement.

- The eye may be affected by conjunctivitis, corneal ulceration, uveitis, scleritis, retinitis and oculomotility abnormalities because of cranial nerve involvement.

8. MISCELLANEOUS DISORDERS

8.1 Thyroid eye disease

The ocular manifestations of Grave's disease may pre-date, coincide or follow the systemic disease. The classic triad is the association of ocular changes with thyroid acropachy and pretibial myxoedema. Eye disease may be divided according to Werner's classification ('NO SPECS'), although it is important to appreciate that there is not a step-like progression from one stage to the next, and not all steps occur in all patients.

No signs or symptoms
Only signs (eg lid retraction/lag)
Soft tissue swelling
Proptosis – orbital fat proliferation and muscle changes; auto-decompresses orbital contents
Extraocular muscle changes – usually affect inferior and/or medial recti; lymphocytic infiltrate
Corneal exposure
Sight loss – secondary to corneal disease or optic nerve compression.

Management of ocular manifestations may be divided into:

- **surface abnormalities**: ocular lubricants, tarsorrhaphy
- **muscle changes**: prisms or patches to control diplopia, surgery after defect stable for minimum of six months
- **optic nerve compression**: systemic steroids, radiotherapy, surgical decompression
- **cosmetic**: improve lid position, remove redundant tissue.

8.2 Myotonic dystrophy

Autosomal dominant condition characterised by failure of relaxation of voluntary muscle fibres.

Ophthalmic features of myotonic dystrophy

- Ptosis, poor lid closure and orbicularis weakness
- Retinal pigmentary changes
- Presenile cataract
- Miotic pupils

8.3 Ocular features of the phacomatoses

This group of disorders affects the nervous system, skin, eye and other organs and they are characterised by the presence of hamartomatous lesions.

Sturge–Weber syndrome

Glaucoma occurs on ipsilateral side to cutaneous angioma in 50%. Cavernous haemangioma may be seen in the choroid.

Neurofibromatosis

- The eyelid may be affected by cutaneous neuroma
- In the anterior segment, iris nodules are seen and glaucoma is more common
- Choroidal naevi may be seen on fundoscopy
- The optic nerve may be affected by glioma, and a pulsatile globe suggests a defect of the greater wing of the sphenoid.

von Hippel–Lindau syndrome

Autosomal dominant condition with incomplete penetrance and variable expressivity, the abnormality being on the short arm of chromosome 3.

- Retinal haemangiomas develop bilaterally in 25% of patients and may leak (producing exudates or a serous retinal detachment), or rupture (leading to vitreous haemorrhage). These are histologically identical to the cerebellar haemangioblastomas which also occur.
- Indirectly, increased intracranial pressure due to posterior fossa haemangioblastoma may lead to papilloedema; hypertensive changes may be seen when phaeochromocytoma is present.

Tuberous sclerosis

- Autosomal dominant condition linked to several chromosomal abnormalities; 50% are new mutations. Ocular features include retinal hamartomas and rarely papilloedema or VIth nerve palsy due to increased intracranial pressure secondary to CNS lesions.

8.4 Sarcoidosis

This multisystem granulomatous disease affects the eye and ocular adnexae in about 30% of cases, and of these 25% will have posterior segment disease.

Ocular effects of sarcoidosis

- **Lids**
  Lupus pernio, cutaneous granuloma
- **Lacrimal glands**
  Granulomatous infiltrate, may cause sicca syndrome (Mikulicz's syndrome when combined with parotid involvement)
- **Uveitis**
  Acute or granulomatous, frequently bilateral, and complicated by glaucoma and cataract
- **Retinal involvement**
  With periphlebitic 'candle wax exudates', haemorrhages, oedema and neovascularisation
- **Choroiditis and choroidal granulomas**
- **Optic nerve granuloma**
- **Disc oedema**
- **Nerve palsies: III, IV, VI**

8.5 Keratoconus

Keratoconus is an ectatic condition of the inferior paracentral cornea. Onset is usually in the teens with progressive myopic astigmatism.

Systemic associations are:

- Atopy
- Down's syndrome
- Turner's syndrome
- Marfan's syndrome
- Ehler–Danlos syndrome.

8.6 Glaucoma

Glaucoma describes the group of conditions in which intra-ocular pressure is sufficient to cause visual damage with a characteristic optic neuropathy. The normal intraocular pressure is <22 mmHg. Aqueous humour is formed by the ciliary body, and passes through the pupil and drains, via the trabecular meshwork, into the venous circulation through the episcleral venous system.

Acute glaucoma

- Rapid decrease in visual acuity associated with severe pain and vomiting
- More common in hypermetropes (long-sightedness)

- Is due to closure of the drainage angle resulting in a massive sudden elevation in intra-ocular pressure
- The cornea appears cloudy (due to oedema) and there is a mid-dilated non-reacting pupil
- Failure to treat pressure rapidly results in permanent visual loss.

Chronic glaucoma

- Insidious asymptomatic disease
- Intraocular pressure elevated (usually not as markedly as in acute glaucoma), resulting in cupping of the optic nerve head and loss of visual field
- Classically an arcuate scotoma develops, which progresses to generalised field constriction
- Familial tendency but no strict inheritance
- More common in women and myopes (short-sighted).

Secondary glaucoma

Glaucoma is a possible complication of almost any ocular disorder.

Secondary glaucomas may be generally classified as follows

- **Pre-trabecular**
  (eg fibrovascular membrane in rubeosis)
- **Trabecular**
  Clogging of meshwork by (eg inflammatory cells in uveitis) meshwork alteration due to inflammation in uveitis or scleritis
- **Post-trabecular**
  Raised episcleral venous pressure preventing outflow (eg carotico-cavernous fistula, or cavernous sinus thrombosis)

8.7 Ocular tumours

Primary tumours

- **Choroidal melanoma:** this is the commonest primary intraocular tumour. It presents as a unilateral lesion with variable pigmentation (amelanotic to dark brown). It may be asymptomatic or can cause reduction in acuity or loss of visual field, depending on the site of the lesion.
- **Choroidal haemangioma:** this appears as a red/orange lesion most frequently seen at the macula. A more diffuse lesion can be seen in Sturge–Weber syndrome, which results in a deep red appearance to the fundus; this may only be appreciated by comparison with the contralateral side.

Secondary tumours

The eye may be affected by metastases to the choroid or orbit and cerebral metastases may affect the visual pathway or cause oculomotility disorders.

- **Choroidal metastases** occur most frequently from breast, bronchial and renal primary tumours. They are frequently multiple and also bilateral. Lesions appear pale and are minimally elevated. They are associated with metastatic disease elsewhere. The effect upon vision depends on the site; macular lesions are most common and can cause marked visual loss. Palliative external beam radiation is usually successful in improving vision.

8.8 Blind registration

Blind registration is completed by ophthalmologists and can facilitate rehabilitation and Social Services support. Monocular vision is not a criterion for registration. Two levels for blind registration exist:

- **partial sight registration**: this is applicable when the visual acuity is ≤6/24 in both eyes, or when there is constriction of visual fields, including hemianopia
- **blind registration**: when the visual acuity is ≤3/60 in both eyes.

Chapter 18
Psychiatry

CONTENTS

Psychiatry

1. SCHIZOPHRENIA

Schizophrenia is characterised by disturbances of thought, perception, mood and personality. These lead to 'positive' symptoms, such as delusions, hallucinations and disorganisation of thoughts and speech, and 'negative' symptoms, including decreased motivation, poor self-care and social withdrawal. Patients do not have a 'split personality'. The lifetime risk is about 1% for men and women, although men consistently have an earlier age of onset. There is strong evidence of genetic predisposition, but not through a simple Mendelian model of inheritance (see box below).

Lifetime risk of schizophrenia in relatives of patients with schizophrenia

Relationship	**Per cent with schizophrenia**
Monozygotic twin	50
Children (both parents schizophrenic)	46
Children	13
Dizygotic twin	10
Sibling	10
Uncles/aunts	3
Unrelated	0.9

Schizophrenia is a heterogeneous condition; signs and symptoms present to a highly variable degree between individuals. Despite this, generalisations can be made about certain 'core features'. Schneider's first-rank symptoms were an attempt to tighten diagnostic practice.

1.1 First-rank symptoms

Originally described by Schneider, these represent an attempt to identify symptoms that occur exclusively in schizophrenia. In clinical practice they occur in approximately 70% of schizophrenic patients and in approximately 10% of manic patients. However, for the purpose of medical examinations, including the MRCP, they *should* be considered to be 'diagnostic of' or 'characteristic of' schizophrenia in the absence of obvious organic brain disease. A mnemonic for first-rank symptoms follows.

First-rank symptoms mnemonic: ATPD – Aim To Pass Definitely

Auditory hallucinations of a specific type:
- Third person (ie two or more voices heard discussing the patient)
- Running commentary
- Thought echo

Thought disorder of a specific type (passivity of thought):
- Thought withdrawal
- Thought insertion
- Thought broadcasting

Passivity experiences (delusions of control):
- Actions/feelings/impulses under external control
- Bodily sensations being due to external influence

Delusional perception (two-stage process):
- Normal perception of commonplace object/sight, leads to...
- Sudden, intense, self-referential delusion (eg finding coin on the ground leads to belief of messianic role)

There are many other important clinical features of schizophrenia, including impaired insight, suspiciousness, flat/blunted or incongruous affect, decreased spontaneous speech, general lack of motivation and poor self-care and abnormalities of motor activity such as dyskinesia and catatonia.

Auditory hallucinations which are not of the type covered by the first-rank symptoms may occur, as can other types of delusions, often bizarre and non-mood-congruent. These symptoms can be divided into two categories, as follows.

Positive symptoms

These include delusions, hallucinations and disorder of the form of thought. Temporal lobe epilepsy is one important differential diagnosis that should be considered in individuals who experience positive symptoms and hence an EEG may be useful in certain patients.

Negative symptoms

These include flat/blunted affect, decreased motor activity and speech, poor motivation and self-care. Patients with schizophrenia who manifest predominantly negative symptoms often have frontal cognitive deficits in attention and executive function (planning, goal-directed behaviour and monitoring of performance). CT and/or MRI studies of the brain in such patients have shown ventricular enlargement and cortical sulcal prominence.

1.2 Principles of treatment

Treatment of schizophrenia involves a biopsychosocial model, but compliance with medication is the best predictor of relapse.

Biological treatments

- **Atypical antipsychotics** (eg clozapine, olanzapine, risperidone) are now considered to be first-line therapeutic agents. They have a preferential side-effect profile, particularly with regard to extrapyramidal side-effects. Use of **traditional antipsychotics** (chlorpromazine, haloperidol, trifluoperazine, etc) is limited by extrapyramidal (tardive dyskinesia occurs in >30% of patients on long-term treatment) and cardiac side-effects. Antipsychotics may be given orally, intramuscularly (im) or depot im; depot preparations aid compliance and are now available in atypical form (risperidone). 'Positive' symptoms respond better than 'negative' symptoms to antipsychotic therapy; the atypical antipsychotics are probably better for negative symptoms. **Electroconvulsive therapy (ECT)** may be needed for catatonic stupor.
- **Psychological treatments**: three independent trials have recently shown that cognitive behavioural therapy (CBT) is a valuable adjunctive treatment for patients with persistent hallucinations and delusions. CBT can also aid compliance.
- **Social interventions**: these should target accommodation, finances and daytime activities. Patients and relatives may both benefit from supportive psychotherapy, counselling and education.

2. MOOD DISORDERS

Mood (affective) disorders are conditions in which a pathologically depressed or elated mood is the core feature. Depression is much more common than mania; those who suffer with mania almost invariably have one or more periods of depression at some stage in the course of their illness. The genetic contribution to mood disorders is strongest for bipolar disorder.

2.1 Hypomania/mania (bipolar affective disorder)

Hypomania and mania are mood disorders characterised by pathologically elated or irritable mood. Lifetime prevalence is about 1% with a slight female predominance. Hypomania is a slightly less severe form of mania and psychotic symptoms are absent. The majority of symptoms in both are 'mood congruent', ie understandable in the context of the pathological mood change. There is usually a previous episode of depression or episodes of depression in the future, hence hypomania/mania is part of a bipolar affective disorder. The main differential diagnoses are usually organic psychoses or schizophrenia. The clinical features of hypomania/mania are listed in the box overleaf.

Clinical features of hypomania/mania

- **Mood**
  Predominantly elevated/elated irritable
  Expansive (but note transient depression common)
- **Speech and thoughts**
  Pressured (fast)
  Flight of ideas
  Inflated self-esteem/grandiosity
  Over-optimistic ideas
  Poor attention, concentration
- **Behaviour**
  Insomnia
  Over-activity
  Loss of normal social inhibitions: over familiar, sexual promiscuity, risk-taking, overspending
  Increased libido
  Increased appetite, decreased weight
- **Psychotic symptoms (mania)**
  Mood-congruent (eg delusions of special ability or status, grandiose delusions or auditory hallucinations)

Perhaps the most crucial decision to make in the management of bipolar disorder is the timing of the introduction of long-term prophylactic mood-stabilising medication (typically lithium or anticonvulsants). There are no hard and fast rules; this is a matter of clinical judgement.

Lithium is the most commonly prescribed mood stabiliser and it is particularly important to remember its therapeutic window. (*See* Chapter 2, Clinical Pharmacology, Toxicology and Poisoning.)

Biological/physical treatments of hypomania/mania

- **Short-term, acute episode**
  Antipsychotics (olanzapine is licensed for the treatment of mania)
  Benzodiazepines
  Lithium (plasma level 1.0 mmol/l)
  ECT
- **Long-term, prophylaxis**
  Lithium (plasma level 0.5 mmol/l)
  Sodium valproate
  Carbamazepine
  Lamotrigine
  Depot antipsychotics

2.2 Depression

Depression occurs with a wide range of severity and has a multifactorial aetiology. Lifetime incidence of depression varies from 1% to 20% according to severity. Evidence for a genetic contribution is most compelling in the most severe illness, whereas mild and moderate depression are usually best explained by psychosocial models. These latter disorders are rarely treated by psychiatrists unless they are complicated by co-morbidity with substance misuse or personality disorder. The variation in severity and symptomatology of depression has led to a number of classification systems:

- endogenous versus reactive (more closely related to precipitating life events)
- melancholic versus neurotic
- unipolar (depression only) versus bipolar (depression with mania).

Clinical features of depression

'Biological' symptoms (shown in italics) are especially important because their presence predicts response to physical treatments. They are also known as 'somatic', 'endogenous' or 'melancholic' symptoms.

- **Mood**
  Loss of reactivity
  Diurnal variation (worse in am)
  Pervasively lowered
  Variable anxiety/irritability

- **Speech and thoughts**
  Slowed speech, low volume
  Reduced attention/concentration
  Reduced self-esteem
  Reduced confidence
  Ideas of guilt, worthlessness, hopelessness
  Bleak, pessimistic outlook
  Ideas and acts of self-harm

- **Behaviour**
  Insomnia (early morning wakening)
  Psychomotor agitation or retardation
  Reduced libido
  Loss of enjoyment (anhedonia)
  Decreased appetite
  Weight loss
  Decreased social interactions
  Reduced energy/increased fatigue
  Decreased activity

- **Psychotic symptoms**
  Mood-congruent
  Delusions of guilt, physical illness
  Auditory hallucinations with derogatory content

2.3 Depression in the elderly

Depression in the elderly is often missed. This is in part due to the prejudice that depression is an inevitable consequence of increasing age, but also because older patients tend to present less with depressed mood and more with physical complaints. It is likely to be associated with social isolation, bereavement, financial problems, physical ill health and chronic pain. The most common presentations are physical symptoms (or hypochondriasis), insomnia (and psychomotor disturbances), most commonly agitation but stupor may occur. Cognitive impairment may mimic dementia (see overleaf).

Treatment of depression on the elderly

Again, a biopsychosocial model is used:

- **Biological**: **selective serotonin re-uptake inhibitors** (SSRIs) are currently the most popular first-line agents. In the elderly, patients may be sensitive to the side-effects of tricyclic agents. **ECT** may be preferable in severe illness.

- **Psychological**: cognitive behavioural therapy.
- **Social**: decrease isolation.

2.4 Differentiation of depression from dementia

The cognitive impairment seen in severe depression, sometimes called depressive pseudodementia, can lead to a misdiagnosis of primary depression, particularly in elderly patients. The table below details differentiating clinical features.

Clinical features of depression and dementia

Clinical features	Depression	Dementia
Family history	Affective disorder	Alzheimer's disease (in some)
Illness duration	Short	Long
Progression	Rapid	Slow
History of previous depression	Yes	No
Biological symptoms of depression	Present	Absent
c/o poor memory	Yes	No
History given	Detailed	Vague
Effort at testing	Poor	Good
Response at test results	Picks on faults	Pleased
Other behaviour	Contrary	Compatible
Examination of concentration/attention	Variable	Consistently poor
Orientation tests	'Don't know'	Poor
Memory loss	Global	Recent
Primitive reflexes	Absent	Present
Apraxias	Absent	Present
Word intrusions	Corrects	Unaware
Neuropsychological tests		
Test performance	Variable	Always poor
Pattern	Nil specific	Verbal IQ > performance IQ

2.5 Principles of treatment

Treatments in depression target the biological, psychological and social aetiologies. If biological symptoms are present then physical treatments are indicated, whatever the apparent psychosocial precipitants. *See also* Section 11, 'Treatments in psychiatry'.

Treatment of depression

- **Biological treatments**
  Antidepressants
  Lithium (for augmentation of antidepressant effect, long-term prophylaxis or in treatment-resistant illness)
  Thyroid hormone (T_3; augmentation therapy in resistant depression)
  ECT (for severe or resistant depression)
  Antipsychotics (if psychotic symptoms present)
- **Psychological treatments**
  Supportive psychotherapy/counselling
  Cognitive therapy
- **Social interventions**
  Accommodation, finances, day-time activities

3. ANXIETY DISORDERS

3.1 Generalised anxiety disorder

The clinical features of generalised anxiety disorder are persistent and generalised, occurring across a range of daily circumstances. Patients never completely return to a baseline level of zero anxiety. Anxiety commonly co-exists with other psychiatric disorders, particularly depression. Organic causes of anxiety disorder include drugs (eg caffeine) and thyrotoxicosis.

Cognitive symptoms

- Apprehension
- Fear of death, losing control or going mad
- Hypervigilance.

Somatic symptoms

- Palpitations
- Shortness of breath and hyperventilation
- Butterflies in the stomach, nausea, loose bowel motions
- Urinary frequency
- Muscle tension
- Headaches, dizziness, lightheadedness, tingling in fingers and around mouth.

Treatment of anxiety disorders

- **Biological**: specific SSRI antidepressants have been shown to be especially useful. Benzodiazepines (with care), beta-blockers, buspirone (5-HT_{1A} partial agonist) and tricyclic antidepressants are also used in the short-term.
- **Psychological**: cognitive behavioural therapy and anxiety management.

3.2 Panic disorder

These patients suffer paroxysms of intense anxiety (panic) interspersed with periods of complete remission. Typical attacks last several minutes and occur without situational cues. Somatic symptoms are prominent. Patients may develop an anticipatory fear of the next attack.

Physical treatment includes short-term use of benzodiazepines with care, and specific serotonin re-uptake inhibitors (SSRIs). Cognitive behavioural therapy is an appropriate psychological treatment.

3.3 Phobic disorders

These patients suffer from intense anxiety which is reliably precipitated by a situational cue. The fear they experience is out of proportion to the situation and cannot be reasoned or explained away. This results in the avoidance of the feared situation and related situations and this, in turn, further reinforces the phobia.

Specific/simple phobias include fear of flying, heights, animals, etc. Agoraphobia is anxiety about being in places or situations from which escape may be difficult; for example, in crowds, on public transport, on a bridge, etc. Social phobia is a persistent fear of humiliation or embarrassment in social situations.

Appropriate physical treatments include SSRIs, β-blockers and occasionally short-term use of benzodiazepines 'with care'. Patients may also benefit from psychological treatments including:

- behavioural psychotherapy: systematic desensitisation (controlled exposure to the feared situation), flooding, modelling
- supportive psychotherapy
- psychodynamic psychotherapy (see Section 11.5, 'The psychotherapies').

4. OBSESSIVE COMPULSIVE DISORDER

Obsessive compulsive disorder may also be called obsessional illness, or obsessional neurosis. Mild obsessional symptoms are very common and may actually be helpful for certain occupations (eg accountancy and medicine). Pathologically severe symptoms may be secondary to other psychiatric or neuropsychiatric disorders (see below). The lifetime prevalence of primary obsessive compulsive disorder is between 2% and 3%, with a slight excess of females affected.

Obsessions are ideas, thoughts (ruminations) or images, that are:

- recurrent
- persistent
- occurring against the patient's will

- regarded as absurd, but insight is maintained
- recognised as a product of the patient's own mind (in contrast to psychosis, the patient recognises that their thoughts are abnormal)
- resisted → anxiety.

Compulsions are:

- irresistible impulses to carry out a particular activity
- usually triggered by an obsessional thought.

OBSESSION	→	**COMPULSION**	→	**RITUAL**
hands dirty		must wash hands		washing

Compulsions and ritualised behaviours are sometimes referred to together as 'compulsions'. There is a large overlap with depressive disorder, and the two conditions often co-exist:

- 30% of patients with obsessive compulsive disorder have associated depression
- 25% of patients with depression develop obsessions.

Other associations include:

- schizophrenia (3–5%)
- anorexia nervosa
- organic brain disease (frontal lobe syndromes, Sydenham's chorea, Tourette's syndrome (obsessional symptoms in 11–80%)).

Treatment of obsessive compulsive disorders

- **Biological**: antidepressants, which increase 5HT neurotransmission (clomipramine, SSRIs), and antipsychotics if the patient is resistant to antidepressant alone. Psychosurgery may be effective for the most severely disabled patients.
- **Psychological**: cognitive behavioural therapy (CBT), which includes habituation training and thought stopping (for obsessions), and exposure with response prevention (for compulsions).

5. UNEXPLAINED PHYSICAL SYMPTOMS

Within a general hospital or general practice setting psychiatric referral may occur because no organic cause is found for physical symptoms. Somatic symptoms may be a manifestation of depression, anxiety or schizophrenia (rare) and these diagnoses should be excluded before a diagnosis of somatoform, conversion or factitious disorder is made.

5.1 Somatoform disorders

In this group of disorders there is repeated presentation of physical symptoms accompanied by persistent requests for medical investigations. If physical disorders are present, they do not explain the nature or extent of symptoms. Repeated negative findings and reassurance have little effect and patients usually refute the possibility of psychological causation. In somatisation disorder the emphasis is on particular symptoms (eg back pain); in hypochondriacal disorder, patients believe they have a specific disease process (eg cancer).

Somatisation disorder

- More than two years of **multiple physical *symptoms*** without adequate explanation
- Persistent refusal to accept advice or reassurance that there is no physical explanation
- Functional impairment due to the nature of symptoms and resulting behaviour
- Affects women much more often than men
- Is accompanied by a tendency to excessive drug use.

Particularly common symptoms include gastrointestinal sensations (pain, belching, vomiting, nausea), abnormal skin sensations (itching, burning, tingling) and sexual and menstrual complaints.

Hypochondriacal disorder

- Persistent belief in presence of at least one **serious physical *illness*** despite repeated negative investigations
- Typical illnesses include cancer, AIDS
- Persistent refusal to accept advice or reassurance
- Fear of drugs and side-effects.

The principles of treatment for somatoform disorders are to exclude an organic basis for the complaint, acknowledge that the symptoms exist and then educate the patient about basic physiology and elicit and challenge the assumptions leading from the symptoms. Self-monitoring (by keeping a diary) can assist with the re-attribution of physical experiences.

5.2 Conversion disorder

This is a **rare** cause of unexplained physical symptoms. The theory is that intolerable psychic anxiety is **unconsciously** 'converted' to physical symptoms. The extent of 'motivation' or voluntary control is usually hard to assess, but there is a clear alteration or loss in physical function which is usually acute, but may be chronic.

Such 'psychogenic' symptoms usually follow an unresolved stressful event and their existence may lead to a reduction in psychological distress ('primary gain') and to a resolution of the stressful event. Although some patients experience the 'secondary gain' of attention from others, others may be indifferent to their loss of function ('la belle indifference'). Isolated conversion symptoms may occur in schizophrenia or depression.

Convincing evidence of psychological causation may be difficult to find. It is vital to exercise caution in making a diagnosis of conversion disorder, especially in the presence of a known CNS or peripheral nervous system disorder.

Treatment involves detection of the underlying conflict (usually through psychotherapy) and may require hypnosis/abreaction.

5.3 Factitious disorder

Also known as Munchausen's syndrome, this is the **intentional** production of physical or psychological symptoms. It is usually associated with severe personality disorder and treatment is extremely difficult.

6. EATING DISORDERS

Anorexia nervosa and bulimia nervosa share many clinical features and patients may satisfy criteria for anorexia or bulimia at different stages of their illness. Eating disorders are much more common in women, but 5–10% of cases of anorexia are male.

Anorexia nervosa is largely restricted to social groups in which thinness is coveted. Presentation is usually in adolescence. The long-term outcome is poor, with only 20% making a full recovery and long-term mortality is around 15–20%.

Bulimia nervosa has a prevalence in young women of 1–2% and usually presents in the 20s. About one-third of patients have a previous history of anorexia. Outcome is highly variable but is worse if there is preceding anorexia or if the bulimia is part of a multi-impulsive personality disorder.

Differentiation of eating disorders

	Anorexia nervosa (restricting subtype)	Anorexia nervosa (bulimic subtype)	Bulimia nervosa
'Nervosa' psychopathology	Yes	Yes	Yes
Behaviour to control weight	Yes	Yes	Yes
Bulimic episodes	No	Yes	Yes
Low weight (<15% average body weight)	Yes	Yes	No
Amenorrhoea	Yes	Yes	Possible

Figure 1 A schematic representation of the relationship between anorexia nervosa and bulimia nervosa. In clinical practice a diagnosis of bulimia is restricted to those with greater than average body weight. Those in the overlap are considered to have anorexia, bulimic subtype

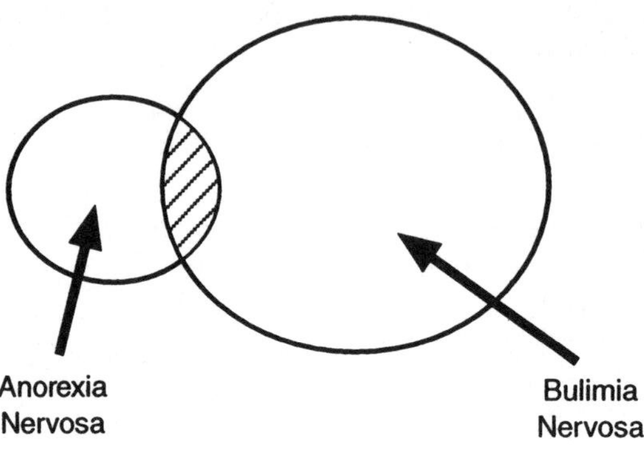

6.1 Anorexia nervosa and bulimia nervosa: diagnostic criteria

Anorexia nervosa: diagnostic criteria	
Loss of (>15%) normal body weight which is self-induced:	Extreme avoidance of foods considered 'fattening' Aggravated by self-induced vomiting, purging or exercise
A specific psychopathology ('nervosa'):	Overvalued idea that fatness is a dreadful state Extremely harsh definition of fatness Will not let weight rise above very low threshold
Specific endocrine associations:	
Female	Amenorrhoea Delayed puberty if very young (primary amenorrhoea)
Male	Loss of sexual interest and potency Delayed puberty if very young; arrest of secondary sexual characteristics

Bulimia nervosa: diagnostic criteria

Key features:

- episodes of binge eating
- persistent preoccupation with eating
- irresistible craving for food.

- **Attempts to counteract the 'fattening' effects of food**
  Self-induced vomiting
  Periods of starvation
  Purgative and diuretic abuse
  Abuse of appetite suppressants
  Abuse of thyroid hormones
  Neglect to use insulin (diabetics)
- **Specific psychopathology ('nervosa')**
  Morbid fear of fatness
  Sharply defined weight threshold
  Earlier episode of anorexia nervosa

6.2 Medical complications of anorexia nervosa

These are mostly physiological adaptations to starvation and usually revert with refeeding.

Medical complications of anorexia nervosa

- **Cardiovascular**
  Bradycardia (87%)
  Hypotension (85%)
  Ventricular arrhythmias
  ECG abnormalities
  Congestive cardiac failure
- **Gastroenterological**
  Eroded dental enamel/caries (secondary to vomiting)
  Enlarged salivary glands (secondary to vomiting)
  Oesophagitis
  Erosions
  Ulcers
  Oesophageal rupture
  Acute gastric dilatation with refeeding
  Decreased gastric emptying
  Constipation
  Duodenal dilatation
  Irritable bowel syndrome
  Melanosis coli (secondary to laxatives)
- **Renal**
  Decreased GFR
  Decreased concentration ability
  Hypokalaemic nephropathy
  Pre-renal uraemia
- **Haematological**
  Pancytopenia
  Hypoplastic marrow
  Low plasma proteins
- **Musculoskeletal**
  Early onset leads to shorter stature
  Osteoporosis
  Pathological fractures
  Proximal myopathy
  Cramps
  Tetany
  Muscle weakness

Continues …

... Continued

- **Metabolic**
  Hypothermia and dehydration
  Electrolyte disturbance (especially hypokalaemia)
  Hypercholesterolaemia and carotinaemia
  Hypoglycaemia and raised liver enzymes

- **Neurological**
  Reversible brain atrophy (on CT scan)
  Abnormal EEG and seizures

- **Endocrine**
  Low follicle-stimulating hormone (FSH), luteinising hormone (LH), oestrogens, testosterone
  Low tri-iodothyronine (T_3)
  Raised cortisol and positive dexamethasone suppression test
  Raised growth hormone (GH)

6.3 Principles of treatment

Biological/physical treatments

- **Anorexia nervosa**
  Restoration of weight as an inpatient, ideally in a specialist eating disorder unit
  Drugs have a limited place in management
  Enteral/parenteral nutrition is rarely indicated

- **Bulimia nervosa**
  Selective serotonin re-uptake inhibitor (SSRI) may be useful reduce bingeing and self-induced vomiting
  Effect not related to the presence of depressive symptoms

Psychological treatments

- **Anorexia nervosa**
  Supportive psychotherapy
  Family therapy
  Cognitive behavioural therapy

- **Bulimia nervosa**
  Cognitive behavioural therapy
  Cognitive analytic therapy
  Self-help manuals

7. DELIBERATE SELF-HARM

A good deal is known about the epidemiology of, and risk factors for, deliberate self-harm, both fatal and non-fatal. These are presented in the following table. A decrease in the rate of suicide, particularly in patients with mental illness, has been the target of many government policies.

Features of suicide and non-fatal self-harm

	Suicide	**Non-fatal self-harm**
Annual incidence in UK	1/10, 000 (5000 total)	20–30/10, 000
Sex	M : F = 3 : 1	F > M
Age	Young males, late middle age	Young <35 years
Socioeconomic class	I, V	IV, V
Childhood	Parental death	Broken home
Physical health	Chronic or terminal illness, handicapped, pain	Nil specific
Mental illness	Depression ~ 60% Alcoholism ~ 20%	Depression ~ 10%
Pre-morbid personality	Usually good	Antisocial, borderline personality disorder
Precipitants	Guilt, hopelessness	Situational
Setting	Premeditated, alone, warnings	Impulsive, others present

The incidence of completed suicide is reduced during wartime and in certain religious groups (eg Roman Catholics). The incidence is increased in springtime, amongst those working in certain high-risk occupations, such as farmers and doctors, and amongst those who are unemployed, have a family history of suicide and have the means available to carry it out (ie weapons/drugs).

- Non-fatal deliberate self-harm is a strong risk factor for eventual completed suicide.
- Approximately 20% of non-fatal deliberate self-harm cases repeat within one year.
- 1–2% per year of non-fatal deliberate self-harm cases will lead to suicide within one year.
- 10–20% eventually commit suicide.

Prevention of the above involves the identification and treatment of mental illness, increased awareness among GPs and in hospital staff, and the removal of the means to commit suicide (firearms restrictions, limit sales of paracetamol, catalytic converters).

8. ORGANIC PSYCHIATRY

Organic brain disorders can mimic any other functional mental disorder. Features that raise the possibility of an organic disorder include visual perceptual abnormalities (illusions or hallucinations), cognitive deficit clearly preceding other symptoms, neurological signs and fluctuating symptoms.

8.1 Acute organic brain syndrome

This is also known as acute confusional state, or delirium. The young and the elderly are especially vulnerable. A breakdown of the blood–brain barrier is implicated. There are multiple possible aetiologies, both intra- and extra-cranial.

Causes of acute organic brain syndrome

- **Extra-cranial**
  Hypoxia (cardiac, respiratory)
  Infection (respiratory, urinary, septicaemia)
  Metabolic (electrolyte imbalance, uraemia, hepatic encephalopathy, porphyria, hypoglycaemia)
  Hypovitaminosis (thiamine, B_{12})
  Endocrine (hypo/hyperthyroid, hypo/hyperparathyroid, diabetes, Addison's/Cushing's, hypopituitarism)
  Toxic (alcohol intoxication, alcohol withdrawal, all other illicit drugs, prescribed drugs (many), heavy metals)
- **Intra-cranial**
  Trauma (head injury)
  Infection (meningitis, encephalitis)
  Vascular disease (TIA/stroke) hypersensitive encephalopathy, subarachnoid haemorrhage
  Space-occupying lesion (tumour, abscess, subdural haemorrhage)
  Epilepsy

Characteristic clinical features of acute organic brain syndrome

- Clouding of consciousness
- Disorientation
- Poor attention (digit span)
- Memory deficits
- Disturbed behaviour (especially at night)
- Mood abnormalities
- Disordered speech and thinking
- Abnormal perceptions (especially visual misperceptions and hallucinations)
- Abnormal beliefs
- Patients may be severely agitated or withdrawn and stuporose

EEG tests for this condition are sensitive but not specific; results may be abnormal (slowing of rhythm, low voltage trace) in the absence of clear cognitive abnormalities.

Principles of treatment are:

- specific – to treat cause of confusional state
- general – to optimise immediate environment and reduce disorientation
- symptomatic – careful use of sedatives if necessary.

8.2 Dementia

Dementia is the global deterioration of higher mental functioning secondary to progressive neurodegenerative disease. Characteristic clinical features of dementia include episodic memory loss, apraxia, deterioration in self-care skills, temporal and topographical disorientation and personality changes in the presence of clear consciousness (cf acute confusional state). Delusions, hallucinations, agitation and aggression may occur with mild to moderate disease severity.

Aetiology

- Alzheimer's disease ~ 50%
- Lewy body dementia ~ 20%
- Vascular dementia (multi-infarct dementia) ~ 20%.

For differentiation of dementia from depression, *see* Section 2.4

Features of Alzheimer's disease and multi-infarct dementia

Clinical feature	Alzheimer's	Multi-infarct dementia
Age of onset	70–90 years	60–80 years
Sex	F > M	M > F
Family history	FAD* less than 1%	–
Aetiology	Genetic + environmental	Embolic
Onset	Insidious	Acute
Presenting symptoms	Cognitive	Emotional
Cognitive impairment	Diffuse	Patchy
Insight	Early loss	Preserved
Personality	Early loss	Preserved
Course of progression	Relentless	Stepwise
Focal neurological signs	Unusual	Common
Previous CVA** or TIA***	–	+++
Hypertension	–	+++
Associated ischaemic heart disease	–	+++
Seizures	+	+++
Most common cause of death	Infection	Ischaemic heart disease
Time to death from diagnosis	2–5 years	4–5 years

*FAD = familial Alzheimer's disease; **CVA = cerebrovascular accident; ***TIA = transient ischaemic attack.

8.3 Physical illnesses particularly associated with mental disorders

Physical illnesses particularly associated with mental disorders

- **Neurological**
  Parkinson's disease (depression, dementia)
  Huntington's disease (personality change, depression, suicide, dementia)
  Neurosyphilis (dementia, depression, grandiosity)
  Epilepsy (depression, psychosis)
  Multiple sclerosis (depression, elation, dementia)
  Wilson's disease (affective disorder, aggression, cognitive impairment)
  Prion diseases (depression, personality changes, dementia)
  Brain tumour (location determines early symptoms)
  Myasthenia gravis (depression)
  Motor neurone disease (depression, dementia)

- **Endocrine**
  Cushing's syndrome: psychiatric disturbance in about 50% of hospital cases, depression, euphoria, confusion, paranoid psychoses, cognitive dysfunction in 66%
  Addison's disease: psychiatric features in virtually 100%, depression, withdrawal, apathy, memory difficulties in up to 75%
  Hyperthyroidism: psychological disturbance in 100%, restlessness, agitation, confusional state (rare), psychosis (very rare)
  Hypothyroidism: mental symptoms universal at presentation, lethargy, cognitive slowing, apathy > depression, irritability, confusional state, dementia, affective or schizophreniform psychosis (very rare)
  Phaeochromocytoma: paroxysmal anxiety

- **Other systemic causes**
  Systemic lupus erythematosus (SLE) (acute confusional state, affective or schizophreniform psychosis) may be further complicated by the effect of steroids
  Vitamin deficiency (B_1: Wernicke–Korsakoff syndrome; B_{12}: acute confusional state, depression)
  Porphyria (especially AIP): acute confusional state, depression, paranoid psychosis
  Paraneoplastic syndrome: depression, psychosis

8.4 Drug-induced mental disorders

Many drugs can lead to psychiatric conditions.

Mental disorders induced by drugs

Anxiety	**Depression**	**Psychotic symptoms**
Amphetamines	Reserpine	Amphetamines
Cocaine	Beta-blockers	LSD
Alcohol	Calcium antagonists	Cocaine
Phencyclidine	Oral contraceptive pill	Marijuana
	Corticosteroids	L-Dopa
	Alcohol	Anti-cholinergic drugs
	Frusemide	Anabolic steroids

9. ALCOHOL ABUSE

The complications of alcohol are wide-ranging and cross social, psychological and neuropsychiatric domains. General medical problems are not covered here.

9.1 Social consequences of alcohol abuse

- Family/marital problems
- Incest
- Absenteeism from work
- Accidents (major factor in ≥ 10% of road traffic accidents)
- Crime (associated with acute abuse)
- Vagrancy.

9.2 Acute withdrawal

Acute withdrawal causes a wide spectrum of symptoms. The fully developed syndrome is known as delirium tremens.

Delirium tremens

- **Definition of full syndrome**
  Vivid hallucinations (often visual)
  Delusions
  Profound confusional state
  Tremor
  Agitation
  Sleeplessness
  Autonomic overactivity (including pyrexia)
- **Other clinical features**
  Associated trauma or infection in 50%
  Prodromal features may occur
  Onset usually after 72 hours of abstinence
  Visual illusions/hallucinations prominent
  Duration ≤3 days in majority
  Hypokalaemia common ± hypomagnesaemia
  Mortality up to 5%

Treatment of alcohol withdrawal

- In-patient
- Rehydration, antibiotics, parenteral high-potency B-complex vitamins, sedation
- Sedative drugs which facilitate GABA-ergic neurotransmission are cross-tolerant with alcohol and have anticonvulsant properties (eg a reducing dose of chlordiazepoxide, chlormethiazole oral/iv (only when patient in hospital)). Phenothiazine should be avoided because of the risk of seizure. If an antipsychotic drug is required, then haloperidol should be used.

9.3 Psychological consequences of alcohol abuse

These include dysphoric mood, pathological jealousy (Othello syndrome) and sexual problems (impotence, decreased libido). Other symptoms are alcoholic hallucinosis and alcohol dependence syndrome.

Alcohol dependence syndrome – seven key features

- Sense of compulsion to drink
- Stereotyped pattern of drinking
- Prominent drink-seeking behaviour
- Increased tolerance to alcohol
- Repeated withdrawal symptoms
- Relief drinking to avoid withdrawal symptoms
- Reinstatement after abstinence

Suicide is more common amongst this group (16% with full dependence syndrome) as is para-suicide (used acutely by 35%).

9.4 Neuropsychiatric consequences of alcohol abuse

The most likely neuropsychiatric consequences of alcohol abuse are Wernicke's encephalopathy and Korsakoff's syndrome/psychosis. This group is also more likely to suffer seizures, head injury and dementia.

Rarer conditions associated with alcohol abuse include cerebellar degeneration, central pontine myelinosis and Marchiafava–Bignami disease (demyelination of the corpus callosum, optic tracts and cerebral peduncles).

Wernicke's encephalopathy (WE)

A disorder of acute onset featuring:

- nystagmus
- abducens and conjugate gaze palsies (96%)
- ataxia of gait (87%)
- global confusional state (90%)
- hypothermia and hypotension.

Note: the 'classic triad' (ocular signs, ataxia and confusional state) of symptoms is not always present.

It is caused by thiamine deficiency, most commonly secondary to alcoholism, but more rarely due to:

- carcinoma of the stomach
- toxaemia
- pregnancy
- persistent vomiting
- dietary deficiency.

Pathology

- **Macroscopic**: petechial haemorrhages
- **Microscopic**: dilatation and proliferation of capillaries, small haemorrhages, pale staining parenchyma, reactive change in astrocytes and microglia, neurones relatively spared.

Structures affected

- Mamillary bodies
- Walls of IIIrd ventricle
- Floor of IVth ventricle
- Periaqueductal grey matter
- Certain thalamic nuclei – med dorsal, anteromedial, pulvinar
- Brainstem
- Cerebellum anterior lobe/vermis
- Cortical lesions rarely seen.

Treatment

Parenteral thiamine. Up to 80% of sufferers go on to develop Korsakoff's syndrome.

Korsakoff's syndrome

A marked memory disorder with good preservation of other cognitive functions.

Clinical features

- Chronic disorder usually following Wernicke's encephalopathy
- Inability to consolidate new information
- Retrograde amnesia of days/years
- Patchy preservation of long-term memory
- Confabulation not complaints of poor memory
- Apathy
- Lack of insight.

Pathology

As for Wernicke's encephalopathy.

Treatment

Thiamine. There may be a response in only 20% of sufferers.

10. SLEEP DISORDERS

10.1 Normal sleep

In normal sleep, drowsiness first gives way to increasingly deep non-REM (rapid eye movement) sleep. The first REM period occurs after 50–90 minutes and lasts for 5–10 minutes. The cycle repeats at approximately 90-minute intervals so that there are four to six REM periods each night. In total, REM occupies 20–25% of a night's sleep.

REM sleep	Non-REM sleep
Asynchronous, mixed frequency EEG	EEG synchronous, with sleep spindles, K-complexes, generalised slowing with delta waves
Bursts of rapid conjugate eye movements	Four stages recognised; stages 3 and 4 characterised as 'slow wave' sleep
Prominent autonomic changes – increased heart rate, blood pressure – penile tumescence	
Decreased muscle tone	
Extensor plantar responses may occur	

Figure 2 Pictorial representation of the adult sleep cycle. Shaded areas indicate REM sleep.

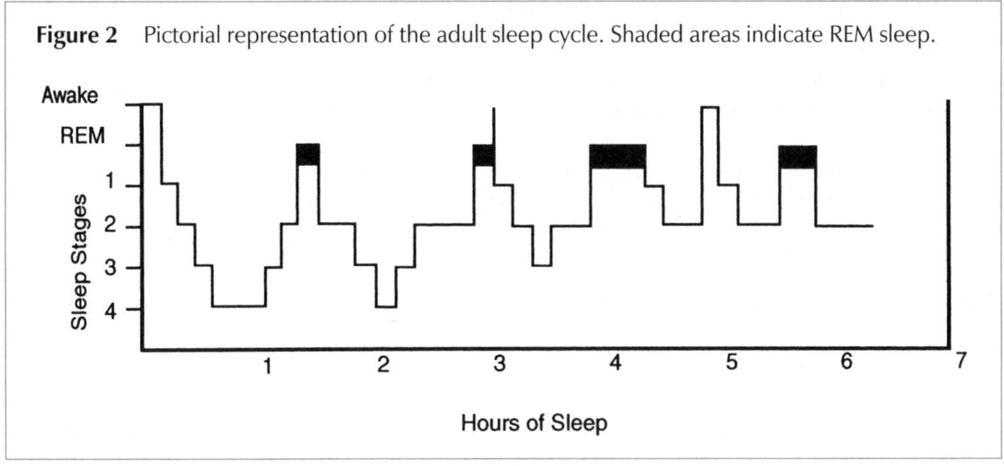

10.2 Insomnia

Insomnia is seen in a wide range of psychiatric and medical disorders. Psychiatric disorders may account for up to 36% of patients with insomnia. Paradoxically sleep deprivation may be used to treat depression and may precipitate mania.

The following box describes the pattern of insomnia in various disorders.

Mental disorders and sleep disturbance

Disorder	**Pattern of insomnia**
Major depression	Initial and late insomnia (early morning waking)
Mania	in up to 80%
Generalised anxiety disorder	Globally reduced sleep
Post-traumatic stress disorder	
Initial and middle insomnia	
Intrusive nightmares about trauma	
Acute confusional state	Disturbed sleep cycle

10.3 Narcolepsy

Narcolepsy is a condition that is often undiagnosed. Typically onset is between the ages of 10 and 20, and the increased risk in a first-degree relative is × 40. **Cataplexy** is a sudden loss of muscle tone leading to collapse; it occurs in response to an emotional stimulus (eg laughing, crying).

- Hypersomnolence 100%
- Cataplexy 90%
- HLA-DR2 positive 99%

- Major affective disorder or personality problems 50%
- Sleep paralysis 40%
- Hypnagogic hallucinations (auditory hallucinations while dropping off to sleep) 30%

In narcolepsy, REM sleep occurs at the **onset** of nocturnal sleep. Daytime attacks also consist of periods of REM sleep occurring out of context.

11. TREATMENTS IN PSYCHIATRY

11.1 Antipsychotics

Antipsychotics are indicated in schizophrenia, mania, other paranoid psychoses and psychotic depression. 'Atypical' antipsychotics have preferable side-effect profiles and are now used as first-line treatment in schizophrenia.

Antipsychotics are most effective against the 'positive' symptoms of schizophrenia. They have an immediate sedative action but the antipsychotic action may be delayed for three weeks. They play an important role in preventing relapse.

Clozapine is effective in treatment-resistant schizophrenia and severe tardive dyskinesia. However, there is increasing evidence that the atypical antipsychotics clozapine, olanzapine and, to a lesser extent, risperidone are linked to hyperglycaemia, impaired glucose tolerance and occasionally to fatal diabetic ketoacidosis.

Side-effects of antipsychotic drugs

Class	Example	Side-effects
Atypical antipsychotics (highly selective blockade of mesolimbic D_2 receptors and serotonin ($5HT_{2A}$) receptors)	Sulpiride/amisulpride	Hyperprolactinaemia
	Olanzapine Risperidone Clozapine	Weight gain Nausea, dyspepsia Blood dyscrasias: neutropenia (3%), agranulocytosis (1%); myocarditis and cardiomyopathy

Continues ...

... Continued

Typical antipsychotics (D_2 receptor antagonists of the mesolimbic, tuberoinfundibular and nigrostriatal systems)		All of the following side-effects can be seen with each of the three classes of typical antipsychotic drugs
Phenothiazines	Chlorpromazine, thioridazine	**Extrapyramidal** – acute dystonia, Parkinsonism, akathisia, tardive dyskinesia
Butyrophenones	Haloperidol, droperidol	
Thioxanthenes	Flupentixol, zuclopenthixol	**Anticholinergic** – dry mouth, constipation, etc **Antiadrenergic** – postural hypotension **Antihistaminergic** – sedation **Endocrine** – hyperprolactinaemia, photosensitivity (especially phenothiazines) **Other** – Lowered seizure threshold Neuroleptic malignant syndrome Prolonged QT_C interval

11.2 Antidepressants

Antidepressants are indicated in depressive illness, anxiety disorders (especially panic disorder and phobic disorders) and obsessional illness.

In depressive illness, antidepressants have a response rate of around 65%, with a delay in action of between 10 days and 6 weeks. The presence of 'biological' symptoms can help in the prediction of response. Antidepressants also play a prophylactic role in recurrent depressive disorders.

Drugs which inhibit 5HT reuptake are particularly useful in obsessional illness. Most antidepressants are associated with hyponatraemia, which is mediated via syndrome of inappropriate ADH (SIADH); elderly females are particularly vulnerable to developing this. Abrupt cessation of paroxetine causes a discontinuation syndrome with flu-like symptoms, dizziness and insomnia.

Class	Example	Side-effects
SSRI*	Citalopram Fluoxetine Fluvoxamine Paroxetine Sertraline	Nausea, sexual dysfunction, headache, sleep disturbance (early), increased anxiety (early)
Tricyclic	Amitriptyline Imipramine Clomipramine	**Anticholinergic** – dry mouth, constipation, etc **Antiadrenergic** – postural hypotension **Antihistaminergic** – sedation Weight gain Lower seizure threshold Cardiac arrhythmias
SNRI**	Venlafaxine	Nausea Hypertension
MAOI	Phenelzine	Anticholinergic Antiadrenergic Hypertensive reaction with tyramine-containing foods Important drug interactions
RIMA***	Moclobemide	Potential tyramine interaction
Presynaptic α_2-antagonist	Mirtazapine	Agranulocytosis

*SSRI = selective serotonin re-uptake inhibitor.
**SNRI = Selective noradrenaline re-uptake inhibitor.
***RIMA = Reversible inhibitor of monoamine oxidase A.

The side-effects and toxicity of lithium are described in detail in Chapter 2, Clinical Pharmacology, Toxicology and Poisoning.

11.3 Benzodiazepines

Benzodiazepines are only indicated for the short-term relief of severe, disabling anxiety. The *British National Formulary* recommends only 2–4 weeks of use. They are not indicated for 'mild' anxiety but can be used as adjunctive treatment for anxiety, agitation and behavioural disturbance in acute psychosis or mania. They are only indicated for insomnia if the condition is severe, disabling or subjecting the patient to extreme distress.

Longer half-life	Diazepam equivalent (mg)*	Half-life (hours)	Shorter half-life	Diazepam equivalent (mg)	Half-life (hours)
Diazepam	5	20–90	Lorazepam	0.5	8–24
Chlordiazepoxide	15	20–90**	Oxazepam	15	6–28
Nitrazepam	5	16–40	Temazepam	10	6–10
Chlorazepate	–	50–100	Alprazolam	–	6–16
Flurazepam	–	50–100			

*Approximate equivalent doses to diazepam 5 mg.
**Includes active metabolites.

Benzodiazepine withdrawal syndrome may not develop for up to three weeks, but can occur within a few hours for short-acting drugs. Symptoms include insomnia, perspiration, anxiety, tinnitus, decreased appetite, decreased weight, perceptual disturbances and tremor.

The recommended withdrawal regime involves transferring the patient to an equivalent dose of diazepam, preferably taken at night. Ideally the dose should be decreased by approximately 1/8 of the daily dose every two weeks. If withdrawal symptoms occur, the dose is maintained until symptoms improve.

11.4 Electroconvulsive therapy (ECT)

ECT is indicated in severe or treatment-resistant depression or where there are psychotic symptoms, life-threatening lack of food and fluid intake, or for stupor and elderly (especially agitated) patients. 'Biological' features help predict the likely response. It is also indicated to treat catatonia associated with schizophrenia and in treatment-resistant cases of mania.

Side-effects of ECT

- **Early**
  Headache
  Temporary confusion
  Impaired short-term memory (bilateral ECT worse than unilateral)
  (Rare) fractures, dislocation, fat embolism
- **Late (6–9 months)**
  No memory impairment detected
  Subjective impairment

Contraindications to ECT

Raised intra-cranial pressure (the only absolute contraindication), cardiac arrest less than 2 years previously, other cardiac disease, pulmonary disease, history of CVA.

ECT has a mortality rate of 3–5 deaths per 100, 000 (cf minor surgery + general anaesthesia). The mortality rate of untreated major depression is 10%.

11.5 The psychotherapies

Type	Frequency	No. of sessions	Indications
Counselling	Weekly-monthly	6–12	Mild depression Anxiety Bereavement
Cognitive behavioural	Weekly	8–12	Depression Anxiety Somatoform disorder Eating disorders
Behavioural	Weekly	6–12	Phobias Anxiety Obsessional illness Sexual dysfunction Dementia
Psychoanalytic	1–5/week	50–indefinite	Neurosis Personality disorders Psychosexual
Group	Weekly	6–12	Anxiety Substance misuse Eating disorders

Chapter 19
Respiratory Medicine

CONTENTS

5. Tumours
- 5.1 Lung cancer
- 5.2 Mesothelioma
- 5.3 Mediastinal tumours

6. Granulomatous and diffuse parenchymal lung disease
- 6.1 Sarcoidosis
- 6.2 Histiocytosis X
- 6.3 Pulmonary fibrosis
- 6.4 Idiopathic pulmonary fibrosis ('usual interstitial pneumonia' – UIP)

7. Pulmonary vasculitis and eosinophilia
- 7.1 Wegener's granulomatosis
- 7.2 Churg–Strauss syndrome
- 7.3 Polyarteritis and Henoch–Schönlein vasculitis
- 7.4 Connective tissue disorders
- 7.5 Pulmonary eosinophilia

8. Miscellaneous respiratory disorders
- 8.1 Pleural effusion
- 8.2 Pneumothorax
- 8.3 Obstructive sleep apnoea/hypopnoea syndrome (OSAHS)
- 8.4 Adult respiratory distress syndrome (ARDS)
- 8.5 Rare lung disorders

Spirometry

- FEV_1 refers to the volume of gas expired in the first second of a forced expiration
- FVC refers to the total volume of gas expired on forced expiration
- The normal ratio of FEV_1/FVC is 70–80%
- A reduction in FEV_1 with a preserved FVC occurs in airways obstruction (eg asthma or COPD). In patients with severe COPD a **slow** vital capacity is a more accurate measurement as it allows time for the lungs to empty fully and hence a true FEV_1/FVC ratio can be determined
- Restriction refers to a reduction in FVC with a preserved FEV_1/FVC ratio and occurs in conditions such as pulmonary fibrosis, neuromuscular disorders, obesity and pleural disease.

Flow volume loops

A flow volume loop is produced by plotting flow on the *y* axis against volume on the *x* axis.

Figure 1 Typical flow volume loop

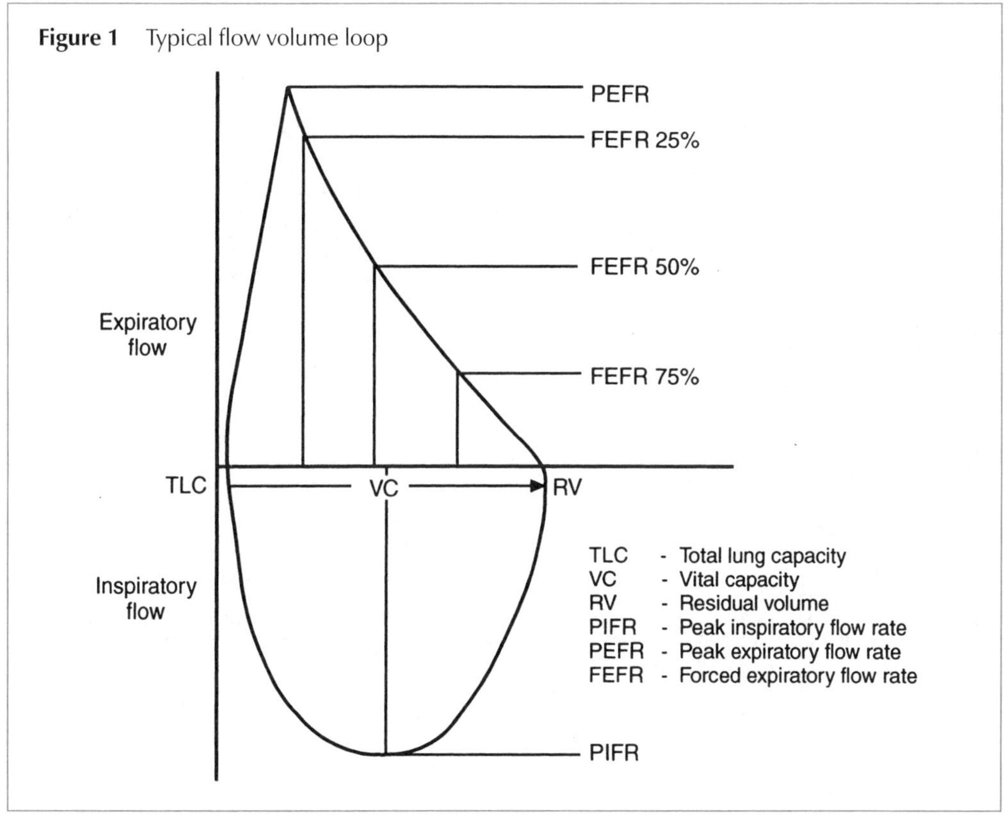

If a subject inspires rapidly from residual volume (RV) to total lung capacity (TLC) and then exhales as hard as possible back to residual volume, a record can be made of the maximum flow volume loop. This loop shows that expiratory flow rises very rapidly to a maximum value, but then declines over the rest of expiration. During the early part of a forced expiration the maximum effort-dependent flow rate is achieved within 0.1 s, but the rise in transmural pressure leads to the airways being compressed and therefore to the flow rate being reduced. The flow rate is then said to be effort-independent.

A great deal can be learned by comparing the form of the loop to that which is normally seen ('triangle sitting on a semi-circle'). Several patterns can be recognised, reflecting various disorders.

Figure 2 Flow volume loops in different disorders

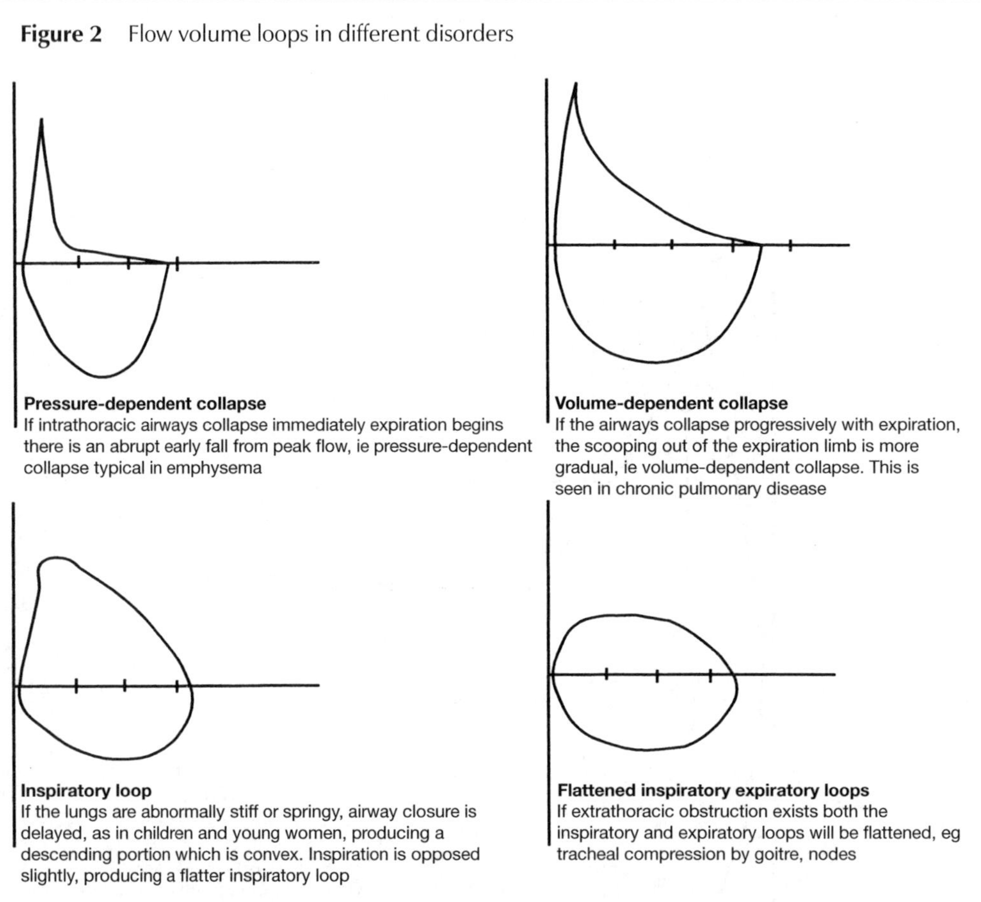

Pressure-dependent collapse
If intrathoracic airways collapse immediately expiration begins there is an abrupt early fall from peak flow, ie pressure-dependent collapse typical in emphysema
Volume-dependent collapse
If the airways collapse progressively with expiration, the scooping out of the expiration limb is more gradual, ie volume-dependent collapse. This is seen in chronic pulmonary disease
Inspiratory loop
If the lungs are abnormally stiff or springy, airway closure is delayed, as in children and young women, producing a descending portion which is convex. Inspiration is opposed slightly, producing a flatter inspiratory loop
Flattened inspiratory expiratory loops
If extrathoracic obstruction exists both the inspiratory and expiratory loops will be flattened, eg tracheal compression by goitre, nodes

Lung volumes

- Tidal volume, inspiratory and expiratory reserve volumes and vital capacity can all be measured by use of a spirometer.
- Total lung capacity, residual volume and functional residual capacity can be measured using a helium dilution method, nitrogen washout or body box.

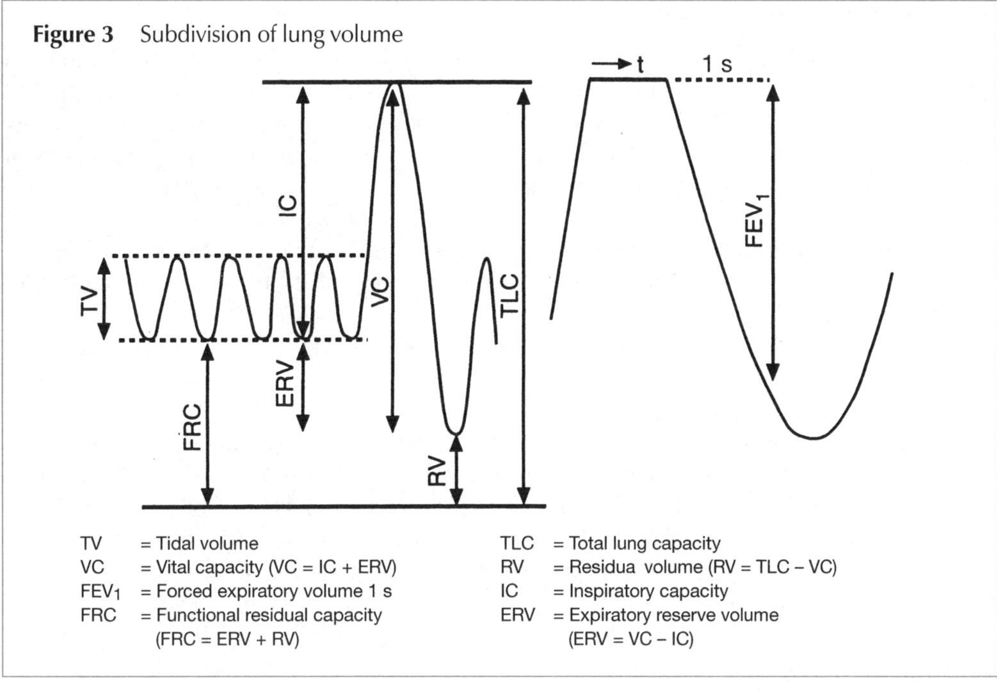

Figure 3 Subdivision of lung volume

1.5 Gas transfer

Transfer of carbon monoxide is solely limited by diffusion and is used to measure gas transfer. Either a single breath hold or a steady-state method can be used. Results are expressed both as total gas transfer (DLCO) or gas transfer corrected for lung volume (KCO, ie KCO = DLCO/VA where VA is alveolar volume).

Causes of hypoxaemia

- **Hypoventilation**
  Opiate overdose
  Paralysis of respiratory muscles
- ***V*/*Q* mismatch**
  Pulmonary embolus
- **Low inspired partial pressure of oxygen**
  High altitude
  Breathing a hypoxic mixture
- **Diffusion impairment**
  Pulmonary oedema
  Fibrosing alveolitis
  Bronchiolar-alveolar cell carcinoma
- **Shunt***
  Pulmonary A-V malformations
  Cardiac right to left shunts

* Hypoxaemia caused by shunt cannot be abolished by administering 100% oxygen

Oxygen and carbon dioxide transport

Oxygen is transported in the blood by combination with the haemoglobin (Hb) in the red cells. A tiny amount is dissolved (0.3 ml/100 ml blood, assuming pO_2 of 100 mmHg). The oxyhaemoglobin dissociation curve is sigmoid in shape. Once oxygen saturation falls below 90% the amount of oxygen carried to the tissues falls rapidly. The *p*50 (the partial pressure at which haemoglobin is 50% saturated) is 26 mmHg.

- The curve is **shifted to the right** by high temperature, acidosis, increased pCO_2 and increased levels of 2,3-diphosphoglycerate (2,3-DPG); this encourages offloading of oxygen to the tissues.
- The curve is **shifted to the left** by changes opposite to those above, and by carboxy-haemoglobin and fetal haemoglobin.

Carbon dioxide is transported in the blood as bicarbonate, in combination with proteins as carbamino compounds, and it is also dissolved in plasma. Carbon dioxide is 20 times more soluble than oxygen and about 10% of all CO_2 is dissolved. CO_2 diffuses into red blood cells where carbonic anhydrase facilitates the formation of carbonic acid which dissociates into bicarbonate and hydrogen ions. Bicarbonate diffuses out of the cell and chloride moves in to maintain electrical neutrality.

Acid–base control

The normal pH of arterial blood is 7.35–7.45. Blood pH is closely regulated and variation outside this pH range results in compensation either by the lung or the kidney to return pH to normal. Failure to excrete CO_2 normally results in a respiratory acidosis; this is usually due to hypoventilation. Hyperventilation causes lowering of the pCO_2 and alkalosis.

pH can also be altered by metabolic disturbance. Metabolic acidosis and alkalosis are considered in Chapter 13, Metabolic Diseases. Mixed respiratory and metabolic acid–base disturbances are common.

Arterial blood gases

Normal values are:

- pH 7.37–7.43
- pO_2 >10.6 kPa (77 mmHg) whilst breathing room air
- pCO_2 4.7–6.0 kPa (35–45 mmHg)
- HCO_3 (bicarbonate) 22–28mmol/l.

When recording blood gases the percentage of inspired oxygen should always be stated. The value in kilopascal (kPa) should be multiplied by 7.6 to convert to mmHg.

1.6 Adaptation to high altitude

The barometric pressure decreases with altitude; at 18, 000 feet it is half the normal 760 mmHg. Hyperventilation, due to hypoxic stimulation of peripheral chemoreceptors, is an early response to altitude. The respiratory alkalosis produced is corrected by renal excretion of bicarbonate.

- Hypoxaemia stimulates the release of erythropoietin from the kidney, and the resultant polycythaemia allows increased carriage of oxygen by arterial blood.
- There is an increased production of 2,3-DPG, which shifts the oxygen dissociation curve to the right, allowing better offloading of oxygen to the tissues.
- Hypoxic vasoconstriction increases pulmonary artery pressure causing right ventricular hypertrophy. Pulmonary hypertension is sometimes associated with pulmonary oedema – altitude sickness.

2. DISEASES OF LARGE AIRWAYS

2.1 Asthma

Asthma is a chronic inflammatory disorder of the airways. In susceptible individuals this inflammation causes symptoms which are associated with widespread but variable airflow obstruction that is reversible either spontaneously or with treatment. There is an increase in airway sensitivity to a variety of stimuli.

The prevalence of asthma has been increasing in recent years, principally among children. Approximately 5.1 million people suffer from asthma in the UK – 1.4 million of these are children. Around 1500 asthma deaths occur annually in the UK.

The development of asthma is almost certainly due to a combination of genetic predisposition and environmental factors. Atopy is strongly associated with asthma. The most important allergens are the house dust mite (*Dermatophagoides pteronyssinus*), dog allergen (found in pelt, dander and saliva), cat allergen (predominantly in sebaceous glands), pollen, grasses and moulds.

Factors provoking asthma attacks

- Exposure to sensitising agents
- Infection
- Drugs, including aspirin, non-steroidal anti-inflammatory agents, beta-blockers
- Exercise
- Gastro-oesophageal reflux
- Cigarette smoke, fumes, sprays, perfumes, etc
- Failure to comply with medication

In patients with asthma the airways are narrowed by a combination of contraction of bronchiolar smooth muscle, mucosal oedema and mucus plugging. In the early stages changes are reversible; however, in chronic asthma structural changes (including thickening of the basement membrane, goblet cell hyperplasia and hypertrophy of smooth muscle) develop and ultimately lead to irreversible fibrosis of the airways. Asthma is regarded as a complex inflammatory condition and mast cells, eosinophils, macrophages, T-lymphocytes and neutrophils are all involved in the pathogenesis. A variety of inflammatory mediators are released including histamine, leukotrienes, prostaglandins, bradykinin and platelet activating factor (PAF).

Chronic asthma

The hallmark of chronic asthma is variable and reversible airflow obstruction. This causes:

- shortness of breath
- chest tightness
- wheeze
- cough.

At times the cough may be productive of sputum which may be clear, or yellow/green, due to the presence of eosinophils. The normal diurnal variation in airway calibre is accentuated in asthmatics and symptoms may be worse at night.

Physical signs of asthma

- Tachypnoea
- Hyperinflation of the chest
- Nasal polyps (particularly in aspirin-sensitive asthmatics)
- Wheezing, most marked in expiration
- Atopic eczema

Diagnosis of asthma

The diagnosis of asthma is clinical and is often confirmed by diary recordings of the peak expiratory flow rate (PEFR). The pattern of lung function tests may be very helpful (see opposite). Challenge tests with histamine or methacholine, or with exercise, can be used to assess airways' responsiveness where the diagnosis is unclear. Responsiveness is expressed as the concentration of provoking agent required to decrease the FEV_1 by 20%.

Typical lung function tests in asthma

- Significant (>25%) diurnal peak expiratory flow rate (PEFR) variability on at least 3 days per week for a minimum of 2 weeks
- Significant improvement in PEFR (>15%) and FEV_1 (at least 400 ml) post bronchodilator or trial of oral or inhaled steroids
- Increased lung volumes
- Reduced FEV_1
- FEV_1/FVC ratio <70%
- Gas trapping

Other clinical features which are helpful in making a diagnosis of asthma are:

- a history of asthma in childhood or of eczema or hay fever
- a family history of asthma
- symptoms of perennial rhinitis, nasal polyps or chronic sinusitis
- history of wheezing associated with aspirin, NSAIDS or β-blockers.

Skin prick tests

Skin prick tests can be used to assess atopy. Many asthmatic subjects make IgE in response to common allergens. A tiny quantity of allergen is introduced into the superficial layers of the dermis and tests are read at 20 min. The diameter of the weal is measured in millimetres, the size of the weal correlating well with bronchial challenge testing. Serum total IgE is commonly raised in asthmatics. Specific IgE may be measured by radio-allergo-sorbent testing (RAST).

Treatment

The mainstay of treatment is inhaled corticosteroid with short-acting β-agonists to relieve symptoms. Treatment is altered in a stepwise fashion as recommended in the BTS/SIGN National Guidelines. The dose of inhaled steroid should initially be low to moderate and subsequently reduced once adequate control has been achieved.

- Long-acting β-agonists (eg salmeterol or eformoterol) should be added in patients who are inadequately controlled on beclomethasone diproprionate (200 mg/day) or an equivalent steroid inhaler.
- Oral theophylline preparations or β_2 agonist tablets are of benefit in some patients.
- Leukotriene receptor antagonists (*see also* Chapter 2, Clinical Pharmacology, Toxicology and Poisoning) may be particularly useful for exercise-induced asthma, and in patients with aspirin sensitivity.
- Long-term oral corticosteroids are reserved for patients with very severe asthma.
- Allergen avoidance may be helpful in reducing the severity of existing disease in patients exposed and sensitised.

All inhalers are now required to be CFC-free.

Acute severe asthma

Asthma symptoms may worsen acutely necessitating prompt treatment to relieve the attack. An immediate assessment is essential, looking for signs of severity which include the following:

- Speech impairment
- Tachycardia (pulse >110 beats/min)
- Respiratory rate >25 breaths/min
- PEFR 33–50% of predicted

Life-threatening asthma is associated with any one of the following:

- hypoxaemia
- PEFR <33% of predicted
- exhaustion
- bradycardia (pulse < 60 beats /min)
- hypotension
- a silent chest
- a normal or raised pCO_2.

Arterial blood gases should be performed if the patient is hypoxic on air (saturations <92%) and a chest X-ray is necessary to exclude pneumothorax.

Management consists of high-flow oxygen therapy, nebulised bronchodilators (β-agonists ipratropium), steroids and, if infection is considered likely, antibiotics. PEFR should be measured regularly to assess the response to treatment.

- If there is no improvement with nebulisers, then intravenous infusions of either salbutamol or aminophylline should be used.
- A single dose of intravenous magnesium can be given to patients who have not had a good response to bronchodilators, or to those with life-threatening asthma.
- If the patient is severely ill, or not improving with treatment, **they should be promptly transferred to an Intensive Care Unit**.

Allergic bronchopulmonary aspergillosis

Most patients with allergic bronchopulmonary aspergillosis are asthmatics but the condition may occur in non-asthmatics. This condition is considered in detail in Section 3.6.

2.2 Chronic obstructive pulmonary disease (COPD)

COPD is defined as a chronic, slowly progressive disease characterised by airflow obstruction that does not markedly change over several months. Most of the lung function impairment is fixed although some reversibility can be produced by bronchodilator therapy. Long-term prognosis is determined by post-bronchodilator FEV_1.

COPD accounts for 6–7% of all UK deaths at present. However the incidence of COPD is increasing and it is likely to become the third commonest cause of death worldwide (it is currently fourth) by 2020.

The diagnosis is made by:

- history of cough with sputum production, wheeze and shortness of breath
- history of frequent winter bronchitis and delayed recovery from viral infections
- reduced FEV_1/FVC ratio.

Causes of COPD

- Smoking (usually a history of at least 20 pack-years)
- Dust exposure
- Alpha-1 antitrypsin deficiency
- Air pollution
- Low birth weight and low socioeconomic status

COPD is due to a combination of chronic bronchitis and emphysema.

Chronic bronchitis is defined as chronic cough and sputum production for at least three months of two consecutive years in the absence of other diseases recognised to cause sputum production.

Emphysema is characterised by abnormal, permanent enlargement of the air spaces distal to the terminal bronchioles, accompanied by destruction of their walls without obvious fibrosis. Emphysema may be centriacinar (predominantly affecting the upper lobes and associated with smoking), panacinar, paraseptal or predominantly localised around scars (scar emphysema).

Signs of COPD

- Hyperinflation
- Weight loss
- Flapping tremor
- Pursed-lip breathing
- Wheeze
- Central cyanosis
- Cor pulmonale: raised JVP, right ventricular heave, loud P2, tricuspid regurgitation, peripheral oedema, hepatomegaly

Investigations

- **PFTs**: FEV_1 <80% predicted, FEV_1/FVC <70%; patients have large lung volumes and reduced gas transfer factor (DLCO) in emphysema. COPD may be graded by the FEV_1:

  Mild COPD: FEV_1 50–80% of predicted
  Moderate COPD: FEV_1 30–50% of predicted
  Severe COPD: FEV_1 < 30% of predicted.

- **Chest X-ray**: may be normal or show evidence of hyperinflation, bullae or prominent vasculature due to pulmonary hypertension.
- **Arterial blood gases**: may indicate type 1 or type 2 respiratory failure.
- **FBC**: possible polycythaemia.
- **ECG**: may show p pulmonale, right axis deviation, right bundle branch block.
- **Sputum culture**: *Haemophilus influenzae, Streptococcus pneumoniae* or less commonly *Staphylococcus, Moraxella catarrhalis* or Gram-negative organisms.

Treatment of COPD

Several recent clinical trials have shown no impact of inhaled steroids on disease progression in COPD. Pulmonary rehabilitation is increasingly recognised as an important part of disease management.

Treatments available for COPD

- Smoking cessation
- Inhaled anticholinergic drugs
- Inhaled short- or long-acting β_2 agonists
- Inhaled or systemic steroids
- Long-term oxygen therapy (LTOT)
- Lung volume reduction surgery (for patients with severe emphysema) or bullectomy
- Theophyllines
- Diuretics
- Pulmonary rehabilitation
- Transplantation

Treatment of acute exacerbations

Antibiotics are indicated for acute exacerbations if two of the following are present:

- increased breathlessness
- increased sputum volume
- increased sputum purulence.

Regular bronchodilator (nebulised or inhaled) are given in addition to short courses of oral steroids and controlled oxygen therapy.

- Patients should be treated along conventional lines for an hour and arterial blood gases then repeated.
- If significant acidosis (pH <7.35) with hypercapnia persists, then non-invasive positive pressure ventilation (NIPPV) should be instituted via a face mask.

2.3 Alpha-1 antitrypsin deficiency

Many different phenotypes of alpha-1 antitrypsin are known, the common ones being designated M, S and ZZ. MM confers 100% protease inhibitor activity while the most severe deficiency is produced by ZZ. Panlobular emphysema develops, which is most marked in the basal areas of the lungs. Emphysema is thought to result from an imbalance in the lung between neutrophil elastase (which destroys elastin) and the elastase inhibitor, alpha-1 antitrypsin (which protects against the proteolytic degradation by elastin). The decline in lung function is accelerated in smokers.

- PFTs show airflow obstruction, large lung volumes and reduced KCO
- cirrhosis of the liver is more common, particularly in those of ZZ phenotype
- smoking cessation is imperative
- replacement therapy with alpha-1 antitrypsin is not routinely given
- lung transplantation may be an option for some patients
- genetic counselling should be offered and siblings of index cases should be genetically tested.

2.4 Long-term oxygen therapy (LTOT)

Two trials have established the benefit of LTOT. In the MRC trial, oxygen via nasal cannulae was given to raise the pO_2 to 8 kPa (60 mmHg) for at least 15 hours per day compared to patients with COPD receiving conventional therapy. After 3 years of treatment, survival was 50% better in the group receiving oxygen.

The NOTT trial compared 12 and 24 hours of continuous oxygen therapy and was terminated prematurely due to better survival in the group receiving 24-hour therapy. Patients are eligible for LTOT if they **exhibit all of the following**:

- pO_2 on air <7.3 kPa (55 mmHg)
- normal or elevated pCO_2
- FEV_1, <1.5 litres
- pO_2 7.3–8 kPa (55–60 mmHg) with evidence of pulmonary hypertension, polycythaemia peripheral oedema or nocturnal hypoxaemia.

Arterial blood gases must be measured when the patient is clinically stable, and on two occasions which are at least 3 weeks apart. pO_2 on oxygen should be >8 kPa (60 mmHg) without an unacceptable rise in pCO_2. Oxygen should be given via a concentrator for at least 15 hours per day. The patient must have stopped smoking before LTOT is considered.

2.5 Respiratory failure

Respiratory failure is an inability to maintain adequate oxygenation and carbon dioxide excretion. There are two recognised types of respiratory failure.

- **Type 1** respiratory failure is present when there is hypoxaemia with normal or low levels of carbon dioxide.
- **Type 2** respiratory failure is hypoxaemia with high pCO_2.

Causes of respiratory failure

- **Reduced ventilatory drive**
  Opiate overdosage, brainstem injury
- **Mechanical problems**
  Chest trauma causing flail chest
  Severe kyphoscoliosis
  Obesity
- **Neurological conditions (affecting chest wall muscles)**
  Guillain–Barré syndrome
  Polio
- **Alveolar problems**
  Barriers to diffusion
  Pulmonary oedema
  Pulmonary fibrosis
  V/Q mismatch
  Pulmonary embolus
  Shunt (cardiac or pulmonary)
  Reduced inspired partial pressure of oxygen
  High altitude
- **Upper airway obstruction**
  Laryngeal tumour
  Obstructive sleep apnoea
- **Lower airway obstruction**
  Bronchospasm
  Sputum retention

- **Type 1 respiratory failure** may be corrected by increasing the inspired oxygen concentration.
- **Type 2 respiratory failure** may require mechanical ventilatory support. Respiratory stimulants such as doxapram may be useful for those with reduced respiratory drive.

2.6 Ventilatory support

This may be invasive or non-invasive.

Non-invasive positive pressure ventilation (NIPPV)

This involves the use of a securely fitting nasal or full face mask. The technique has been used to provide long-term respiratory support in the community for patients with respiratory failure due to conditions such as severe chest wall deformity or old polio.

- It is used increasingly to manage episodes of acute respiratory failure due, for example, to exacerbations of COPD – as an alternative to (and often more appropriate than) ventilation on the Intensive Care Unit (ICU).
- NIPPV can be carried out on general wards using portable bi-level pressure support ventilators. Regular monitoring of blood gases is necessary and the ventilator settings are altered in response. As the patient improves, time spent off the ventilator is lengthened until the patient is weaned.
- When NIPPV treatment is instituted, a decision as to whether ICU referral would be appropriate if the patient were to deteriorate should be clearly stated in the case notes.

Positive pressure ventilation

Conventional ventilation requires access to the airway, by means of either an endotracheal tube or tracheostomy. Indications for positive pressure ventilation include the following.

- Type 2 respiratory failure from any cause
- Paralysis of respiratory muscles (eg Guillain–Barré syndrome)
- Multiple organ failure
- Trauma cases, including injury to the chest or cervical spine
- Inability to maintain a clear airway
- Reduced conscious level – Glasgow coma scale <5
- During and after certain surgical procedures

Ventilation should be considered when there is failure to maintain oxygenation (pO_2 <8 kPa (60 mmHg)) despite high inspired oxygen concentrations (usually associated with hypercapnia and acidosis). It is often necessary in patients with multiple organ dysfunction associated with sepsis or trauma.

Continuous positive airways pressure (CPAP)

CPAP is delivered through a tightly fitting face mask or it may be used in conjunction with conventional ventilation. It provides a pneumatic splint to the airway and is the treatment of choice for obstructive sleep apnoea. CPAP improves oxygenation in patients requiring high concentrations of oxygen by the recruitment of collapsed airways. It may, however, cause hypotension, the rise in mean intrathoracic pressure inhibiting venous return and reducing cardiac output.

3. LUNG INFECTIONS

HIV/AIDS-associated respiratory disease is covered in Chapter 8, Genito-urinary Medicine and AIDS.

3.1 Pneumonia

Pneumonia is an acute inflammatory condition of the lung usually caused by bacteria, viruses or, rarely, fungi. The chest X-ray will show consolidation, the hallmark of which is an air bronchogram.

Community-acquired pneumonia

The incidence is 5–11/1000 adult population per year, and this is much more common in the elderly. Causal organisms are given overleaf.

Causes of pneumonia

- *Streptococcus pneumoniae* (60–70%)
- Atypical organisms, including *Mycoplasma pneumoniae* (5–15%), *Legionella pneumophila*, *Chlamydia psittaci*, *Chlamydia pneumoniae* and *Coxiella burnetii* (Q fever)
- *Haemophilus influenzae*
- *Staphylococcus aureus*
- Gram-negative organisms
- Viruses, including influenza, varicella-zoster, CMV

General investigations for patients admitted to hospital with pneumonia

These include FBC, biochemical profile (including liver function test), CRP, arterial blood gases, chest X-ray and blood and sputum cultures.

- Paired serological tests for atypical organisms and viruses should be used in selected cases.

Signs of severe pneumonia (CURB–65 criteria)

- ***C***onfusion (<8/10 score on abbreviated mental test (AMT))
- ***U***rea >7 mmol/l
- ***R***espiratory rate >30 breaths/minute
- ***B***P systolic <90 mmHg and/or diastolic <60 mmHg
- Age >65.

Patients with three or more CURB criteria are at high risk of death and are regarded as having **severe community-acquired pneumonia**.

- Hypoxaemia (pO_2 <8 kPa despite oxygen therapy) and multilobe involvement also confer a worse prognosis.
- The presence of coexisting disease is a bad prognostic factor.

Specific pneumonias

Streptococcus pneumoniae

There is an abrupt onset of illness, with high fever and rigors. Examination reveals crackles or bronchial breathing, and herpetic cold sores may be present in >1/3 cases.

- Elderly patients may present with general deterioration or confusion.
- Capsular polysaccharide antigen may be detected in serum, sputum, pleural fluid or urine.
- Increasing incidence of penicillin resistance, particularly in countries such as Spain.
- Vaccine available.

Mycoplasma pneumoniae

Mycoplasma pneumoniae tends to affect young adults; it occurs in epidemics every 3–4 years. There is typically a longer prodrome, usually of 2 or more weeks, and the white cell count may be normal. Cold agglutinins occur in 50%; the mortality is low.

- Extrapulmonary complications include: peri/myocarditis, erythema multiforme, erythema nodosum, Stevens–Johnson syndrome, haemolytic anaemia, DIC, thrombocytopenia, meningo-encephalitis, cranial and peripheral neuropathies, bullous myringitis, hepatitis and pancreatitis.

Legionella pneumophila

Outbreaks are usually related to contaminated water cooling systems, showers, or air conditioning systems, but sporadic cases do occur. Legionnaire's disease usually affects the middle-aged and elderly, patients often having underlying lung disease. Males are affected more than females (3:1). Diagnosis is by direct fluorescent antibody staining or serological tests; antigen may be detected in the urine.

Clinical and laboratory features

- Gastrointestinal upset common; diarrhoea, jaundice, ileus and pancreatitis may occur
- WCC often not elevated with lymphopenia; thrombocytopenia/pancytopenia may occur
- Hyponatraemia due to SIADH
- Headache, confusion and delirium are prominent and focal neurological signs may develop
- Abnormal liver and renal function in approximately 50%
- Acute renal failure, interstitial nephritis and glomerulonephritis may develop

Staphylococcus aureus

Staphylococcus aureus pneumonia may follow a viral illness; it has a high mortality (30–70%). The disease is more common in intravenous drug addicts.

Specific features include:

- toxin production with extensive tissue necrosis
- staphylococcal skin lesions may develop
- chest X-ray shows patchy infiltrates with abscess formation in 25% and empyema in 10%
- >25% of patients have positive blood cultures.

Treatment of pneumonia

All patients should be given appropriate concentrations of oxygen and they may require intravenous fluids if circulating volume is depleted. Treatment is with oral amoxicillin and erythromycin for non-severe cases requiring hospitalisation and with a third-generation cephalosporin and clarithromycin intravenously in severe cases.

- A single antibiotic can be used for community patients or those admitted to hospital for non-medical reason.
- Newer fluoroquinolones (eg moxifloxacin) provide an alternative for patients who are allergic to penicillin or macrolides.

- Intravenous treatment should be stepped down to oral treatment after 48 hours provided the patient is improving.
- If a specific organism is isolated the appropriate antibiotic is given.

Treatment should continue for 7–10 days depending upon response. Up to 21 days of treatment is recommended for *Legionella* pneumonia.

Nosocomial (hospital-acquired) pneumonia

This is defined as pneumonia that develops 2 or more days after admission to hospital (0.5–5% of hospitalised patients). The organisms usually involved include:

- *Staphylococcus aureus*
- Gram-negative bacteria: *Klebsiella, Pseudomonas, E. coli, Proteus* spp., *Serratia* spp., *Acinetobacter* spp.
- anaerobes
- fungi
- *Streptococcus pneumoniae* (and other streptococci) are less common.

Treatment is with broad-spectrum agents (eg third-generation cephalosporins).

Aspiration pneumonia

Aspiration pneumonia may complicate impaired consciousness and dysphagia. Particulate matter may obstruct the airway, but also chemical pneumonitis may develop from aspiration of acid gastric contents, leading to pulmonary oedema.

- Anaerobes are the principal pathogens, arising from the oropharynx.
- There are typically two to three separate isolates in each case.
- Multiple pulmonary abscesses or empyema may result.
- Treat with metronidazole in combination with broad-spectrum agent (eg third-generation cephalosporin).

Cavitation may develop in certain lung infections.

Cavitations associated with lung infections

- *Staphylococcus aureus*
- *Klebsiella pneumoniae*
- *Legionella pneumophila* (rare)
- Anaerobic infections
- *Pseudomonas aeruginosa*
- *Mycobacterium tuberculosis* and atypical mycobacterial infections

Lung abscess

This may be suspected when the patient is slow to improve from a pneumonia. A chest X-ray will show single or multiple fluid-filled cavities. Prolonged courses of antibiotics are needed, sometimes with percutaneous drainage.

3.2 Empyema

A collection of pus in the pleural space may complicate up to 15% of community-acquired pneumonias and is more common when there is a history of excess alcohol consumption, poor dentition, aspiration or general anaesthesia.

- A diagnosis of empyema is suspected if a patient is slow to improve, has a persistent fever or elevation of the white cell count or CRP, and has radiological evidence of a pleural fluid collection. The pH of pleural fluid is <7.2.
- Untreated, extensive fibrosis occurs in the pleural cavity, weight loss and clubbing develop and the mortality rate is high.
- The mainstay of treatment is drainage of the pleural space combined with continuous high-dose intravenous antibiotic treatment. Daily intra-pleural administration of streptokinase has been shown to liquefy the pus and facilitate percutaneous drainage with improved resolution rates.
- For those who fail to resolve with medical therapy, thoracotomy and decortication of the lung may be necessary.

3.3 Tuberculosis

The number of new cases of tuberculosis (TB) declined in the UK throughout the 20th century mainly due to the improvement in living standards. In recent years, however, the incidence of TB has begun to increase again. Those at risk include:

- those on low incomes
- homeless people
- alcoholics
- HIV-positive individuals
- immigrants from countries with a high incidence of TB.

The most commonly involved site is the lung – with lymph node, bone, renal tract and GI tract being less common. Tuberculous meningitis is the most serious complication.

Primary TB

Primary infection occurs in those without immunity. A small lung lesion known as the Ghon focus develops in the mid or lower zones of the lung and is composed of tubercle-laden macrophages. Bacilli are transported through the lymphatics to the draining lymph nodes which enlarge considerably and caseate. Infection is often arrested at this stage and the bacteria may remain dormant for many years. The peripheral lung lesion and the nodes heal and may calcify. The entire process is often asymptomatic; however, specific immunity begins to develop and tuberculin skin tests become positive.

Post-primary TB

Organisms disseminated by the blood at the time of primary infection may reactivate many years later. The most common site for post-primary TB is the lungs, with bone and lymph node sites being less common. Reactivation may be precipitated by a waning of host immunity, for example due to malignancy or immunosuppressive drugs including steroids.

Clinical picture

Primary infection is often asymptomatic, but may cause mild cough and wheeze or erythema nodosum. Clinical features of reactivation or re-infection are described in the following box.

Features of TB reactivation or re-infection

- Persistent cough
- Night sweats
- Pleural effusion
- Meningitis
- Weight loss
- Haemoptysis
- Pneumonia
- Lymphadenopathy

Miliary TB

This is caused by widespread dissemination of infection via the bloodstream. It may present with non-specific symptoms of malaise, pyrexia and weight loss. Eventually hepatosplenomegaly develops and choroidal tubercles may be visible on fundoscopy. The chest X-ray shows multiple rounded shadows a few millimetres in diameter. It is universally fatal if left untreated.

Diagnosis of TB

- **Chest X-ray**
  May show patchy shadowing in the upper zones with volume loss and cavitation, and ultimately fibrosis
- **Pleural fluid aspiration and biopsy**
- **Bronchoscopy and lavage**
  Used for those unable to expectorate; transbronchial biopsy if miliary disease is a possibility
- **Early morning urine specimens**
  For renal tract disease
- **Liver biopsy**
- **Lymph node biopsy**
- **Bone marrow aspirate**
- **Morning sputum collections**
  For acid–alcohol fast bacilli smear
- **CSF culture**

Specimens are examined for AAFB using Ziehl–Neelsen or auramine stains and then cultured on Löwenstein–Jensen medium. Cultures are continued for at least 6 weeks as the organism is slow growing. PCR for tuberculous DNA can be used to provide a rapid diagnosis.

Treatment

(*See also* Section 3.2 in Chapter 11 Infectious Diseases.) This is with a combination of four drugs:

- rifampicin
- isoniazid
- pyrazinamide
- ethambutol.

Short courses of treatment for 6 months are now standard. All drugs are given for 2 months and isoniazid and rifampicin are continued for a further 4 months.

- Sensitivity testing will identify drug resistance and all four drugs are continued until sensitivities are known.
- If pyrazinamide has to be discontinued due to side-effects, a 9-month regime is necessary.
- Second-line agents (eg ethionamide, propionamide, streptomycin, cycloserine) may be needed.
- Compliance can pose major problems and directly observed therapy (DOT – larger doses of drugs administered three times per week) is used when poor compliance is anticipated.

Multi-drug resistant TB (MDR-TB) signifies resistance to rifampicin and isoniazid and currently accounts for 2% of tuberculous infections. It is mainly concentrated in the London area.

Side-effects of antituberculous treatment

Side-effects are common:

- **hepatitis**: may be caused by rifampicin, isoniazid and pyrazinamide
- **optic neuritis**: may be caused by ethambutol **visual acuity** should be checked before treatment is initiated
- **peripheral neuropathy**: may be due to isoniazid; 10 mg of pyridoxine daily is given in those at particular risk of this complication (eg alcoholics, diabetics and in patients with renal failure).

Prevention

BCG vaccination is given to most children aged 13 years provided that a Heaf test shows grade 0–1 reactivity. BCG provides approximately 70% protection against TB and prevents disseminated disease developing. In infants at particular risk, vaccination is given at birth. **Chemoprophylaxis** (isoniazid for 6 months or rifampicin and isoniazid for 3 months) is given to those with evidence of recent infection (Heaf conversion) but no clinical or radiological disease. Patients with pulmonary TB (particularly those who are sputum smear positive for AAFB) are potentially infectious and close contacts should be screened for disease. Once 2 weeks of antituberculous chemotherapy has been completed, the patient is considered to be non-infectious.

TB is a notifiable disease.

Opportunistic mycobacterial infections

These account for 10% of all mycobacterial infections. Causative organisms include the following:

- *Mycobacterium kansasii*
- *Mycobacterium xenopi*
- *Mycobacterium malmoense*
- *Mycobacterium avium intracellulare*.

These organisms cause disease which is clinically and radiologically identical to TB. Pulmonary disease, lymphadenitis (in children) and disseminated infection are the commonest clinical problems. The organisms are ubiquitous in the environment and are low-grade pathogens. Opportunistic mycobacterial infections constitute a relatively higher proportion of mycobacterial infections in AIDS patients.

- The onset of symptoms is usually gradual.
- Treatment programmes are generally longer than for TB, and are often continued for 18 months to 2 years.
- Rifampicin and ethambutol are the mainstay of treatment, but for those not responding, streptomycin, clarithromycin or ciprofloxacin may be added.
- Opportunistic infections do not need to be notified.
- Contact tracing is unnecessary as person to person infection is very rare.

3.4 Bronchiectasis

This is the permanent dilatation of sub-segmental airways which are inflamed, tortuous, flabby and partially/totally obstructed by secretions. Bronchiectasis may be cystic, cylindrical or varicose. The obstruction often leads to post-obstructive pneumonitis so that the lung parenchyma may be temporarily or permanently damaged.

Causes of bronchiectasis

- Congenital
- Post-infective (eg following episodes of childhood measles, pneumonia or pertussis)
- Immune deficiency
- Post-tuberculosis
- Allergic bronchopulmonary aspergillosis (ABPA) – proximal
- Complicating sarcoidosis or pulmonary fibrosis
- Idiopathic – 60%
- Distal to an obstructed bronchus (or a bronchus severely compressed from encroaching lymph nodes)
- Secondary to bronchial damage resulting from a chemical pneumonitis (eg inhalation of caustic chemicals)
- Mucociliary clearance defects: primary ciliary dyskinesis or associated with situs inversus (Kartagener's syndrome) or associated with azoospermia and sinusitis in males (Young's syndrome)

Clinical features

There is a history of chronic sputum production which is often mucopurulent and accompanied by episodes of haemoptysis. Occasionally bronchiectasis can be 'dry' with no sputum production but episodic haemoptysis. Exertional dyspnoea and wheeze may be associated. Patients complain of malaise and fatigue; one-third have symptoms of chronic sinusitis. There may be few abnormal clinical findings other than occasional basal crackles or wheeze on chest examination; clubbing may be present.

Investigations

- **Sputum microbiology**: most commonly shows *Haemophilus influenzae, Streptococcus pneumoniae* or *Pseudomonas aeruginosa*; mycobacteria and fungi may also be seen.
- **Chest X-ray**: may be normal or may show thickening of bronchial walls and in *cystic* bronchiectasis, ring shadows ± fluid levels. The upper lobes are most frequently affected in ABPA, cystic fibrosis, sarcoidosis and tuberculosis.
- **Pulmonary function tests**: may be normal or show an obstructed/restricted pattern (or both).
- **High-resolution CT scanning**: is diagnostic in >90% of cases.
- **Immunoglobulin levels (or antibody response following vaccination, eg *H. influenzae*** or pneumococcus): may demonstrate deficiency of humoral immunity.

Conditions associated with bronchiectasis

- Rheumatoid arthritis
- Sjögren's syndrome
- Yellow nail syndrome and primary lymphoedema
- Infertility
- Malignancy (childhood acute lymphoblastic leukaemia, adult chronic lymphocytic leukaemia)
- Inflammatory bowel disease (usually ulcerative colitis)

Treatment

As far as possible the aetiology of the bronchiectasis should be established in every case. If there is an underlying immune deficiency state, treatment with intravenous gamma globulin replacement therapy is beneficial. Regular physiotherapy with postural drainage and using 'the active cycle of breathing' helps to clear the airways.

- Inhaled bronchodilators are often used.
- **Antibiotics** are usually given in response to an exacerbation, but some patients require continuous oral therapy, which usually consists of three antibiotics in monthly rotation.
- Nebulised antibiotics can be used to reduce the microbial load and they are particularly useful when a patient is colonised with pseudomonas.
- Adequate hydration is important but mucolytics are generally not helpful.
- Surgery is reserved for those with localised severe disease; lung transplantation has been successful.

Complications

Infective exacerbations are the principal problem. Haemoptysis usually settles with treatment of the infection but occasionally embolisation of the bleeding vessel is required. Chest pain over an area of bronchiectatic lung is not uncommon. In the long term, systemic amyloid may result.

3.5 Cystic fibrosis

Cystic fibrosis is the most common fatal autosomal recessive condition in the Caucasian population, affecting 1 in 2500 live births; 1 in 25 adults are carriers of the gene. The cystic fibrosis gene has been localised to the long arm of chromosome 7 and codes for the cystic fibrosis transmembrane conductance regulator protein (CFTR), which functions as a chloride channel (*see also* Chapter 7, Genetics). Over 800 mutations have been identified, the most common being Δ508. The basic defect involves abnormal transport of chloride across the cell membrane; in the sweat gland there is a failure to reabsorb chloride and in the airway there is failure of chloride secretion. Diagnosis is made by detection of an abnormally high sweat chloride (>60 mEq/l) and by genetic analysis.

Pulmonary disease

A significant inflammatory infiltrate may be identified in the lungs at a very early age. The airways become obstructed by thick mucus due to decreased chloride secretion and increased sodium reabsorption, and so bacterial infection becomes established in early life.

Infection occurs in an age-related fashion: infants and young children become colonised with *Staphylococcus aureus* and subsequently *Haemophilus influenzae*. In the teenage years infection with *Pseudomonas aeruginosa* occurs.

The other major pathogens involved are:

- *Streptococcus pneumoniae*
- *Burkholderia cepacia* complex

- *Mycobacterium tuberculosis*
- atypical mycobacteria
- *Aspergillus fumigatus*
- viruses.

Chronic infection and inflammation causes lung damage with bronchiectasis affecting predominantly the upper lobes. Patients have breathlessness and reduced exercise tolerance, cough with chronic purulent sputum production, and occasional haemoptysis. Physical signs include clubbing, cyanosis, scattered coarse crackles and occasional wheeze. Slight haemoptysis is often associated with infection but major haemoptysis may occasionally necessitate pulmonary arterial embolisation.

- Pulmonary function tests show airflow obstruction; chest X-ray may show hyperinflation, atelectasis, visible thickened bronchial walls, fibrosis and apical bullae; pneumothorax occurs in up to 10% of patients.
- In the terminal stages of disease, respiratory failure develops; 90% of deaths are attributable to respiratory failure. The average life expectancy has increased into the fourth decade of life.

Gastrointestinal tract

Pancreatic insufficiency is present in over 90% of patients. Malabsorption causes bulky offensive stools, with weight loss and deficiency of fat-soluble vitamins (A, D, E and K). Babies may present with meconium ileus and adults may develop an equivalent syndrome with obstruction of the small bowel due to poorly digested intestinal contents causing abdominal pain, distension, vomiting and severe constipation.

- Obstruction of the biliary ductules in the liver may eventually lead to cirrhosis with portal hypertension, splenomegaly and oesophageal varices.
- Gallstones (in 15% of patients), peptic ulcer and reflux oesophagitis are all more prevalent.
- Pancreatitis may develop in older patients.

Involvement of other systems

- **Diabetes**: eventually occurs in up to 1/3 of patients. There is a gradual loss of pancreatic islet cells with fibrosis developing. Ketoacidosis is very uncommon.
- **Upper airway disease**: nasal polyps occur frequently (up to 1/3 of patients); chronic purulent sinusitis may develop.
- **Fertility**: virtually all males are infertile due to abnormal development of the vas deferens and seminiferous tubules, but fertility in women is only slightly reduced. Although many women with cystic fibrosis have had successful pregnancies, pregnancy may lead to life-threatening respiratory complications.
- **Osteoporosis** is more common with an increased risk of fractures.

Treatment of cystic fibrosis

Care for patients with cystic fibrosis is best given in a specialist unit which can provide extensive multidisciplinary input.

Antibiotics and respiratory treatments

In the UK most centres give antibiotics when sputum becomes increasingly purulent, pulmonary function tests are deteriorating or the patient is generally unwell with weight loss. Most patients become chronically colonised with *Pseudomonas aeruginosa* and so two different antibiotics (eg ceftazidime and tobramycin) are used in combination to prevent resistance developing.

- Up to 25% of patients become colonised with *Burkholderia cepacia*, an organism which is highly transmissible from one individual to another and associated with a worse prognosis. These patients are therefore segregated from patients colonised with *Pseudomonas*, in hospital, at outpatient clinics and also socially.
- Most patients need continuous anti-staphylococcal treatment.

Nebulised antibiotics reduce the microbial load and are useful in those who need frequent courses of intravenous antibiotics; colistin or tobramycin are used continuously in a twice daily regimen.

- DNase helps to liquefy viscous sputum and is helpful in some patients. Bronchodilators and inhaled steroid are given to treat airflow obstruction. Physiotherapy, using the active cycle of breathing technique, should be tailored to individual needs.

Pancreatic enzyme supplements

Given with main meals and snacks to those with pancreatic insufficiency. Meconium ileus equivalent is treated with vigorous rehydration and regular oral gastrografin. Good nutritional status is associated with improved prognosis; supplementary overnight feeding with nasogastric tube or via gastroenterostomy can help to maintain body weight.

Transplantation

Either double-lung or heart-lung transplantation may be appropriate for some patients with terminal respiratory failure. Non-invasive positive pressure ventilation may be utilised to support a patient before transplantation. The timing of lung transplantation is difficult and must be assessed in each individual case. Liver and pancreas transplants are also frequently carried out.

Future developments in cystic fibrosis

Screening of newborns for cystic fibrosis will soon be practised throughout the UK. Extensive research is being carried out into gene therapy, although this is still a long way from having a clinical application.

3.6 Aspergillus and the lung

Aspergillus causes three distinct forms of pulmonary disease:

Allergic bronchopulmonary aspergillosis

Most patients with allergic bronchopulmonary aspergillosis are asthmatics but the condition may occur in non-asthmatics.

The disease is due to sensitivity to *Aspergillus fumigatus* spores mediated by specific IgE and IgG antibodies. The allergic response results in airways becoming obstructed by rubbery mucus plugs containing Aspergillus hyphae, mucus and eosinophils; plugs may be expectorated. The following changes may be found on investigation:

- lobar or segmental collapse of airways occurs
- fleeting chest X-ray shadows due to intermittent obstruction of airways
- positive skin-prick tests and RAST to *Aspergillus*
- positive precipitins to *Aspergillus fumigatus*
- raised serum IgE > 1000 ng/ml
- peripheral blood and pulmonary eosinophilia
- the condition may result in proximal bronchiectasis.

Treatment is with oral corticosteroids which may be required long-term; itraconazole is also useful and may allow the dose of steroid to be reduced.

Colonising aspergillosis

Fungal colonisation of cavities in the lung parenchyma, of dilated bronchi or the pleural space.

A mass or ball of fungus develops known as an aspergilloma. *A. fumigatus* is usually responsible, but occasionally *A. niger, A. flavus* or *A. nidulans* may be implicated. Cavities due to TB, sarcoidosis, cystic fibrosis or pulmonary neoplasms may be colonised. Cough and sputum production often occur and are features of the underlying disease. Haemoptysis is a common complication, and this may be massive.

- An aspergilloma is usually suspected by chest X-ray which demonstrates a cystic space containing a rounded opacity. An air space is visible between the fungal mass and the cavity wall – the 'halo' sign.
- Precipitating antibodies are nearly always present but response to skin testing is variable.
- Sputum examination may reveal fungal hyphae.

Many aspergillomas require no specific treatment. Treatment is indicated for recurrent haemoptysis, systemic symptoms and where there is evidence of fungal invasion of surrounding tissue. Intra-cavity instillation of amphotericin paste is sometimes useful, and systemic treatment with the newer azoles (eg voriconazle) may be helpful in some cases. Surgical resection of the affected area of lung may be curative.

Invasive aspergillosis

Fungal infection spreads rapidly through the lung causing granulomas, necrosis of tissue and suppuration. It occurs most commonly in the immunosuppressed host and may be rapidly fatal. Progressive chest X-ray shadowing (which may cavitate), associated with fever, chest pain and haemoptysis which does not settle promptly with antibacterial agents, suggests invasive aspergillosis.

- Cough with copious sputum production, often with haemoptysis, is usual.
- Examination of sputum or bronchio-alveolar lavage fluid may demonstrate fungal hyphae. High-resolution CT scanning shows pulmonary infiltrates with the 'halo' sign. Treatment is with systemic antifungal agents

4. OCCUPATIONAL LUNG DISEASE

4.1 Asbestos-related disease

Exposure to asbestos was previously commonplace in many occupations including ship building, laggers, building, dockers and factories engaged in the manufacture of asbestos products.

Effects of asbestos on the lung

Pleural plaques

These appear 20 or more years after low-density exposure. They develop on the parietal pleura of the chest wall, diaphragm, pericardium and mediastinum, and commonly calcify. Pleural plaques are usually asymptomatic but they may cause mild restriction.

Diffuse pleural thickening

This can extend continuously over a variable proportion of the thoracic cavity, but is most marked at the lung bases. It causes exertional dyspnoea; PFTs show restriction, decreased compliance, reduced total lung capacity, but the KCO is normal.

Pleural effusions may occur in asbestos-related disease, usually within 15 years of exposure. They often resolve spontaneously, leaving thickening of the visceral pleura.

Asbestosis

The onset of asbestosis is usually >20 years after exposure (but with higher levels of exposure fibrosis occurs earlier). Fibrotic changes are more pronounced in the lower lobes; patients present with slowly worsening exertional dyspnoea and clinical examination reveals fine inspiratory crackles in the lower zones. Clubbing may occur.

- Chest X-ray shows small irregular opacities, horizontal lines and, in more advanced disease, honeycomb and ring shadows.
- High-resolution CT (HRCT) confirms fibrosis associated with pleural disease.
- PFTs show a restrictive defect with reduced KCO.

- There is an increased risk of lung cancer (see below).
- The disease is untreatable and death is usually due to respiratory failure or malignancy.

Lung cancer

Asbestosis is associated with a substantially increased risk of lung cancer (see later section), and the predisposition is synergistic with smoking. The risk of mesothelioma is also markedly increased.

Compensation claims for occupational lung disease

Patients with all of the above asbestos-related diseases (except pleural plaques) are entitled to state compensation and a disability pension. Patients can also claim against their employers for negligently exposing them to asbestos for any of the above asbestos-related conditions (including pleural plaques). They should be advised to begin legal action within 3 years of being told that they have an asbestos-related condition.

- The same applies for patients with coal workers' **pneumoconiosis** and **occupational asthma** and a small number of other industrial diseases.

4.2 Coal workers' pneumoconiosis (CWP)

The incidence of this pneumoconiosis is related to total dust exposure. Dust particles 2–5 μm in diameter are retained in the respiratory bronchioles and alveoli. Simple CWP is characterised by small rounded opacities (<1.5 mm in diameter) on chest X-ray, and is associated with focal emphysema. The lesions are asymptomatic.

Progressive massive fibrosis (PMF)

Progressive massive fibrosis involves the development of larger opacities (>3 cm in diameter) on a background of simple CWP.

- PMF lesions are usually in the upper zones and may cavitate.
- Cough, sputum production and dyspnoea occur with reduced life expectancy, deaths occurring from progressive respiratory failure.
- PFTs show a mixed obstructive/restrictive pattern with reduced KCO.

Coal mining is recognised as a cause of **COPD**.

Caplan's syndrome is the development of multiple round pulmonary nodules in patients with rheumatoid arthritis and a background of coal workers' pneumoconiosis. Nodules may develop before the joint disease, and occur in crops in the periphery of the lung. They may be associated with pleural effusion and may ultimately calcify.

4.3 Silicosis

This is caused by inhaling silicon dioxide, a highly fibrogenic dust; those commonly affected are quarry workers, hard rock miners and civil engineers, amongst the groups exposed. Silicosis was commonly associated with TB in the first half of the 20th century.

- An acute illness characterised by dry cough and breathlessness occurs within a few months of exposure to very high levels of dust.
- With more chronic exposure silicotic nodules form, which are 3–5 mm in diameter and predominantly affect the upper lobes.
- Eggshell calcification occurs around enlarged hilar glands.
- Gradually worsening breathlessness is associated with restrictive lung physiology and a fall in gas transfer.
- There is no effective treatment (other than lung transplantation in patients with respiratory failure), but the disease is compensatible.

4.4 Berylliosis

The inhalation of fumes from molten beryllium causes an acute alveolitis. However, most cases of berylliosis are due to chronic low level exposure, causing a tissue reaction similar to sarcoidosis. Non-caseating granulomata form in the lungs and lymph nodes surrounded by fibrous tissue; the chest X-ray shows fine nodulation evenly distributed throughout the lung fields with bilateral hilar lymphadenopathy.

- A positive blood and BAL beryllium lymphocyte proliferation assay is strongly associated with the presence of chronic beryllium disease.
- Interstitial fibrosis develops with shrinking of the lungs.
- Patients develop progressive breathlessness with death ultimately occurring due to respiratory and right heart failure.

4.5 Byssinosis

This is caused by exposure to cotton dust, flax and hemp. Acute exposure causes airways narrowing in 1/3 of affected individuals. However, chronic byssinosis develops after years of heavy exposure to cotton dust; symptoms are worse on the first day back after a break from work, and include chest tightness, cough, dyspnoea and wheeze.

- There is a progressive decline in FEV_1 during the working shift, most marked on the first day of the week.
- Prevention is by reducing the levels of cotton dust to which employees are exposed.
- Bronchodilators may provide some relief of symptoms.

4.6 Occupational asthma

Occupational asthma is now the commonest industrial lung disease in developed countries. A large number of agents encountered at work cause asthma and are officially recognised for industrial compensation. These include the following.

Causes of occupational asthma

- Isocyanates
- Platinum salts
- Stainless steel welding
- Epoxy resins
- Azodicarbonamide (PVC, plastics)
- Glutaraldehyde
- Wood dust
- Laboratory animals and insects
- Dyes
- Acid anhydride and amine hardening agents
- Resin used in soldering flux
- Proteolytic enzymes
- Pharmaceuticals
- Many other chemicals
- Any known sensitising agent in the workplace
- Flour/grains

Occupational asthma develops after a period of asymptomatic exposure to the allergen, but usually within two years of first exposure. Detection depends on a careful history, and PEFR monitoring both at work and at home. Once occupational asthma has developed, bronchospasm may be precipitated by other non-specific triggers such as cold air, exercise, etc. Occupational asthma may develop in workers with previously diagnosed asthma. In order to identify the substance involved specific IgE levels may be measured or occasionally bronchial provocation testing may be performed. Early diagnosis and removal of the individual from exposure to the allergen is essential if they are to make a full recovery. Asthma symptoms may persist despite termination of exposure.

4.7 Reactive airways dysfunction syndrome (RADS)

This reactive airways dysfunction syndrome refers to bronchial hyper-responsiveness following the inhalation of high concentrations of irritant gas, aerosols or particles. Asthma-like symptoms usually develop within minutes to hours after exposure and airways hyper-reactivity persists over a prolonged period of time. 'Irritant asthma' occurs following multiple exposures to lower concentrations of irritants.

4.8 Extrinsic allergic alveolitis (hypersensitivity pneumonitis)

This is a hypersensitivity pneumonitis caused by a specific immunological response (usually IgG-mediated) to inhaled organic dusts.

- **Farmers' lung** is due to the inhalation of thermophilic actinomycetes (usually *Micropolyspora faeni* and *Thermoactinomyces vulgaris*), when workers are exposed to mouldy hay.

- **Bird fanciers' lung** is caused by inhaled avian serum proteins, present in excreta, and in the bloom from feathers; it primarily affects those who keep racing pigeons and those keeping budgerigars as pets.
- **Ventilation pneumonitis** occurs in inhabitants of air-conditioned buildings where thermophilic actinomycetes grow in the humidification system.
- **Bagassosis** is due to exposure to *Thermoactinomyces sacchari* in sugar cane processors.
- **Malt workers' lung** is due to the inhalation of *Aspergillus clavatus*.
- **Mushroom workers' lung** is due to the inhalation of *Thermophilic actinomycetes*.

Clinical features of extrinsic allergic alveolitis

The clinical features depend on the pattern of exposure. An acute allergic alveolitis develops several hours after exposure to high concentrations of dust. Breathlessness and 'flu-like' symptoms occur, sometimes associated with fever, headaches and muscle pains. The symptoms are short-lived and usually resolve completely within 48 hours.

- Inspiratory crackles may be heard on chest auscultation.
- The disease may present in a sub-acute or chronic form characterised by cough, breathlessness, fatigue and weight loss.
- Clubbing may occur in association with irreversible pulmonary fibrosis.

Investigation and treatment

The diagnosis of extrinsic allergic alveolitis is made by establishing a history of exposure to antigen and the demonstration of precipitating antibodies in the patient's serum.

- **Chest X-ray** may show a generalised haze sometimes associated with nodular shadows. In chronic cases, progressive upper zone fibrosis and loss of lung volume occurs.
- **Spirometry** becomes restrictive and gas transfer is reduced.
- **Histology** of lung biopsy tissue shows a mononuclear cell infiltrate with the formation of non-caseating granulomas.
- Fluid obtained from **BAL** has a high lymphocyte count.
- **Precipitins**: the demonstration of specific IgG antibodies in serum against the identified antigen. Precipitins may be present in the absence of clinical disease.

Once the diagnosis is established the patient should be isolated from the antigen; if this is impossible respiratory protection should be worn. Corticosteroids accelerate the rate of recovery from an acute attack but are generally not helpful once established fibrosis develops.

Pulmonary fibrosis in extrinsic allergic alveolitis

Multiple episodes of acute exposure to agents causing extrinsic allergic alveolitis (EAA), or long-term low-grade exposure, as occurs in budgerigar owners, can lead to irreversible lung fibrosis. These chronic cases present with progressive dyspnoea, weight loss and fatigue. The chest X-ray will show lung shrinkage but calcification or cavitation does not develop. High resolution CT (HRCT) demonstrates reticular, nodular and ground glass opacities. Prompt diagnosis of EAA is important as the disease is reversible when diagnosed early.

5. TUMOURS

5.1 Lung cancer

Lung cancer is the most prevalent cancer worldwide and accounts for 1:3 cancer deaths in men and 1:6.5 cancer deaths in women. Female mortality from lung cancer now exceeds that from breast cancer. Twenty per cent of smokers will develop lung cancer. The prognosis is poor, with a mean survival of less than 6 months. The five-year survival rate is 10–13%.

Causes of lung cancer

- **Smoking**
  Over 90% of lung cancers occur in current or ex-smokers
- **Atmospheric pollution**
  Persistently higher lung cancer rates in urban populations; passive smoking
- **Industrial exposures**
  Asbestos fibre, aluminium industry, arsenic compounds, benzoyl chloride, beryllium
- Increased incidence in patients with cryptogenic fibrosing alveolitis and systemic sclerosis

Smoking is the leading cause of lung cancer. Although smoking rates have declined amongst adult men and to a lesser extent among women, there is an increasing number of teenage smokers, particularly girls.

Histological types of lung cancer

- **Squamous cell** (20–30%): usually arises from a central airway.
- **Small cell** (20%): arises in central airways and grows rapidly producing both intra-thoracic and metastatic symptoms.
- **Adenocarcinoma** (30–40%): may be peripheral and slow-growing. Now the commonest form of lung cancer.
- **Undifferentiated large cell** (10%).
- **Bronchiolar-alveolar** cell carcinoma (5%).

Clinical features of lung cancer

Patients commonly present with cough, breathlessness, haemoptysis, chest pain or weight loss. Lung cancer should be suspected if a pneumonia fails to resolve radiologically. Occasionally an asymptomatic lesion will be noted on a routine chest X-ray.

Intra-thoracic complications of lung cancer

- Collapse of lung distal to obstructing tumour
- Recurrent laryngeal nerve palsy causing hoarseness
- Dysphagia due to compression of the oesophagus by enlarged metastatic lymph nodes or tumour invasion
- Pericarditis with effusion
- Phrenic nerve palsy with raised hemidiaphragm
- Pleural effusion
- Superior venacaval obstruction causing headache, distension of the veins in the upper body, fixed elevation of the JVP, facial suffusion with conjunctival oedema
- Rib metastases
- Spontaneous pneumothorax

Metastases can occur throughout the body but the most commonly involved sites are:

- Supraclavicular and anterior cervical lymph nodes, adrenals, bones, liver, brain and skin.

Haemoptysis is one of the common presenting symptoms of lung cancer.

Causes of haemoptysis

- **Common causes**
  Carcinoma of the bronchus
  Pneumonia/acute bronchitis
  Bronchiectasis
  Pulmonary tuberculosis
  Pulmonary embolus
  Mitral valve disease
  Infective exacerbation of COPD
- **Rarer causes**
  Vascular malformations
  Mycetoma
  Connective tissue disorders
  Vasculitis
  Goodpasture's syndrome
  Cystic fibrosis
  Bleeding diathesis
  Idiopathic pulmonary haemosiderosis

Paraneoplastic syndromes

- **Syndrome of inappropriate ADH (SIADH)**: chiefly associated with small cell lung cancer. May resolve with chemotherapy but recurs with tumour progression. Treatment involves fluid restriction initially and demeclocycline for resistant cases.
- **Ectopic ACTH**: mainly associated with small cell lung cancer.
- **Hypercalcaemia**: usually associated with multiple bony metastases from squamous cell carcinoma; ectopic parathyroid hormone (PTH) secretion occurs in a few squamous cancers.
- **Gynaecomastia**: associated with large cell carcinoma and adenocarcinoma; may be painful.
- **Hyperthyroidism**: rare (due to ectopic thyroid-stimulation hormone (TSH)) – squamous cell lung cancer.

- **Lambert–Eaton syndrome**: almost exclusively associated with small cell lung cancer; produces a proximal myopathy, reduced tendon reflexes and autonomic features.
- **Clubbing**: occurs in 10–30% of lung cancers; may resolve after resection (see box below).
- **Hypertrophic pulmonary osteoarthropathy (HPOA)**: produces periostitis, arthritis and gross finger clubbing. HPOA is most commonly associated with adenocarcinoma and least frequently with small cell carcinoma. It involves the long bones (tibia/fibula, radius/ulna or femur/humerus). It is associated with subperiosteal new bone formation visible on plain X-ray and is often painful.

Pulmonary causes of clubbing

- Carcinoma of the bronchus
- Asbestosis
- Lung abscess
- Cystic fibrosis
- Tuberculosis
- Cryptogenic fibrosing alveolitis
- Bronchiectasis
- Empyema
- Mesothelioma

Pancoast's syndrome

This is due to a tumour of the superior sulcus. The most common presenting complaint is pain (due to involvement of the eighth cervical and first thoracic nerve roots) extending down the medial side of the upper arm to the forearm and hand. The small muscles of the hand may atrophy. Horner's syndrome may develop. Chest X-ray demonstrates a shadow at the extreme apex, and there may be destruction of the first and second ribs.

Diagnosis of lung cancer

Wherever possible, the histological type of lung cancer should be confirmed and the patient should be staged, usually by CT scanning. Non-small cell lung cancers are staged using the TNM classification whilst small cell lesions are classified as either limited stage (confined to one hemithorax) or as extensive disease. An assessment of performance status is important prognostically.

Diagnosis of lung cancer

- Sputum cytology
- CT thorax
- Percutaneous CT-guided biopsy of peripheral nodules
- Bronchoscopy
- Biopsy of metastatic deposit (including lymph nodes)
- Resection of peripheral nodules.

Treatment of lung cancer

Surgery offers the best chance of cure. At the time of presentation only 10–20% of patients with non-small cell lung cancer will be operable. The 5-year survival rate depends on the clinical stage (60% for stage I tumours but only 7% for stage IIIb tumours, when disease is locally advanced). Patients whose tumour is technically operable, but who are unfit for surgery due to coexisting medical conditions or poor lung function, may be treated with **radical radiotherapy**.

- **Palliative radiotherapy** is very effective in relieving pain from bony metastases, controlling haemoptysis and cough. Dyspnoea and dysphagia due to oesophageal compression by lymph nodes respond well to radiotherapy.
- **Superior vena caval obstruction** can also be treated with radiotherapy; however, stenting provides more immediate relief of symptoms.
- **Chemotherapy** for non-small cell lung cancer offers only a very small survival benefit but has been shown to provide effective palliation.
- **Unresectable tumours** which compromise the trachea or large airways may be palliated by local techniques to maintain airway patency. These include brachytherapy (intraluminal radiotherapy), laser therapy, airways stents and/or photodynamic therapy.

Small cell lung cancer is associated with an extremely poor prognosis if left untreated, with a median survival of only 8 weeks. The tumour is, however, much more sensitive than other types of lung cancer to chemotherapeutic agents, and cycles of combination chemotherapy can result in remission in up to 80% of cases.

- Median survival is now 14–20 months for limited disease and 8–13 months for extensive disease.
- Once the disease has relapsed, mean survival is 4 months.

5.2 Mesothelioma

This is most common in men between the ages of 50 and 70 years. The lesion arises from mesothelial cells of pleura, or less commonly, the peritoneum. **Asbestos exposure** is responsible for at least 85% of malignant mesotheliomas, and the risk of mesothelioma increases with the dose of asbestos received. Crocidolite (blue) is more potent than amosite (brown) and both are more potent than crysotile (white asbestos) in causing mesothelioma.

There is usually a latent period of >30 years between asbestos exposure and development of mesothelioma. The tumour arises from the visceral or parietal pleura, and expands to encase the lung. Pleural mesothelioma presents with chest pain, weight loss and dyspnoea and may cause pleural effusion.

- Annual incidence of mesothelioma in the UK exceeds 1300 cases. Controls over asbestos exposure only came into force in the 1970s, and the incidence of mesothelioma is rising and is expected to peak around 2020. A detailed occupational history is essential.
- Chest X-ray and CT thorax usually show an effusion with underlying lobulated pleural thickening and contraction of the hemithorax.

- Diagnosis is made by pleural biopsy often done as a VATS procedure (see Section 6.4); the main differential diagnosis is adenocarcinoma of the pleura or benign pleural thickening.
- **Treatment** is unsatisfactory; radical surgical procedures are occasionally performed. Radiotherapy is helpful for pain relief and for prevention of seeding of biopsy track. Randomised trials of chemotherapy for mesothelioma are currently ongoing. Pleural effusions should be drained and talc pleurodesis considered once a tissue diagnosis has been made. Involvement of the palliative care team is often helpful.
- Median survival from presentation is 8–14 months for pleural mesothelioma and 7 months for peritoneal mesothelioma.
- Patients with mesothelioma may be eligible for industrial compensation.

5.3 Mediastinal tumours

Mediastinal tumours are often asymptomatic and they may be an incidental finding on a routine chest X-ray. In adults, 90% are benign. Clinical presentation is with stridor, superior venacaval obstruction, dysphagia, Horner's syndrome, hoarseness or pericardial effusion. The causes can be divided according to situation in the mediastinum.

- **Anterior mediastinum**: thymoma, retrosternal thyroid, lymphoma, teratoma, fibroma, lipoma, seminoma and choriocarcinoma.
- **Middle mediastinum**: aortic arch aneurysm, left ventricular aneurysm and pericardial cysts.
- **Posterior mediastinum**: neurogenic tumours (neurofibroma, neuroblastoma, neurolemoma, chemodectoma and phaeochromocytoma), oesophageal tumours and diaphragmatic hernia.

The initial investigation is usually chest X-ray which will be followed by CT scan. Occasionally radionucleotide scans are needed to confirm the presence of functioning thyroid tissue. MRI scanning may be used to define tissue planes and operability.

6. GRANULOMATOUS AND DIFFUSE PARENCHYMAL LUNG DISEASE

6.1 Sarcoidosis

Sarcoidosis is a multisystem granulomatous disorder primarily affecting young adults. The aetiology is unknown. The prevalence varies among different populations but in the UK it is 20–30 /100, 000, being highest among West Indian and Asian immigrants. The characteristic histological lesion is the granuloma composed of macrophages, lymphocytes and epithelioid histiocytes which fuse to form multinucleate giant cells. The disease may present acutely with erythema nodosum and bilateral hilar lymphadenopathy on the chest X-ray (good prognosis with most patients showing radiological resolution within a year) or insidiously with multi-organ involvement. Ninety per cent of patients have intra-thoracic involvement.

Chest X-ray changes are graded as:

- **stage 0**: clear chest X-ray
- **stage 1**: bilateral hilar lymphadenopathy (BHL)
- **stage 2**: bilateral hilar lymphadenopathy and pulmonary infiltration
- **stage 3**: diffuse pulmonary infiltration.

Patients may have no respiratory symptoms or complain of dyspnoea, dry cough, fever, malaise and weight loss. Chest examination is frequently normal; finger clubbing is rare.

Diffuse parenchymal lung involvement may progress to irreversible fibrosis; the mid and upper zones of the lungs are most frequently affected. Calcification of the hilar nodes or the lung parenchyma may occur with chronic disease. Pleural effusion is rare.

Upper airway involvement (infrequent): the nasal mucosa may become hypertrophied and cause obstruction, crusting and discharge; perforation of the nasal septum and bony erosion are rare.

Extra-pulmonary disease

- **Lymphadenopathy**: painless, rubbery lymph node enlargement is more common in Black patients; the cervical and scalene lymph nodes are most frequently affected.
- **Splenomegaly** (25%).
- **Liver involvement**: this is common but, apart from liver enlargement, is often subclinical (derangement of liver function tests). Liver biopsy is of diagnostic value in 90% (typical sarcoid granulomata).
- **Skin**: erythema nodosum (most commonly in Caucasian females) in disease with BHL; skin plaques, subcutaneous nodules and lupus pernio (violaceous lesions on the nose, cheeks and ears) seen in chronic disease.
- **Acute anterior uveitis (25%)**: chronic iridocyclitis affects older patients and responds poorly to treatment.
- **Heerfordt–Waldenstrom syndrome**: consists of parotid gland enlargement, uveitis, fever and cranial nerve palsies.
- **Neurological manifestations** (uncommon): cranial nerve palsies (facial nerve most often affected), meningitis, hydrocephalus, space-occupying lesions and spinal cord involvement; granulomata infiltrating the posterior pituitary may produce diabetes insipidus, hypothalamic hypothyroidism or hypopituitarism.
- **Cardiac sarcoid** may result in cardiac muscle dysfunction or involve the conducting system, producing arrhythmias, bundle-branch block or complete heart block.
- **Renal involvement**: renal impairment may be associated with hypercalcaemia. Acute renal failure can be due to granulomatous interstitial nephritis. Glomerulonephritis is a rare complication (*see also* Chapter 15, Nephrology).
- **Bone cysts**: with overlying soft tissue swelling occur most often in the phalanges, metacarpals, metatarsals and nasal bones; arthritis is common.
- **Hypercalcaemia**: this occurs in at least 5% of cases of sarcoidosis and it is due to excess production of vitamin D and gut activity (calcium reabsorption) to vitamin D.

Diagnosis

The combination of BHL with erythema nodosum (EN) in a young adult is virtually diagnostic of acute sarcoidosis. The combination of BHL, EN in association with fever and arthralgia is known as Löfgren's syndrome. The main differential diagnoses are TB and lymphoma, and every effort should be made to confirm the diagnosis of sarcoidosis histologically.

- **Thoracic C-T** appearances are often characteristic showing hilar and mediastinal lymphadenopathy, nodules along bronchi, vessels and in subpleural regions, ground glass shadowing, parenchymal bands, cysts and fibrosis.
- **Tissue biopsy** (transbronchial and endobronchial biopsy) can demonstrate non-caseating granulomata in 85–90% of cases with respiratory involvement.
- Elevated serum angiotensin-converting enzyme (ACE) and calcium are consistent with the diagnosis but are non-specific. The 24-hour urinary calcium excretion is often raised.
- The Kveim–Siltzbach test (intradermal injection of extract of spleen from patient with active sarcoidosis with skin biopsy at 4–6 weeks demonstrating a granulomatous response) **is no longer used**.
- Anergy to Heaf testing favours a diagnosis of sarcoid but patients who are HIV-positive or who have overwhelming TB may also be anergic.

Treatment of sarcoidosis

The best prognosis is associated with acute sarcoidosis which frequently undergoes complete remission without specific therapy.

- Stage 0 and 1 disease usually resolves spontaneously.
- With stage 2 disease, lung function tests should be performed serially and treatment instituted if there is evidence of progressive deterioration.
- Steroids are the mainstay of therapy for chronic disease but response is unpredictable.

Steroid therapy is definitely indicated for hypercalcaemia and hypercalciuria which persists despite dietary calcium restriction, and also for ophthalmological and neurological complications such as sarcoidosis. Other immunosuppressive agents (eg azathioprine and methotrexate) may be used as steroid-sparing agents.

6.2 Histiocytosis X

Three clinical entities are recognised:

- **Eosinophilic granuloma**: solitary bone lesions occurring in children and young adults. Lung disease is known as Langerhan's cell histiocytosis.
- **Letterer–Siwe disease**: a diffuse multisystem disorder of infancy which is rapidly lethal.
- **Hand–Schuller–Christian disease**: characterised by exophthalmos, bony defects and diabetes insipidus (in children and teenagers). Diffuse nodular shadows occur in the lung with hilar lymphadenopathy.

In adults histiocytosis is often confined to the lung. It is rare and most likely in young adults.

Patients present with non-productive cough and breathlessness. The chest examination is usually normal.

- Strongly associated with smoking.
- Chest X-ray shows multiple ring shadows on a background of diffuse reticulo-nodular opacities mainly in the upper and mid-zones; the lung bases are spared.
- With disease progression larger cysts and bullae form and interstitial fibrosis develops. Spontaneous pneumothorax occurs in 25%. Lung volumes are preserved.
- Diagnosis is by high-resolution CT scanning and lung biopsy.
- **Treatment** includes smoking cessation and steroids; spontaneous remission occurs in 25% of patients; however, in a further 25% the disease may be rapidly fatal. Patients may progress to end-stage fibrotic lung disease.

6.3 Pulmonary fibrosis

Interstitial lung disease is associated with many conditions including the connective tissue diseases (particularly systemic lupus erythematosus (SLE) and systemic sclerosis), rheumatoid arthritis and sarcoidosis. When pulmonary fibrosis develops without obvious cause it is known as idiopathic pulmonary fibrosis. Extrinsic allergic alveolitis also causes diffuse interstitial fibrosis.

6.4 Idiopathic pulmonary fibrosis ('usual interstitial pneumonia' – UIP)

This is a specific form of lung fibrosis characterised by UIP on lung biopsy. It accounts for around 80% of patients with interstitial lung fibrosis. The prevalence is increasing (currently 20–30 per 100, 000 in some areas). It is a disease of the middle-aged and elderly, more common in men, and is possibly the result of an inhaled environmental antigen; metal and wood dusts have been implicated but no causal relationship has been identified. There may be an association with Epstein–Barr virus (EBV). Patients present with a dry cough and breathlessness, and signs include cyanosis, finger clubbing and fine late inspiratory crackles.

- **Lung function tests**: small lung volumes, with reduction in gas transfer and restrictive spirometry.
- **Blood gas analysis**: typically shows type 1 respiratory failure with hypoxaemia and a normal or low pCO_2.
- **Chest X-ray**: reveals small lung volumes and interstitial shadowing most marked at the bases and peripheries. High-resolution CT scanning (HRCT) is useful to determine the degree of inflammatory change and the likelihood of response to steroids.
- **VATS** (video-assisted thoracoscopic surgery) or open lung biopsy can be used to confirm the diagnosis and histology shows variable degrees of established fibrosis and acute inflammation.

Treatment of idiopathic pulmonary fibrosis

Steroids and other immunosuppressive agents have been used; patients with established honeycomb fibrosis on HRCT do not usually respond. Single lung transplantation should be considered in patients below the age of 60 years. Patients may benefit from pulmonary rehabilitation, oxygen therapy and, in terminal cases, morphine in order to palliate symptoms.

Other forms of interstitial lung disease

The following conditions are recognised subtypes of interstitial lung disease:

- non-specific interstitial pneumonia (NSIP)
- desquamative interstitial pneumonia (DIP)
- acute interstitial pneumonia (AIP)
- respiratory bronchiolitis associated interstitial lung disease (RBILD)
- lymphocytic interstitial pneumonitis (LIP).

NSIP, DIP and RBILD are more steroid responsive and carry a better prognosis. AIP carries the same poor prognosis as adult respiratory distress syndrome (ARDS).

Extrinsic allergic alveolitis (EAA or hypersensitivity pneumonitis)

(This is covered in Section 4, Occupational lung disease.)

Drugs causing pulmonary fibrosis

- **Amiodarone**
  Causes an alveolitis (which may be reversible on drug cessation), progressing to diffuse fibrosis; commoner when higher doses are used
- **Sulfasalazine**
- **Methotrexate**
- **Busulfan**
- **Bleomycin**
- **Cyclophosphamide**
- **Nitrofurantoin**
- **Gold**
- **Melphalan**

Causes of reticular-nodular shadowing on chest X-ray

- **Upper zone**
  Extrinsic allergic alveolitis
  Sarcoidosis
  Coal workers' pneumoconiosis
  Silicosis
- **Basal zone**
  Idiopathic pulmonary fibrosis
  Lymphangitis carcinomatosis
  Drugs
  Connective tissue disorders

Causes of calcification on chest X-ray

- **Lymph node calcification**
  Sarcoidosis
  Silicosis
  Tuberculosis

- **Parenchymal calcification**
  Healed tuberculous lesions
  Healed fungal infections
  Previous varicella pneumonia
  Mitral stenosis*
  Chronic left ventricular failure*
  Hyperparathyroidism
  Chronic renal failure

- **Parenchymal calcification (cont.)**
  Vitamin D intoxication
  Benign tumours
  Busulfan lung
  Caplan's syndrome
  Alveolar microlithiasis

- **Pleural calcification**
  Calcified pleural plaques following asbestos exposure, and pleural calcification due to previous haemothorax (pleural)

* Results in secondary pulmonary haemosiderosis

7. PULMONARY VASCULITIS AND EOSINOPHILIA

7.1 Wegener's granulomatosis

Small/medium-sized arteries, veins and capillaries are involved with a granulomatous inflammation. Ninety per cent of Wegener's cases present with upper or lower respiratory tract symptoms. Upper airway involvement includes crusting and granulation tissue on the nasal turbinates producing nasal obstruction and a bloody discharge; collapse of the nasal bridge produces a saddle-shaped nose; c-ANCA is present is 90% of cases (*see also* Chapter 10, Immunology; Chapter 15, Nephrology and Chapter 20, Rheumatology).

- Respiratory **symptoms**: cough, haemoptysis, breathlessness and pleurisy.
- Large rounded shadows may be visible on the chest X-ray and these often cavitate. Pleural effusions and infiltrates may develop.
- Seventy-five per cent develop glomerulonephritis and eye and joint involvement are common. Patients may have a typical vasculitic skin rash and mononeuritis multiplex may also develop.
- **Prognosis**: untreated the median survival is 5 months. Treatment with cyclophosphamide and steroids has now reduced mortality to around 10%.

7.2 Churg–Strauss syndrome

A syndrome of necrotising vasculitis, eosinophilic infiltrates and granuloma formation, there is often a prior history of asthma and sometimes allergic rhinitis. Peripheral blood eosinophilia occurs with eosinophilic infiltrates of the lungs and often the gastrointestinal tract. Vasculitic lesions appear on the skin (purpura, erythema or nodules).

- p-ANCA is positive in 50%.
- Chest X-ray shows nodular or confluent shadows without cavitation.
- Treatment is with steroids and/or cyclophosphamide.

7.3 Polyarteritis and Henoch–Schönlein vasculitis

- Microscopic polyangiitis (MPA) may involve the lungs to produce pulmonary haemorrhage, haemoptysis and occasionally pleurisy; granulomas are not a feature.
- Lung involvement is uncommon in polyarteritis nodosa; it consists of pulmonary infiltrates (composed mainly of neutrophils) without granuloma formation.
- Pulmonary involvement is a rare feature in Henoch–Schönlein purpura (HSP). The disorder can be associated with streptococcal or hepatitis B (less often with viral or fungal) infections.

7.4 Connective tissue disorders

- **Rheumatoid disease**: has many pulmonary associations which include bronchiectasis, obliterative bronchiolitis, bronchiolitis obliterans organising pneumonia (BOOP), pulmonary fibrosis, nodules, Caplan's syndrome and pleurisy with effusion.
- **SLE**: pulmonary fibrosis, BOOP, pleural effusion and shrinking lung syndrome can all occur.
- **Systemic sclerosis**: associated with bronchiectasis, pulmonary fibrosis and aspiration pneumonia (due to dysphagia).

All may cause pulmonary hypertension.

Pulmonary vasculitis occurs in association with

- Ulcerative colitis
- Takayasu's disease
- Multiple pulmonary emboli
- Giant cell arteritis
- Behçet's disease
- Infection

7.5 Pulmonary eosinophilia

This describes a group of disorders characterised by peripheral blood eosinophilia and eosinophilic infiltrates in the lungs.

Causes of pulmonary eosinophilia

- Churg–Strauss syndrome
- Löffler's syndrome
- Drug induced (eg nitrofurantoin, sulfasalazine, imipramine, phenytoin)
- Allergic bronchopulmonary aspergillosis (ABPA)
- Chronic eosinophilic pneumonia
- Hypereosinophilic syndrome
- Acute eosinophilic pneumonia
- Tropical pulmonary eosinophilia (associated with parasite infection, eg *Strongyloides stercoralis*, *Toxacara canis*)

Löfflers syndrome (simple pulmonary eosinophilia)

Transient radiographic shadows and peripheral blood eosinophilia are seen in association with the passage of parasites (commonly *Ascaris lumbricoides*) through the lungs. The illness usually lasts less than 2 weeks and the eosinophilia is moderate. Symptoms are mild and include cough, rhinitis, night sweats and fever. The condition usually resolves spontaneously.

Chronic eosinophilic pneumonia

Peripheral blood eosinophilia and persistent pulmonary infiltrates occur without any obvious cause.

- The **chest X-ray** is often described as a 'reverse batwing' being the photo-negative appearance of pulmonary oedema.
- **Lung biopsy** shows airspace consolidation with an eosinophilic inflammatory infiltrate.
- **Symptoms** are more severe than in simple pulmonary eosinophilia. The condition responds to steroids.

Hypereosinophilic syndrome

Characterised by very high eosinophil counts (mean 20×10^9/l), the syndrome has clinical manifestations (weight loss, fever, night sweats, hepatomegaly and lymphadenopathy) similar to chronic eosinophilic pneumonia. Cardiac involvement occurs in 60% (producing arrhythmias and cardiac failure).

- Thrombo-embolism occurs in two-thirds of patients.
- Other organ involvement: central nervous system (intellectual deterioration and peripheral neuropathies), GI tract and the kidney (proteinuria and hypertension).
- Steroids are effective.

Acute eosinophilic pneumonia

Patients present with an acute illness with fever, myalgia, pleurisy and respiratory failure. The chest X-ray shows diffuse infiltrates, but these are not usually peripheral. The blood eosinophil count is usually normal although the eosinophil count in fluid obtained from BAL is very high. Treatment is with high-dose steroids and ventilatory support.

8. MISCELLANEOUS RESPIRATORY DISORDERS

8.1 Pleural effusion

Transudates are usually clear or straw-coloured, whereas exudates are often turbid, bloody and may clot on standing. Fluid protein content should be examined: protein levels >30 g/l (or fluid to serum ratio >0.5) and lactic dehydrogenase (LDH) levels >200 IU (fluid to serum ratio of >0.6) are consistent with an exudate. pH <7.1 also suggests an exudate.

- Low concentrations of glucose in the pleural fluid compared to serum glucose are found in infection and with rheumatoid arthritis.
- In pancreatitis the amylase level may be higher in pleural fluid than in blood.
- **Cell content should be examined**. Transudates contain <1000 white cells made up of a mixture of polymorphs, lymphocytes and mesothelial cells. Exudates usually have a much higher white cell count. In bacterial infection this is usually polymorphs but in TB, lymphocytes predominate.
- Malignant cells from a primary bronchial carcinoma or from metastatic disease may be found in approximately 60% of malignant pleural effusions.
- Any patient with pneumonia who develops a pleural effusion should have the fluid analysed for pH. A pH of <7.2 suggests a developing empyema.

Causes of pleural effusion

Transudates

Common	**Uncommon**
LVF	Myxoedema
Cirrhosis of the liver	Pulmonary emboli
Nephrotic syndrome	Sarcoidosis
Acute glomerulonephritis	Peritoneal dialysis
Other causes of hypoproteinaemia	

Exudates

Common	**Uncommon**
Pulmonary embolism	
Infections	
Bacterial pneumonia	Fungal
TB	Viral
	Parasitic
Malignancy	
Primary carcinoma of bronchus	Lymphoma
Metastatic carcinoma	Pleural tumours
Connective tissue disorders	
Rheumatoid arthritis	Wegener's granulomatosis
Systemic lupus erythematosus	Sjögren's syndrome
	Immunoblastic lymphadenopathy
Subdiaphragmatic	
Pancreatitis	Hepatic abscesses
Subphrenic abscess	
Trauma	
Haemothorax	Ruptured oesophagus
Chylothorax	

continued overleaf

Causes of pleural effusion (cont'd)

Other rare causes
Meigs syndrome
Asbestos exposure
Familial Mediterranean fever
Yellow nail syndrome
Post-thoracotomy syndrome
Dressler's syndrome

8.2 Pneumothorax

Pneumothorax may be classified as either primary or secondary, the latter complicating underlying lung disease. Presenting symptoms are of pleuritic chest pain and breathlessness and the degree of dyspnoea relates to the size of the pneumothorax. Primary spontaneous pneumothorax usually occurs at rest and the peak age of presentation is in patients in their early 20s. Pneumothorax is much more common in smokers.

Clinical signs of pneumothorax

- Diminished breath sounds
- Decreased chest excursion on the affected side
- Hyper-resonance of percussion note
- Auscultatory 'clicks'

Signs of tension

- Severe breathlessness
- Hypotension
- Mediastinal shift
- Cardiac arrest (often electro-mechanical dissociation)

Diagnosis

This is made when a visceral pleural line is seen on chest X-ray. In patients with emphysema it must be differentiated from large, thin-walled bullae. In general, the pleural line is convex towards the lateral chest wall in pneumothorax, whereas a large bulla tends to be concave towards the lateral chest wall. CT scan can be used to differentiate between these two conditions.

Treatment

- In a patient who has no underlying lung disease and with no clinical distress accompanying a small pneumothorax, no specific therapy is required but follow-up chest X-ray should be arranged to ensure lung re-expansion.
- In all other patients, aspiration of the pneumothorax should be attempted first, except if there are signs of a tension pneumothorax, when a drain should be inserted immediately.

- If the pneumothorax recurs despite aspiration, a small-bore chest drain should be inserted.
- If the lung fails to re-expand within a few hours then suction should be applied to the drain. Chest drains should not be clamped. Once the lung has been fully re-inflated for 24 hours, and bubbling has ceased, the suction can be discontinued. Provided that the lung remains fully inflated, the drain can then be removed. Removal of the drain too early is likely to result in recurrence of the pneumothorax.
- If the lung does not re-expand with chest drain and suction then the patient should be referred for thoracic surgery.
- Patients with recurrent pneumothorax on the same side will also need thoracic surgical intervention.

8.3 Obstructive sleep apnoea/hypopnoea syndrome (OSAHS)

It is estimated that approximately 1–2% of adult men and 0.5–1% of women suffer from obstructive sleep apnoea. The cardinal symptom is daytime somnolence due to the disruption of the normal sleep pattern. This leads to poor concentration, irritability and personality changes and a tendency to fall asleep during the day. Road traffic accidents are more frequent in this group of patients. The problem is exacerbated by night-time alcohol intake and sedative medication.

Pathogenesis

During sleep, muscle tone is reduced and the airway narrows so that airway obstruction develops between the level of the soft palate and the base of the tongue. Respiratory effort continues but airflow ceases due to the obstructed airway; eventually the patient arouses briefly and ventilation is resumed. The cycle is repeated several hundreds of times throughout the night.

- Over 80% of men with OSAHS are obese (BMI >30). Hypothyroidism and acromegaly are also recognised causes. Retrognathia can cause OSAHS, and large tonsils may obstruct the airway. Patients with OSAHS have higher blood pressure than matched controls.
- Patients (or their partners) give a history of loud snoring interrupted by episodes of apnoea. There may be a sensation of waking up due to choking. Sleep is generally unrefreshing.
- Patients suspected of suffering from OSAHS have some measure of daytime somnolence made (eg using the Epworth scoring system). Mental concentration is impaired.
- Diagnosis is made by demonstration of desaturation (SaO_2 below 90%) associated with a rise in heart rate and arousal from sleep, together with cessation of airflow. The frequency of apnoeic/hypopnoeic episodes per hour is used to assess disease severity. The diagnosis can be made in most patients by home pulse oximetry recordings or by limited sleep studies, but where the diagnosis is in doubt, full polysomnography (sleep studies) may be needed.

Treatment of sleep apnoea

- Nocturnal continuous positive airways pressure (CPAP) administered via a nasal mask
- Tonsillectomy if enlarged tonsils are thought to be the cause
- Correction of underlying medical disorders (eg hypothyroidism)
- Weight loss for individuals who are obese
- Anterior mandibular positioning devices are useful in some patients
- Tracheostomy (only as a last resort)

Uvulopalatopharyngoplasty is not generally of benefit.

Once a patient has been diagnosed as suffering from OSAHS, and if they are suffering from excessive daytime somnolence, then the Licensing Authorities should be informed and the patient should refrain from driving. Patients may resume driving once their OSAHS has been satisfactorily treated. Holders of HGV licences may also have their licence reinstated once they have been adequately treated.

8.4 Adult respiratory distress syndrome (ARDS)

This is a syndrome comprising:

- arterial hypoxaemia
- bilateral fluffy pulmonary infiltrates on chest X-ray
- non-cardiogenic pulmonary oedema (pulmonary capillary wedge pressure <18 cmH_2O)
- reduced lung compliance.

Causes of ARDS

- Sepsis
- Burns
- DIC
- Pneumonia
- Aspiration of gastric contents
- Near drowning
- Drug overdoses (eg diamorphine, methadone, barbiturates, Paraquat)
- Trauma
- Pancreatitis, uraemia
- Cardiopulmonary bypass
- Pulmonary contusion
- Smoke inhalation
- Oxygen toxicity

Management

No specific treatment is available and management is essentially supportive. Supplemental oxygen is given and patients frequently require mechanical ventilation. Pressure-controlled inverse ratio ventilation is used as this lowers peak airway pressure, reduces barotrauma and creates better distribution of gas in the lungs. With the addition of positive end-expiratory pressure (PEEP) there is greater alveolar recruitment, increased functional residual capacity, better lung compliance and reduced shunt. Turning the patient into the prone position intermittently allows those dependent parts of the lung which are susceptible to atelectasis to re-expand and improves blood flow to the ventilated parts of the lung.

- Inhaled nitric oxide (NO) is a potent vasodilator which causes selective vasodilatation of the ventilated areas of the lung when inhaled at low concentrations.
- Use of exogenous surfactant in adult patients has no proven value.
- Corticosteroids have been shown to be beneficial in the latter stages of ARDS that is characterised by progressive pulmonary interstitial fibro-proliferation.

8.5 Rare lung disorders

Lymphangioleiomyomatosis

This affects young/middle-aged women and is characterised by non-neoplastic proliferation of atypical smooth muscle resulting in airways and vascular obstruction, cyst formation and progressive decline in lung function. It may occur spontaneously or as part of the tuberose sclerosis complex. Fifty per cent of patients have renal angiomyolipomas.

- Patients present with progressive breathlessness, pneumothorax or chylous effusions.
- The chest X-ray may appear normal initially but HRCT shows thin-walled cysts. The condition must be differentiated from histiocytosis X.
- Pregnancy and oestrogen replacement are associated with more rapid disease progression.
- The only known cure is lung transplantation. Hormonal therapy with progesterone is used to slow disease progression.
- Average survival is 10–20 years.

Alveolar proteinosis

A disorder characterised by the accumulation of phospholipid and proteinaceous material in the alveoli and distal airways. The male:female ratio is 3:1, with age of onset 30–50 years. Patients present with dyspnoea of effort and cough; occasionally constitutional symptoms (fever, weight loss and malaise) develop. Haemoptysis and chest pain may occur.

- Chest X-ray shows bilateral infiltrates with air bronchograms in a butterfly pattern.
- Bronchoalveolar lavage establishes the diagnosis, yielding milky fluid.
- Treatment consists of interval whole lung lavage under general anaesthesia.

Pulmonary amyloidosis

The lungs are frequently involved in systemic amyloidosis (most often in primary amyloidosis); either the lung parenchyma or the tracheobronchial tree may be predominantly affected. The diagnosis is usually confirmed by biopsy. (*See also* Chapter 15, Nephrology.)

- **Bronchial tree**: plaques visible on bronchoscopy; leads to breathlessness, wheezing, stridor and haemoptysis.
- **Nodules**: may develop throughout the lung parenchyma or a solitary nodule may occur.
- **Diffuse parenchymal amyloidosis**: may develop with amyloid deposited along the alveolar septa and around blood vessels; this form is extremely rare.

Idiopathic pulmonary haemosiderosis

This condition is of unknown cause and is characterised by recurrent episodes of alveolar haemorrhage, haemoptysis and secondary iron deficiency anaemia. It may present in childhood with chronic cough, pallor and failure to thrive. Generalised lymphadenopathy and hepatosplenomegaly may occur.

- In the early stages the chest X-ray shows transient blotchy shadows.
- Eventually **pulmonary fibrosis** develops, and this is associated with chronic dyspnoea and finger clubbing. Steroids are unhelpful and patients die of *cor pulmonale* or of massive bleeding.

Chapter 20
Rheumatology

CONTENTS

Rheumatology

1. RHEUMATOID FACTOR

Rheumatoid factors (RF) are antibodies to human IgG, usually reacting with the Fc portion. Routine hospital tests detect IgM rheumatoid factors, but RF may be of any immunoglobulin isotype (IgM/IgG/IgA).

- **Agglutination tests (Latex/SCAT)**: detect only IgM RF.
- **RIA/ELISA tests**: can detect any class of RF (IgA, IgG, IgM).

IgM RF is found in

- **Normal population**
  (4% overall; 25% of the elderly)
- **Chronic infections**
  (usually low titre)
  Syphilis 10%
  Leprosy 50%
  Bacterial endocarditis 25%
  Pulmonary tuberculosis 5–20%
- **Other 'immunological' diseases**
  Autoimmune liver disease
  Sarcoidosis
  Paraproteinaemias
  Cryoglobulinaemias
  Transplant recipients
- **Connective tissue disorders**
  (often high titre, ie >1/160)
  Rheumatoid arthritis 70%
  Rheumatoid arthritis with extra-articular features 100%
  Sjögren's syndrome >75%
  Systemic lupus erythematosus (SLE) 20–40%
  Scleroderma 30%
  Polyarteritis nodosa 0–5%
  Dermatomyositis 0–5%
- **Miscellaneous**
  Relatives of rheumatoid arthritis patients
  Increasing age
  Transiently during acute infections

In rheumatoid arthritis, the RF is an assessment of prognosis rather than a diagnostic test.

2. RHEUMATOID ARTHRITIS

Rheumatoid arthritis (RA) is a chronic symmetrical inflammatory polyarthritis. It characteristically involves small joints, and can be both erosive and deforming. Soft tissues and extra-articular structures may also be involved in the disease process. RA is the most common form of inflammatory arthritis. It affects 1–3% of the population in all racial groups, with a female:male ratio of 3:1. It may start at any age but onset is most commonly in the 40s.

The cause is not known but both genetic and environmental factors are thought to play a part, with genetic factors accounting for 10–30% of the risk of developing RA. There is an association with HLA-DR4 and patients with DR4 tend to have more severe disease.

Prognosis is variable and difficult to predict in individual cases:

- 50% are too disabled to work 10 years after diagnosis
- 25% have relatively mild disease
- there is excess mortality.

The following are associated with a worse prognosis:

- positive rheumatoid factor
- extra-articular features
- HLA-DR4
- female sex
- early erosions
- insidious onset
- severe disability at presentation.

2.1 Clinical features

The onset of disease may take several forms:

- insidious (weeks/months) 55–70%
- intermediate 15–20%
- acute (days) 8–15%.

Other rare patterns of onset:

- **palindromic**: episodic with complete resolution between attacks
- **systemic**: presentation with systemic/extra-articular features
- **polymyalgic**: symptoms initially similar to polymyalgia rheumatica.

2.2 Musculoskeletal features

Joints

Symmetrical metacarpophalangeal (MCP) joint and wrist arthritis is characteristic but any synovial joint can be involved. RA tends to start in the hands and feet but, in time, most joints of the upper and lower limbs become affected. The cervical spine is involved in more than 30%. Hip or distal interphalangeal (DIP) joint involvement is unusual in early disease.

Characteristic deformities

- Ulnar deviation of MCP joints
- Swan-neck deformities of fingers
- Boutonnière deformities of fingers
- Z deformity of thumbs

Soft tissue involvement in RA

- **Tenosynovitis**
  Tendon rupture (extensor more frequently than flexor)
  Carpal tunnel syndrome (common)
- **Ligament laxity**
  Atlanto-axial subluxation (most are asymptomatic)
  Sub-axial subluxation
- **Lymphoedema**
  Rare

2.3 Extra-articular manifestations

Extra-articular features may arise in several ways:

- true extra-articular manifestations of the rheumatoid process
- non-articular manifestations of joint/tendon disease (not specific to RA)
- systemic effects of inflammation (not specific to RA) (eg amyloidosis)
- adverse drug effects.

True extra-articular manifestations of rheumatoid disease:

- present in approximately 30% of patients with RA
- rheumatoid factor is always positive
- arthritis tends to be more severe.

Rheumatoid nodules are the most characteristic extra-articular feature.

Rheumatoid nodules

- 20–30% of cases
- Rheumatoid factor always positive
- Any site – most commonly subcutaneous at extensor surfaces and pressure points
- Mimic malignancy in the lung and may cavitate
- Associated with more severe arthritis
- Sometimes induced by methotrexate therapy
- The pathology of a rheumatoid nodule involves a central area of fibrinoid necrosis surrounded by pallisading macrophages with a fibrous capsule on the outer periphery

Eye involvement is common; 20–30% of patients have keratoconjunctivitis sicca (Sjögren's syndrome). Episcleritis (painless reddening of the eye lasting about a week) is likely to be as common but usually goes unnoticed. Scleritis (reddening and pain) is a manifestation of vasculitis and is uncommon. Repeated attacks of scleritis produce scleromalacia (blue sclera) and the eye may perforate (scleromalacia perforans). This is very rare. In contrast to the spondyloarthropathies, iritis is not a feature.

Vasculitis is usually benign, manifesting as nail fold infarcts and mild sensory neuropathy in association with active joint disease. The much rarer systemic rheumatoid vasculitis carries a significant mortality. Its features include cutaneous ulceration, mononeuritis multiplex and involvement of the mesenteric, cerebral and coronary arteries. Renal vasculitis is unusual.

Cardiorespiratory manifestations: pleural and pericardial disease are common (30%) but asymptomatic in all but a few cases. Less common features include interstitial lung disease and the very rare, and often rapidly fatal, obliterative bronchiolitis. Caplan's syndrome (massive lung fibrosis in RA patients with pneumoconiosis) is very rare.

Felty's syndrome (splenomegaly, neutropenia and RA) is rare. Patients with Felty's syndrome usually have a positive ANA and may have associated leg ulcers, lymphadenopathy and anaemia.

Systemic effects of inflammation

- Malaise, fever, weight loss, myalgia
- Anaemia of chronic disease
- Osteoporosis (immobility also contributes)
- Lymphadenopathy
- Amyloidosis

Non-articular manifestations of joint/tendon disease

- Entrapment neuropathy, most commonly carpel tunnel syndrome, may occur in up to 30% of patients, but is usually mild. It may be the first symptom of RA
- Cervical myelopathy due to atlanto-axial subluxation (rare, but high mortality)
- Hoarseness and stridor due to cricoarytenoid arthritis (rare, but dangerous).

Adverse drug effects

- **Skin rashes**: may be due to NSAIDs or disease-modifying drugs. Rashes occur in about 10% of patients treated with gold or penicillamine.
- **Renal impairment**: due to prostaglandin inhibition, or the much rarer acute interstitial nephritis, may be due to NSAIDs. Proteinuria occurs in about 10% of patients receiving gold or penicillamine but only a few develop nephrotic syndrome. The proteinuria usually resolves after cessation of treatment.
- **Gastrointestinal**: NSAIDs commonly cause peptic and intestinal ulceration. Gold may cause stomatitis (common) and enterocolitis (rare). Diarrhoea is common with leflunomide.
- **Hypertension**: this can occur with NSAIDs, ciclosporin A and leflunomide.

Other extra-articular features/associations of RA

- Palmar erythema (common)
- Recurrent respiratory infections
- Pyoderma gangrenosum
- Depression (30%)

2.4 Investigations

The diagnosis of RA is based primarily on the history and examination. Laboratory tests and X-rays may be helpful but are rarely diagnostic in early disease. In clinical studies, RA can be diagnosed when four or more of the following are present:

- Morning stiffness >1 hour for more than 6 weeks
- Arthritis of hand joints (wrist, MCP or PIP) for more than 6 weeks
- Subcutaneous nodules
- Characteristic X-ray findings
- Arthritis of three or more joint areas for more than 6 weeks
- Symmetric arthritis for more than 6 weeks
- Positive rheumatoid factor

Radiology

- **Early changes**
  Soft tissue swelling
  Juxta-articular osteoporosis
- **Intermediate changes**
  Joint space narrowing (due to cartilage loss)
- **Late changes**
  Bone and joint destruction
  Subluxation
  Ankylosis (rare nowadays)

Laboratory studies

- Rheumatoid factor is positive in 70%.
- Most laboratory abnormalities are secondary to active inflammation or drug effects and are not specific to RA. They are used to monitor disease activity and screen for adverse drug effects.
- Erythrocyte sedimentation rate (ESR), C-reactive protein (CRP) and plasma viscosity reflect disease activity.
- Alkaline phosphatase is often mildly raised in active disease.
- If the aspartate transaminase (AST) and alanine aminotransferase (ALT) are raised, this is more likely to be drug-induced rather than a result of the disease process.
- Anaemia is common and may be:
  Iron deficient: gastric blood loss from NSAIDs
  Normochromic: with active disease (often with thrombocytosis)
  Aplastic: rare drug effect (eg aurothiomalate, NSAIDs)
  Haemolytic: rare as a manifestation of RA, but mild forms common with sulfasalazine.
- Immunoglobulin levels may be raised.
- Complement levels are usually normal, or elevated as an acute phase response.
- Ferritin may be elevated in an acute phase response and cannot be used to assess iron status.
- Synovial fluid examination is rarely helpful in diagnosis but is often done to exclude other diagnoses (eg sepsis, gout). Rheumatoid effusions, like those of most other inflammatory arthropathies, contain large numbers of polymorphs.

2.5 Drug therapy

Drugs used in the treatment of RA fall into two categories: **symptom-modifying** and **disease-modifying**. The disease-modifying drugs are also referred to as slow-acting anti-rheumatic drugs or second-line drugs; the newer **biologic agents also fall into this category**.

- **Symptom-modifying drugs**: these will reduce pain, stiffness and swelling (eg NSAIDs).
- **Disease-modifying drugs** have additional actions and will:
  Reduce pain, swelling and stiffness
  Reduce ESR and CRP
  Correct the anaemia of chronic disease
  Possibly slow disease progression.

Other extra-articular features do not respond to disease-modifying drugs, though nodules may regress. Methotrexate is unusual in that it can increase the formation of rheumatoid nodules.

Disease-modifying drugs in common use are listed below, together with the necessary parameters for monitoring.

Disease-modifying drugs in common use

Drug	Monitoring
Antimalarials (chloroquine/hydroxychloroquine)	Ophthalmological
Sulfasalazine*	Full blood count (FBC), liver function tests (LFT)
Methotrexate	FBC, LFT
Leflunomide	FBC, LFT, blood pressure (BP)
Azathioprine	FBC, LFT
Gold (sodium aurothiomalate)	FBC, urinalysis
D-Penicillamine	FBC, urinalysis
Ciclosporin A	FBC, urea and electrolytes (U&Es), BP

Tumour necrosis factor α (TNFα) blockers (infliximab, adalimumab, etanercept) – see below
IL-1 blockers (anakinra) – see below

* In the UK, sulfasalazine is the usual first-choice disease-modifying agent, with methotrexate reserved for patients who are intolerant or refractory to sulfasalazine

Biologic disease-modifying agents

Tumour necrosis factor α (TFNα) blockers (infliximab, adalimumab, etanercept)
IL-1 blockers (anakinra).

These agents are used in severe active rheumatoid arthritis when standard disease-modifying therapy has failed. This means failure to respond to methotrexate and at least one other disease-modifying drug. These drugs block the action of cytokines, either TNFα or IL-1. The onset of clinical effects is rapid compared with traditional disease-modifying drugs (usually apparent with two weeks).

- **Corticosteroids**: although effective at reducing the acute phase response and synovitis, are not thought to be truly 'disease-modifying'.

TNFα blockers

These consist of infliximab, adalimumab and etanercept.

- **Infliximab**: chimeric (human-mouse) monoclonal antibody against TNFα – administered intravenously.
- **Adalimumab**: human monoclonal antibody against TNFα – administered subcutaneously.
- **Etanercept**: TNFα receptor fusion protein consisting of a dimer of the extracellular portion of two p75 receptors fused to the Fc portion of human IgG1 – administered subcutaneously.

IL-1 blockers

Anakinra is a recombinant form of the human IL-1 receptor antagonist which binds to the IL-1 type 1 receptor (IL-1 R1) and competitively prevents binding of IL-1. It is administered intravenously.

Infliximab and anakinra are usually given in combination with methotrexate. Biologic disease-modifying agents are also effective in psoriatic arthritis, ankylosing spondylitis and juvenile arthritis. Several specific **adverse effects** are recognised:

- Immunosuppression: severe infections (mostly respiratory but also disseminated tuberculosis can occur). Live vaccines are contraindicated in patients receiving these agents.
- Injection site reactions (common but rarely significant).
- Worsening of heart failure.
- Anti-nuclear antibodies develop in about 10% of patients, but clinical lupus is rare.
- Demyelination (rare).

3. SPONDYLOARTHROPATHIES (HLA-B27-ASSOCIATED DISORDERS)

This group of disorders is characterised by seronegative (ie rheumatoid factor negative) inflammatory arthritis and/or spondylitis. The peripheral arthritis is typically asymmetrical, involving larger joints, especially the knees and ankles. Characteristic articular features include enthesitis (inflammation at sites of tendon insertion), sacroiliitis and dactylitis. These arthropathies should not be confused with seronegative RA, which is a symmetrical small joint arthritis.

The spondyloarthropathies include:

- Ankylosing spondylitis
- Reiter's syndrome/reactive arthritis
- Undifferentiated spondyloarthropathy
- Psoriatic arthritis
- Enteropathic arthritis (with ulcerative colitis or Crohn's disease)

Associated conditions:

- Psoriasis
- Anterior uveitis (independently associated with HLA-B27)
- Inflammatory bowel disease
- Erythema nodosum

There is an association with HLA-B27 and a tendency for relatives to have other conditions within the group.

Prevalence of HLA-B27 in spondyloarthropathies	(%)
Normal Caucasian population	8
Ankylosing spondylitis	90
Reiter's syndrome	70
Enteropathic spondylitis	50
Psoriatic arthritis	20
Psoriatic arthritis with sacroiliitis	50

3.1 Ankylosing spondylitis

Typically begins with the insidious onset of low back pain and stiffness in a young man. The age of onset is usually between 15 and 40 years and the male:female ratio is about 5:1. It is less common than RA, with a prevalence of about 0.1%. The prognosis is good.

Clinical features of ankylosing spondylitis

- **Articular**
  Sacroiliitis is the characteristic feature, but radiological changes may not be evident for several years
  Spondylitis (100%)
  Peripheral joints (35%)
  Inter-vertebral discitis (rare)
- **Extra-articular**
  Anterior uveitis (25%)
  Aortic incompetence (4%)
  Apical lung fibrosis (rare)
  Aortitis (rare)
  Heart block (rare)
  Amyloidosis (rare)

Investigations:

- ESR/CRP may be elevated
- normochromic anaemia
- alkaline phosphatase often mildly elevated.

HLA-B27 in diagnosis

This should not be a routine test in back pain. Although a negative result makes ankylosing spondylitis unlikely, a positive result is of little help.

Radiology

- **Sacro-iliac joints**
  Irregular/blurred joint margins
  Subchondral erosion
  Sclerosis
  Fusion
- **Spine**
  Loss of lumbar lordosis
  Squaring of vertebrae
  Romanus lesion (erosion at the corner of vertebral bodies)
  Bamboo spine (calcification in anterior and posterior spinal ligaments)
  Enthesitis (calcification at tendon/ligament insertions into bone)

Treatment

- Physiotherapy and regular home exercises
- NSAIDs
- Disease-modifying drugs (eg sulfasalazine, methotrexate) help peripheral arthritis but are less effective for spinal disease
- Anti-TNFα therapy can be effective for disease that is refractory to other treatment
- Surgery (joint replacement, spinal straightening) in end-stage disease.

3.2 Reiter's syndrome

Reiter's syndrome is a form of reactive arthritis characterised by a triad of arthritis, conjunctivitis and urethritis. A reactive arthritis usually begins 1–3 weeks after an initiating infection at a distant site. Antigenic material from the infecting organism may be identified in affected joints but complete organisms cannot be identified or grown, and the arthritis does not respond to treatment with antibiotics.

Reiter's syndrome is said to be 20 times more frequent in men than in women. This is likely to be an overestimate because cervicitis may go unrecognised. The true male:female ratio is more likely to be 5:1. Post-dysenteric reactive arthritis has an equal sex distribution. The age of onset is 15–40 years.

Recognised precipitating infections:

- **post-urethritis** (*Chlamydia trachomatis* – 50%)
- **post-dysenteric** (*Yersinia*, *Salmonella*, *Shigella*, *Campylobacter*).

Clinical features of Reiter's syndrome

- **Classical triad**
  Arthritis
  Conjunctivitis
  Urethritis
- **Rare features**
  Heart: pericarditis, aortitis, conduction defects
  Lung: pleurisy, pulmonary infiltrates
  CNS: meningoencephalitis, peripheral neuropathy
- **Other features**
  Circinate balanitis (25%)
  Buccal/lingual ulcers (10%)
  Keratoderma blenorrhagica (10%)
  Iritis (chronic cases only – 30%)
  Plantar fasciitis/Achilles tendonitis
  Fever/weight loss

Prognosis

- Complete resolution, no recurrence in 70–75%
- Complete resolution, recurrent episodes in 20–25% (usually B27 +ve)
- Chronic disease in <5% (usually B27 +ve).

Treatment

- Mild disease: NSAIDs
- Chronic disease may need disease-modifying drugs
- Prominent systemic symptoms may need corticosteroids.

3.3 Psoriatic arthritis

Chronic synovitis occurs in about 8% of patients with psoriasis. The arthritis may precede the diagnosis of psoriasis in 1 in 6 of these patients. Males and females are equally affected.

Patterns of psoriatic arthritis

- Polyarthritis similar to RA (most common type)
- Distal interphalangeal joints (5–10%)
- Sacroiliitis and spondylitis (20–40%)
- Asymmetric oligoarthritis (20–40%)
- Arthritis mutilans (<5%)

Characteristic features of psoriatic arthritis

- Nail pitting and onycholysis
- DIP joint arthritis
- Telescoping fingers in arthritis mutilans
- Paravertebral calcification
- Dactylitis

Drug treatment

The same approach is adopted as for treatment of rheumatoid arthritis:

- symptom-modifying drugs (analgesics, NSAIDs)
- disease-modifying drugs (eg sulfasalazine, methotrexate)
- anti-TNFα therapy for refractory disease.

4. INFLAMMATORY CONNECTIVE TISSUE DISORDERS

4.1 Autoantibodies in diagnosis

This topic is covered in detail in Chapter 10, Immunology.

Anti-double-stranded DNA antibodies

(See also the section on anti-nuclear antibodies (ANA), Chapter 10, Immunology.)

- Specific for systemic lupus erythematosus (SLE) (except low titres on ELISA assay)
- Present in approximately 80% of patients with SLE.

Antibodies to extractable nuclear antigens (ENA)

Many ENA antibodies have been described in the literature; they are covered in Chapter 10, Immunology.

Anti-phospholipid and anti-neutrophil antibodies

These are covered in Chapter 10, Immunology.

4.2 Systemic lupus erythematosus (SLE)

A multi-system inflammatory connective tissue disorder with small vessel vasculitis and non-organ-specific autoantibodies. It is characterised by skin rashes, arthralgia and antibodies against double-stranded DNA. Young women are predominantly affected with a female:male ratio of 10:1. It is more common in West Indian populations. Ten-year survival exceeds 90%.

Clinical features of SLE

- **Common** (>80% of cases)
  Arthralgia or non-erosive arthritis
  Rash (malar, discoid or photosensitive)
  Fever

- **Others**
  Serositis (30–60%): pericarditis, pleurisy, effusions
  Renal: proteinuria (30–60%), nephrotic syndrome less common, glomerulonephritis (15–20%) – *see also* Chapter 15, Nephrology
  Neuropsychiatric (10–60%): psychosis, seizures
  Haematological (up to 50%): leukopenia, thrombocytopenia, haemolysis
  Alopecia (up to 50%)
  Raynaud's phenomenon (10–40%)
  Oral or nasal ulcers (10–40%)
  Respiratory (10%): pneumonitis, shrinking lung syndrome
  Cardiac (10%): myocarditis, endocarditis (Libman–Sacks)

Investigations for SLE

FBC may show:

Abnormalities of FBC in SLE

- Anaemia of chronic disease (normal mean cell volume (MCV))
- Neutropenia
- Thrombocytopenia
- Haemolytic anaemia (high MCV, reticulocytosis)
- Lymphopenia
- Aplastic anaemia (rare)

ESR reflects disease activity, whereas CRP may not. This discrepancy can be used to differentiate between a flare of SLE and intercurrent infection.

Low C3 and C4 suggest lupus nephritis.

Antibodies

- ANA-positive in 95% of cases, usually with a homogeneous staining pattern
- Anti-double-stranded DNA antibodies in high titre are very specific for SLE
- Anti-Sm antibodies are found in only 20% but are very specific for lupus
- Anti-Ro or anti-La are found in ANA-negative subacute cutaneous lupus
- Antiphospholipid antibodies (or false-positive VDRL) occur in 40%, but only a minority have thrombotic events

Lupus variants

Drug-induced lupus is more common in men than in women. It is usually mild and always resolves on stopping the drug. CNS and renal disease are rare. ANA is positive but antibodies to double-stranded DNA are not usually present. The pathogenesis is not known, and antibodies to the drug do not occur. The drugs commonly implicated (procainamide, isoniazid and hydralazine) all have active amido groups. *See also* Chapter 2, Clinical Pharmacology, Toxicology and Poisoning.

Antiphospholipid antibody syndrome (Hughes' syndrome): recurrent venous or arterial thromboses, fetal loss and thrombocytopenia. Libman–Sacks endocarditis and focal neurological lesions (such as cerebrovascular accident (CVA) or transient ischaemic attack (TIA)) in lupus are usually due to antiphospholipid antibodies.

Treatment of lupus depends on severity and organ involvement.

Treatment of SLE

- **Sunscreens**
  Sunburn can provoke a generalised flare in disease
- **Plasma exchange**
  In difficult cases with most aggressive disease
- **NSAIDS and anti-malarials**
  (eg hydroxychloroquine) used for arthritis and skin-limited disease
- **Corticosteroids and immunosuppressive drugs**
  For vital organ involvement (eg *see* Chapter 15, Nephrology for treatment of lupus nephritis)
- **Anticoagulation**
  For thrombotic features

4.3 Dermatomyositis and polymyositis

Polymyositis is an idiopathic inflammatory disorder of skeletal muscle. When associated with cutaneous lesions it is called dermatomyositis. These conditions are rare (5 cases per million). Five-year survival is 80% with treatment. Myositis may also occur with other connective tissue disorders.

Clinical features of dermatomyositis and polymyositis

- **Muscle disease**
  Proximal weakness
  Swelling and tenderness of muscles
- **Others**
  Pulmonary muscle weakness
  Interstitial lung disease
  Oesophageal dysfunction
  Arthralgia
  Weight loss
  Fever
- **Skin rash**
  Heliotrope discoloration of the eyelids
  Gottron's papules (scaly papules over MCP/PIP joints)
  Periungual telangiectasia
  Erythematous macules

Juvenile dermatomyositis differs from the adult form. Vasculitis, ectopic calcification and lipodystrophy are commonly present.

Malignancy

The elderly with dermatomyositis and polymyositis have a higher prevalence of malignancy than would be expected by chance and this is most pronounced in dermatomyositis. There is no association between dermatomyositis/polymyositis and malignancy in children or adults of young and middle age.

Laboratory tests in dermatomyositis/polymyositis

- **Muscle**
  Elevated muscle enzymes:
  Creatine kinase (CK), aspartate transaminase (AST), lactate dehydrogenase (LDH)
  Abnormal EMG
  Biopsy showing inflammation, muscle fibre necrosis and regeneration
- **Autoantibodies**
  Antinuclear antibodies may be present
  Anti-Jo-1 is associated with a specific syndrome of: acute-onset myositis; interstitial lung disease; fever; arthritis; Raynaud's phenomenon; mechanics' hands (fissuring of the digital pads without ulceration and periungual infarcts)

Treatment

- **Corticosteroids**: CK falls rapidly but muscle power takes many weeks to improve.
- **Immunosuppressives**: methotrexate or cyclophosphamide can be used in resistant cases.

4.4 Systemic sclerosis

Systemic sclerosis is a connective tissue disorder characterised by thickening and fibrosis of the skin (scleroderma) with distinctive involvement of internal organs. It is a rare condition, occurring in all racial groups, with an incidence of 4–12/million per year. It is more common in women (female:male ratio 4:1) and may start at any age.

Some cases may be due to exposure to substances such as vinyl chloride.

Clinical features of systemic sclerosis

- **Raynaud's phenomenon**
  Initial complaint in 70%
  Associated digital ulcers and calcinosis (very unusual in primary Raynaud's phenomenon)
- **Musculoskeletal**
  Arthralgia
  Erosive arthritis in about 30%
  Myositis (usually mild, often asymptomatic with raised CK)
  Flexion deformities of fingers due to skin fibrosis
- **Pulmonary**
  Fibrotic interstitial lung disease
  Pulmonary hypertension
- **Renal**
  Scleroderma renal crisis (malignant hypertension, rapid renal impairment with 'onion skin' intra-renal vasculature) – *see also* Chapter 15, Nephrology
- **Scleroderma**
  Early oedematous phase
  Later indurated and hidebound
  Affected areas may become pigmented and lose hair
- **Gastrointestinal**
  Motility can be impaired at any level (smooth muscle atrophy and fibrosis)
  Oesophagus (reflux, dysphagia, peptic strictures)
  Gastric dilatation
  Intestine (bacterial overgrowth, malabsorption, steatorrhoea, pseudo-obstruction
  Colon (constipation)

Laboratory tests include:

- **Elevated ESR or CRP**
- **Autoantibodies**
  Rheumatoid factor positive in 30%
  Antinuclear factor positive in 90% (homogeneous, speckled or nucleolar staining)
  Anticentromere and Anti-Scl-70 are quite specific
  Anticentromere positive in 50–90% of limited and 10% of diffuse scleroderma
  Anti-Scl-70 (anti-topoisomerase-I) positive in 20–40%.

Disease patterns

- **Limited scleroderma with systemic involvement – CREST**
  Scleroderma limited to the face, neck and limbs distal to the elbow and knee
  Usually begins with Raynaud's phenomenon
  CREST (Calcinosis, Raynaud's, oEsophageal dysmotility, Sclerodactyly, Telangiectasia)
  Anti-centromere antibody positive in most
  Renal crisis rare, pulmonary hypertension more common
  Better prognosis (70+% 10-year survival).

- **Diffuse scleroderma with limited involvement**
  Scleroderma involving trunk and proximal limbs as well as face and distal limbs
  Usually begins with swelling of fingers and arthritis
  Anti-Scl-70 antibodies 20–40%
  Pulmonary hypertension rare, renal crisis more common
  Worse prognosis (50% 10-year survival).

- **Scleroderma without internal organ disease**
  Plaques: morphoea
  Linear: coup de sabre.

Treatment

- **Supportive**
  NSAIDs for arthralgia/arthritis
  Proton pump inhibitors for reflux
  Intermittent antibiotics for bacterial overgrowth in the small bowel
  Vasodilators for Raynaud's phenomenon
  Prostacyclin or iloprost infusions for severe Raynaud's phenomenon and digital ischaemia

- **Specific**
  D-Penicillamine can slow the progression of skin disease
  Steroids and immunosuppressives for interstitial lung disease
  Steroids do not help the skin

4.5 Sjögren's syndrome

A connective tissue disorder characterised by lymphocytic infiltration of exocrine glands, especially the lacrimal and salivary glands. The reduced secretions produce the dry eyes and dry mouth of the sicca syndrome. Secondary Sjögren's syndrome describes the presence of sicca syndrome and either RA or a connective tissue disorder. About 30% of rheumatoid patients have secondary Sjögren's syndrome.

Clinical features of Sjögren's syndrome

- **Dryness from atrophy of exocrine glands**
  Eyes (xerophthalmia) which may allow corneal ulceration
  Mouth (xerostomia) with increased dental caries
  Respiratory with hoarseness, dysphagia, respiratory infections
  Vaginal, producing dyspareunia
- **Arthralgia or arthritis**
  Which may be erosive
- **Raynaud's phenomenon**
- **Lymphadenopathy**
- **Gland swelling**
  In the early stages (eg parotid)
- **Vasculitic purpura**
- **Neuropathies**
- **Renal tubular acidosis (30%)**
- **Pancreatitis**

Laboratory tests

- Anaemia and leukopenia are common
- ANA frequently present
- Anti-Ro or anti-La present in primary Sjögren's syndrome
- ESR and CRP reflect disease activity
- Rheumatoid factor positive in most cases
- Polyclonal hypergammaglobulinaemia

Treatment

- **Artificial tears**: plugging of lacrimal punctae in severe cases
- **Moistening sprays**: for the mouth
- **NSAIDs**: and sometimes hydroxychloroquine for arthritis.

4.6 Mixed connective tissue disease/overlap syndromes

Some patients have features of more than one connective tissue disorder and are said to have overlap syndromes. One specific overlap syndrome, mixed connective tissue disease, is associated with anti-RNP antibodies. The clinical features are Raynaud's phenomenon, swollen hands and other features from at least two connective tissue disorders (SLE, scleroderma or polymyositis).

- **Prognosis**: the 10-year survival is 80%. Patients who have features mainly of scleroderma and polymyositis fare much worse, with a 10-year survival as low as 30%.

5. VASCULITIS

5.1 Overview of vasculitis

Systemic vasculitis usually presents with constitutional symptoms such as general malaise, fever and weight loss, combined with more specific signs and symptoms related to specific organ involvement. The diagnosis is based on a combination of clinical and laboratory findings, and is usually confirmed by biopsy and/or angiography.

Aetiology

Infections, malignancy and drugs may all produce vasculitic illness but, in many cases, the trigger for endothelial injury is unknown. The following mechanisms of endothelial cell injury have been proposed in the pathogenesis of vasculitis:

- **immune complex deposition**: hepatitis-B-associated polyarteritis nodosa
- **direct endothelial cell infection**: HIV
- **anti-endothelial cell antibodies**: Kawasaki's disease, Behçet's disease
- **ANCA-mediated neutrophil activation**: Wegener's granulomatosis
- **T-cell-dependent injury**: giant cell arteritis.

Clinical features of vasculitis

- **General**
  Constitutional (fever, weight loss, fatigue, anorexia)
  Musculoskeletal (arthralgia, arthritis, myalgia)
  Skin (livedo reticularis, urticaria)
- **Related to specific organ involvement**
  Kidney (proteinuria, hypertension, glomerulonephritis)
  Respiratory (alveolitis, infiltrates, haemorrhage, sinusitis)
  Neuropathy (mononeuritis multiplex, sensory neuropathy)
  Gastrointestinal (diarrhoea, abdominal pain, perforation, haemorrhage)
  Cardiovascular (jaw or extremity claudication, angina, myocardial infarction)
  Central nervous system (headache, visual loss, stroke, seizures)

5.2 Classification of vasculitis

The vasculitides are classified according to the size of vessel involved and the pattern of organ involvement.

- **Large vessels**
  Takayasu's arteritis
  Giant cell/temporal arteritis
  Aortitis associated with ankylosing spondylitis
- **Small/medium-sized vessels**
  Granulomatous:
    Wegener's granulomatosis
    Churg–Strauss syndrome
    Granulomatous angiitis of the CNS
  Non-granulomatous:
    Polyarteritis nodosa
    Kawasaki disease
    Arteritis/vasculitis of RA, SLE, Sjögren's syndrome
    Microscopic polyangiitis
- **Small vessel vasculitis**
  Leukocytoclastic vasculitis: allergic or hypersensitivity vasculitis
  Henoch–Schönlein syndrome
  Cryoglobulinaemia
  Drug-induced vasculitis
  Vasculitis of RA, SLE, Sjögren's syndrome
  Microscopic polyangiitis
- **Others**
  Behçet's syndrome (vasculitis and venulitis)

Laboratory tests:

- ESR/CRP are invariably elevated in active disease
- Normochromic anaemia and leukocytosis (usually a neutrophilia) are common
- Eosinophilia is characteristic of Churg–Strauss syndrome but may occur in any vasculitis
- Serum creatinine and urinary protein assessments are essential if vasculitis is suspected since renal involvement is one of the most important factors affecting prognosis
- Autoantibodies:
  cANCA is useful in identifying Wegener's disease and microscopic polyangiitis
  pANCA may be positive in any vasculitis
  ANCA titres may reflect the activity of vasculitis and titres may begin to rise before a flare in disease activity.

Treatment

- **Large vessel group**: corticosteroids only for most cases
- **Medium/small vessels**: corticosteroids and immunosuppressives (cyclophosphamide and/ or azathioprine)
- **Small vessel group**: some conditions benign, corticosteroids and immunosuppressives in some cases.

Prognosis

The size of vessel involved and presence of renal involvement are the most important factors determining prognosis. Despite treatment with immunosuppressive agents and steroids, up to 20% of patients with systemic vasculitis of the small/medium vessel group die within one year of diagnosis. Patients with large or small vessel vasculitis have a much more favourable outlook.

5.3 Polymyalgia rheumatica, giant cell and other large vessel arteritis

Giant cell arteritis is a vasculitis of large vessels, usually the cranial branches of arteries arising from the aorta. Polymyalgia rheumatica is not a vasculitis, but is found in 40–60% of patients with giant cell arteritis. Both are disorders of the over 50s and both are relatively common. Polymyalgia has an incidence of 52/100, 000 people aged over 50, and giant cell arteritis of 18/100, 000 people over 50. Treatment is with corticosteroids.

Features of polymyalgia rheumatica and giant cell arteritis

- **Polymyalgia rheumatica**
  Female:male ratio 3:1
  Age >50 years
  Proximal muscle pain (shoulder or pelvic) *without* weakness
  Early morning stiffness
  Raised acute phase response (ESR/CRP)
  Abnormal liver function tests (alkaline phosphatase/gamma glutamyl transpeptidase (GGT))
  CK normal
  Synovitis of knees, etc may occur
  Response to corticosteroids is dramatic and prompt (within 24–48 hours)
- **Giant cell arteritis**
  General malaise, weight loss, fever
  Temporal headache with tender, enlarged non-pulsatile temporal arteries
  Scalp tenderness
  Jaw claudication
  Visual disturbance/loss
  Polymyalgia rheumatica
  Positive temporal artery biopsy (patchy granulomatous necrosis with giant cells)

Takayasu's arteritis (pulseless disease)

This rare condition presents with systemic illness such as malaise, weight loss and fever. The main vasculitic involvement is of the aorta and its main branches, producing arm claudication, absent pulses and bruits. Thirty per cent of patients have visual disturbance. Diagnosis is by angiography and treatment involves corticosteroids.

5.4 Wegener's granulomatosis

A rare disorder (incidence 0.4/100, 000) characterised by a granulomatous necrotising vasculitis. Any organ may be involved but the classical Wegener's triad includes:

- **upper airways (sinuses, ears, eyes)**: saddle nose, proptosis
- **respiratory**: multiple pulmonary nodules
- **renal**: focal proliferative glomerulonephritis often with segmental necrosis.

Treatment is with corticosteroids and immunosuppressives. cANCA is present in 90% of cases (*see also* Chapter 10, Immunology and Chapter 15, Nephrology).

5.5 Churg–Strauss syndrome (allergic angiitis and granulomatosis)

A rare systemic vasculitis with a similar pattern of organ involvement to polyarteritis nodosa but with associated eosinophilia and asthma. Though corticosteroids are required, the condition of most patients can be controlled without immunosuppressives. In some cases, the disease is triphasic. *See also* Chapter 19, Respiratory Medicine.

- **Prodromal**: allergic features of asthma, rhinitis.
- **Eosinophilia**: with eosinophilic pneumonia or eosinophilic gastroenteritis.
- **Systemic vasculitis**.

5.6 Polyarteritis nodosa

Primary necrotising vasculitis of small/medium-sized vessels with formation of micro-aneurysms. It is uncommon with an incidence of 5–9 per million, but it may be as much as 10 times more frequent in areas where hepatitis B is endemic. Presentation is usually with constitutional symptoms. Any organ may be involved but commonly skin, peripheral nerves, kidney, gut and joints are affected. Treatment is with corticosteroids and immunosuppressives.

- Hepatitis B surface antigen is present in 30% of cases world-wide, but <10% in the UK.
- Mild eosinophilia may be present.
- LFTs often abnormal.
- ANCA is positive in <10%.
- Renal disease is manifest by accelerated phase hypertension, but not glomerulonephritis (*see* Chapter 15, Nephrology).

5.7 Microscopic polyangiitis (microscopic polyarteritis)

Usually presents between the ages of 40 and 60 with constitutional illness and renal disease. Though classified with the medium/small vessel disorders, microscopic angiitis tends to affect small arteries and arterioles of the kidney. Organs involved include:

- **kidney**: glomerulonephritis as for Wegener's disease
- **skin**: palpable purpura
- **lung**: infiltrates, haemoptysis, haemorrhage
- **gut, eye or peripheral nerves** can also be involved.

ANCA is positive in most cases: pANCA in 60% and cANCA in 40% (*see also* Chapter 10, Immunology and Chapter 15, Nephrology).

5.8 Kawasaki disease

An acute febrile illness with systemic vasculitis which mainly affects children less than five years old. The peak onset is at 1.5 years and it has an incidence of about 6/100, 000 in the under-fives. It is more common and more severe in males. The cause is not known but its occasional occurrence in mini-epidemics suggests an infectious agent. (*Rickettsia* has been implicated.)

Clinical features of Kawasaki disease

- **Fever**
  (Followed by thrombocytosis)
- **Mucocutaneous**
  Rashes, red cracked lips, strawberry tongue, conjunctivitis
- **Vasculitis**
  With coronary aneurysm formation
  Myocardial infarctions in 2.5%
- **Lymphadenopathy**
  (Especially cervical)

Treatment differs from most other vasculitides. Corticosteroids are contraindicated since they increase coronary aneurysms. Anti-inflammatory doses of aspirin are used during the acute febrile phase and anti-platelet doses once the fever resolves and thrombocytosis occurs. Intravenous immunoglobulin is also effective.

5.9 Behçet's syndrome

Behçet's syndrome is a rare condition most commonly found in Turkey and the eastern Mediterranean where there is a strong association with HLA B5. There is an equal sex ratio but the disease is more severe in males. The pathological findings are of immune-mediated occlusive vasculitis and venulitis. The diagnosis is based on clinical features.

- **Main clinical features**
  Recurrent oral ulceration (100%)
  Recurrent painful genital ulceration (80%)
  Recurrent iritis (60–70%)
  Skin lesions (60–80%)
- **Other features**
  Cutaneous vasculitis
  Thrombophlebitis
  Pathergy reaction (red papules >2 mm at sites of needle pricks after 48 hours)
  Erythema nodosum
  Arthritis (usually non-erosive, asymmetrical, lower limb)
  Neurological involvement (aseptic meningitis, ataxia, pseudobulbar palsy)
  Gastrointestinal involvement

6. CRYSTAL ARTHROPATHIES AND OSTEOARTHRITIS

6.1 Gout

Hyperuricaemia is common and usually asymptomatic, but in some individuals uric acid crystals form within joints or soft tissues to produce a variety of diseases.

Clinical features of gout

- **Acute crystal arthritis**
  Particularly affecting the small joints of the feet (eg first MTP usually recurrent)
- **Gouty nephropathy**
  Tubulo interstitial disease due to parenchymal crystal deposition
  Acute intratubular precipitation resulting in acute renal failure
  Urate stone formation (radiolucent)
- **Chronic tophaceous arthritis**
  These are aggregations of urate crystals affecting articular, periarticular and non-articular cartilage (eg ears)

Aetiology

Uric acid is a breakdown product of purine nucleotides. Purines can be synthesised from precursors, but significant amounts are ingested in normal diets and released at cell death. Hyperuricaemia arises because of an imbalance in uric acid production/ingestion and excretion.

Causes of gout

- **Primary (innate)**
  Idiopathic (90% of these are due to under-excretion of uric acid)
  Rare enzyme deficiencies: eg hypoxanthine-guanine phosphoribosyltransferase (HGPRT) deficiency (Lesch–Nyhan syndrome)

- **Secondary hyperuricaemia**
  Increased uric acid production/intake
  Myeloproliferative and lymphoproliferative disorders
  High purine diet, eg purines in beer (even non-alcoholic)
  Cytolytic therapy
  Acidosis, eg the ketosis of starvation or diabetes
  Extreme exercise, status epilepticus
  Psoriasis
  Decreased uric acid excretion
  Renal failure (*see also* Chapter 15, Nephrology)
  Drugs (diuretics, low-dose aspirin, ciclosporin, pyrazinamide)
  Alcohol
  Lead intoxication (saturnine gout)
  Down's syndrome

Diagnosis

- Negatively birefringent needle-shaped crystals must be identified in joint fluid or other tissues for a definitive diagnosis.
- In chronic tophaceous gout the X-ray appearances (large punched-out erosions distant from the joint margin) are characteristic and may allow diagnosis.
- In clinical practice, a characteristic history with hyperuricaemia is often thought sufficient, but there are pitfalls: uric acid may fall by up to 30% during an acute attack; hyperuricaemia is common and may be coincidental.

Treatment of gout

- **Acute attack**
  NSAIDs, (colchicine or steroids may be used if NSAID intolerant)

- **Prophylaxis**
  Allopurinol, a xanthine oxidase inhibitor, is the drug of first choice. It may precipitate acute attacks at the outset of treatment unless an NSAID or colchicine is given
  Probenecid and sulfinpyrazone are less effective

Indications for prophylaxis

- Recurrent attacks of arthritis
- Tophi
- Uric acid nephropathy
- Nephrolithiasis
- Cytolytic therapy
- HGPRT deficiency.

6.2 Calcium pyrophosphate deposition disease (CPDD)

This is a spectrum of disorders ranging from asymptomatic radiological abnormalities to disabling polyarthritis. The underlying problem is the deposition of calcium pyrophosphate crystals in and around joints. This is most commonly idiopathic and age-related, but may occur in metabolic disorders especially those with hypercalcaemia or hypomagnesaemia. Calcium pyrophosphate forms positively birefringent brick-shaped crystals – 'pseudogout'.

Variants:

- **asymptomatic**: radiological chondrocalcinosis (30% of over 80s)
- **acute monoarthritis**: pseudogout (usually knee, elbow or shoulder)
- **inflammatory polyarthritis**: mimicking RA (10% of CPDD)
- **osteoarthritis**: often of hips and knees but with involvement of the index and middle MCP joints (rarely seen in primary osteoarthritis).

Causes of CPDD	**Treatment of CPDD**
Hyperparathyroidism	Chondrocalcinosis alone needs no treatment
Wilson's disease	NSAIDs for arthritis
Bartter's syndrome	Correction of metabolic disturbances (if possible)
Hypomagnesaemia	
Haemochromatosis	
Hypophosphatasia	
Ochronosis	

6.3 Osteoarthritis

Osteoarthritis (OA) is the most common joint disease. It is characterised by softening and disintegration of articular cartilage, with secondary changes in adjacent bone. The prevalence of OA on X-ray rises with age and affects 70% of 70-year-olds. Many individuals with radiological OA, however, are asymptomatic.

Common joints involved are:

- distal interphalangeal joints (Heberden's nodes)
- proximal interphalangeal joints (Bouchard's nodes)
- base of thumb (first carpometacarpal joint)
- hips
- knees
- spine.

Metacarpophalangeal joint OA suggests a secondary cause (eg CPDD disease).

OA subsets

- **Primary**
  Localised (one principal site, eg hip)
  Generalised (eg hands, knees, spine)
- **Secondary**
  Dysplastic disorders
  Mechanical damage (eg osteonecrosis, post-meniscectomy)
  Metabolic (eg ochronosis, acromegaly)
  Previous inflammation (eg sepsis, gout, RA)

Treatment of osteoarthritis

This includes the following:

- exercise
- physiotherapy
- occupational therapy
- analgesics including NSAIDs
- intra-articular injection (steroid or hyaluronic acid)
- surgery.

7. ARTHRITIS IN CHILDREN

Classifications:

- juvenile idiopathic arthritis (previously termed 'juvenile chronic arthritis' (JCA))
- systemic connective tissue disease
- reactive arthritis (eg rheumatic fever)
- other (psoriatic, viral, leukaemic).

Juvenile idiopathic arthritis

Juvenile idiopathic arthritis is persistent arthritis of more than 3 months' duration in children under the age of 16. It is one of the more common chronic disorders of children and is a major cause of musculoskeletal disability and eye disease. The cause is not known. A number of distinct clinical patterns of onset are recognised.

Clinical patterns of onset of juvenile idiopathic arthritis

	Systemic	Polyarticular	Pauciarticular
Frequency (%)	10	30	60
Number of joints	Variable	5 or more	4 or less
Female:male ratio	1:1	3:1	5:1
Extra-articular	Prominent	Moderate	Rarer
Uveitis (%)	Rare	5	20
Rheumatoid factor (%)	Rare	15	Rare
Antinuclear factor (%)	10	40	85
Prognosis	Moderate	Moderate	Good

Systemic (classical Still's disease)

The hallmark is a high spiking fever which, with the salmon pink evanescent rash, is virtually diagnostic. There is usually visceral involvement with hepatosplenomegaly and serositis. Initially the arthritis may be flitting as in rheumatic fever, but in 50% of cases this develops into a chronic destructive arthropathy. This is usually a disease of the under-fives, but adult cases do occur.

Polyarticular

Arthritis of more than four joints. This is probably two distinct disorders. Younger children with negative rheumatoid factor have a symmetrical arthritis of large joints (especially the knees), though the small joints can be affected. Older children, usually teenagers, with a positive rheumatoid factor have, in fact, early-onset rheumatoid arthritis.

Pauciarticular

Arthritis of between one and four joints. Again there are two distinct groups. Older boys with sacroiliitis and HLA-B27 who probably have juvenile-onset ankylosing spondylitis, and younger girls, usually ANA positive who may have uveitis. Regular ophthalmological screening is required in this group.

Treatment of arthritis in children

- Physiotherapy
- Splintage
- NSAIDs
- Disease-modifying agents (eg methotrexate) in persistent polyarticular disease
- Corticosteroids may be needed for systemic disease
- Anti-TNFα therapy for refractory disease

Chapter 21
Statistics

CONTENTS

Statistics

1. STUDY DESIGN

1.1 Research questions

A research study should always be designed to answer a particular research question. The question usually relates to a specific population. For example:

- Does taking folic acid early in pregnancy prevent neural tube defects?
- Is a new inhaled steroid better than current treatment for improving lung function amongst cystic fibrosis patients?
- Are those who smoke more likely to develop cancer?

Random samples of the relevant groups are taken. For example, pregnant women, cystic fibrosis patients, those who do and do not smoke.

Based on the outcome in the samples, inferences are made about the populations from which they were randomly sampled. Statistical analysis enables us to determine what inferences can be made.

Studies are either experimental or observational.

1.2 Experimental studies

In experimental studies, individuals are assigned to groups by the investigator. For example, pregnant women will be assigned to take either folic acid or a placebo; cystic fibrosis patients will be assigned to either the new or current treatment. In both of these examples the second group is known as a control group.

Note that a control group does not necessarily consist of normal healthy individuals. In the second example the control group comprises cystic fibrosis patients on standard therapy.

Individuals should be randomised to groups to remove any potential bias. Randomisation means that each patient has the same chance of being assigned to either of the groups, regardless of their personal characteristics. Note that random does not mean haphazard or systematic.

Experimental studies may be:

- **Double-blind**: none of the patient, the researcher assessing the patients, or the treating clinician knows which treatment the patient has been randomised to receive
- **Single-blind**: either the patient or the researcher/clinician does not know (usually the patient)
- **Unblinded** (or open): both the patient and the researcher/clinician know

Clinical trials are experimental studies

1.3 Crossover studies

In a crossover study, each patient receives treatment and placebo in a random order. Fewer patients are needed because many between-patient confounders may be removed. For example, even though pairs of cystic fibrosis patients may be chosen and randomised to groups on the basis of their disease severity this does not ensure that the groups will be of similar age or sex.

Crossover studies are only suitable for chronic disorders that are not cured but for which treatment may give temporary relief. There should be no carryover effect of the treatment from one treatment period to the next.

1.4 Observational studies

In observational studies the groups being compared are already defined (eg smokers and non-smokers) and the study merely observes what happens.

Case control, cross-sectional and **cohort** are particular types of observational studies that, respectively, consider features of the past, the present and the future to try to identify differences between the groups.

- If we take groups of individuals with and without cancer with the aim of identifying different features in their past that might explain a causal route for the cancer this is a **case control** study.
- If we take groups of smokers and non-smokers and follow them forward in time to see whether one group is more prone to cancer then this is a **cohort** study.

1.5 Confounding

Confounding may be an important source of error. A confounding factor is a background variable (ie something not of direct interest) that:

- is different between the groups being compared

and

- affects the outcome being studied.

For example, in a study to compare the effect of folic acid supplementation in early pregnancy on neural tube defects, age will be a confounding factor if:

- either the folic acid or placebo group tends to consist of older women

and

- older women are more, or less, likely to have a child with a neural tube defect.

When studying the effects of a new inhaled steroid against standard therapy for cystic fibrosis patients, disease severity will be a confounder if:

- one of the groups (new steroid/standard therapy) consists of more severely affected patients

and

- disease severity affects the outcome measure (lung function).

In the comparison of cancer rates between smokers and non-smokers, diet will be a confounder if:

- smokers eat less fruit and vegetables

and

- eating more fruit and vegetables reduces the risk of contracting cancer.

If a difference is found between the groups (folic acid/placebo, new steroid/standard therapy and smokers/non-smokers) we will not know whether the differences are, respectively, due to folic acid or age, to the potency of the new steroid or the severity of disease in the patient, or to smoking or diet.

Confounding may be avoided by matching individuals in the groups according to potential confounders. For example, we could age-match folic acid and placebo pairs or deliberately recruit smokers and non-smokers with similar fruit and vegetable consumption. We could find pairs of cystic fibrosis patients of similar disease severity and randomly allocate one of each pair to receive the new steroid while the other receives standard therapy.

2. DISTRIBUTIONS

2.1 Types of data

Data may be either categoric (qualitative) or numeric (quantitative).

- With **categoric** variables each individual lies in one category
- **Numeric** data are measured on a number scale.

Ranks give the order of increasing magnitude of numeric variables. For example:

Sample of seven readings:

2.3	5.0	3.9	1.3	–2.1	1.3	4.2

In order of magnitude:

-2.1	1.3	1.3	2.3	3.9	4.2	5.0

Ranks:

1	2.5	2.5	4	5	6	7

Note that there are seven values in the sample and the largest value has rank 7. Where there are ties (for example, the two values 1.3), the ranks are averaged between the tied values.

The **mode** is the value that occurs most often. In the example above:

Mode = 1.3.

The **median** is the middle value when the values are ranked. In the example above:

Median = 2.3.

The **mean** is the arithmetic average. In the example above:

$$\text{Mean} = \frac{2.3+5.0+3.9+1.3-2.1+1.3+4.2}{7} = \frac{15.9}{7} = 2.27.$$

2.2 Skewed distributions

The distribution of a set of values may be asymmetric or skewed.

Figure 1 (a) Negative or downward or left skew (b) Positive or upward or right skew

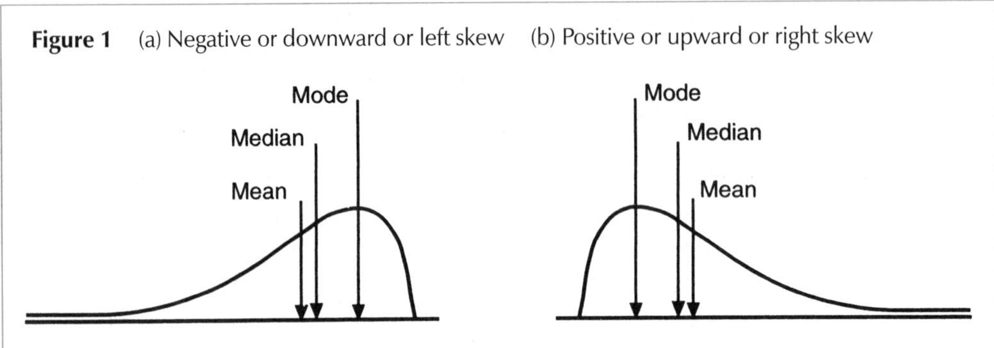

In a sample of this type the mean is 'pulled towards' the values in the outlying tail of the distribution and is unrepresentative of the bulk of the data.

Note that the skew is named according to the direction in which the tail points. In the left-hand diagram (a), the tail points to the left, to negative values and downwards.

If the distribution is skewed then the median is preferable as a summary of the data.

2.3 Normal distribution

The Normal distribution is symmetric and bell-shaped. The Normal distribution is sometimes called the Gaussian distribution.

Figure 2 Normal distribution

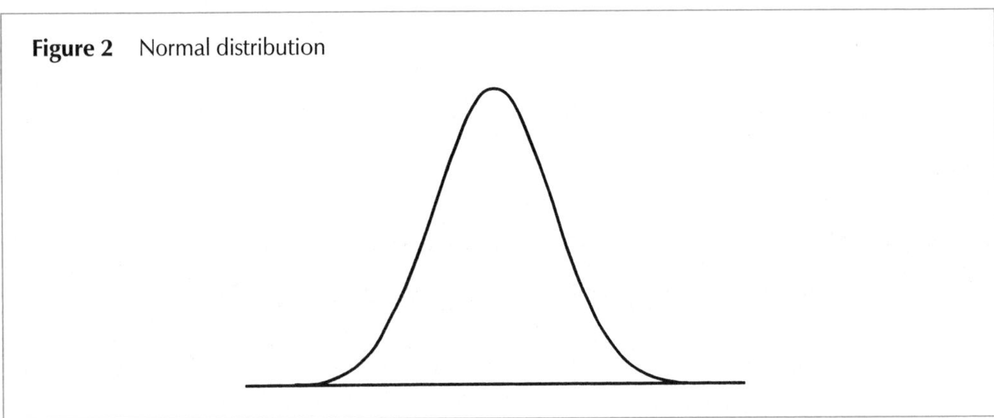

2.4 Standard deviation

The standard deviation (= $\sqrt{\text{variance}}$) gives a measure of the spread of the distribution values. The smaller the standard deviation (or variance) the more tightly grouped the values.

Figure 3 (a) Small standard deviation (b) Large standard deviation

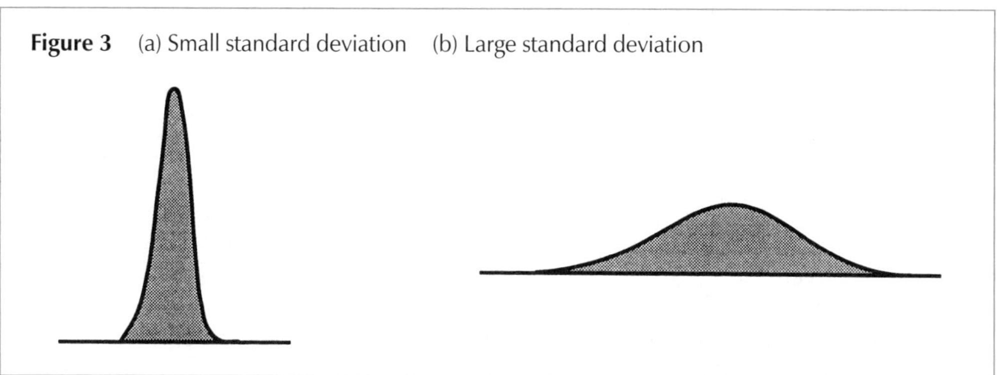

If the values are normally distributed, then:

- approximately 68% of the values lie within ±1 standard deviation of the mean
- approximately 95% of the values lie within ± 2 standard deviations of the mean
- exactly 95% of the values lie within ± 1.96 standard deviations of the mean (hence 2.5% lie in each tail).

3. CONFIDENCE INTERVALS

3.1 Standard error (SE or SEM)

This is a measure of how precisely the sample mean approximates the population mean.

$$\text{Standard error} = \frac{\text{standard deviation}}{\sqrt{n}}, \text{ where } n \text{ is the sample size}$$

The standard error is smaller for larger sample sizes (i.e. as n increases, SEM decreases). The more observations in the sample (the bigger the value of n) the more precisely the sample mean estimates the population mean (ie the less the error).

The SEM can be used to construct **confidence intervals.**

- The interval (mean ± 1.96 SEM) is a 95% confidence interval for the population mean.
- The interval (mean ± 2 SEM) is an approximate 95% confidence interval for the population mean.
- The interval (mean ± 1.64 SEM) is a 90% confidence interval for the population mean.

There is a 5%, or 0.05, or a 1 in 20 chance that the true mean lies outside the 95% confidence interval.

- 'We are 95% confident that the true mean lies inside the interval.'

There is a 10%, or 0.1, or 1 in 10 chance that the true mean lies outside the 90% confidence interval.

- 'We are 90% confident that the true mean lies inside the interval.'

Note the difference between the standard deviation and the standard error.

- Standard deviation (SD) gives a measure of the spread of the data values.
- Standard error (SE) is a measure of how precisely the sample mean approximates the population mean.

For example, FEV_1 is measured in 100 students. The mean value for this group is 4.5 litres with a standard deviation of 0.5 litres. If the values are normally distributed then:

approximately 95% of the values lie in the range (4.5 ± 2(0.5))
= (4.51 ± 1)
= (3.5, 5.5 litres)

$$\text{Standard error} = \frac{0.5}{\sqrt{100}} = \frac{0.5}{10} = 0.05.$$

An approximate 95% confidence interval for the population mean FEV_1 is given by:

(4.5 ± 2(0.05)) = (4.5 ± 0.1) = (4.4 – 4.6) litres

ie we are 95% confident that the population mean FEV_1 of students lies in the range 4.4–4.6 litres.

Confidence intervals can similarly be constructed around other summary statistics; for example, the difference between two means, a single proportion or percentage, the difference between two proportions. The standard error always gives a measure of the precision of the sample estimate and is smaller for larger sample sizes.

4. SIGNIFICANCE TESTS

Statistical significance tests, or hypothesis tests, use the sample data to assess how likely some specified null hypothesis is to be correct. The measure of 'how likely' is given by a probability (p) value. Usually, the null hypothesis is that there is 'no difference' between the groups.

4.1 Null hypotheses and p values

To answer the research questions in Section 1 we test the following null hypotheses:

- There is no difference in the incidence of fetuses with neural tube defects between the groups of pregnant women who do and do not take folic acid supplements.
- Lung function is similar in cystic fibrosis patients who receive the new inhaled steroid when compared with the patients on current treatment.
- Smokers and non-smokers have equal chances of contracting cancer.

Even if these null hypotheses were true we would not expect the averages or proportions in our sample groups to be identical. Because of random variation there will be some difference. The ***p* value** is the probability of observing a difference of that magnitude if the null hypothesis is true.

Since the p value is a probability, it takes values between 0 and 1. Values near to zero suggest that the null hypothesis is unlikely to be true. The smaller the p value the more significant the result:

- $p = 0.05$, the result is significant at 5%.
  The sample difference had a 1 in 20 chance of occurring if the null hypothesis were true.
- $p = 0.01$, the result is significant at 1%.
  The sample difference had a 1 in 100 chance of occurring if the null hypothesis were true.

Statistical significance is not the same as clinical significance. Although a study may show that the results from drug A are statistically significantly better than for drug B we have to consider the magnitude of the improvement, the costs, ease of administration and potential side-effects of the two drugs, etc before deciding that the result is clinically significant and that drug A should be introduced in preference to drug B.

4.2 Significance, power and sample size

The study sample may or may not be compatible with the null hypothesis. On the basis of the study results, we may decide to disbelieve (or reject) the null hypothesis. In reality, the null hypothesis either is or is not true.

	Null hypothesis:	
	True	False
Decision based on study results: 'Accept' null hypothesis	OK	(II)
'Reject' null hypothesis	(I)	OK

The study may lead to the wrong conclusions:

- A low (significant) *p* value may lead us to disbelieve (or reject) the null hypothesis when it is actually true – Box (I) above. This is known as a **type I error**.
- The *p* value may be high (non-significant) when the null hypothesis is false – Box (II) above. This is known as a **type II error**.

The **power** of a study is the probability (usually expressed as a percentage) of correctly rejecting the null hypothesis when it is false.

Larger differences between the groups can be detected with greater power. The power to identify correctly a difference of a certain size can be increased by increasing the sample size. Small samples often lead to type II errors (ie there is not sufficient power to detect differences of clinical importance).

In practice there is a grey area between accepting and rejecting the null hypothesis. The decision will be made in the light of the *p* value obtained. We should not draw different conclusions based on a *p* value of 0.051 compared with a value of 0.049. The *p* value is a probability. As it gets smaller the less likely it is that the null hypothesis is true. There is no sudden changeover from 'accept' to 'reject'.

4.3 Parametric and non-parametric tests

Statistical hypothesis tests are either parametric or non-parametric. Choosing the appropriate statistical test depends on:

- the type of data and their distribution
- whether the data are paired or not.

Parametric tests usually assume the data are normally distributed. Examples are:

- *t*-test (sometimes called 'Student's *t*-test' or 'Student's paired *t*-test')
- Pearson's coefficient of linear correlation

An unpaired (or 2-sample) *t*-test is used to compare the average values of two independent groups (eg patients with and without disease, treated versus placebo, etc).

A paired (or 1-sample) *t*-test is used if the members of the groups are paired. For example, each individual with disease is matched with a healthy individual of the same age and sex; in a crossover trial the measurements made on two treatments are paired within individuals.

Non-parametric tests are usually based on ranks. Examples are:

- Wilcoxon
- Sign
- Mann-Whitney *U*
- Kendall's *S*
- Spearman's Rank Correlation
- Chi-squared (χ^2)

Chi-squared is used to compare proportions (or percentages) between two groups.

5. CORRELATION AND REGRESSION

Sometimes measurements are made on two continuous variables for each study subject, eg CD4 count and age, blood pressure and weight, FRC and height. The data can be displayed in a scatterplot.

Figure 4 Scatterplot of CD4 count versus age

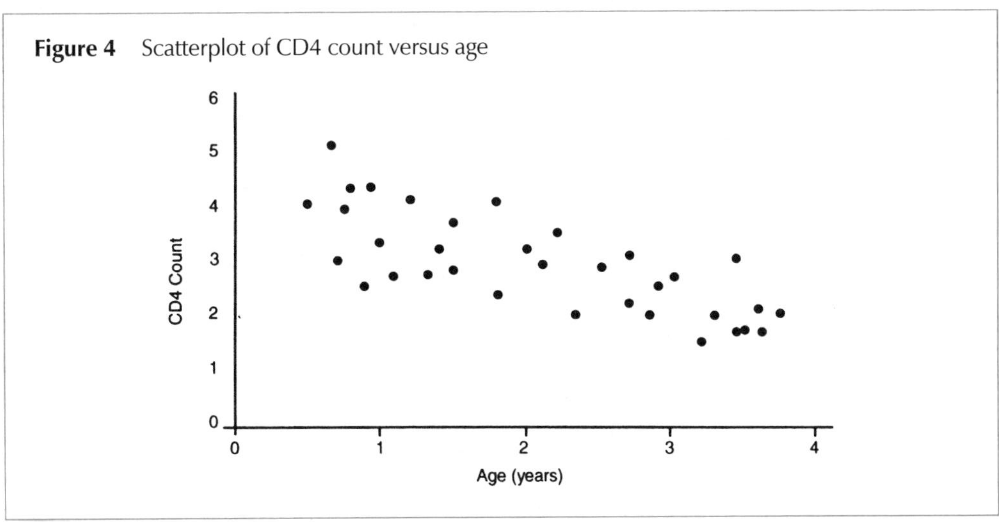

5.1 Correlation coefficients

The correlation coefficient (sometimes called Pearson's coefficient of linear correlation) is denoted by r and indicates how closely the points lie to a line.

r takes values between –1 and 1, the closer it is to zero the less the linear association between the two variables. (Note that the variables may be strongly associated but not linearly.)

Negative values of r indicate that one variable decreases as the other increases (eg CD4 count falls with age).

Values of –1 or +1 show that the variables are perfectly linearly related, ie the scatterplot points lie on a straight line.

Figure 5 Scatterplots with different correlation coefficients

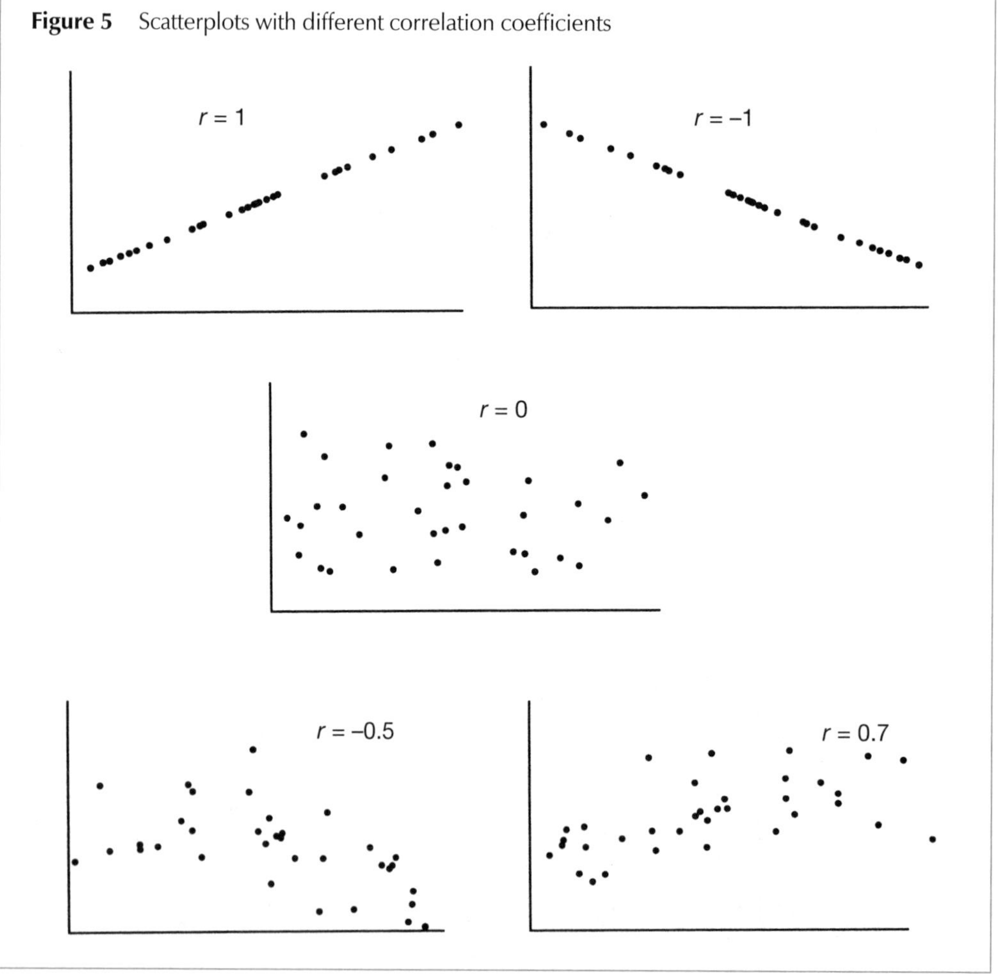

Correlation coefficients:

- show how one variable increases or decreases as the other variable increases
- do not give information about the size of the increase or decrease
- do not give a measure of agreement.

Pearson's *r* is a parametric correlation coefficient. Spearman's Rank Correlation and Kendall's *S* are non-parametric correlation coefficients.

- Parametric correlation coefficients quantify the extent of any linear increase or decrease.
- Non-parametric correlation coefficients quantify the extent of any tendency for one variable to increase or decrease as the other increases (for example, exponential increase or decline, increasing in steps, etc).

A *p* value attached to a correlation coefficient shows how likely it is that there is no linear association between the two variables.

A significant correlation does not imply cause and effect.

5.2 Linear regression

A regression equation ($Y = a + bX$) may be used to PREDICT one variable from the other.

Figure 6 Linear regression line

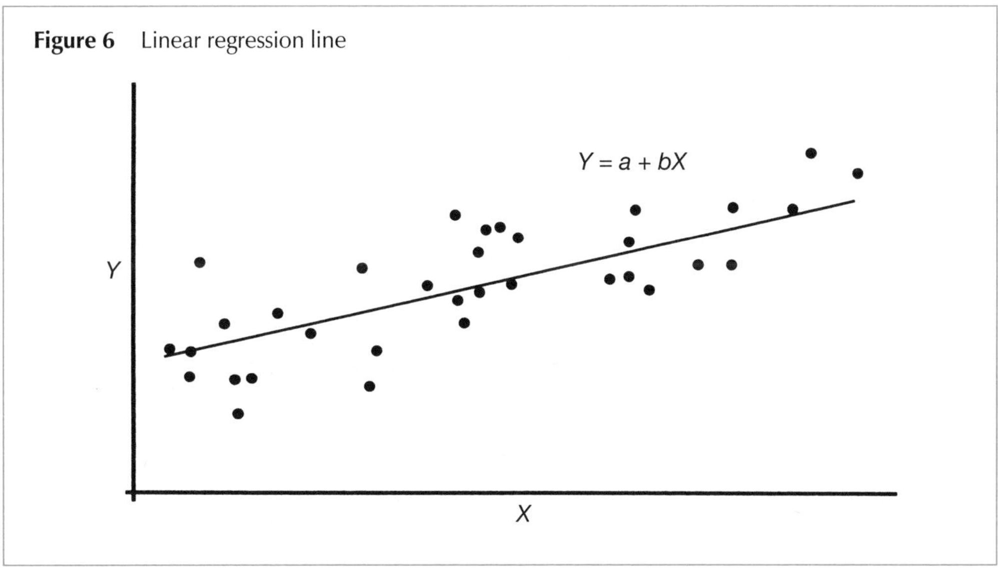

- *'a'* is the intercept – the value *Y* takes when *X* is zero.
- *'b'* is the slope of the line – sometimes called the **regression coefficient**. It gives the average change in *Y* for a unit increase in *X*.
- If *'b'* is negative then *Y* decreases as *X* increases.

Figure 7 CD4 count versus age

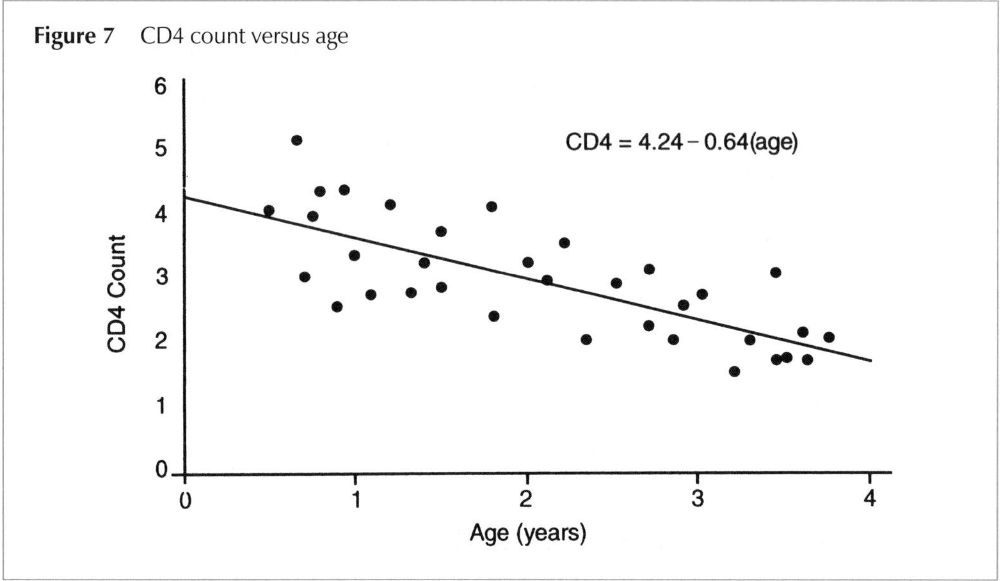

If the units of measurement change then so will the regression equation. For example, if age is measured in months rather than years then the value of the slope (the average change in CD4 for a unit increase in age) will alter accordingly.

6. SCREENING TESTS

Screening tests are often used to identify individuals at risk of disease. Individuals who are positive on screening may be investigated further to determine whether they actually have the disease.

- Some of those who screen positive will not have the disease.
- Some of those who have the disease may be missed by the screen (ie test negative).

Screening test result:	Diseased	Disease-free
Positive – indicating possible disease	a	b
Negative	c	d

- **Sensitivity** is the proportion of true positives correctly identified by the test

  $$=\frac{a}{a+c}$$

- **Specificity** is the proportion of true negatives correctly identified by the test

  $$=\frac{d}{b+d}$$

- **Positive predictive value** is the proportion of those who test positive who actually have the disease

  $$=\frac{a}{a+b}$$

- **Negative predictive value** is the proportion of those who test negative who do not have the disease

  $$=\frac{d}{c+d}$$

Note that the positive and negative predictive values depend on the **prevalence** of the disease and may vary from population to population.

Likelihood ratios

- The **likelihood ratio (LR) for a positive test result, LR+** $=\frac{\text{sensitivity}}{1-\text{specificity}}$.

- The **likelihood ratio for a negative test result, LR–** $=\frac{1-\text{sensitivity}}{\text{specificity}}$.

Likelihood ratios may be multiplied by pre-test odds to give post-test odds. They are not prevalence-dependent.

Example

A screening test is applied to patients with and without disease *X*. Of 100 who have the disease, 60 test positive; of 200 without the disease, only 20 test positive.

The following table may be constructed:

Screening test result	Disease X	Disease-free
Positive (indicating possible disease)	60	20
Negative	40	180

Therefore, the following are true:

- sensitivity = 60/100 = 0.6 or 60%
- specificity = 180/200 = 0.9 or 90%
- LR+ = 0.6/(1–0.9) = 6
- LR– = (1–0.6)/0.9 = 0.44
- the positive predictive value is 60/(60 + 20) = 0.75 or 75% (ie 75% of those who test positive actually have the disease in this sample)
- the prevalence of the disease in this sample is 100/(100 + 200) =+ 0.33 or 33%.

If a particular patient had a prior odds of 1.5 of having the disease (meaning that he or she is 1.5 times more likely to have the disease than not to have it) then 1.5/2.5 (or 60%) of patients of this type will have the disease. The **posterior odds** of the patient having the disease will thus be determined by the result of the screening test:

- if the test is positive then the odds of having the disease will be 1.5×6 = 9
- if the test is negative, the odds will be 1.5×0.44 = 0.66.

Note that, as expected, the odds of having the disease rise if the test is positive and fall if the test is negative.

A posterior odds of 9 means that the patient is nine times more likely to have the disease than not, which equates to a probability of 9/10 or 0.9 (as opposed to 0.6 before testing). A posterior odds of 0.66 equates to a probability of 0.66/1.66, or 0.4 (as opposed to 0.6 before testing).

Index

Where more than one page number appears against a heading, page numbers in bold indicate the main treatment of a subject.